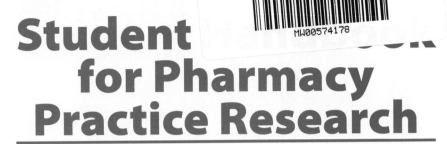

Student Handbook for Pharmacy Practice Research

Notice

Medicine is an ever-changing science. As new research and clinical experience broaden our knowledge, changes in treatment and drug therapy are required. The authors and the publisher of this work have checked with sources believed to be reliable in their efforts to provide information that is complete and generally in accord with the standards accepted at the time of publication. However, in view of the possibility of human error or changes in medical sciences, neither the authors nor the publisher nor any other party who has been involved in the preparation or publication of this work warrants that the information contained herein is in every respect accurate or complete, and they disclaim all responsibility for any errors or omissions or for the results obtained from use of the information contained in this work. Readers are encouraged to confirm the information contained herein with other sources. For example and in particular, readers are advised to check the product information sheet included in the package of each drug they plan to administer to be certain that the information contained in this work is accurate and that changes have not been made in the recommended dose or in the contraindications for administration. This recommendation is of particular importance in connection with new or infrequently used drugs.

Student Handbook for Pharmacy Practice Research

A COMPANION BOOK TO CONDUCT PRACTICE-BASED RESEARCH IN PHARMACY

Editors

Rajender R. Aparasu, MPharm, Phd, FAPhA
Mustafa and Sanober Lokhandwala Endowed Professor
Department Chair
Department of Pharmaceutical Health Outcomes and Policy
College of Pharmacy
University of Houston
Houston, Texas

John P. Bentley, RPh, PhD, FAPhA, FNAP
Professor of Pharmacy Administration
Research Professor in the Research Institute of Pharmaceutical Sciences
Director of the Center for Pharmaceutical Marketing and Management
School of Pharmacy
University of Mississippi
University, Mississippi

Adam N. Pate, PharmD, BCPS
Clinical Associate Professor of Pharmacy Practice
Department of Pharmacy Practice
School of Pharmacy
University of Mississippi
University, Mississippi

New York • Chicago • San Francisco • Athens • London • Madrid • Mexico City • Milan
New Delhi • Singapore • Sydney • Toronto

To Amma, Anasuya Aparasu—My strength and inspiration
Aparasu

To my mom, Delphine Bentley—A kinder person I have never met
Bentley

To my wife, 3 children, and all the mentors and teachers
who have helped me along the way
Pate

Contents

Chapter Three. Research Infrastructure in Pharmacy Settings 47
Joshua T. Swan and Lan N. Bui

Chapter Four. Formulating Practice-Based Research
Questions and Hypotheses. 71
Marion K. Slack

SECTION II: CONDUCTING PRACTICE-BASED RESEARCH

Chapter Eight. Case Reports and Case Series in Pharmacy 185
Katie E. Barber and Jamie L. Wagner

Chapter Nine. Intervention Research in Pharmacy Settings 203
Divya A. Varkey and Elisabeth M. Wang

Chapter Ten. Implementation Science in Pharmacy Settings. 223
Douglas Thornton

Chapter Eleven. Survey Research in Pharmacy Settings 245
Anandi V. Law and Sun Lee

Chapter Twelve. Patient-Reported Outcomes Research in Pharmacy 269

Nalin Payakachat and Amy M. Franks

Chapter Thirteen. Quality Improvement Research in Pharmacy Settings. 295

Ana L. Hincapie and Elizabeth Schlosser

Chapter Fourteen. Secondary Data Research in Pharmacy Settings 327

Sujith Ramachandran and Kaustuv Bhattacharya

Chapter Fifteen. Qualitative Research in Pharmacy Settings. 355
Kimberly M. Kelly and Trupti Dhumal

Chapter Sixteen. Drug Utilization Research in Healthcare 377
Varun Vaidya

Chapter Nighteen. Narrative and Scoping Reviews in Pharmacy Settings .445

Marie Barnard

Chapter Twenty. Systematic Reviews and Meta-Analysis in Pharmacy 461

Wei-Hsuan Lo-Ciganic and Juan M. Hincapie-Castillo

Chapter Twenty-Four. Research Manuscripts 547
Jordan R. Covvey and Spencer E. Harpe

Chapter Twenty-Five. Peer Review and the Publication Process . . .587
Shane P. Desselle

About the Editors

Rajender R. Aparasu, MPharm, PhD, FAPhA, is the Mustafa and Sanober Lokhandwala Endowed Professor and Founding Chair of the Department of Pharmaceutical Health Outcomes and Policy at the University of Houston College of Pharmacy. He is a renowned scholar and educational leader with over 25 years of experience in the areas of pharmaceutical outcomes research and policy. He started his academic career at South Dakota State University – College of Pharmacy in 1995 after obtaining his PhD from the University of Louisiana – Monroe. He joined as Professor at the University of Houston – College of Pharmacy in 2006. He was the inaugural Chair of the College of Pharmacy's new department, Pharmaceutical Health Outcomes and Policy. He has taught various professional and graduate courses in pharmacy. He served as a mentor for over 25 graduate students and post-doctoral fellows for the past 10 years. His primary areas of research interest include outcomes research and pharmacoepidemiology, with particular emphasis on improving the quality of pharmaceutical care in older adults. His research group focuses on evaluating medication safety in older adults using real-world data based on novel methodological approaches in observational research.

Dr. Aparasu has continuous research funding from Federal sources, including R01, R15, R56, and R03, to generate real-world evidence. His non-Federal funding sources include pharmaceutical companies and other organizations. He has published nearly 150 peer-reviewed manuscripts and has over 250 presentations in national and international meetings. He was listed among the World's Top 2% Scientists in Geriatrics based on various citation metrics as per PLOS Biology. In 2012, he was recognized by his peers as a Fellow of the American Pharmacists Association (FAPhA) for his exemplary professional achievements and outstanding service and contribution to the pharmacy profession. In 2016, Dr. Aparasu was selected for the *Fulbright Specialist* Roster and visited Indonesia to mentor pharmacy and medical faculty in research. In 2022, he was honored by the American Association of Colleges of Pharmacy (AACP) as the recipient of the Paul R. Dawson Award for Excellence in Patient Care Research. He is a grant reviewer for the *American Heart Association (AHA), Patient-Centered Outcomes Research Institute*

(PCORI), and *National Institutes of Health (NIH)*. He was recently invited to serve on the *Disease Control and Prevention (CDC) – National Center for Health Statistics (NCHS)* Board of Scientific Counselors NAMCS Workgroup.

John P. Bentley, RPh, PhD, FAPhA, FNAP, is a Professor of Pharmacy Administration, a Research Professor in the Research Institute of Pharmaceutical Sciences, and the Director of the Center for Pharmaceutical Marketing and Management at the University of Mississippi School of Pharmacy, with a joint appointment in the Department of Marketing in the School of Business Administration. He previously served as the Program Coordinator for the University's Graduate Minor in Applied Statistics. In the pharmacy curriculum, Dr. Bentley teaches elements of research design, biostatistics, epidemiology, and drug literature evaluation. At the graduate level, he teaches several applied statistics courses, including general linear models, multivariate statistics, and elective courses focusing on the application of modern longitudinal data analysis methods and principles of statistical mediation and moderation. He has conducted research projects in a variety of areas, including: patient-reported outcomes; medication use, misuse, and outcomes; pharmacoepidemiology; healthcare quality assessment; measurement of adherence to medications; pharmaceutical marketing and patient behavior; patients' evaluation of healthcare providers; pharmacy practice management; health behaviors among college students; and ethics and professionalism. His statistics interests include latent variable analysis, longitudinal data analysis, the analysis of statistical interactions (i.e., moderation analysis), and the statistical analysis of mechanisms of effects (i.e., mediation analysis).

Dr. Bentley has been a member of many interdisciplinary research teams, consulted with numerous researchers concerning statistical analysis, and served on the MS or PhD committees of over 170 students from various disciplines. He was named a Fellow of the American Pharmacists Association in 2009 and the National Academies of Practice in 2019. He has been recognized as a Thelma Cerniglia Distinguished Teaching Scholar at the University of Mississippi School of Pharmacy and has received the Excellence in Graduate Teaching and Mentoring Award from the University of Mississippi Graduate School, the University of Mississippi's Faculty Achievement Award for Outstanding Teaching and Scholarship, and the Outstanding Article of the Year Award for a paper published in *Quality of Life Research*. He has served as a member and chair of the University of Mississippi Institutional Review Board (IRB), a peer reviewer for many journals, and an Associate Editor for the *Journal of the American Pharmacists Association*. Dr. Bentley received his BS in pharmacy and MBA from Drake University, his MS and PhD in pharmacy administration from the University of Mississippi, and his MS and PhD in biostatistics from the University of Alabama at Birmingham (UAB).

Adam N. Pate, PharmD, BCPS, is a Clinical Associate Professor of Pharmacy Practice at the University of Mississippi School of Pharmacy. He has practiced pharmacy in both internal medicine and ambulatory care and has conducted research projects in a variety of areas. His primary research interests and publications have been in educational research and the scholarship of teaching and learning.

Dr. Pate has worked with a number of students and residents on research projects, including being the research advisor for the University of Mississippi School of Pharmacy Community residency program and actively participating as a residency preceptor at his practice site with North Mississippi Medical Center. In 2019, he was named an American Association of Colleges of Pharmacy Emerging Teaching Scholar and has consistently been involved in mentoring and developing research projects with students, including participation as an American Association of Colleges of Pharmacy (AACP) Walmart Scholar Mentor. He has served as a peer reviewer for multiple journals, including serving on the editorial board and being named the 2019 #1 reviewer for the *American Journal of Pharmaceutical Education.* Dr. Pate has also served in a variety of roles and committees within AACP, including serving as the 2019-2020 AACP Pharmacy Practice Section Chair. He has also served on the National Association of Boards of Pharmacy – North American Pharmacist Licensure Examination (NAPLEX) Review Committee for a number of years, including attending a multitude of NAPLEX item writing workshops. Dr. Pate received his BS in Pharmaceutical Sciences and PharmD from the University of Mississippi. He subsequently completed a PGY-1 Pharmacy residency, including completing requirements for a residency teaching certificate at the University of Arkansas for Medical Sciences in Little Rock, Arkansas.

Contributors

Katie E. Barber, PharmD
Associate Professor of Pharmacy Practice
School of Pharmacy
University of Mississippi
Jackson, Mississippi

Marie Barnard, PhD
Assistant Professor of Pharmacy Administration
Research Assistant Professor in the Research
    Institute of Pharmaceutical Sciences
School of Pharmacy
University of Mississippi
University, Mississippi

Kaustuv Bhattacharya, PhD
Research Assistant Professor, Center for
    Pharmaceutical Marketing and Management
Assistant Professor, Department of Pharmacy
    Administration
School of Pharmacy
University of Mississippi
University, Mississippi

Lan N. Bui, PharmD, MPH, BCPS
Assistant Professor of Pharmacy Practice
McWhorter School of Pharmacy
Samford University
Birmingham, Alabama

Jordan R. Covvey, PharmD, PhD, BCPS
Associate Professor of Pharmacy
    Administration
Division of Pharmaceutical, Administrative
    and Social Sciences
School of Pharmacy
Duquesne University
Pittsburgh, Pennsylvania

Shane P. Desselle, RPh, PhD, FAPhA
Professor
Editor, *Research in Social and Administrative
    Pharmacy*
Editor, *Exploratory Research in Clinical and
    Social Pharmacy*
Department of Social, Behavioral and
    Administrative Sciences
Touro University California College of
    Pharmacy
Vallejo, California

Trupti Dhumal, MS
PhD Student
Department of Pharmaceutical Systems
    and Policy
School of Pharmacy
West Virginia University
Morgantown, West Virginia

Amy M. Franks, PharmD
Chair and Associate Professor of Pharmacy
    Practice
Department of Pharmacy Practice
College of Pharmacy
University of Arkansas for Medical Sciences
Little Rock, Arkansas

Spencer E. Harpe, PharmD, PhD, MPH,
FAPhA
Professor of Pharmacy Practice
College of Pharmacy
Midwestern University
Downers Grove, Illinois

Ana L. Hincapie, PhD MS
Associate Professor
Division of Pharmacy Practice and
    Administrative Sciences
College of Pharmacy
University of Cincinnati
Cincinnati, Ohio

Juan M. Hincapie-Castillo, PharmD,
MS, PhD
Assistant Professor
Department of Epidemiology
Gillings School of Global Public Health
University of North Carolina
Chapel Hill, North Carolina

Kimberly Illingworth, PhD, RPh, FAPhA
Assistant Dean for Learning and Assessment
Associate Professor of Pharmacy Practice
Director, Purdue University Academic and
    Ambulatory Care Fellowship Program
Faculty Associate, Center for Aging and the
    Life Course
College of Pharmacy
Purdue University
West Lafayette, Indiana

Khalid M. Kamal, MPharm, PhD
Professor and Chair
Department of Pharmaceutical Systems and
    Policy
School of Pharmacy
West Virginia University
Morgantown, West Virginia

Kimberly M. Kelly, PhD, MS
Professor
Department of Pharmaceutical Systems and
    Policy
School of Pharmacy
West Virginia University
Morgantown, West Virginia

Mandy King, MS
Director of Research Integrity and
    Compliance
Office of Research and Sponsored Programs
University of Mississippi
University, Mississippi

Anandi V. Law, BPharm, MS, PhD,
FAPhA
Professor, Department of Pharmacy Practice
    and Administration
Associate Dean for Assessment
Director, ACCP-peer reviewed Fellowship in
    Health Outcomes
College of Pharmacy
Western University of Health Sciences
Pomona, California

Sun Lee, PharmD
Assistant Professor of Social and
    Administrative Sciences
Department of Clinical Sciences
Fred Wilson School of Pharmacy
High Point University
High Point, North Carolina

Wei-Hsuan "Jenny" Lo-Ciganic,
MSPharm, MS, PhD
Associate Professor
Department of Pharmaceutical Outcomes
   and Policy
College of Pharmacy
University of Florida
Gainesville, Florida

Bryan L. Love, PharmD, MPH, FCCP,
BCPS (AQ ID)
Associate Professor
Department of Clinical Pharmacy and
   Outcomes Sciences
College of Pharmacy
University of South Carolina
Columbia, South Carolina

Molly A. Nichols, PharmD
Hook Drug Foundation Fellow in Community
   Practice Research
Post Doctoral Fellow
College of Pharmacy
Purdue University
Indianapolis, Indiana

Lauren G. Pamulapati, PharmD,
BCACP
Assistant Professor, Ambulatory Care
School of Pharmacy
Virginia Commonwealth University
Richmond, Virginia

Nalin Payakachat, BPharm, MSc, PhD
Adjunct Professor, Division of Pharmaceutical
   Evaluation and Policy
College of Pharmacy
University of Arkansas for Medical Sciences
Little Rock, Arkansas

Sujith Ramachandran, PhD
Assistant Professor of Pharmacy
   Administration
Department of Pharmacy Administration
Assistant Director, Center for Pharmaceutical
   Marketing and Management
School of Pharmacy
University of Mississippi
University, Mississippi

Elizabeth Schlosser, PharmD, BCPS,
BCACP
Clinical Assistant Professor
Division of Pharmacy Practice and
   Administrative Sciences
College of Pharmacy
University of Cincinnati
Cincinnati, Ohio

Marion K. Slack, PhD
Professor Emeritus
Department of Pharmacy Practice and Science
College of Pharmacy
University of Arizona
Tucson, Arizona

Margie E. Snyder, PharmD, MPH, FCCP,
FAPhA
Associate Professor of Pharmacy Practice
Co-Director, Community Pharmacy Programs
College of Pharmacy
Purdue University
Indianapolis, Indiana

Joshua T. Swan, PharmD, MPH, FCCM,
BCPS
Scientist and Associate Professor of Surgery
   in Outcomes Research
Program Director, Clinical Pharmacy
   Fellowship in Outcomes Research

Department of Surgery
Houston Methodist
Houston, Texas

Douglas Thornton, PharmD, PhD, BCPS
Assistant Professor
Director PREMIER Center
Department of Pharmaceutical Health
  Outcomes and Policy
College of Pharmacy
University of Houston
Houston, Texas

Varun Vaidya, PhD
Professor and Director, Health Outcomes and
  Socioeconomic Sciences
Director, BSPS Pharmacy Administration
College of Pharmacy and Pharmaceutical
  Sciences
University of Toledo, Health Science Campus
Toledo, Ohio

Divya A. Varkey, PharmD, MS
Clinical Associate Professor
Department of Pharmacy Practice and
  Translational Research
College of Pharmacy
University of Houston
Houston, Texas

Jamie L. Wagner, PharmD, BCPS
Clinical Associate Professor of Pharmacy
  Practice
School of Pharmacy
University of Mississippi
Jackson, Mississippi

Matthew A. Wanat, PharmD, BCPS,
BCCCP, FCCM
Clinical Associate Professor
Director, Fellowship in Academic Pharmacy
Department of Pharmacy Practice and
  Translational Research
College of Pharmacy
University of Houston
Houston, Texas

Elisabeth M. Wang, PharmD, BCCP
Clinical Assistant Professor
College of Pharmacy
University of Houston
Houston, Texas

Erin Hickey Zacholski, PharmD, BCOP
Assistant Professor, Hematology and
  Oncology
School of Pharmacy
Virginia Commonwealth University
Richmond, Virginia

Preface

Clinical and translational research will play an increasingly important role in health-care and the profession of pharmacy, including pharmacy education. The 2008 report from the American Association of Colleges of Pharmacy (AACP) task force on educating clinical scientists detailed the content areas and competencies needed for the PharmD curriculum.[1,2] These competencies included identifying opportunities across the research spectrum, from identifying research problems and gaps to conducting the research and disseminating the research findings. The latest standards from the Accreditation Council for Pharmacy Education (ACPE) require pharmacy education and training to incorporate various elements of research, including foundational, applicational, and translational components of clinical research.[3] In recent years, there has been a greater focus from a variety of stakeholders on practice-based research for generating evidence and translating this evidence to direct patient care. Pharmacists and student pharmacists are increasingly involved in or have the opportunity to be involved in this clinical and translational research across the research and practice continuum. Although initially practice-based research was limited to those with advanced training or degrees, today's student pharmacists increasingly have opportunities to be involved in research during their professional training. Pharmacy schools are also intensifying the focus on preparing students to conduct research via encouraging or mandating research during professional education and training in elective and required courses or capstone programs.

---

[1] Carter BL, Blouin RA, Chewning BA, et al. Report of the AACP Educating Clinical Scientists Task Force II. *Am J Pharm Educ.* 2008;72(Suppl):S10.

[2] Figg WD, Chau CH, Okita R, et al. 2008. Pharm. D. Pathways to biomedical research: The National Institutes of Health special conference on pharmacy research. *Pharmacotherapy.* 2008;28(7):821–833.

[3] Accreditation Standards and Key Elements for the Professional Program in Pharmacy Leading to the Doctor of Pharmacy Degree. STANDARDS 2016. Accessed August 29, 2021. https://www.acpe-accredit.org/pdf/Standards2016FINAL.pdf

In discussing the challenges that are inherently specific to PharmD and residency research, this book became a natural extension of our previous book, *Principles of Research Design and Drug Literature Evaluation* (Aparasu and Bentley). The previous book emphasized principles and execution of scientific research with a focus on a detailed discussion of clinical research designs, statistical analysis, and evidence-based medicine principles that readers could use to carry out research and apply evidence to patient care. However, there was a need for a book that can help our student pharmacists and residents who are beginning their journeys as researchers. The vision for this book evolved over discussions about the challenges and successes of PharmD and residency research projects at our respective institutions. This book speaks directly to the challenges of PharmD and residency research and provides novice researchers and their mentors with a practical and systematic framework that can be used for conducting practice-based research in pharmacy settings.

The goal of this companion book is to provide student pharmacists and residents a practical and systematic framework or a "how-to and hands-on" focus for initiating and conducting practice-based research in pharmacy settings. The concepts and components found in this book have evolved over years of refinement in facing challenges and experiencing successes in teaching and mentoring student pharmacists and residents during their research projects. It is designed for student pharmacists and residents who undertake a capstone or standalone research project as part of their professional training, and we hope it serves as a valuable resource to enhance the research quality of PharmD and residency projects. This book focuses on practical approaches and considerations for conducting practice-based research highlighting how to leverage existing resources and infrastructure at academic institutions and practice settings to enhance a research project. There is a special emphasis on learner-involved research in each chapter, highlighting the application of concepts in the chapter through example research that involved or was conducted by students or residents (or both).

This book is divided into three sections. Section I covers critical elements in the planning of practice-based research. Section II provides practicalities of conducting practice-based research in pharmacy settings. Section III gives readers a dissemination framework for practice-based research in pharmacy.

Chapters 1 through 7 in Section I are intended to be a guide to assist learners as they create and establish their practice-based research. This section starts with a chapter on the concepts of practice-based research and its role in pharmacy (Chapter 1). The next two chapters cover topics on how to identify a research mentor and maximize that relationship (Chapter 2) and commonly used research and support infrastructure, including layered learning models (Chapter 3). Generalized approaches for identifying research questions and hypotheses (Chapter 4) and selection of research methods and designs for practice-based research (Chapter 5) are also detailed. Additionally, readers will find that the other chapters in this section cover required practical considerations such as human subjects protections and institutional review board (IRB) approval (Chapter 6) as well as technical considerations such as data management, planning for statistical analysis, and the process of collaborating with statisticians (Chapter 7). We hope that learners and mentors who read these chapters will find valuable advice in setting up their research projects for success.

Section II includes fourteen chapters covering the variety of pharmacy practice-based research that learners may be engaged in clinical and academic settings. The first three chapters discuss commonly used learner-involved research projects in clinical settings, from case reports/case-series (Chapter 8) and intervention research (Chapter 9) to implementation research (Chapter 10). The next two chapters describe research involving self-reports like survey research in general (Chapter 11) and patient-reported outcomes research in specific (Chapter 12). Quality improvement research (Chapter 13) and generalized approaches for secondary data research (Chapter 14) are also detailed. Furthermore, this section explains qualitative approaches (Chapter 15) and often used drug utilization research (Chapter 16) in pharmacy. With the increasing use of epidemiology and economic concepts in pharmacy, the research process for pharmacoepidemiology (Chapter 17) and pharmacoeconomic research (Chapter 18) are also described. There are two chapters focusing on literature reviews; the details for conducting both narrative/scoping (Chapter 19) and systematic review and meta-analysis (Chapter 20) are described. This section ends with a chapter on educational research in pharmacy (Chapter 21).

Each chapter in Section II addresses critical considerations for learners to conduct specific types of practice-based research. These chapters are intended to orient novice researchers to the type of research described, including common research questions, practical and technical considerations, mentorship and expertise, and the dissemination framework. Each chapter also uses a learner-involved research project as an example to demonstrate the concepts discussed in the chapter. It is our hope that readers can use this section and the content of these chapters to serve as a quick reference to begin considerations for specific research projects. Additionally, we included open-ended discussion questions in each of these chapters to facilitate conversations around key concepts between learner and mentor.

The final section of the book focuses on best practices in disseminating research findings. It includes chapters covering best practices and practical considerations in abstract and poster presentations (Chapter 22) and best methods for podium and other oral presentations (Chapter 23). This section also details critical considerations and techniques for manuscript preparation (Chapter 24) and successfully navigating the peer-review process along with decision-making processes commonly utilized by editors (Chapter 25).

We hope that this book will help student pharmacists, residents, and fellows interested in conducting practice-based research in pharmacy. We hope that all mentees and mentors can use this text as a resource and a guide to developing better research questions, designing better studies, and ultimately making a greater impact on patient care and student learning. This book can also be an excellent resource for undergraduate students in the pharmaceutical sciences, graduate students in pharmacy-related disciplines, and research fellows. Faculty members advising student pharmacists can use the book along with *Principles of Research Design and Drug Literature Evaluation* for a capstone course or standalone project/course supplemented by research articles. The contents of this book should also be very useful for PharmD programs with capstone or senior/honors research projects. This book would also be ideal for elective research courses and should be a valuable resource to residents and residency preceptors in helping to manage the research component (i.e., completion of a research study or a quality improvement project) of residency training.

Chapter authors are experts specializing in pharmacy practice research. Each chapter includes learning objectives, key terminology, review questions, online resources, and references. The chapters were developed from the learner's perspective to provide practical and technical considerations for conducting practice-based research. In addition to figures and tables, each chapter provides an example of learner-involved research. We greatly appreciate feedback from students and faculty for future editions. All research is considered a work in progress, including the contents of this book.

Rajender R. Aparasu, PhD, FAPhA
John P. Bentley, RPh, PhD, FAPhA, FNAP
Adam N. Pate, PharmD, BCPS

Acknowledgments

We sincerely thank all of the authors for patiently working with us in developing the chapter content and updating the chapters. We believe that mentorship and guidance are the foundation for high-quality research, and we greatly appreciate our authors sharing their expertise and experiences in mentoring for this book. Our gratitude also goes to all of our mentees who provided feedback, encouragement, and insight that has helped us to become better mentors. We also would like to thank our respective university and college/school faculty colleagues and administration teams for providing us the time and encouragement to complete this project. We are most appreciative of the editorial assistance provided by the production staff at McGraw Hill and would like to specifically recognize the efforts and support of Himanshu Abrol with MPS Limited. We are so grateful for the help and support provided by the publishing team at McGraw Hill, especially Michael Weitz and Peter J. Boyle. Most of all, we are thankful for our families and their unwavering support, in particular Anu, Sandy, and Kristen.

Rajender R. Aparasu, PhD, FAPhA
John P. Bentley, RPh, PhD, FAPhA, FNAP
Adam N. Pate, PharmD, BCPS

I

PLANNING FOR PRACTICE-BASED RESEARCH

Chapter One

Introduction to Practice-Based Research in Pharmacy

Rajender R. Aparasu, PhD, FAPhA

Chapter Objectives

- Define translational and practice-based research in pharmacy
- Discuss the conceptual basis of practice-based research in pharmacy
- Describe the goals and characteristics of practice-based research in pharmacy
- Identify the scientific approach to practice-based research in pharmacy
- Define mentorship and the role of mentors for practice-based research
- Understand challenges for learner-involved practice-based research
- Discuss the dissemination framework for practice-based research

Key Terminology

Practice-based research, translational research, population-based research, patient-oriented research, practice-based research networks, structure, process, outcome, mentorship

Introduction

Over the years, scientific contributions and therapeutic innovations have contributed immensely to the growth of the pharmacy profession. Basic research in biomedical sciences lays the foundation to develop applications in pharmaceutical sciences. Applied research

3

helps in developing pharmaceutical products for further evaluation in clinical and translational research. Clinical and translational research is instrumental for drug development and patient care. It provides scientific evidence for new therapeutic discoveries and existing therapies, especially comparative effectiveness and safety. This evidence forms the core of evidence-based medicine. Clinical and translational research also involves the incorporation of new evidence into clinical care. However, research has found that it takes an average of 17 years for 14% of the new discoveries to enter clinical practice.[1] This gap in new discoveries in clinical care provides great opportunities for clinical and translational research to shorten the timeline and improve the uptake of new discoveries in clinical practice.

Innovation and applied research have been critical to the success and growth of both the pharmaceutical industry and pharmacy practice. Similarly, improving and expanding the scope of pharmacy practice will require further research into novel practice models. Over the years, several practice changes have been introduced and successfully implemented to improve patient outcomes. These include therapeutic drug monitoring, generic substitution, and other therapeutic deliveries in inpatient care. Outpatient practice improvements include medication therapy management, collaborative practice agreements, patient counseling, immunizations, and others. These practice innovations required practice-based research to develop the scientific evidence. This chapter will define practice-based research and discuss the conceptual basis of practice-based research, including the scope, goals, and characteristics of practice-based research. This chapter also discusses the scientific approach for practice-based research and the importance of mentorship for learner-involved research. Finally, the challenges for learner-led research and dissemination framework for practice-based research are detailed.

Practice-Based Research

Clinical research involves patient-oriented research, epidemiological and behavioral research, and outcomes research.[2] In the last decade, there has been an increasing focus on translational research to move science from bench to bedside. **Translational research** includes "two areas of translation: The first area is the process of applying discoveries generated during research in the laboratory, and in preclinical studies, to the development of trials and studies in humans. The second area of translation concerns research aimed at enhancing the adoption of best practices in the community."[3] Clinical research is much broader than translational research and encompasses much of the patient-care research. Over the years, clinical research has focused on applying discoveries, the first part of translational research. The second area aiming to implement best practices requires a strong understanding of both clinical practice and healthcare policy.

Translational research has been redefined as "the multidirectional integration of basic research, patient-oriented research, and population-based research, with the long-term aim of improving the health of the public."[4] There are three components of translational research. The first component of translational research "expedites the movement between basic research and patient-oriented research that leads to new or improved scientific understanding or standards of care." The second component "facilitates the movement between patient-oriented research and population-based research that leads to better patient outcomes, the implementation of best practices, and improved health status in communities." The third component "promotes interaction between laboratory-based research and population-based research to stimulate a robust scientific understanding of human health and disease."[4]

Translational research requires the structure of clinical practice to successfully achieve the translational aims of moving science from bench to bedside and vice versa. Practice settings are also needed for drug development to conduct clinical trials and to translate research evidence to patient care. Translational research helps solve issues of provision of care while incorporating evidence into practice. The practice settings can also provide an understanding of the dynamics of patient care to develop solutions involving basic and applied sciences.

Practice-based research is a component of clinical and translational research that occurs in clinical practice settings to improve patient outcomes. In pharmacy, it occurs in community and institutional practices where patients receive pharmaceutical care and services. Practice-based research can: (1) identify problems in translating evidence to patient care, (2) evaluate the gap in efficacy and effectiveness, and (3) improve efficiencies in diagnosis, treatment, and monitoring to improve patient outcomes.[5] Practice-based research can also involve a variety of research designs and methods, including clinical trials, observational studies, surveys, secondary data studies, and qualitative research. According to Potter et al., practice-based research is a cycle involving two intentions: (1) findings from practice-based research should inform theory development, and (2) the reuptake of the research evidence should inform and improve practices and policies.[6] The practice-based research cycle involves several phases, with each phase informing the next phase and cycle of research repeating to optimize the healthcare practices and policies (see Figure 1–1). The phases of practice-based research include (i) assessment research, (ii) effectiveness research, (iii) evidence synthesis, (iv) implementation research, and (v) change in practice, policy, and theory.

Both patient-oriented and population-based research can be conducted in pharmacy practice settings. Patient-oriented research involves "studies that include a group of patients or healthy individuals that are designed to understand the mechanisms of disease and health, to determine the effects of a treatment, or to provide a decision analysis

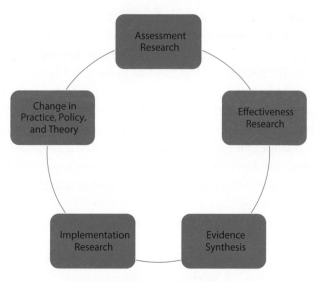

Figure 1–1. Cycles of practice-based research.

of care trajectories of patients."[7] **Population-based research** involves "studies involving epidemiology, social and behavioral sciences, public health, quality evaluation, and cost-effectiveness."[4] Although one practice site is sometimes enough for some types of practice-based research, others might require multiple sites and networks. There is also an increasing interest among researchers to conduct research involving multiple sites using similar settings for prospective and retrospective research.

Practice-based research networks (PBRNs) consist of a group of clinicians or practitioners involved in translational research who adopt best practices and conduct clinical research.[8] PBRNs have a long history in clinical research involving physician practices, mainly primary care physicians. With the support of the Agency for Healthcare Quality and Research, there has been significant growth of PBRNs. Although PBRNs started in primary care, they now involve several disciplines or disease-specific networks. According to the American College of Clinical Pharmacy (ACCP), PBRN is one of the first clinical pharmacy-based research networks involving over 1,000 clinical pharmacists in inpatient and outpatient settings.[9] Several pharmacy-based PBRNs have developed over the years, including state-based PBRNs.[10] These networks rely on members to contribute to research activities such as research ideas, patient enrollment, data collection, and dissemination. The practice-based research training networks (PBRTN) have also been initiated to provide research training and mentorship mechanisms to residents to improve research and associated outcomes.[11]

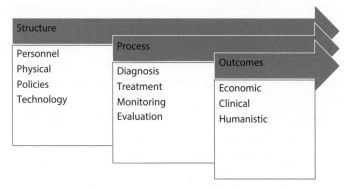

Figure 1–2. Donabedian conceptual model for pharmacy practice research.

Conceptual Framework for Practice-Based Research

Practice-based research can be conceptualized using the Donabedian Model (see Figure 1–2).[12] According to Avis Donabedian, the domains to assess and improve healthcare quality are based on the structure, process, and outcomes of healthcare. The structure refers to healthcare resources, including physical, personnel, and policies and procedures. The assumption is that healthcare practices with necessary human and material resources and other structural support can deliver quality healthcare. In pharmacy, the structure can include pharmacists, technicians, equipment, and pharmacy policies. Structural measures reflect the available infrastructure and capacity to provide healthcare and do not ensure performance involving these resources to achieve the outcome. The process refers to the performance or actions undertaken by the providers to achieve the outcome. The assumption is that if the right actions are performed in clinical practice, it will lead to optimal outcomes. In pharmacy, the process can include all pharmacist activities to deliver pharmaceutical care. The process should have strong evidence to be incorporated into regular practice. Process measures are the core of quality improvement practices and research. The outcomes refer to effects or final results obtained from utilizing the structure and processes of healthcare. The patient is often the focus of the outcome and can include the patient's clinical status, behavior, or satisfaction with care. In the Medical Model, good health is the absence of five Ds—*Death, Disability, Disease, Discomfort, Dissatisfaction*; these are often measured as patient outcomes for practice-based research.[13] According to the Economic, Clinical, Humanistic Outcomes (ECHO) Model,[14] the outcomes are classified as: *Clinical outcomes*—mortality, morbidity, and clinical measures associated with an intervention; *Economic outcomes*—medical and nonmedical costs averted due to intervention; and *Humanistic outcomes*—patients' self-evaluation of the effects—satisfaction or quality of life. Most practice-based research involves one or more of these outcomes.

The outcome evaluation is considered the gold standard in practice-based research since it is the end result of healthcare provision. The effect of structure and process can be intermediate or long term as long as there is a link between them. The time horizon for the development of the outcome dictates the selection of specific intermediate or long-term outcomes. Both structure and process can have variable time horizons for the manifestation of outcomes. For example, medication therapy management may require over a year to have influence on morbidity and mortality, whereas intermediate outcomes such as blood pressure and blood glucose can be used to evaluate the short-term effects of care. These considerations should be carefully incorporated when conducting practice-based research.

According to the Institute of Medicine (IOM), all stakeholders in healthcare should pursue the following six aims in the delivery of quality healthcare.[15] Quality healthcare should be (1) safe: avoid harm to patients from the delivery of healthcare; (2) effective: deliver care that benefits patients; (3) patient-centered: care that is individualized based on patient preferences and values; (4) timely: ensure timely, needed care and avoid delays; (5) efficient: care that maximizes the use of healthcare resources; and (6) equitable: care that does not vary due to personal characteristics—race or ethnicity—and minimizes healthcare disparities at the individual and population level. These aims have been the focus of the recent efforts by federal and non-federal agencies to provide value-based care. National agencies such as the Pharmacy Quality Alliance and National Committee for Quality Assurance have developed various quality of care measures using these aims.

Practice-based research can address the IOM aims in the continuum of pharmacy practice using the measures of structure, process, and outcomes (see Dimensions of Healthcare Quality in Table 1–1). Most of the clinical and translational research, including pharmacy practice research, involves addressing questions to evaluate the effects of structure and process on outcomes. The evaluation of structural measures includes

TABLE 1–1. **DIMENSIONS OF HEALTHCARE QUALITY**

Quality Aims	Quality Measures		
	Structure	Process	Outcomes
Safe			
Effective			
Patient-centered			
Timely			
Efficient			
Equitable			

studies involving pharmacists, pharmacy technicians, pharmacy infrastructure and policies, and state policies. Significant pharmacy practice-based research involves the evaluation of process activities by pharmacists. These may include medication therapy, patient counseling, immunization, and other services. The process can also include the provision of specific medications for real-world effectiveness studies.

Goals and Characteristics of Practice-Based Research

GOALS OF PRACTICE-BASED RESEARCH

The goals of practice-based research can be conceptualized within the four dimensions of scholarship by Ernest Boyer.[16] The four dimensions of scholarship for practice-based research include: (1) Scholarship of Discovery, (2) Scholarship of Teaching, (3) Scholarship of Integration, and (4) Scholarship of Application (see Figure 1–3). The scholarship of discovery involves the generation of new knowledge. This has been the traditional and mainstream of scholarship through publication, patents, and other dissemination modes. The healthcare and pharmaceutical industries are driven by the generation of new knowledge regarding prevention, diagnosis, and treatment. The scholarship of teaching involves traditional and innovative approaches for transmission of knowledge and skills. Any professional education, including pharmacy, relies on novel approaches to teaching and learning. In recent years, there is an increasing emphasis on the scholarship of teaching to enhance academic delivery for professional growth in pharmacy colleges.

The scholarship of integration involves bringing knowledge across disciplines to provide connections and context to understand the real world. This is especially important in healthcare as there is an integration of diverse sciences and disciplines to develop and provide innovative solutions to patient care. For example, health services research

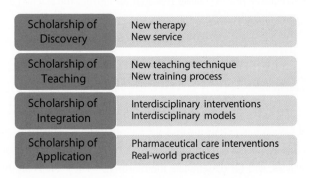

Scholarship of Discovery	New therapy New service
Scholarship of Teaching	New teaching technique New training process
Scholarship of Integration	Interdisciplinary interventions Interdisciplinary models
Scholarship of Application	Pharmaceutical care interventions Real-world practices

Figure 1–3. Dimensions of pharmacy practice research.

involves multiple disciplines from basic to applied sciences to examine "access to, and the use, costs, quality, delivery, organization, financing, and outcomes of healthcare services to produce new knowledge about the structure, processes, and effects of health services for individuals and populations."[17] The scholarship of application involves diverse methods and techniques to apply science and theory for practical applications. For example, the concept of pharmaceutical care required extensive work to apply and develop solutions and models for solving real-world problems using the scholarship of application.

CHARACTERISTICS OF PRACTICE-BASED RESEARCH

There are eight basic characteristics that capture the core values of practice-based research: (1) scholarly, (2) rigorous, (3) practical, (4) ecological, (5) methodologically diverse, (6) collaborative, (7) equitable, and (8) translational.[5] Practice-based research requires principles of scientific inquiry for developing and incorporating evidence. These include empiricism, objectivity, theory, and ethical standards.[18] The rigor of practice-based research is based on the scientific conduct using existing norms and peer evaluation for dissemination. Practice-based research must be practical as it involves the development and application of evidence to solve real-world problems and improve patient care. An ecological paradigm is needed to conduct practice-based research as it involves healthcare practices that consider the health of individuals within a multidimensional context involving biological, familial, social, environmental, and policy factors.

Practice-based research involves diverse methods, including quantitative and qualitative approaches to address the how and why of developing and implementing evidence. Highly collaborative efforts are needed to conduct practice-based research as it involves practitioners, scientists, and others who understand the science and practice of healthcare. Healthcare also requires equitable provision and access to minimize healthcare disparities at the individual and population levels. The practice-based research should develop and implement evidence that is equitable across all populations. The translation of the evidence requires practice-based research for moving the science from bench to bedside to improve and advance patient care.

Scientific Approach for Practice-Based Research

Practice-based research generally involves the following steps: (1) pose a research question and hypothesis, (2) develop and implement a research plan, (3) perform data collection and analysis, and (4) disseminate the research.[19] These steps are more aligned with quantitative research, but the process can be used for qualitative research also.

Practice-based research can involve a mixed approach, involving both quantitative and qualitative approaches. Although each of the steps is discussed in detail in our previous book *Principles of Research Design and Drug Literature Evaluation*,[20] these steps are discussed to help conduct learner-involved practice-based research with resource and time constraints.

The first step in practice-based research is to develop a research question and hypothesis. The commonly used sources include improvements in current practices, ongoing practice initiatives by the administrators, previous research by the mentor's team, replication studies based on the literature, and new ideas based on the existing settings and research infrastructure. The learners have to be keenly aware of the practical considerations to answer the research questions. These include funding, expertise, environment, and access to patient-care data, and others. Good practice-based clinical research questions can be developed using the patient, intervention, comparator, outcomes, timeline, and settings (PICOTS) framework.[21] The PICOTS framework requires the research question to identify the population to be studied, intervention to be applied, comparator to be used, outcomes to be evaluated, timeline to evaluate the outcomes, and healthcare setting of interest. Hypothesis for practice-based research questions can be based on the existing theories, the pathophysiology of a disease, or the pharmacology of a medication. Descriptive or exploratory research does not require a research hypothesis. Most of the evaluation research in pharmacy practice focuses on questions addressing the effect of structure and process on outcomes.

To implement practice-based research, learners should have an understanding of research design and methods. The research designs can be experimental or observational. Experimental designs can include randomized controlled trials, and observational research can include cohort, case-control, or cross-sectional studies. The observational research approaches are more practical than experimental studies for ease of implementation and requirements of institutional approvals and resources. The methods to collect data are either primary or secondary. Primary methods are used to collect data specifically for the research question using techniques such as surveys. Qualitative research requires primary data collection involving interviews and focus groups. Secondary methods involve the use of existing data and can include medical charts or other institutional data sources. Secondary data sources require less time and resources than primary data and are usually preferred by learners. See Table 1–2 for examples of common designs and methods for learner-involved research.

Data collected from primary and secondary sources should be formatted to conduct appropriate statistical analyses. Both quantitative and qualitative research requires robust analytical approaches. Statistical analysis involving descriptive and inferential statistics provides quantitative answers to the research question. Qualitative research requires a thick description and thematic analysis. Research findings are often disseminated as

TABLE 1–2. EXAMPLES OF LEARNER-INVOLVED RESEARCH

Publication	Question/Objective	Design	Methods	Analysis
Jano E, Aparasu RR. Healthcare outcomes associated with beers' criteria: a systematic review. *Ann Pharmacother.* 2007 Mar;41(3):438-447	To examine healthcare outcomes associated with Beers' criteria of inappropriate medication use based on a literature review	Literature Review	Narrative review of studies evaluating inappropriate medications use	Literature synthesis of studies evaluating inappropriate medications use
Aparasu RR, Mort JR, Brandt H. Psychotropic prescription use by community-dwelling elderly in the United States. *J Am Geriatr Soc.* 2003 May;51(5):671-677.	To examine psychotropic prescription use in community-dwelling elderly in the United States and its association with predisposing, enabling, and need factors	Cross-section Study	Retrospective analysis of the 1996 Medical Expenditure Survey	Descriptive and multivariable analyses
Bentley JP, Thacker PG. The influence of risk and monetary payment on the research participation decision making process. *J Med Ethics.* 2004 Jun;30(3):293-298	To determine the effects of risk and payment on subjects' willingness to participate, and to examine how payment influences subjects' potential behaviors and risk evaluations	3 × 3 randomized factorial design	Survey of students enrolled in pharmacy schools	Two factor analysis of covariance
Bentley JP, Stroup LJ, Wilkin NE, Bouldin AS. Patient evaluations of pharmacist performance with variations in attire and communication levels. *J Am Pharm Assoc (2003).* 2005 Sep-Oct;45(5):600-607	To determine whether the attire of a pharmacist has any effect on how he is evaluated when a patient also considers the pharmacist's performance and to assess whether attire and performance interact to influence patients' evaluations	Randomized, cross-sectional, three-factor design	Online surveys	Principal component analysis and three-way analysis of variance
Pearson SC, Eddlemon T, Kirkwood M, Pate A. Are fishbowl activities effective for teaching pharmacotherapy and developing postformal thought in pharmacy students? A pilot study. *Curr Pharm Teach Learn.* 2018 Aug;10(8):1070-1075. doi: 10.1016/j.cptl.2018.05.009; Epub 2018 Jun 6. PMID: 30314543	To use fishbowl activities in large lecture environments to improve post-formal thought and critical thinking skills in pharmacy students	Pre- and Post-design	Online surveys	Wilcoxon signed rank test
Elizabeth B. Hearn, Laurie W. Fleming, Adam N. Pate, et al. Evaluation of a novel process for selecting advanced pharmacy practice experiences. *Curr Pharm Teach Learn.* 2021;13(10):1300-1305. https://doi.org/10.1016/j.cptl.2021.07.020	To evaluate both students and preceptors' satisfaction with the Selective Tiered Optimization process and to identify ways for improvement	Cross-sectional design	Online surveys	Descriptive and bivariate analyses involving *t*-tests

12

posters, podiums, and hopefully publications. The scientific discourse and scrutiny are more for publications than posters and podiums. Although communication format may vary, the core content for dissemination is based on the introduction, methods, results, and discussion (IMRaD).[22] The introduction provides relevant context to examine the research question based on existing literature on the subject. The methods include details of the study design, methods, and analysis. Results present the descriptive and inferential findings based on the analyses. Lastly, the discussion interprets and explains the findings by providing appropriate context based on what is known and not known about the research question.

Research Mentorship and Importance of a Mentor

Research requires knowledge, skill, and experience for study implementation. Most learners may have a knowledge base about research methods, design, and analysis but often lack the skills and experience to successfully implement the research. Novice researchers require the guidance of a mentor to maneuver the intricacies of research. Mentorship is critical for students, residents, and fellows to learn to practice and implement practice-based research. **Mentorship** is defined as "a collaborative learning relationship and working alliance based on intentionality, trust, and shared responsibility for the interactions in that relationship and the effectiveness of those interactions."[23]

Mentors help to transfer the skills and experiences to mentees, and mentees learn to practice the skills while conducting the research. Most learner-involved research, especially in a professional program, involves a single mentor because of the size and scope of the research. Mentorship in graduate education, residency, or fellowship can involve multiple mentors based on the expertise and guidance needed. The mentoring team often involves diverse members with expertise in clinical care, research design and methods, statistics, and others based on the needs of the research. Mentorship involves both formal and informal means to achieve the mentee's goals.

Mentorship for practice-based research can also be considered in the framework of the Donabedian Model. (see Figures 1–4)[12] In order to achieve the outcomes of mentorship, such as the research knowledge, skills, and practices, there needs to be structure and process for mentees to learn and implement research. The structural components can include fiscal, physical, personnel, and policies and procedures. These are provided by the institutions of learning. Fiscal resources are sometimes needed for learner-involved research for resources such as instrumentation, patient incentives, fees, supplies, data, software tools, travel, printing, and others. Both internal and external support can be used to obtain these resources. The physical resources

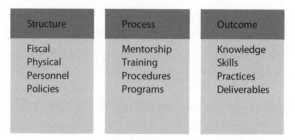

Structure	Process	Outcome
Fiscal	Mentorship	Knowledge
Physical	Training	Skills
Personnel	Procedures	Practices
Policies	Programs	Deliverables

Figure 1–4. Donabedian model for mentorship in research.

include access to patients, people to conduct the research, resources for study implementation, access to data, development of analytical files, assistance with statistical analysis, and other research resources. Most academic and clinical settings have some resources to implement practice-based research. In addition to the mentorship team, learner-involved research needs other supporting systems such as information technology, institutional review board (IRB), and other research support. Finally, the policies and procedures at institutions for research in general and learner-involved research in specific are critical to providing the necessary framework. This can include documents and guides for learners to conduct practice-based research. Finally, time is an important resource that must be a factor as most learners have limited time to conduct research. These structural components are utilized by the mentor to support the research needs of the mentees.

Both formal and informal processes are needed to implement the mentorship process to impart the knowledge, skills, and practices of research. These include necessary training in research techniques and the dissemination process. Institutions and mentors are vital in ensuring that effective processes are in place for learners. Recent studies have highlighted programmatic barriers for effective implementation of mentoring programs such as lack of leadership support, limited expertise and mentors, organized mentoring process, sustainable incentives for mentors, and competing priorities.[24] Therefore, consistent support and processes are needed for effective mentoring. However, the ultimate responsibility falls on the mentoring team to ensure the implementation of the research mentoring process. The goals of mentorship are to provide the knowledge, skills, and practices of research; however, effective mentorship results in deliverables such as presentations, posters, podiums, thesis, and publications. Studies have found barriers in knowledge and practice of the publication process by pharmacy trainees.[24] Therefore, there should be concerted efforts in collaborative learning to achieve the publication deliverables within the given time and resources. Finally, there need to be strong assessments to ensure the mentorship is effective in meeting the needs of both mentors and mentees. Often formal evaluations are needed to evaluate the mentorship to achieve the collaborative learning goals.

Challenges for Learner-Involved Practice-Based Research

There are several challenges for learners to conduct practice-based research. The following discussion presents common challenges and suggestions for novice researchers to conduct practice-based research. These include mentorship, time and research constraints, research resources, and administrative approvals.

Mentors provide guidance, support, and expertise to conduct the research. They also serve as a role model, advisor, and sponsor by providing the necessary support structure involving other mentors and peers. Therefore, there should be strong institutional support for research mentoring programs and mentors. The availability of mentors and their acceptance can be a challenge for learners. In addition, some mentors are highly sought by learners. Therefore, learners should plan ahead in seeking their guidance much before they start the research. This should be based on mutual interests and the academic and professional goals of learners.

Most students, residents, and fellows have limited time to conceptualize, design, implement and complete research projects. Often there is less than a year to conduct and complete the practice-based research. Time considerations are critical in planning and executing the research. Therefore, time management is important, and the mentor–mentee should come up with a timeline for each of the research steps. Time considerations are critical in all aspects of research, including research question and design, money and resources, and institutional approvals.

Learners should carefully consider the time factor in developing the research question, planning the research design and data collection, analysis, and final dissemination of practice-based research. These considerations start with the research question. For example, research to evaluate utilization patterns of medications for any disease will take less time and effort to execute than the research to evaluate the comparative effectiveness of medications. Generally, descriptive research will provide a good starting question for learners. Learners should have a good understanding of the research process, especially research design and methods, as these have to be decided prior to the study implementation. It is critical that learners have the requisite knowledge regarding research design and methods. With respect to design, cross-sectional studies generally take less time and effort than longitudinal studies. Observational research will also take less time and resources than experimental research. Similarly, retrospective studies are not as time-intensive and are less susceptible to small sample size limitations as prospective studies for data collection. Finally, descriptive analyses are easier and time-friendly than multivariate/multivariable analyses. The timeline for sharing the research work involving posters, podiums, and publications should also be carefully planned because of the efforts needed for each.

Practice-based research requires significant resources and sometimes money to implement the research. The learner-developed research question should be answered based on the available resources/infrastructure or the possibility of imminent resources. Learners should have a reasonably good understanding of the available research resources and support for executing the research. This can include access to patients, people to support/conduct the research, access to data, analytical file development, statistical analysis assistance, and other research resources. Most institutions have existing resources for learners. However, sometimes funds are needed to support these resources. There are some funding sources for learners, such as professional organizations, practice sites, universities and colleges, and research mentors. External funding requires more time and effort for proposal preparation and funding considerations.

Most practice-based research requires several approvals to conduct the research. Any research-based existing literature such as narrative, scoping, or systematic reviews generally does not require institutional approvals. The extent of approvals needed is based on the type of research. Often, these approvals require considerable time and effort for the paperwork. Generally, these approvals include IRB to ensure the protection of human subjects and administrative approvals to minimize disruptions for organizational activities. In addition to the university IRB, approvals may be required at the practice site if it involves patients or data sources from the practice. Practice sites may require administrative approvals by the leadership, such as hospital administrators, if the research is conducted in these settings. These approvals often require mentorship support and detailed proposals with careful justifications to conduct practice-based research.

Dissemination of Practice-Based Research

Dissemination of practice-based research is critical to showcase the learning by students, residents, and fellows. This is also important to share the findings of the practice-based research with others. In general, learner-involved research often leads to abstracts, posters, podiums, publications, and others. There is also an expectation from the mentors for defined deliverables as part of the collaborative learning. The dissemination formats can be classified into many ways: (1) print and oral, (2) peer-reviewed and non-peer-reviewed, and (3) internal and external audience. Print formats can include posters, publications, brochures, newsletters, and nonscientific publications. Oral formats include class/institutional presentations, podiums in scientific meetings, and other talks. There is often a peer-review process for printed material such as research abstracts published in scientific meetings and for publications in scientific journals. Most of the other formats, such as newsletters and nonscientific publications, will not follow a peer-review approach. The audience for print and oral formats can be internal or external. The internal audience for oral/print formats can be fellow learners, mentors, teachers, and academic/institution personnel. The presentations at regional and national meetings will have an external audience.

Learners often disseminate their research using abstracts, posters, podiums, publications, social and news media, and others. However, studies have found that pharmacy residency projects have resulted in more abstracts and posters than full publications.[25,26] The publication rate has been found to be generally low (<5%). Therefore, concerted efforts are needed to disseminate the research via peer-reviewed publications. There are often prescribed formats and best practices for most dissemination formats. The content for most dissemination formats is based on the IMRaD. The posters involving large format prints are often presented in scientific meetings after acceptance of the research abstract. It is important to present the poster content involving graphics and text material to share the research in the required format by the meeting organizers and other best practices for posters. Podiums are oral presentations to internal and external audiences. The podiums at respective institutions are usually longer than podiums at scientific meetings. Oral presentations for institutional administrators can help translate the evidence from practice-based research. The goal of these podiums is to share the research succinctly by adhering to the best practices for oral presentations.

Learner-involved research can be published in peer-reviewed publications. In addition to original scientific research, learners have opportunities to publish their research in special sections for residents and fellows. Over the years, there have been numerous reporting guidelines and formats for publishing research rather than the simplistic IMRaD approach. There are guidelines for each study design, such as randomized trials, observational research, and qualitative research, to standardize research reporting. Most publications now require the manuscript to be drafted using these standardized reporting formats. The learners should be aware of these reporting guidelines to present and publish the research work. These reporting guidelines and formats are highly beneficial as they provide the structure for developing the content for the publications. The best resource to get these reporting guidelines and formats is the EQUATOR Network. It is an "umbrella" organization that brings all stakeholders with a mutual interest in improving the quality of reporting in research publications.[27] The CONSORT and other guideline developers initiated the EQUATOR in 2006 with initial funding from the UK National Health Service (NHS) National Knowledge. Later, four national centers were launched in the United Kingdom, Canada, France, and Australia to expand EQUATOR activities.

In recent times, social media has played an important and increasing role in sharing research findings because of their wider visibility and acceptance. These include LinkedIn, Facebook, Twitter, Instagram, Tumblr, YouTube, and others. The content for these social media can be specifically created to attract attention from followers. The links for posters, podiums, and publications can also be embedded while sharing. Often national meetings and journals are also sharing some of the research content using social media tools. Although the content for social media may not require best practices, sharing links from standardized formats like publications and abstracts can give greater visibility for the research.

Other dissemination forms can include brochures, newsletters, blogs, and others. These are usually designed for nonscientific communications but can be used effectively to reach different audience groups. These require both content and creativity to develop and disseminate scientific content. These are effectively used to disseminate scientific findings to both lay and learned audiences. Although these are not recommended formats for scientific communications, they can be part of collaborative learning to showcase creativity to reach different audiences. With increased interest in the dissemination of research, multiple formats and mediums are needed for the acceptance and translation of research.

Summary and Conclusions

Practice-based research is vital for the growth of the healthcare profession and for expanding the scope of pharmacy practice. It provides much-needed evidence for advancing therapeutic and practice innovations. Most national pharmacy practice and educational organizations emphasize the need for research competence for pharmacy practitioners, with practice-based research being a major component of advanced pharmacy education. Increasingly, pharmacy students are also involved in conducting research as part of capstone or elective coursework. Learners should have the knowledge, skills, and experiences to practice the art and science of practice-based research. This starts with a strong understanding of translational and practice-based research in pharmacy. Practice-based research can be conceptualized using the structure, process, and outcomes adopted from the Donabedian Model. The practice-based research often focuses on generating evidence for the structure and process of pharmacy practice to improve patient care outcomes and deliver quality healthcare using the six aims of the IOM.

There are four different dimensions of scholarship for practice-based research, along with the eight basic characteristics that capture the core values of practice-based research. Research requires knowledge, skill, and experience for study implementation.

Therefore, mentors are critical for students, residents, and fellows to learn to practice and implement practice-based research. Dissemination of practice-based research is also important to showcase the learning by students, residents, and fellows. These can include posters, podiums, publications, and others based on best practices. Learners also face various challenges from time and resource constraints to scientific considerations to conduct practice-based research. However, strong mentorship involving a collaborative learning structure and process can help overcome the challenges to achieve the mentee's goals.

Key Points and Advice

- Understanding the conceptual basis of practice-based research is vital to learning and implementing research in pharmacy settings.
- There is significant scope for practice-based research, including the scholarship of discovery, teaching, integration, and application for needed breadth for research innovation.
- Learning a scientific approach to practice-based research requires mentors for guidance to implement research.
- There needs to be a strong research infrastructure and resources along with an effective mentorship process for learners to gain the knowledge, skills, and practices of research.
- Although there are challenges for learner-involved research, collective and concerted efforts by mentees and mentors help overcome the challenges.
- In addition to learning, there are often expectations in mentorship to disseminate the research via presentations, podiums, and publications.

Chapter Review Questions

1. Define translational and practice-based research in pharmacy.
2. Explain the conceptual basis of practice-based research in pharmacy, citing examples.
3. Describe the goals of practice-based research in pharmacy and provide an example from the literature.
4. Using a recent study from pharmacy literature, describe the steps in the scientific approach involved in practice-based research.
5. Define mentorship and explain the mentorship process.
6. Using a recent study from pharmacy literature, identify the challenges to conducting research at your institution.

Online Resources

- ASHP Foundation Research Resources. http://www.ashpfoundation.org/MainMenu Categories/ResearchResourceCenter/ResearchResources
- American College of Clinical Pharmacy (ACCP) Research Institute. http://www.accpri.org/
- University of Washington's Institute for Translational Health Sciences Clinical and Translational Sciences. Research Toolkit. http://www.researchtoolkit.org/
- American Pharmacists Association. Conducting Research Projects. https://www.pharmacist.com/conducting-research-projects
- Interpreting and Conducting Practice-Based Research: An Overview of Real-World Evidence. https://www.amcp.org/Resource-Center/real-world-evidence-research/interpreting-and-conducting-practice-based-research

REFERENCES

1. Balas EA. From appropriate care to evidence-based medicine. *Pediatr Ann.* 1998 Sep;27(9):581-584.
2. Eunice Kennedy Shriver National Institute of Child Health and Human Development (NICHD). *Overview of responsibilities for ClinicalTrials.gov: Compliance with Public Law 110-85 The Food and Drug Administration Amendments Act Title VIII Clinical Trial Databases.* Clinical Research Policy Guidance Document. NICHD;2010. https://www.nichd.nih.gov/sites/default/files/grants-funding/policies-strategies/policies/Documents/NICHD_ClinicalTrials_gov_Policy_final.pdf
3. Alan I. Leshner, Sharon F. Terry, Andrea M. Schultz, Catharyn T. Liverman, eds. *The CTSA Program at NIH. Opportunities for Advancing Clinical and Translational Research.* Washington, DC: National Academies Press, Institute of Medicine; 2013.
4. Rubio DM, Schoenbaum EE, Lee LS, et al. Defining translational research: implications for training. *Acad Med.* 2010 Mar;85(3):470-475.
5. Westfall JM, Mold J, Fagnan L. Practice-based research—"Blue Highways" on the NIH roadmap. *JAMA.* 2007 Jan 24;297(4):403-406.
6. Potter MA, Quill BE, Aglipay GS, et al. Demonstrating excellence in practice-based research for public health. *Public Health Rep.* 2006 Jan–Feb;121(1 suppl):1-16.
7. Nathan DG. The several Cs of translational clinical research. *J Clin Invest.* 2005 Apr;115(4):795-797.
8. Agency for Health Research and Quality. Practice-Based Research Networks (PBRNs). Accessed August 29, 2018. https://pbrn.ahrq.gov/
9. Marinac JS, Kuo GM. Characterizing the American College of Clinical Pharmacy practice-based research network. *Pharmacotherapy.* 2010 Aug;30(8):865.
10. Planas LG, Desselle SP, Cao K. Valuable lessons for pharmacist PBRNs: insights and experiences from physician PBRN members. *Pharmacy (Basel).* 2019 Aug 27;7(3):123.

11. Pruchnicki MC, Rodis JL, Beatty SJ, et al. Practice-based research network as a research training model for community/ambulatory pharmacy residents. *J Am Pharm Assoc. (2003)*. 2008 Mar–Apr;48(2):191-202.

12. Donabedian A. *The Definition of Quality and Approaches to Its Management, vol 1: Explorations in Quality Assessment and Monitoring*. Ann Arbor, Mich: Health Administration Press; 1980.

13. Lohr KN. Outcome measurement: concepts and questions. *Inquiry*. 1988;25:37-50.

14. Kozma CM, Reeder CE, Schulz RM. Economic, clinical, and humanistic outcomes: a planning model for pharmacoeconomic research. *Clin Ther*. 1993 Nov–Dec;15(6): 1121-1132;discussion 1120. PMID: 8111809.

15. Committee on Quality of Health Care in America. Institute of Medicine of the National Academies. *Crossing the Quality Chasm: A New Health System for the 21st Century*. Washington, DC: National Academies Press; 2001.

16. Boyer E. *Scholarship Reconsidered: Priorities of the Professoriate*. Princeton, NJ: Princeton University Press; 1990.

17. Institute of Medicine (US) Committee on Health Services Research. In: Thaul S, Lohr KN, Tranquada RE, eds. *Training and Work Force Issues*. Washington, DC: National Academies Press; 1994.

18. Kerlinger FN. *Foundations of Behavioral Research*. 3rd ed. New York: Holt, Rinehart and Winston; 2006.

19. Aparasu RR. Scientific approach to pharmaceutical policy research. In: Aparasu RR, ed. *Research Methods for Pharmaceutical Practice and Policy*. Binghamton, NY: Pharmaceutical Product Press; 2010.

20. Aparasu RR, Chatterjee S. Scientific approach to research and practice. In: Aparasu Rajender R, Bentley John P, eds. *Principles of Research Design and Drug Literature Evaluation*. 2nd Edition. New York, NY: McGraw Hill; 2020.

21. Velentgas P, Dreyer NA, Nourjah P, Smith SR, Torchia MM, eds. *Developing a protocol for observational comparative effectiveness research: A user's guide*. AHRQ Publication No. 12(13)-EHC099. Rockville, MD: Agency for Healthcare Research and Quality. 2013. https://effectivehealthcare.ahrq.gov/sites/default/files/related_files/user-guide-obser-vational-cer-130113.pdf

22. Pakes GE. Writing manuscripts describing clinical trials: A guide for pharmacotherapeutic researchers. *Ann Pharmacother*. 2001;35(6):770-779.

23. National Academies of Sciences, Engineering, and Medicine; Policy and Global Affairs; Board on Higher Education and Workforce; Committee on Effective Mentoring in STEMM; Dahlberg ML, Byars-Winston A, eds. *The Science of Effective Mentorship in STEMM*. Washington, DC: National Academies Press; 2019.

24. Morbitzer KA, McLaughlin JE, Devanathan AS, Ozawa S, McClurg M Roth. How-to guide for overcoming barriers of research and scholarship training in Pharm. D. and pharmacy residency programs. *JACCP*. 2021;4 (6):743-753.

25. O'Dell KM, Shah SA. Evaluation of pharmacy practice residents' research abstracts and publication rate. *J Am Pharm Assoc (2003)*. 2012 Jul–Aug;52(4):524-527.
26. Weathers T, Ercek K, Unni EJ. PGY1 resident research projects: publication rates, project completion policies, perceived values, and barriers. *Curr Pharm Teach Learn*. 2019 Jun;11(6):547-556.
27. The EQUATOR NETWORK. Enhancing the Quality and Transparency of health Research. https://www.equator-network.org/

2

Chapter Two

Research Mentorship

Lauren G. Pamulapati, PharmD, BCACP and Erin Hickey
Zacholski, PharmD, BCOP

Chapter Objectives

- Identify approaches to find a research mentor
- Describe the mentor–mentee relationship
- Explain the benefits, expectations, and responsibilities of a mentor
- Explain the benefits, expectations, and responsibilities of mentees
- Discuss benefits and resources for developing a career development plan (e.g., NIH Career Development plan)
- Describe general approaches for managing conflicts

Key Terminology

Mentor, mentee, mentorship, research contract, mentoring-up, career development plan, win-win negotiation, residency, fellowship

Introduction

Undertaking a research project for the first time can feel daunting; however, you do not have to begin this process alone. With the assistance of one or several mentors, you can be guided through the research process. A **mentor** is defined as a trusted counselor or guide, whereas a mentee is the one who is being mentored.[1] In healthcare professions, we often refer to mentorship as a dynamic, bidirectional, reciprocal relationship in which guidance is provided by an experienced individual (mentor) to a less experienced individual (mentee), most often a trainee, to develop their professional skills and knowledge.[2,3] This can be done in an informal or formal process, but in either case, the mentor acts as an information provider, facilitator, role model, assessor, planner, and resource developer.[4]

Traditionally, mentorship was thought of as dyadic, a relationship between one mentor and one mentee. However, mentorship has evolved to include many individuals and structures to support the mentee's development, which will be discussed in more detail later in the chapter. To better address the changes in mentorship beyond a dyadic relationship, the National Academies of Sciences, Engineering, and Medicine (NASEM) proposed a definition of mentorship as a "professional, working alliance in which individuals work together over time to support the personal and professional growth, development, and success of the relationship partners through the provision of career and psychosocial support."[5] This definition better encompasses the many facets of mentorship and the resulting benefits that effective mentoring can provide to not just the mentee, but the mentor, as well. A great example of this multilevel dynamic relationship is that of a co-pilot (e.g., the mentee) and a pilot (e.g., the mentor) developing and executing a flight plan. The two individuals will work together to guide the plane to their destination; however, when turbulence (e.g., obstacles in the mentor relationship) occurs, the control tower (e.g., institutional leaders or others involved in the mentoring relationship) will lend a hand to ensure the pilots successfully and safely complete their flight. In the mentoring relationship, this may entail linking the pair to others in their network or providing development opportunities that will optimize their relationship.[5]

Similar to other fields of science, mentorship has become integral in all areas of our pharmacy careers, whether it be clinical practice development, or for the purpose of this chapter, research development.[6] Effective research mentorship is important, as research experiences offered early in one's pharmacy career have been shown to improve critical thinking skills, increase interest in future research, and increase marketability in one's career search.[7] Research mentorship will enable the mentee to broaden their skillset and confidence within pharmacy, better preparing them for various career paths by deepening their learning experiences beyond the classroom.[8] This chapter will present the science of mentorship, define the mentorship process, discuss the benefits of mentorship, provide conflict management strategies for common mentor–mentee conflicts, and detail tools and tips in career development planning.

Science of Mentorship

Mentorship often seems simplistic, but there are several theoretical frameworks of mentorship that help ground discussions of the concepts discussed throughout this chapter. There are six primary theoretical models for mentorship that can apply to science, technology, engineering, mathematics, and medicine (STEMM) careers: (1) ecological systems theory, (2) social cognitive career theory, (3) tripartite integration model of social influence, (4) social exchange theory, (5) social capital theory, and (6) social network theory.[5]

The ecological systems theory states that the mentoring relationship is influenced by five levels of systems, namely one-on-one level, faculty level, university-community level, national and global level, and changes over time. This theory emphasizes the importance of accounting for personal factors and environmental systems that impact the mentoring relationship. In short, the mentor and mentee must consider environmental factors (e.g., competing practice site or residency priorities) that may impact their individual behaviors in the mentorship relationship. The social cognitive career theory relies on self-efficacy beliefs, the belief that individuals possess the innate ability to successfully overcome challenges, and outcome expectations. This belief seeks to explain an individual's motivation and persistence in goal achievement in relation to the individual's belief regarding the likelihood that a specific behavior will lead to the desired outcome. Applying this theory to research mentorship, a mentor should consider providing a mentee with learning experiences that can improve their self-efficacy and subsequently aid in career decisions. Within STEMM careers, the tripartite integration model of social influence explains how an individual finds their identity within the science community and then integrates into that community. This theory suggests that a mentor should serve as a role model for the mentee, demonstrating the attitudes and behaviors that are necessary for success in their area of pharmacy practice/research. The social exchange theory focuses on the mentoring relationship more transactionally and evaluates the cost–benefit for both the mentor and mentee. One central assumption of social exchange theory is that the relationship is reciprocal or else it will not flourish, i.e., if the costs outweigh the benefits, one will not engage in the relationship. The social capital theory is situated around the concept that dominant groups reproduce social inequality. Effective mentorship in this model should impart knowledge and resources tailored to the needs of the mentee in order to enable them to find their individual research fit, thus promoting mobility within the field. Lastly, the social network theory discusses the influence of social structure on human behavior. Those with larger, diverse social networks will experience greater upward mobility and adaptability than those with smaller, undiversified social networks. This theory emphasizes the importance of mentorship relationships moving beyond dyadic relationships into larger mentorship networks.[5]

Mentorship Process

With a brief overview of the theoretical models for mentorship, one is better positioned to begin to consider the process of how to find a mentor or a group of mentors that will be the best fit for their specific needs. One way to be proactive in finding a mentor is to manage-up, or mentor-up. **Mentoring-up** is a concept adapted from the business concept of managing up, in which the mentee is an active participant in their mentoring relationship and shifts emphasis from a mentor-only responsibility to a shared responsibility between the mentor and mentee.[3,9] In Figure 2–1, you can see there are several steps in the mentoring-up process: initiation, cultivation, separation, and redefinition.[3,9]

INITIATION PHASE

In the initiation phase, the mentee is responsible for self-identifying career goals and expectations for the research, work style and habits, knowledge and skills gaps, and specific opportunities that are being sought. Additionally, the mentee should write down short- and long-term goals to ensure the research project and mentor are capable of meeting these goals.

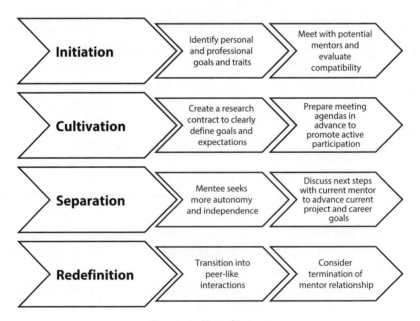

Figure 2–1. Mentorship stages.

Mentees often approach mentoring relationships for a variety of reasons. Some seek out research mentors as a learner to enhance their competitiveness for future career paths, such as those pursuing residency or fellowship or a career in academia. **Residencies** are organized, directed, postgraduate training programs in a defined area of pharmacy practice, whereas **fellowships** are a directed, highly individualized, postgraduate program designed to prepare the participant to become an independent researcher.[10] Research experience often sets candidates apart in the competitive application process for either of these postgraduate training opportunities.[11] Residents or fellows may seek out research mentors as they are looking to their next career step, especially those interested in academia who may seek out additional research opportunities to gain experience in their future job area, or build skills in areas they may be expected to fulfill on their own, post-training. For others, such as early pharmacy students, embarking on a research project may be a way of exploring different possible career paths within the pharmacy profession. Alternatively, some pharmacy students may approach research mentoring as a curricular requirement (e.g., research capstones or other required research courses) in which they may have limited options of choosing a mentor or area of research interest.[12] Knowing one's motivation for pursuing research can help in establishing a mentor relationship and may impact the type of mentor you have access to.

After identifying your motivation and goals for engaging in research, the mentee can start identifying potential mentors that may fulfill these goals. Mentors may come from a variety of places, including people you already know, such as faculty members or preceptors. Finding a good fit in a mentor is important for establishing a mentor–mentee relationship. The "3 As": attraction, affect, and action is a useful tool to help young mentees assess mentor compatibility and fit.[2] Attraction means that the mentee looks up to the mentor in some way, and conversely, the mentor sees potential in the mentee. Next, evaluate the mentor's affect—the mentor should have a supportive, encouraging affect, that the mentee believes will help facilitate their growth through this new process. Even if a mentor meets the attraction and affect domains, action A will help mentees avoid a common pitfall in research mentorship, which is the time commitment. This arises when mentors and mentees lack the necessary time and attention required to put the relationship into action; thus, both must be willing to invest time and respond in a timely manner.[2]

After identifying suitable mentors using the "3 As" it is often helpful to formalize your goals of the relationship with a self-assessment. The best way to do this is to ask yourself and your potential mentor several questions.[13]

1. Why am I pursuing this research opportunity?
2. Do my career and research goals align with the current career and research agenda of the mentor?
3. Is my potential research mentor someone I look up to and want to emulate in my career?

4. Are our personal work styles similar?

5. Am I willing and able to commit the needed time and effort to this research project?

6. What expectations do I have of a mentor? What expectations does the mentor have of me?

After this self-reflection, the mentee should ask to meet with potential mentors with a clearly defined purpose for each meeting. Mentees should be prepared to discuss their background and clearly define their individual goals and needs so the mentor can ensure they have the time and expertise needed to meet these goals. These meetings will not only help mentees in selecting the right mentor fit but also serve as an opportunity to market yourself and play into helping evaluate the cost benefits associated with the relationship based on the social exchange theory that the benefits should outweigh the costs for both the mentor and the mentee. At the end of the meeting, it is appropriate to ask for recommendations from other potential mentors, as this can help mentees start building a network of potential mentors. While this process can feel daunting, the key is perseverance. It is better to have too many potential mentors than none, and this will facilitate your development of a personal board of directors, which is discussed later in the chapter.[9]

CULTIVATION PHASE

After identifying a mentor, the next step is to begin cultivating the relationship. This is your time to manage-up, or mentor-up, by taking ownership of your relationship and clearly articulating your needs, and managing information flow. First, it is important to identify how the mentor and mentee would like to receive communication. This helps both parties tailor deliverables and meetings to each other's preferred communication style. Next, be prepared for all mentor–mentee meetings. Mentees should prepare meeting agendas and share them with their mentor in advance of meetings. They should also ask for feedback regarding tasks completed on the agenda, then evaluate upcoming tasks, including identifying new deadlines for these tasks within a reasonable timeframe.[9]

SEPARATION PHASE

As a mentee becomes more comfortable with their research project, they will approach the separation phase, in which the mentee should seek more autonomy and independence. At this phase, it is appropriate to discuss with your mentor how your relationship will continue, evolve, or close after the research project is complete. Mentees should use this time to discuss personal achievements and progress during the project as well as appropriate next steps regarding professional or career goals. This is also an ideal time to ask a mentor if they have recommendations or could help connect you with new mentors.[9]

REDEFINITION PHASE

The last phase of a mentor–mentee relationship is redefinition. This is when the mentor and mentee transition into colleagues and have a more peer-like interaction. It is presumed that the relationship is no longer one of formal mentorship as the mentee should have obtained the skill sets or met their predefined goals for the relationship at this phase of their career. Additionally, it is not uncommon for the mentee to now find themselves serving as a mentor, imparting their newly formed knowledge and skills onto others.[5]

Mentor–Mentee Characteristics and Expectations

In the process of finding a mentor, you must be realistic about what characteristics you are seeking and defining expectations for both you and the mentor. Effective research mentorship is centered on finding the right mentor–mentee fit, and thus carefully considering needs and expectations from a mentor is critical.

MENTOR CHARACTERISTICS AND EXPECTATIONS

To promote a successful mentorship relationship, the mentor should have adequate time, experience, and compatible psychosocial characteristics. The first and likely most important consideration is time. Using the ecological systems theory framework, the mentor and mentee must recognize the substantial investment of time the mentoring relationship will require and balance this with competing time demands. This should be one of the first things a mentee assesses when seeking out a mentor for a research project because competing priorities for either the mentor or mentee can result in unanswered inquiries, lack of availability for meetings, and ultimately a less than effective mentor–mentee relationship. Highlighting the competing priorities, a mentor should also assist in setting deadlines for the research project depending on the mentees' previous research experiences; the mentee likely may not be able to establish an appropriate research timeline alone. An effective mentor will be able to assess a mentee's baseline knowledge at the beginning of the relationship and help set realistic expectations for a research project. This should include providing feedback regarding a mentee's research proposal, timeline, and research goals, including assisting with developing targeted tasks for a mentee to work on between meetings.[2,6,14,15]

As mentioned previously, the goal of mentorship is to aid in the professional development of skills and knowledge. This means that your mentor should be experienced in the type and topic of research you are interested in. Before seeking out a mentor, consider if their career interests and goals align with yours. For example, if you are interested in bench research, you will likely be seeking out one of the basic science professors at your school, such as those in the pharmaceutics or medicinal chemistry departments. Additionally, depending on an institution's resources, you may reach out to pharmacokinetic researchers, such as those working in infectious diseases. Alternatively, if a mentee is more interested in practice-based research, they should seek out a member of the pharmacy practice department, ideally already involved in an area of research of interest to the mentee. Misaligning your research and career goals with those of your mentor can lead to feeling overwhelmed or disengaged from the project.[2,6,14,15]

Finally, mentees should consider several psychosocial characteristics when looking for a mentor. Mentor–mentee compatibility regarding personality, shared interests, and working style will help foster a collegial relationship and establish a firm foundation for the mentor–mentee relationship. Self-reflection on the part of a mentee concerning how you learn best and if you need structured directed guidance, or gentle supervision, will allow a mentee to better assess fit with potential mentors based on their teaching and communication styles. Another way to assess fit is to consider interactions you have had with the individual up to this point. Did you find yourself wanting to learn more from them and interested in carrying on the conversation later? This may be a good clue into your mentorship compatibility. Along with compatibility, an effective mentor should be engaged, enthusiastic about teaching, patient, and respectful. As a novice, you are not going to know all the answers right away; thus, finding a mentor who understands your limitations and helps you overcome these barriers in your research journey will make the experience much more enjoyable.[2,6,9,14,15]

MENTEE CHARACTERISTICS AND EXPECTATIONS

Many of the traits noted for mentors can be reciprocated by mentees, as outlined in Table 2-1. Just like good communication is needed on behalf of mentors, the same is expected from mentees. The mentee should be an active participant in their learning, demonstrating an ability to speak up regarding their research or career needs. They should be self-directed and engaged in learning, demonstrating independence in between research meetings. Additionally, mentees should be receptive and welcoming of feedback when tasks are completed ensuring that continuous improvement can be enacted by the mentee.[2]

Setting clear guidelines regarding project timelines and deliverables will help ensure the mentee is meeting mentor expectations and is important for establishing open communication for the mentoring relationship. Sometimes, a mentor may provide a small

TABLE 2-1. BIDIRECTIONAL MENTOR AND MENTEE CHARACTERISTICS

Domain	Mentor Characteristics	Mentee Characteristics
Meetings and communication	Accessible and available	Adaptable
	Responsive to inquiries	Proactive in reaching out when help is needed
	Sufficient time for mentoring	Good time management for completing research tasks
Expectations and feedback	Provides timely constructive feedback	Receptive and open to feedback
		Enacts changes based on feedback given
	Outlines realistic expectations and goals	Takes responsibility for assigned tasks
		Prepares in advance of meetings
		Follows up on meeting tasks
	Effective conflict resolution skills	Receptive to negotiations
Career development	Able to counsel and advise about career paths	Self-identification of career goals
	Expertise in the topic area	Self-directed learner
	Assist in the development of new skills	
	Acknowledge contributions of the mentee	Appreciation of time and effort from mentor
	Foster self-reflection	Self-reflective
	Advocate for the mentee	Communicate in a straight-forward manner on behalf of oneself
Research support	Knowledge of scholarly process	Responsive to new ideas
	Sufficient experience in research, publication, and presentations	Initiative for learning new concepts and ideas
Psychosocial support	Engaged, active listener	Speaks up on behalf of oneself
	Enthusiastic and motivating	Desire for personal growth and development
	Patient and self-less	Team player
	Interpersonal compatibility: Shared interests and working style to that of the mentee	Interpersonal compatibility: Shared interests and working style to that of mentor
	Respectful and understanding	Respectful and open

set of tasks, such as conducting a literature review, to assess responsiveness and level of determination on behalf of the mentee before embarking on a full mentored research project with them.[16] This enables the mentor to better evaluate appropriate individual mentee expectations, while giving the mentee the opportunity to demonstrate their initiative in the project.

If an individual has decided to serve as your mentor, one method commonly used to formally outline expectations is a **research contract**, a document detailing the obligations and commitments between a mentor and mentee over the course of a research project. An example research contract can be found in Figure 2–2. This contract may be referenced when determining if the effort matches what was outlined at the beginning of the research project to avoid over and underinclusive authorship practices, as well as defining authorship order, keeping in mind the criteria outlined by the International Committee of Medical Journal Editors (ICMJE) that should be met for authorship, which is discussed further in Chapter 24.[17] To avoid authorship surprises at the time of manuscript and/or poster preparation, the research contract allows these expectations to be discussed upfront, and possibly written into the research contract, with criteria outlined for the mentee to follow to ensure their place in the predetermined authorship order.[18]

Introduction:
Participating in [insert research activity here] can be mutually beneficial for both the mentee and mentor alike. To ensure that mentees have the proper intention for participating in this activity and to ensure clearly defined expectations for the research project, this form should be completed prior to starting the research mentoring relationship.

Prerequisites:

Personal attributes
1. What are your professional goals for conducting research or other scholarly activities?
2. Considering your academic/residency workload, how much time can you dedicate to the research project each week?
3. What is your preferred method of communication (e.g., virtual versus in-person)?
4. How do you prefer to receive feedback (e.g., modality and frequency)?

Research considerations
5. Submit evidence of completion of CITI modules (check with your mentor first to see if this is required for your project).
6. Write a short description of the research or scholarly activity proposed.
7. Write objectives for completing the research or portion of the project. Note: these should be specific to the project outlined by your mentor. Examples include conducting a literature search, perform data collection, write poster abstract, etc.
8. Write out the proposed timeline for completing the above-mentioned tasks (e.g., IRB, literature search, data collection, data analysis, poster,and/or manuscript submission).

Agreement Statements:
Acknowledge that as a **mentee**, I take on the primary role and responsibility for meeting all agreed upon deadlines and objectives for the research project or scholarly activity. I will communicate my progress to my mentor as appropriate and seek guidance when necessary.

_____   _____
Mentee Signature   Date

Acknowledge that as a **mentor**, I commit to providing research or scholarly training to the mentee through discussions, self-directed learning opportunities, and feedback on various assignments. I will communicate expectations, set reasonable goals and deadlines, and follow standard practices and procedures while mentoring them through the scholarly process.

_____   _____
Mentor Signature   Date

Figure 2–2. Example research contract.

TABLE 2-2. MENTEE AND MENTOR BENEFITS

Mentee Benefits	Mentor Benefits
— Feeling of empowerment and self-efficacy	— Personal fulfillment
— Attainment and enhancement of skills (e.g., project management, critical thinking)	— Assistance with projects
	— Increased productivity and outputs
— Increased job competitiveness	— Leadership development

SHARED MENTOR AND MENTEE CHARACTERISTICS

As described above, there are common characteristics of mentors and mentees that promote a successful mentorship relationship. These characteristics can be broken into five domains: (1) meetings and communication; (2) expectations and feedback; (3) career development; (4) research support; and (5) psychosocial support.[7] Within each of these domains, characteristics can be defined for both mentors and mentees, further representing the bidirectional relationship of the mentor–mentee relationship (Table 2–1).[2,6,14,15]

Benefits of Mentorship

Mentorship continues to be a vital part of research, with benefits observed for both the mentee and the mentor (Table 2–2). For both the mentee and mentor, there is often a sense of personal fulfillment and empowerment, especially when the research leads to outputs, such as posters, publications, and funding opportunities. For mentees or students, Henchey and colleagues found that mentored student research resulted in increased student confidence, especially in regard to the ability to review and evaluate medical literature.[19] Furthermore, students have indicated that research exposure made them more competitive for jobs and postgraduate training, thus enhancing mentee marketability.[7,19,20] This complements previous studies that have shown mentorship for pharmacy students and residents has led to increased publication rates and abstract presentations at professional meetings, while enhancing learner experiences in all areas of the research process from study design to publication.[7] These direct outputs of presentations and publications, as well as increased confidence and skillsets gained, may translate to enhanced career opportunities, thus extrinsic benefits for both the mentor and the mentee.

Types of Mentors

While you may find a single mentor for certain aspects of research, you will also form relationships with multiple mentors. These mentors may work within your department or institution, or you may look for mentors outside your institution. Additionally, some mentors are assigned, while others are fostered through personal connections.

INTRA-INSTITUTIONAL MENTORS

As a trainee, you are most likely going to be exposed to intra-institutional mentors, or those who are affiliated with your institution, whether it be your school of pharmacy or place of work for residency or fellowship. Residency programs will utilize different approaches for matching mentees with research mentors. Some mentors are selected by the mentee based on compatible mentor and mentee research interests and available projects. The advantage of this approach is that the mentee can better align their research interests with those of the available mentors and projects, as well as choose a mentor based on previously described characteristics. Alternatively, some residency programs assign mentors to the mentee based on projects that are already started in the previous residency year. This model typically means that there are a defined number of residency projects with set mentors; thus, the new residents are restricted to those available projects. While the alignment of research or career interests within this model may be limited, this approach does enable the resident to focus on data collection and analysis skills rather than getting bogged down in research design, which can often delay a project and risk it not being completed in the defined residency period.

For pharmacy students, you are often embarking on research with faculty members at your school, whether through an assigned course, such as a research capstone and research elective course, or through the identification of a research mentor, as described above. The assigned approach has downfalls in that it may not match your interests, or the mentor may not be compatible with your learning style; however, as an early learner, this approach may be effective in providing early exposure to the research process and still helps with building a network of mentors. Another intra-institutional mentor that students often do not consider are their peers in the form of near-peer mentoring, in which senior-level students mentor junior-level students with oversight by a faculty member or preceptor.[15,21] Near-peer mentoring has demonstrated the ability to decrease stress and anxiety among junior-mentees, thus increasing satisfaction with their experience and increasing retention on projects.[15] Lee and colleagues demonstrated an increase in research productivity in the form of more poster presentations and manuscripts through the utilization of near-peer teaching.[21] Near-peer teaching has also demonstrated the ability to enhance the mentee's educational and career opportunities.[8] The success of near-peer teaching is often attributed to cognitive confluence, which relates to the concept that senior-level learners are better able to understand issues brought forth by the junior-level learners, thus enabling them to better explain the concepts and manage problems that arise.[21]

INTER-INSTITUTIONAL RELATIONSHIPS

Less often in your training experience, you may have a research mentor from outside of your organization, thus an inter-institutional relationship. These mentor relationships may develop through networking at professional organizational meetings or through internships. This type of relationship is rare as a learner but may become more common as you progress through your pharmacy career and build your network. The advantage of these inter-institutional relationships is having an outside perspective and being able to learn from others outside your institution, thus increasing your exposure to different research and practice approaches.

PERSONAL BOARD OF DIRECTORS

As discussed previously, you likely will not find all of the characteristics you are looking for in one mentor; thus, finding a complement of multiple mentors is recommended.[9] Multiple mentors can take the form of a personal board of directors (PBOD), a group of individuals who advise you in different aspects of your career.[22] From a research perspective, individuals you may consider including in your PBODs include: someone who is in or has been in your circumstance (e.g., a near-peer mentor), someone in your field (e.g., a junior-level mentor), someone who is a leader in the area you aspire to grow or succeed (e.g., a senior-level mentor), and someone who can introduce you to others in the profession (e.g., a junior or senior level mentor).[22] Junior level mentors can be of complement to senior-level mentors, as they may have more time to commit to the mentee, whereas senior-level mentors can serve as connectors to others in the field.[9] Near-peer mentors can also help connect you to others. For example, you may find a fellow student or resident who has successfully developed a mentoring relationship with a faculty member or preceptor you feel would be a good personal fit for you. Further exploring career interests and guidance with this fellow student or resident and discussing their mentor–mentee relationship may provide you the opportunity to approach the mentor with an idea for a research project and begin establishing a mentor–mentee relationship of your own.

Managing Conflicts

COMMON CHALLENGES IN MENTOR–MENTEE RELATIONSHIPS

Despite one's best efforts to identify an ideal mentor, conflicts will inevitably still arise. To maximize the bidirectional benefits from the research mentor–mentee relationship, avoiding and resolving common conflicts are essential. Due diligence in appropriately selecting a mentor is often the first step in avoiding common challenges. Utilizing the "3 As," described previously, is one strategy to assess fit and avoid conflicts.[2] Even after using due diligence in selecting a research mentor, many challenges or conflicts arise spontaneously during the mentoring relationship simply due to the demanding nature of training programs and professional careers. Challenges reported in the health sciences mentoring literature include difficulty maintaining the relationship, perceived lack of commitment by one party, and perceived bias of the mentor.[14,23] These challenges to productive and harmonious mentor–mentee relationships often are the result of competing priorities and/or misaligned expectations. Understanding and anticipating these challenges and planning resolution approaches may allow for the preservation of the relationship and research progress.

Competing Priorities

No matter the type of mentor, both the mentor and mentee contribute a large amount of time and effort to learning, teaching, and conducting high-quality research. Practice-based researchers who commit to mentor–mentee relationships may have mixed professional responsibilities, managing their pharmacy practices, teaching didactically or experientially, and supporting administrative and service duties. Mentors are likely also advising multiple students or may even be engaged as a mentee themselves. Likewise, mentees may be engaged in demanding curricula or residency or fellowship programs with a range of other demands. These examples only encompass professional responsibilities and don't include personal responsibilities or commitments which also compete for the limited resource of individual time.

Competing priorities are an unavoidable reality and are potentiated by the propensity of both mentors and mentees involved in practice-based research to overcommit their time and energy. Trainees involved in research are typically motivated and eager to learn and contribute to research to improve the health system or patient outcomes. Likewise, mentors are commonly empathetic individuals invested in the development of their mentees.[6] When a mentor and mentee agree to work together on a research project, they are consciously or unconsciously placing the project and relationship at a certain rank on their priority list. As the project progresses, differences in prioritization will reveal themselves, potentially causing conflict. Practical strategies for avoiding this challenge include an initial meeting to discuss priorities of both parties, with defined goals and tasks, and the scheduling of regular meetings with defined agendas.[2] Both the mentor and mentee should be transparent about the time commitment and expected timeline for a research project. Prior to committing to a research opportunity, it can be helpful for mentees and mentors to be forthcoming about other professional and personal demands. Participating in a research contract can be a useful tool in providing a venue to consider and discuss project responsibilities and conflicting demands. Clear communication surrounding competing demands and priorities is key to maintaining the professional relationship and ensuring project success. When competing priorities are identified as a conflict, a research mentor may be able to transition into a career-mentoring role, guiding the mentee in prioritizing professional responsibilities, declining new opportunities that may not fit the mentee's long-term goals, and offering resources and psychosocial support for stress management.

Misaligned Expectations

Mentors and mentees enter into a mentoring relationship with the potential to benefit from the experience. With this potential comes preconceived expectations and goals for the relationship and, in this case, the research experience and product. In many settings, such as research mentoring relationships occurring within formal didactic research courses taken for student credit or a fellowship program with defined objectives and timelines, these expectations are clearly delineated. For example, a residency program may have the requirement that a research manuscript suitable for publication in a peer-reviewed journal be submitted prior to successful completion of the program. Other times, the research mentoring relationship occurs outside of strict requirements, and these goals and expectations are not clearly delineated. It is the responsibility of the mentor and mentee to clarify expectations and set short- and long-term research goals together. A research contract may be beneficial in helping to clarify expectations upfront. Ideally, this conversation will happen formally prior to entering into the mentoring relationship. However, even formative discussion of expectations if a conflict arises may lead to increased listening, understanding, and win-win negotiations (Table 2–3).[24]

Conflict Resolution

Avoiding and managing conflicts within research mentoring relationships centers on preemptively communicating and aligning expectations and finding win-win negotiation of outcomes when possible. Negotiation is defined as the process of resolving conflicts between individuals or parties through dialogue and problem solving, whereas a **win-win negotiation** is a technique where parties focus on making certain that both parties are satisfied.[24] A mentoring relationship can be a longstanding professional connection, and practice with these conflict management scenarios and techniques may benefit both parties as well as the research progress.

TABLE 2–3. COMMON RESEARCH MENTORING RELATIONSHIP CHALLENGES AND PROPOSED RESOLUTIONS

Challenge	Situation	Background	Approaches to Resolution
Misaligned expectations	Tamara is a Doctor of Pharmacy student who just began working with a faculty member, Dr. Smith, on a retrospective clinical study. Lately, Dr. Smith has been slow to respond to Tamara's emails to meet, and Tamara is frustrated.	— Tamara is in her fourth year of pharmacy school. She does not have prior experience with research. She is equally eager to gain introductory research experience and present a research poster to strengthen her residency application. She has three months until applications are due. — Dr. Smith is a new faculty member starting a clinical practice amid teaching and service responsibilities. Her father is sick, and she is the primary caregiver. Her goal is to complete this project by the end of Tamara's academic year.	**How to Avoid:** This conflict could have been avoided by discussing priorities and goals at the start of the research mentor–mentee relationship. Tamara's priority is to present a poster in three months, but Dr. Smith's timeline for this project does not fit Tamara's goals. Dr. Smith could have offered an alternative project that fits Tamara's timeline, or directed her to another research mentor. **How to Resolve:** It is not too late for both parties to share their goals for the project openly. At their next meeting, Tamara can clarify that she would like this research project to be among her top priorities to facilitate a poster presentation. Dr. Smith can be honest about her situation. Together, they can determine if there is an aspect of the research project that can be presented in poster format within three months, leaving the remainder of the project to be completed within the year time frame.
Competing priorities	Dr. Booth is a postgraduate Year 1 (PGY1) residency research advisor for Neil. It is the end of Neil's residency year and he has yet to submit a draft manuscript to Dr. Booth. Dr. Booth is disappointed because Neil signed a research contract confirming that he would submit a draft manuscript by the end of the year.	— Neil is a PGY1 resident completing his residency in a few weeks. He is working 80-hour weeks to complete rotation activities and projects and knows that he is behind on his research manuscript. — Neil is eager to move onto a postgraduate Year 2 (PGY2) at another institution, where he will be busy with demanding clinical duties, adjusting to a new city, and starting another research project. He is concerned about his ability to continue to engage with his PGY1 research project after moving on to PGY2.	**How to Avoid:** — This mentor–mentee pair took steps to enable them to effectively approach situations like these by creating a research contract. However, clearly specifying the consequences for an incomplete manuscript would be helpful in determining productive next steps. Consequences for broken contracts may include the inability to graduate residency or the removal/rearrangement of authorship. — Neil and his mentor could have set smaller deadlines for his manuscript with frequent check-ins. If a mentoring relationship had been in place, Neil could have been more proactive about being behind and asked for help earlier. **How to Resolve:** Engaging in a conversation where the interests and positions of both parties are heard and understood could lead to a productive outcome. An example of a win-win negotiation could be for Neil's mentor to help arrange for Neil to be able to take a day from rotation to complete his manuscript. The pair could agree upon a modified authorship order if Neil is unable to continue work on this manuscript after his PGY1 residency.

PGY1, Postgraduate Year One; PGY2, Postgraduate Year Two

Career Development Planning

Working on research with a mentor, intra- or inter-institutionally, can result in a professional relationship that transcends a time-bound project. Mentoring relationships often evolve to focus on non-research topics such as academic advising, networking, and career development planning. Approaching a "career development plan" (CDP) is an important trainee process that requires the dedication of an invested mentor and has many benefits for the mentee.

THE NIH CAREER DEVELOPMENT PLAN

Early understanding of the trainee's "career development plan" is advantageous for successful practice-based research at the student, resident, or fellow level. The CDP is a training plan designed to provide knowledge and skills to conduct research and prepare for future career.[25] When discussed formally, it constitutes a portion of the National Institutes of Health (NIH) Career Development (K) award grant application for postdoctoral fellows or faculty-level candidates. It describes specific training areas needed to achieve short- and long-term goals and mechanisms for gaining this training throughout the award period. Obtaining a K award grant can provide individual research development opportunities by allocating funding and protected time, and increasing competitiveness for acquiring future grant support, like the "R01" grant.[25] In the CDP, the mentor and the applicant describe specific training areas needed (e.g., advanced statistics didactic training), why this training is required to achieve short- and long-term goals, and how this training will be gained throughout the award period. This level of planning cannot be achieved without introspective goal setting, understanding strengths and weaknesses, and ultimately research mentorship.[25,26]

Trainees interested and involved in practice-based research in pharmacy have diverse career paths and goals. Trainees and mentors, at any stage of their development, should investigate how much of their future job will include conducting research, identify their ideal balance of job activities, and seek skills accordingly. Deliberate career development planning, as it pertains to research development, is especially essential to discover, clarify, and communicate one's research goals and identify skills and resources needed to achieve those goals. Though not all trainees are ready or eligible to seek grant-funding opportunities like the NIH K awards, introducing and discussing the CDP in the formal and informal contexts may have many benefits, such as:

1. Discovering career pathways involving practice-based research
2. Strengthening mentor–mentee relationships
3. Expanding the professional research network or
4. Identifying opportunities for research training or funding.

CAREER DEVELOPMENT PLANNING RESOURCES

There are a variety of general tools that may be applicable to trainees involved in pharmacy research. As pharmacy practice-based research opportunities can be as diverse and expansive as the profession itself, career exploration is the first step in career development planning. Several tools are available to both mentors and mentees to help guide career planning discussions.

Career Pathway Assessment Tools

The American Pharmacists Association (APhA) Career Pathway Evaluation Program is an assessment tool that may help both mentors and mentees learn about the various career options in pharmacy that may be a fit for a mentee's individual interests and skills.[27,28] Many of the pathways represented involve varying levels of practice-based research across settings, from conducting research and development within the pharmaceutical industry to an economic and administrative sciences faculty member at a school or college of pharmacy.[29] The APhA Career Pathway assessment can serve as a valuable tool for students, residents, and fellows in planning or reassessing their long-term goals pertaining to careers involving research.[27,28]

Though not pharmacy-focused, the American Association for the Advancement of Science's Individual Development Plan is a similar publicly available, free, interactive assessment tool to help science trainees identify goals and discuss career planning with their mentors. Trainees complete a series of three self-assessments ranking their skills, interests, and values, which are used to help define suitable career matches.[30]

Resident and Fellow Career Development Planning

Postgraduate Year 1 (PGY1) and Postgraduate Year 2 (PGY2) residencies can provide unparalleled opportunities for exposure to practice-based research. To achieve the purpose of a residency, trainees gain further expertise in medication management within broad (PGY1) or specialized (PGY2) patient populations.[10] Trainees seeking or enrolled in residency programs who are interested in practice-based research should recognize that these training experiences typically require completion of a residency research project within one year, while demanding a high level of direct patient care and clinical leadership, among a range of other activities to meet program and accrediting body residency objectives.[31] According to the American Society of Health System Pharmacists (ASHP) Accreditation Standards for PGY1 Pharmacy Residency Programs, residents work to "demonstrate the ability to evaluate and investigate practice, review data, and assimilate scientific evidence to improve patient care and/or the medication-use system." This may include a quality improvement or research project, but program practices may vary due to this wide description according to program and preceptor capabilities.[31] Therefore, there are no uniform requirements for formal research training programs or peer-reviewed publication for ASHP-accredited residencies, and residents should expect variability in research expectations, a prime opportunity for mentor support, during residency.

Recognizing that the ability to conduct independent research is essential for many pharmacists after residency training, the development of local research certificate programs and practice-based research networks have been instituted with success at many programs.[26,32] For example, Pruchnicki and colleagues instituted a multiprogram, multisite practice-based research network for community/ambulatory pharmacy practice residents, including the residency program director, research director, research faculty, and preceptor and resident members. After the implementation of this program, the publication to resident ratio increased from 0.25 to 0.56.[26] Residency programs have mechanisms to improve the learning experience and the impact of the residency research experience. For example, many programs have research committees, which may pre-approve research project ideas prior to resident adoption, and institute formal deadlines to ensure research progress through the year. Modified research timelines have been evaluated to better align with trainees' abilities and skills and fit a meaningful research project into the brief residency timeline. One example of this is the "flipped residency research model," in which residents onboard to an institutional review board–approved project at the start of their year, completing data collection, analysis, and presentation by January before proposing and designing a new project to involve the oncoming resident in.[32] Students interested in developing the ability to conduct independent practice-based pharmacy research after residency should seek programs with robust structured research processes, opportunities, and mentor availability. It is worth noting that many residency-trained pharmacists seek post-residency masters, fellowship, or doctoral programs to gain more training in conducting high-quality practice-based research.[33]

Whereas residencies adopt a clinical postgraduate training focus, the typical focus of pharmacy fellowships is to prepare the trainee to conduct independent research upon completion of the program. Fellowships develop expertise in each portion of the scientific research process: conceptualizing, designing, conducting, and reporting research.[10] A range of organizations offer a diverse array of fellowship experiences for qualified candidates, including schools and colleges of pharmacy, the pharmaceutical industry, and professional organizations. Fellowship may offer the ability to engage in formal didactic training in research methodology and allow the trainee to devote more time to research than a residency. Consequently, fellows are more likely to subspecialize in a specific research area. Graduates of fellowship programs typically enter careers in academia with a large distribution of effort conducting research or enter the pharmaceutical industry. The research mentor in a fellowship is often a more formalized role predetermined before acceptance into a program, and these mentors commonly take on coaching and sponsoring roles in addition to a research advisor.[6] In these settings, fellows are encouraged to discuss and formulate an NIH CDP.

PROFESSIONAL PHARMACY ORGANIZATION RESOURCES

Many professional pharmacy organizations offer learner development and grant programs to further research skills. For example, the American College of Clinical Pharmacy (ACCP) supports research skill development through the Future Grants: Mentored Developmental Research Awards for students, trainees, and early-career members.[34] Likewise, ASHP supports Pharmacy Resident Research Grants, targeting PGY1 and PGY2 residents, and New Practitioner Pharmacist Leadership Development Grants, aimed at practitioners within five years of their pharmacy degree undertaking research projects focused on leadership competency development.[35,36] Early mentored experience with grant writing may prepare learners for larger grant and development opportunities as new practitioners, such as participation in the professional organization supported early-career researcher development programs like ACCP's Focused Investigator Training and Mentored Research Investigator Training programs.[35] Specialty practice pharmacy organizations, as well as state-level organizations, may also offer professional development and grant support opportunities for learners. Involvement in professional organizations, particularly those with committees and subsections dedicated to practice-based research, can allow for research project identification, collaboration, and mentor identification at any learner stage.

Summary and Conclusions

Mentorship is a bidirectional, reciprocal relationship in which guidance is provided by an experienced individual (mentor) to a less experienced (mentee) individual to develop their professional skills and knowledge. There are many intrinsic and extrinsic benefits for both the mentor and mentee, such as personal satisfaction and career development. When searching for a mentor, one should consider their own professional goals and how they relate to those of the mentor, as well as the time commitment involved in the research project. To ensure expectations are clearly defined from the start of the mentoring relationship, a mentor may ask the mentee to complete a research contract. Despite best efforts in establishing a mentor–mentee relationship, conflicts may still arise, such as competing priorities or misaligned expectations. Therefore, win-win negotiation techniques should be employed to ensure the conflict is resolved with both parties' interests in mind. Finally, to ensure one is continually moving forward, mentors and mentees may also discuss a CDP that may help define specific steps needed to achieve one's short and long-term goals. Finally, as you embark on your research career, there are many resources available through professional organizations and government agencies to assist in career development; such tools to identify strengths and weaknesses and funding opportunities for early-career research projects can be very helpful.

Key Points and Advice

- Mentorship is a bidirectional, reciprocal relationship.
- Mentorship is not restricted to one individual and mentees may benefit from building a group of individuals to advise them, known as a personal board of directors.
- Expectations for a specific research project should be clearly defined between a mentor and mentee, which may be facilitated through a research contract.
- Conflicts may arise during a mentorship relationship, thus effective conflict resolution skills should be employed by the mentor and mentee.
- Residency and fellowships offer opportunities for further research experience after pharmacy school.
- Career development planning may benefit the mentee in discovering new career pathways involving practice-based research including opportunities for research training or funding, strengthening mentor–mentee relationship, and expanding one's professional network.

Chapter Review Questions

1. Considering your own career interests, what individual(s) would you approach to form your own personal board of directors?
2. What steps are recommended for mentees to take to form, find, and foster a relationship with a research mentor?
3. Consider a time when a mentoring relationship did not go as you expected. Which conflict resolution techniques could you have implemented?
4. Name three strategies that residency programs can use to standardize and structure research training.
5. What self-assessment tools are available to trainees to help guide the fit of a research-oriented career?

Online Resources

- American Pharmacist Association Career Pathway Evaluation Program. https://www.pharmacist.com/Career/Career-Pathways
- American Association for the Advancement of Science's Individual Development Plan. https://myidp.sciencecareers.org/
- Center for the Improvement of Mentored Experiences in Research (CIMER): Materials for Mentors and Mentees. https://cimerproject.org/online-resources/

REFERENCES

1. Dictionary. Merriam-Webster. Accessed January 1, 2021. https://www.merriam-webster.com/
2. Burgess A, van Diggele C, Mellis C. Mentorship in the health professions: a review. *Clin Teach.* 2018;15(3):197-202. doi:10.1111/tct/12756
3. National Research Mentoring Network. Glossary of NRMN Terms. Accessed January 1, 2021. https://nrmnet.net/blog/2019/05/08/glossary-of-nrmn-terms/
4. Fulton J. Mentorship: excellence in the mundane. *BJ HCA.* 2013;7(3):142-144.
5. National Academies of Sciences, Engineering, and Medicine. *The Science of Effective Mentorship in STEMM.* Washington, DC: The National Academies Press; 2019.
6. Barlow B, Barlow A. Identifying the different types of professional relationships: are you my mentor? *Am J Health Syst Pharm.* 2020;77(18):1463-1465. doi:10.1093/ajhp/zxaa134
7. Deal EN, Stranges PM, Maxwell WD, et al. The importance of research and scholarly activity in pharmacy training. *Pharmacotherapy.* 2016;36(12):e200-e205. doi:10.1002/phar.1864
8. National Academies of Sciences, Engineering, and Medicine. Chapter 5: The Role of Mentoring. In: Gentile J, Brenner K, Stephens A, eds. *Undergraduate Research Experiences for STEM Students: Successes, Challenges, and Opportunities.* Washington, DC: The National Academies Press; 2007:129-146.
9. Zerzan JT, Hess R, Schur E, Phillips RS, Rigotti N. Making the most of mentor: a guide for mentees. *Acad Med.* 2009;84(1):140-144. doi:10.1097/ACM.0b013e3181906e8f
10. Beckett RD, Linn DD. Development of an evidence-based residency preparation checklist using a Delphi process. *Am J Health-Syst Pharm.* 2020;77:356-364. doi:10.1093/ajhp/zxz338
11. Wuller CA. A capstone advanced pharmacy practice experience in research. *Am J Pharm Educ.* 2010;74(10):180. doi:10.5688/aj7410180
12. van Schalkwyk G, Katz RB, Resignato J, van Schalwyk SC, Rohrbaugh RM. Effective research mentorship for residents: meeting the needs of early career physicians. *Acad Psychiatry.* 2017;41:326-332. doi:10.1007/s40596-016-0625-9

13. Anderson L, Silet K, Fleming M. Evaluating and giving feedback to mentors: new evidence-based approaches. *Clin Transl Sci.* 2012 Feb;5(1):71-77. doi:10.1111/j.1752-8062.2011.00361.x

14. Kowtko C, Watts LK. Mentoring in health sciences education: a review of the literature. *J Med Imaging Radiat Sci.* 2008 Jun;39(2):69-74. doi:10.1016/j.jmir.2008.04.003

15. Chopra V, Arora VM, Saint S. Will you be my mentor? – four archetypes to help mentees succeed in academic medicine. *JAMA Intern Med.* 2018;178(2):175-176.

16. International Committee of Medical Journal Editors. Recommendations for the conduct, reporting, editing, and publication of scholarly work in medical journals. Updated December 2019. Accessed January 5, 2021. http://www.icmje.org/icmje-recommendations.pdf

17. Minshew LM, McLaughlin JE. Authorship considerations for publishing in pharmacy education journals. *Am J Pharm Educ.* 2019;83(6):7463. doi:10.5688/ajpe7463

18. Henchey C, Keefe K, Munger MA, Witt DM. Fotsering PharmD skills related to research and quality improvement through mentored projects. *Am J Pharm Educ.* 2020;84(9):7940. doi:https://doi.org/10.5688/ajpe7940

19. Osborne KW, Woods KM, Maxwell WD, McGee K, Bookstaver PB. Outcomes of student-driven, faculty-mentored research and impact on postgraduate training and career selection. *Am J Pharm Educ.* 2018;82(4):6246. doi:10.5688/ajpe6246

20. Lee BJ, Rhodes NJ, Scheetz MH, McLaughlin MM. Engaging pharmacy students in research through near-peer teaching. *Am J Pharm Educ.* 2017;81(9):6340. doi:10.5688/ajpe6340

21. Barrington L. Everyone needs a person board of directors. Forbes. Published February 20, 2018. Accessed January 10, 2021. https://www.forbes.com/sites/forbescoachescouncil/2018/02/20/everyone-needs-a-personal-board-of-directors/?sh=2708e8f92bbc

22. Tuma T, Adams J, Hultquist B, Dolan E. The dark side of development: a systems characterization of the negative mentoring experiences of doctoral students. *CBE Life Sci Educ.* 2021 Jun;20:ar16. doi:10.1187/cbe20-10-0231

23. Holdford DA. *Leadership for Pharmacists: Facilitating change in pharmacy practice.* Washington, DC: American Pharmacists Association; 2018.

24. National Institutes of Health: Research Training and Career Development. Accessed January 10, 2021. https://researchtraining.nih.gov

25. Pruchnicki MC, Rodis JL, Beatty SJ, et al. Practice-based research network as a research training model for community/ambulatory pharmacy residents. *J Am Pharm Assoc.* 2008;48(2):191-202. doi:10.1331/JAPhA.2008.07136

26. Schommer JC, Sogol EM, Brown LM. Career pathways for pharmacists. *J Am Pharm Assoc.* 2007;47(5):563-564. doi:10.1331/JAPhA.2007.07074

27. American Pharmacist Association Career Pathway Evaluation Program: Accessed January 10, 2021. https://www.pharmacist.com/Career/Career-Pathways

28. Suggestions for a Good Career Development Plan. National Institute of Neurological Disorders and Stroke website. Published October 8, 2020. Accessed January 17, 2021. https://www.ninds.nih.gov/Funding/Training-Career-Awards/Mentored-Career-Awards/ Suggestions-Good-Career-Development-Plan#_ftn1

29. Fuhrmann CN, Hobin JA, Lindstaedt B, et al. MyIDP Science Careers website. American Association for the Advancement of Science. Accessed January 10, 2021. https://myidp. sciencecareers.org/

30. American Society of Hospital Pharmacists. Definitions of pharmacy residencies and fellowships. *Am J Hosp Pharm*. 1987;44:1142-1144.

31. ASHP Commission on Credentialing. Required Competency Areas, Goals, and Objectives for Postgraduate Year 1 (PGY1) Pharmacy Residencies. American Society of Health System Pharmacists. Published online March 2020.

32. Morbitzer KA, Rao KV, Rhonet DH, et al. Implementation of the flipped residency research model to enhance residency research training. *Am J Health Syst Pharm*. 2019;76(9):608-612. doi:10.1093/ajhp/zxz064

33. Helling D, Johnson S. The future of specialized pharmacy residencies: time for postgraduate year 3 subspecialty training. *Am J Health Syst Pharm*. 2014;71:1199-1203. doi:10.2146/ ajhp140115

34. American College of Clinical Pharmacy Foundation. Investigator Development. Accessed January 1, 2021. https://www.accpfoundation.org/investigator/index.aspx

35. American Society of Health-System Pharmacists Foundation. Pharmacy Resident Research Grant. Accessed January 1, 2021. https://www.ashpfoundation.org/Grants-and-Awards/ Research-Grants/Pharmacy-Resident-Research-Grant

36. American Society of Health-System Pharmacists Foundation. New Practitioner Pharmacist Leadership Development Grants. Accessed January 1, 2021. https://www.ashpfoundation. org/Grants-and-Awards/Research-Grants/New-Practitioner-Pharmacist-Leadership-Development-Grant

3

Chapter Three

Research Infrastructure in Pharmacy Settings

Joshua T. Swan, PharmD, MPH, FCCM, BCPS and
Lan N. Bui, PharmD, MPH, BCPS

Chapter Objectives

- Identify the appropriate people needed for practice-based research in pharmacy
- Identify necessary systems and health information technology to conduct practice-based research in pharmacy
- Discuss the necessary support structure for conducting practice-based research in pharmacy
- Identify approaches for learning about opportunities and available projects for practice-based research in pharmacy
- Describe appropriate timelines for the conduct of learner-involved practice-based research in pharmacy
- Discuss the "layered learning" model for conducting learner-involved research

Key Terminology

Layered learning model, onboarding, orientation, training sites

Introduction

Pharmacists play an important role in creating new knowledge and expanding the current knowledge in clinical practice through conducting high-quality practice-based research.[1] Before being independent researchers, pharmacy learners obtain fundamental research skills during pharmacy school and develop their skills through postgraduate training and education. Different priorities in pharmacy curricula and postgraduate training programs allow pharmacy learners to focus on developing research and scholarly skills.[2–4] As a result, pharmacy learners who are interested in practice-based research should learn how to effectively identify the opportunities, people, and resources to conduct research projects that align well with their interests and training programs' expectations.[5] In addition, pharmacy learners need to learn to set appropriate and realistic expectations and deliverables when planning for their practice-based research projects. High-quality projects require a significant amount of time, and graduate and postgraduate training programs may have a strict timeline for completion.

The purpose of this chapter is to provide an overview of how to identify the expertise, resources, time, and environmental considerations needed to conduct practice-based research in pharmacy and focuses on how to incorporate learners into project teams. Examples are provided to demonstrate how to successfully integrate learners into practice-based research in pharmacy using a layered learning model. The chapter also describes appropriate timelines and expectations for conducting learner-involved, practice-based research in pharmacy.

Research Opportunities Within Pharmacy Learner Programs

Pharmacy learners can engage in practice-based research in pharmacy through various pharmacy learner programs during pharmacy school and postgraduate training. During pharmacy school, learners can participate in practice-based research during their Introductory Pharmacy Practice Experiences (IPPEs), Advanced Pharmacy Practice Experiences (APPEs), research projects that may or may not be part of an academic course or rotation. Postgraduate year 1 (PGY1) and postgraduate year 2 (PGY2) residency training provides additional opportunities to lead major and minor research projects at practice institutions. Pharmacy fellowships provide further opportunities to lead and engage in complex and high-impact studies, including multicenter and externally funded studies.

Depending on availability and learners' experiences and preferences, the size and scope of practice-based projects can vary significantly. Some learners work with a single pharmacy preceptor on a small scope research project. Some learners are involved with an interprofessional research team on a multicenter large-scale project. There are also many cases in between. Each situation has its pros and cons. Small projects with a small study team allow learners to have a high level of autonomy of the study's design, execution, and timeline. However, learners may not receive much support and guidance; thus, the study's data and results can be of low quality. Large projects with large study teams challenge the learner's knowledge and skills and expand their professional networking. The quality of these projects is usually higher as many checks and balances are coming from the large team. However, pharmacy learners may feel overwhelmed with the project's complexity and have difficulty navigating the study team's many personalities and conflicting schedules. Pharmacy learners should clearly define the study's scope and their specific roles before committing to a research project.

IPPE ROTATIONS

IPPE rotations provide pharmacy students with up to 300 hours of interprofessional practice and direct patient care activities during the first three years of pharmacy school. In IPPE rotations, students observe pharmacists practicing in various settings and practice models.[4] Due to students' limited clinical experience at this early point of their training and the limited time dedicated to IPPE rotations, students' opportunities to fully participate in practice-based research may be limited. However, IPPE rotations are excellent opportunities for students to identify their areas of research interest, meet potential research mentors, and develop plans for future research projects. Students interested in research should seek IPPE rotations with preceptors who are known to be strong research mentors or at institutions where research experiences are commonly available for pharmacy learners.

APPE ROTATIONS

APPE rotations allow students to apply and advance their knowledge and skills in various pharmacy practice settings.[4] The duration of APPE rotation is commonly four to six weeks, which provides 160 to 240 hours of training. In APPE rotations, students have many opportunities to collaborate with clinicians and researchers at various health systems. Pharmacy learners can engage in research training for 40 to 60 hours during clinical APPE rotations and 160 to 240 hours during research APPE rotations. Pharmacy students should review rotation syllabi before enrolling as there could be significant variability in the research experiences available among preceptors. Students who desire to continue working on an existing project with a specific preceptor or training site may have the option to create an elective APPE. Training sites are institutions where learners obtain their clinical practice or research training.

STUDENT RESEARCH PROJECTS

Many schools/colleges of pharmacy require a major research project or provide elective research opportunities for students that increase student engagement in research and related scholarly activities.[6-8] These projects provide opportunities to work with a faculty mentor, generate research posters at local, regional, or national conferences, and may lead to co-authorship on a publication. The school/college usually provides guidelines on the types of eligible studies (e.g., literature review vs. chart review study), required deadlines, and deliverables (e.g., study report).[6-11]

RESIDENCY

Postgraduate pharmacy residencies develop essential clinical pharmacy skills and knowledge for patients with a wide range of conditions during PGY1 training and develop independent pharmacy practitioners in specific practice areas during PGY2 training. Most residency programs are accredited by the American Society of Health-System Pharmacists (ASHP), which requires residents to demonstrate their ability "to evaluate and investigate practice, review data, and assimilate scientific evidence to improve patient care and/or the medication use system."[12] Pharmacy residents commonly fulfill this requirement by completing a research study or quality improvement project.[12-14] Residents may devote 200 to 500 hours toward completion of major research projects under the supervision of preceptors (who are usually clinical pharmacists) that commonly yield posters at regional/national conferences and may yield manuscripts in peer-reviewed medical journals.[14-17] It is difficult to execute a high-quality project within a one-year time frame of the residency given the many competing responsibilities assigned to the resident.[16] Therefore, residents should work with research preceptors within the first few months of residency training (and in some cases after the match but prior to starting the program) to develop project plans and identify opportunities to leverage existing infrastructure, such as existing data sets and institutional review board (IRB)–approved applications.[5] Residents who remain at the same institution for PGY1 and PGY2 training can start to develop their PGY2 project during the end of their PGY1 year and may gain efficiency from their knowledge of the institution, experience with the research topic, and existing network of collaborators.[17]

FELLOWSHIP (UNIVERSITY, HEALTH SYSTEM, OR INDUSTRY)

Pharmacy fellowships are research-focused training programs that provide advanced research skills for a particular research topic, care setting, or study design under the supervision of scientists. There are multiple types of fellowships: industry-based, academia-based, health-system-based, or combinations. The duration of a fellowship training range from one to three years and provide 1,500 to 4,500 hours of research training, including didactic coursework, regulatory training, independent hypothesis generation, active research participation, grant writing, and abstract and manuscript completion.[18] Fellows may collaborate on a large portfolio of projects that may yield numerous conference presentations at regional/national conferences, manuscripts in peer-reviewed medical journals, and successful applications for external research funding.

Longitudinal Experiences and the Layered Learning Model

MAXIMIZE RETURN ON INVESTMENT THROUGH LONGITUDINAL EXPERIENCES

As detailed later in this chapter (see "Getting a Badge"), a learner must complete comprehensive administrative onboarding and credentialing at each training site for practice-based research. An effective strategy to reduce this administrative burden is to engage in a sequence of learning experiences at the same institution during pharmacy school and when transitioning from pharmacy school to postgraduate training. Learners can coordinate with the office of experiential education to identify opportunities to complete rotations (IPPE and APPE) and formal P4 student research projects at the same institution, and ideally under the same preceptor and research mentor. Students can also apply for paid internships at the institution where the research will be conducted. Some institutions offer longitudinal experiences, programs that provide a sequence of experiential rotations that allow students to spend most of their experiences at a single site. These competitive programs often offer mentorship and training to prepare learners for competitive postgraduate pharmacy training programs.[19] Additionally, the relationships and reputation established as a student researcher can help the learner be more competitive for postgraduate training (residencies and fellowship) at the same institution. Early commitment and promotion between postgraduate training programs at the same institution (PGY1 to PGY2 or resident to fellow) allow learners to develop proposals and obtain IRB approval prior to the training program's start date. This early planning provides the efficiency needed to execute more complex projects or to meet conference abstract deadlines that occur early in the training program. Examples of consolidated training approaches that were successfully used by chapter co-authors Dr. Swan (faculty) and Dr. Bui (learner at the time) are provided as case studies at the end of this section.

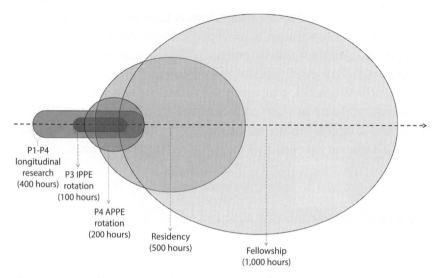

Figure 3–1. Longitudinal experiences and the layered learning model. The sizes of the bubbles depict the amount of time and effort dedicated to research activities for learners at different learning levels. Overlapping regions depict opportunities for learners to collaborate on research experiences using the layered learning model. Students who engage in a longitudinal research experience have the most opportunity to collaborate with a variety of learners.

LAYERED LEARNING MODEL

A layered learning model allows for learners with different experiences and responsibilities to collaborate on a research project under a faculty mentor/supervisor (Figure 3–1). The faculty assesses the skills of each trainee across multiple domains, including clinical pharmacy workflow, project management, epidemiology, biostatistics, database management software (e.g., Microsoft Excel, Microsoft Access, REDCap), navigation of the electronic healthcare record, and clinical research regulatory systems (e.g., IRB application). The faculty then assigns that learner to study activities that fit their skills and desired training experiences. The following case studies illustrate how learners at different levels collaborated on research projects through longitudinal research experiences.

CASE STUDIES

The CHG-BATH Trial

This single-center, investigator-initiated, randomized trial was conducted at Houston Methodist Hospital ("hospital"). The principal investigator, the chapter author Joshua Swan, was a faculty member at Texas Southern University ("university") and had a clinical practice and training site at the hospital. Approximately 20 pharmacy learners supported study design, enrollment, and data collection over a span of four years, which included students (P2, P3, and P4), residents (PGY1 and PGY2), and research fellows. Funding from a research grant at the hospital and from multiple summer research programs at the university was used to pay stipends to cover some of the student support; however, many students supported the study during APPE rotations or provided volunteer support. Some pharmacy students engaged in data collection during clinical and research APPE rotations that were used to generate posters at medical conferences and final reports for P4 research seminar projects at the university. However, several key learners were able to engage in a sequence of learning experiences to support the study over several years and earned authorship on the final publication (see Chapters 2 and 24 for additional discussion of criteria for authorship). As the most remarkable example, chapter author, Lan Bui, was able to sequence together learning experiences from pharmacy school (P2, P3, and P4), PGY1 residency, and fellowship that generated three publications[20-22] and several published abstracts and conference posters. Due to her longitudinal involvement with the study, Lan gained expertise that allowed her to serve in managerial roles where she was responsible for orienting, training, and overseeing the work of upper-level students and residents. For example, as a P3, she provided orientation and training to P4 APPE students who supported data collection. As a P4, she provided orientation and training to PGY2 critical care pharmacy residents who adjudicated adverse events for the study. A second noteworthy learner started supporting the study during her P4 critical care APPE at the hospital and voluntarily supported the study during the summer of her P4 year prior to starting PGY1 training, where she helped develop critical standard operating procedures for study outcome assessment. Even though she completed PGY1 training at another institution near the hospital, she was able to obtain an unpaid postgraduate fellowship appointment at the hospital that allowed her to retain her badge and hospital access to continue supporting the study, and she was able to earn authorship on the final publications.[21-23]

The MENDS2 Trial

This multicenter randomized trial enrolled patients at multiple hospitals across the United States, including Houston Methodist Hospital ("hospital"). At the time of participation, the study site principal investigator, Joshua Swan, was an employee of the hospital. Approximately 30 research learners supported enrollment and data collection over a span of four years, which included P4 pharmacy students, three pharmacy research fellows, and one medical research fellow. Federal funding was used to pay salary support for the pharmacy and medical research fellows. The P4 pharmacy students were all enrolled in four-month longitudinal APPE programs at the hospital and engaged in data collection as core activities during six-week research APPE rotations or as elective activities during four-week hospital and health services APPE rotations, and many students continued to voluntarily support data collection during the remainder of their longitudinal APPE program. During this study, Dr. Swan was the primary preceptor for two concurrent pharmacy learner programs: (a) a PGY1 drug information rotation (1–2 residents per month) and (b) hospital and health services APPE rotation (2–4 students per month). Using a layered learning approach, the residents oversaw hospital pharmacy training for the students, and the fellows oversaw a research topic discussion and journal club series on ICU sedation that was relevant for the MENDS2 trial. The fellows provided orientation, training, and quality assurance on the screening and data collection efforts for the APPE students who elected to participate in research activities. Due to the confidentiality of this multicenter study, none of the learners were able to present research abstracts on preliminary data at medical conferences. However, several key trainees were able to engage meaningfully and earned authorship on the final publication in the *New England Journal of Medicine*.[24]

Human Rabies Immune Globulin Study

This single-center, investigator-initiated, retrospective study was conducted at Houston Methodist Hospital ("hospital"). At the time of participation, the study site principal investigator, Joshua Swan, was an employee of the hospital. Six pharmacy learners supported study design, data collection, and analysis over a span of two years, which included two P4 students, a PGY1 resident, and three research fellows. Research funding from the industry was used to pay salary support for the pharmacy research fellows. The P4 pharmacy students were enrolled in a four-month longitudinal APPE program at the hospital and engaged in data collection as core activities during six-week research APPE rotations, and both continued to voluntarily support data collection during the remainder of their longitudinal APPE program. Using a layered learning approach, the primary preceptors for these six-week APPE rotations were the pharmacy research fellows, which provided the fellows with opportunities to manage orientation, training, oversight, and evaluation of the APPE students. After the pharmacy fellows helped obtain research funding and IRB approval, this project was aligned with a PGY1 resident for a major research project, and this resident supported this project longitudinally over an eight-month period. Due to the significant groundwork and support of the fellowship program and integration of P4 students using a layered learning model, a manuscript from this study was accepted for publication in January (the seventh month of residency training), which is the earliest time to publication for a PGY1 major project at the hospital. All learners earned authorship on the final publication, and the PGY1 resident and one fellow shared co-primary authorship roles.[25] The P4 students and the resident were able to present research abstracts at medical conferences. This publication helped the P4 students and the PGY1 resident successfully compete for their desired postgraduate residency and fellowship training.

Identifying Practice-Based Research Mentors

Pharmacy learners have the opportunity to conduct research with a variety of different mentors during their education and training. Chapters 1 and 2 provide general information on mentorship and the establishment of a mentor–mentee relationship. The following section describes important considerations in the selection of a practice-based research mentor. Pharmacy learners must evaluate the capability of potential research mentors based on the mentor's background training, scholarship profile, research interest, availability for mentoring, relationship with health systems, and teaching styles before formally committing to a mentor–mentee relationship.

NONCLINICAL FACULTY LABORATORIES AT THE SCHOOL/COLLEGE

Nonclinical faculty at schools/colleges of pharmacy (e.g., pharmaceutical sciences faculty) are excellent scientists and are experienced with study design, methodology, and statistical analysis. In addition, they may have more time and resources (i.e., access to funding, research materials, staff, and other assets to perform research) dedicated to research compared to practice-based faculty. Working with nonclinical faculty can be a great option for first- (P1) and second-year (P2) pharmacy students to conduct nonclinical research in the laboratory setting. However, these nonclinical faculty members may not have any clinical pharmacy experience and may not have access to a health system to conduct practice-based research.

ECONOMIC, SOCIAL, AND ADMINISTRATIVE PHARMACY (ESAP) FACULTY

Faculty in the ESAP discipline conduct research on a broad range of topics such as healthcare systems, pharmacoeconomics, pharmacoepidemiology, pharmacy law and regulatory affairs, practice management, professional development, and the social and behavioral aspects of practice. They are excellent scientists, and many are knowledgeable about healthcare systems and practice-based research. Working with ESAP faculty is an excellent option for pharmacy learners to gain experience in survey research, health outcomes research, pharmacoeconomics, and health behavior research. However, ESAP faculty may have limited clinical pharmacy experience and may not have access to a health system to conduct research using patient-specific data.

UNIVERSITY-BASED PHARMACY PRACTICE FACULTY AND THEIR AFFILIATED HEALTH SYSTEM

Pharmacy practice faculties at schools/colleges of pharmacy are excellent clinicians, and many are experienced in navigating complex health systems and conducting practice-based research. Working with clinical faculty is a great option for pharmacy students at all levels to involve with practice-based research. One limitation of university-based pharmacy practice faculty is that they may not be formally trained in study methodology and statistical analyses. As a result, they may have limited experience in obtaining funding and managing high-quality, large-scale studies. However, many university-based pharmacy practice faculty who have completed fellowship or additional research training (e.g., those with PhD, MPH, MS) are proficient in obtaining funding and managing their own studies. Since pharmacy practice faculty usually have competing duties related to clinical APPE rotations and patient care assignments, they may not have the time and resources dedicated to research teaching compared to nonclinical or ESAP faculty.

ADJUNCT FACULTY AND/OR CLINICIANS AND THEIR AFFILIATED HEALTH SYSTEM

Adjunct faculty and/or clinicians and scientists are partially or fully paid by their affiliated health system (instead of pharmacy schools/colleges). They are excellent clinicians and have full access to data and resources at their health systems to conduct practice-based research. Depending on their background training and experience, some adjunct faculty and/or clinicians are more experienced with research methodology and analysis than others. Many adjunct faculty and clinicians take students for short- and long-term internships as well as IPPE and APPE rotations. They are great research mentors and resources for pharmacy learners at all levels. However, as they have competitive clinical duties and administrative assignments given by their institution, they may not have had the time and formal capacity to work with pharmacy students throughout the academic year.[26] Adjunct faculty and clinicians are usually more available to pharmacy residents and fellows employed by the same health systems than pharmacy students.

AFFILIATION AGREEMENTS BETWEEN UNIVERSITIES AND HEALTH SYSTEMS

An affiliation agreement between the university and health systems is the first step of the administrative paperwork that allows pharmacy students to come on-site, receive a badge, and access the electrical medical record (EMR). Establishing an affiliation agreement between institutions can be time-consuming and acts as a rate-limiting step for pharmacy learners to start the research at the health system.

Getting a Badge: Additional Steps Needed to Conduct Research

When pharmacy learners are paired with a research mentor for a practice-based research project, the next steps are for the learners to complete the onboarding and orientation process to the research training site. The onboarding process includes human resources onboarding, biomedical ethics training, research credentialing, and (laboratory) safety training. Orientation includes a general overview of the site and a specific introduction of the research team and project. The steps are essential for the trainee to familiarize themselves with the research training site's policies and culture. The trainees are responsible for keeping the training requirements up to date and following the research training site's policies and regulations. Any delay or violation can result in a suspension or termination of the trainee's access to the institution and research training site.

HUMAN RESOURCES ONBOARDING

To protect patients and other workers, pharmacy learners must undergo background checks, drug testing and have updated vaccination records before gaining access to the health system. The onboarding process is usually coordinated through the university's Experiential Experience (EE) office for pharmacy students and the health system's Human Resources (HR) department for pharmacy residents and fellows. The learners' responsibility is to keep track of their onboarding paperwork and respond promptly to the EE and/or HR department to resolve any issues. Learners also need to keep their research mentor updated with their onboarding process timeline. This would allow the mentor to plan for the training and research activities accordingly.

BIOMEDICAL ETHICS TRAINING AND RESEARCH CREDENTIALING

As required by many IRBs, practice-based research investigators have to complete baseline and periodic training and credentialing in biomedical ethics and human-subject research-related topics. One commonly used credential party is the Collaborative Institutional Training Initiative (CITI Program).[27] Certificates from the CITI Program usually last two to three years, and renewal is needed if the investigators are still involved with research projects at the time their certificates expire. For students who are doing practice-based research at a site that is not part of the institution where their school/college of pharmacy is based, this may mean completing multiple training programs (although some institutions will accept training requirements from other institutions). Another major component of research credentialing is compliance with the Health Insurance Portability and Accountability Act (HIPAA).[28] Practice-based research investigators frequently interact with protected health information (PHI), and HIPAA dictates steps and precautions that the investigators need to abide by to protect patient's privacy and data confidentiality.

(LABORATORY) SAFETY TRAINING

To protect learners, patients, and other workers from dangerous and hazardous situations, pharmacy learners must complete Occupational Safety and Health Administration (OSHA) training related to the areas where they perform their research (e.g., pharmacy, patient unit, laboratory).[29] Most practice-based research projects do not require laboratory safety training for onboarding research learners unless their research projects handle biological specimens or utilize laboratory space.

ORIENTATION TO THE INSTITUTION

Each institution has its own unique culture and sets of policies. Pharmacy learners usually receive online and/or in-person orientation in the first couple of days before they start working on their project. The orientation sessions introduce learners to the institution's general information and specific requirements for the location(s) where the learners conduct the research. Learners should stay engaged in the orientation session and ask questions to understand their rights and responsibilities at the research training site clearly.

Understanding Practice for Conducting Research

PHARMACY PRACTICE MODELS IN HEALTH SYSTEMS

Understanding pharmacy practice models in health systems will optimize pharmacy learners' research planning and execution. In the United States, there are two main types of pharmacy practice models: centralized pharmacy model and decentralized/comprehensive model. In the centralized pharmacy practice model, clinical pharmacists perform mostly clinical pharmacy activities while staff pharmacists perform mostly operational pharmacy activities. In decentralized/comprehensive models, the clinical and staff pharmacists performed a mix of both clinical and operational pharmacy activities.[30-32] In both models, clinical pharmacists usually have more time and responsibility dedicated to practice-based research compared to staff pharmacists.[33]

PHARMACY POLICY AND PROCEDURES

Each institution has its own policy and procedures governing pharmacy administrative, operational, and clinical functions. Pharmacy learners should review the general and specific policies and procedures that are relevant to their research areas. General policy and procedures may include personnel safety, emergency preparedness, medical emergencies, immunization, and substance abuse. Specific policy and procedures may include safe and proper use of investigational drugs or Collaborative Practice Agreements.[34] A Collaborative Practice Agreement is a voluntary written agreement where a prescriber (e.g., physician) authorizes a pharmacist to perform certain patient care activities under his/her authority. The agreement describes activities pharmacist is allowed to perform, under what conditions, and any limitations.[30,35]

PHARMACY AND NONPHARMACY PERSONNEL

Pharmacy learners who participate in practice-based research projects have the opportunity to interact and work with various interprofessional team members. Knowing the role and daily responsibilities of pharmacy and nonpharmacy personnel will allow learners to optimize their research activities and expand their professional networking. Pharmacy personnel includes administrative pharmacists, clinical pharmacists, staff pharmacists, technicians, pharmacy residents, fellows, and students. Nonpharmacy personnel includes clinicians (e.g., physicians, nurses, dietitians, case managers), researchers (e.g., scientists, statisticians, research assistants), and administrative staff (e.g., secretaries, phone operators, HR personnel).[34] All of these individuals can play a role in the conduct of pharmacy practice-based research.

HEALTH INFORMATION SYSTEMS

As technology applications in healthcare continue to grow and mature, pharmacy learners need to learn to navigate different health information systems available at their research training sites. These systems are not only designed to support clinical care but also contain important data that are often critical for practice-based research. Health information systems include many electronic and software applications that are designed to streamline, optimize, and promote the safety of medication prescribing, dispensing, and administration. The common health information systems that pharmacy learners interact with include EMRs, clinical decision support (CDS), bar-coding at medication dispensing, automated dispensing machines (ADM), electronic medication administration records (eMAR), and bar-coding at medication administration (BarA or BCMA).[36,37]

STRUCTURED DATA FOR DISEASE, PROCEDURES, AND MEDICATIONS

In addition to health information systems, pharmacy learners need to familiarize themselves with a different structural coding system for diseases, procedures, and medications. Coding is the practice of abstracting the information from medical records or medications to the appropriate systematic codes that can be used for insurance billings, quality reports, and research. The coding systems that are commonly used for organizing medical diagnoses and procedures are the Diagnosis-Related Group (DRG),[38] International Classification of Diseases (ICD),[39] and Current Procedural Terminology (CPT).[40] DRGs classify and group medical diagnoses that use similar hospital resources and have similar costs.[38] Under each DRG, patients receive a list of ICD codes for specific diagnoses and procedures obtained from the medical charts. There are several versions of the ICD classification; the Tenth Revision (ICD-10) is currently used in U.S. health systems. However, many retrospective studies still use the Ninth Revision (ICD-9) for diagnosis queries.[39,41] CPT is similar to ICD coding, except that it reports clinicians' medical services and procedures rather than the diagnoses.[40]

The classification systems commonly used for organizing medications are National Drug Code (NDC),[42] American Hospital Formulary Service (AHFS), Pharmacologic-Therapeutic Classification,[43] and RxNorm.[44] Published by the U.S. Food and Drug Administration (FDA), the NDC serves as a universal product identifier for drugs and contains information regarding labeler, product, and trade package size.[42] Developed and maintained by ASHP, the AHFS Pharmacologic-Therapeutic Classification groups medications with similar pharmacologic, therapeutic, and/or chemical characteristics into a four-tier hierarchy.[43] Developed by the National Library of Medicine, RxNorm is a standardized coding system that contains information on the medications along with ingredients, strengths, and forms.[44] These medication classifications can be used alone or with conversion mapping tables to each other.

In addition to coding systems for medical diagnoses, procedures, and medications, pharmacy research learners may also come across systems to organize clinical equivalence. Examples for these systems include Anatomical Therapeutic Chemical—Defined Daily Dose (ATC-DDD),[45] Morphine Milligram Equivalent (MME),[46] and National Cancer Institute (NCI) emetic risks of oncologic agents.[47] Recommended by the World Health Organization (WHO), ATC-DDD is used as the international standard for drug utilization studies. Using the ATC-DDD system, clinicians and researchers convert different medication doses to DDDs and quantify drug utilization for a patient or a patient population.[45] The MME system is designed specifically for quantifying opioid doses and the NCI emetic risks of oncologic agents group chemotherapy agents into low, moderate, and high emetic risks.[46,47]

ELECTRONIC DATA CAPTURE SYSTEMS

An Electronic Data Capture (EDC) system is a software that stores patient data collected in research projects. Depending on the research project's nature, pharmacy learners can interact with EDC systems with different complexity and sophistication levels. Most readily available EDC systems are Microsoft Excel and Microsoft Access.[48] Survey Monkey[49] and Qualtrics[50] are free and paid online survey platforms are commonly used for survey studies. One relatively new EDC is Research Electronic Data Capture (REDCap), a free web-based EDC designed to be user friendly, comprehensive, and compliant with electronic data integrity and confidentiality standards such as HIPAA, FDA 21 Code of Federal

Regulation (CFR) Part 11, Federal Information Security Management Act (FISMA), and General Data Protection Regulation (GDPR).[51,52]

INFRASTRUCTURE ACROSS PRACTICE SETTINGS

Research infrastructure for pharmacy practice research varies across community, ambulatory, and hospital settings. Although many pharmacists in various settings express interest in practice-based research, there is still limited involvement and reluctance of pharmacists to engage in research activities, especially in the community setting. The major limiting factors for research involvement in the community setting include competing time for research with other responsibilities as well as lack of training and support for pharmacy staff.[53-55] Hospital and ambulatory settings usually have more pharmacy research expertise and resources as clinical research has been established as one of the practice standards for clinical pharmacists.[26,56]

Obtaining Access to Resources

HUMAN EXPERTISE

Clinical research is a team sport that requires collaboration among administration, investigators, clinicians, and patients (Figure 3–2). The principal investigator at the study site will coordinate with the sponsor/funding agency, regulatory agencies, legal and contracting teams, and study finance teams to execute study funding contracts, confidentiality agreements, and material/data transfer agreements. Learners are rarely able to see these interactions, except for learners in dedicated research training programs (e.g., APPE/resident research rotation or research fellowship). Learners may be able to support IRB applications and may need to seek guidance from regulatory specialists to ensure that research biomedical ethics policies are being appropriately followed. During study design, data collection, and analysis, the learner may desire to seek guidance from data scientists and biostatisticians; however, access to these resources may be limited due to research budgets or lack of need for small-scale projects. Subsequent chapters explore the needed expertise depending on the content area being investigated.

OFFICE SPACE

Dedicated office space is needed for learners to be productive and effective in their research work. Office space in the practice training site allows easy access to patients,

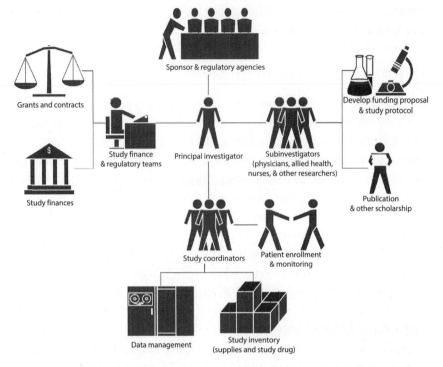

Figure 3–2. Clinical research model. Clinical research is a "team sport" that requires collaboration among administration, investigators, clinicians, and patients. The principal investigator at the study site will coordinate with the sponsor/funding agency, regulatory agencies, legal and contracting teams, and study finance teams to execute study funding contracts, confidentiality agreements, and material/data transfer agreements.

clinicians, and other resources needed for research-related activities. Learners should talk with their preceptors about where they should base their work and if remote access is available if learners cannot go to the training site.

LABORATORY SPACE AND EQUIPMENT

Learners who work at the laboratory should have proper training on laboratory safety, access to appropriate personal protective equipment (PPE), and receive up-to-date manuals and technical support on equipment operation.

COMPUTER EQUIPMENT AND RELEVANT SOFTWARE

Through their affiliation with the practice training site, learners can access computers, software, and intranet that can enhance their research work. Desktops and laptops provided by the practice are equipped with up-to-date configurations and encrypted to ensure HIPAA compliances. Software made available by the practice training site may include reference manager software (e.g., EndNote, RefWorks), project management software (e.g., Microsoft OneNote, Smartsheet), and data analysis software (e.g., STATA, SAS, MiniTab). The practice training site's intranet houses the latest policy and procedures and allows learners to access medical library resources to obtain full-text copies of journal articles.

INFORMATION TECHNOLOGY ACCESS (ON-SITE AND REMOTE)

Preferably, learners should work on the research on-site. However, in certain circumstances, such as natural disasters or unsafe workplace environments (e.g., COVID-19 pandemic), pharmacy learners may obtain remote access to EMRs and research files.

STUDY DATA

Some research projects collect primary data (i.e., data collected directly from sources such as interviews, surveys, laboratory experiments). In contrast, others utilize secondary data (i.e., data collected indirectly, such as reviewing EMRs, data queries) or a combination of primary and secondary data. Pharmacy learners should work with their preceptors and/or data specialist at the practice training site to determine the most appropriate data sources, data collection tools, and methods for their research.

CLINICAL STAFF WORKFLOW

Practice-based research may require the assistance or involvement of both pharmacy and medical staff. Pharmacy learners should build a good rapport with the hospital workers with whom they interact and work. It is also a good idea to observe the clinical staff workflow at the beginning of the research to better understand who has the best knowledge and access to certain data and information. For example, a nurse would be most knowledgeable of patients' daily progress and medication administration records, and a case manager would be most helpful with the patient's discharge plan.

PATIENTS

As part of practice-based research, pharmacy learners may participate in direct patient research activities such as obtaining consent, conducting interviews, collecting biospecimens, and providing education to patients and their families. Learners should be trained appropriately before independently communicating with patients and patient's families. Learners need to have a good understanding of the patient's current medical condition and plan of care. Mistakes in communications such as revealing confidential medical information can negatively affect the current medical care plan for the patients and the institution's overall image.

CONSUMABLE RESOURCES

In certain study designs, such as a clinical trial, learners may work with consumable resources, including communication material, stipends for participants, investigational medications, laboratory specimens, and monitoring. The trainee should be oriented and have access to PPEs, the study's latest standards of operating procedures, laboratory supplies, equipment, and storage. If the practice-based preceptors are not familiar with the training, he/she should be able to arrange the appropriate training and orientation for the learners.

Communication Material

Communication materials such as printed leaflets and handouts are commonly used to recruit and educate patients and their families on a study's purpose and details. Pharmacy learners who are involved with patient recruitment and/or education may help design, produce, and distribute these communication materials. Intranet phones and pagers are also sometimes used for communication of the study's urgent issues. At a minimum, the research learner should have an institution-based email address to communicate PHI.

Stipends for Participants

It should be communicated clearly to a study's participants if they are compensated for the study and how much the stipends are at the time of recruitment. Pharmacy learners may help with distributing the stipend and billing the study for it. It should also be made clear if the learner gets paid for the time they dedicated to the study. There is usually limited funding for research; the research mentor should communicate with learners on the amount and duration of the stipend. In many cases, learners dedicate many hours to the research that are not compensated due to limited funding.

Investigational Medications

If research learners work with investigational medications, they are expected to troubleshoot and answer general questions regarding the products' distribution and monitoring. Most importantly, learners should understand the concept of blinding and avoid revealing the patient's randomized assignment.

Materials Consumed During Laboratory Activities

Laboratory monitoring and specimen collection can be a part of the patient's standard care or used specifically for the research. Pharmacy learners may help with collecting, processing, monitoring, and billing laboratory specimens.

Timelines and Project Management

SETTING INITIAL PROJECT GOALS AND TIMELINE

The study sponsor/funding agency or the pharmacy learner program sets external, non-negotiable deadlines and milestones outlined in the research agreement or training program's curriculum. Internal deadlines are negotiated between the research team and the principal investigator. All project timelines must ensure that project work is completed, reviewed, and approved by the principal investigator in time to achieve external deadlines and milestones. It is essential that learners set realistic expectations for internal deadlines that account for competing requirements of their pharmacy learner programs and the availability of key members of their research team. During repetitive tasks, such as data collection, it is advisable to track the time needed to complete each task early to estimate the remaining time required to complete a project. For example, a trainee records time for the data collection on the first ten patients that averages to be 1 hour per patient. Since the study will include 100 patients, the trainee can then negotiate a project plan with the mentor to ensure that at least 90 hours of protected time are provided to complete data collection. Drafting scholarly documents such as research abstracts, posters, reports, and manuscripts frequently requires more time than a trainee might estimate, especially if the trainee is writing this type of scholarly output for the first time. Research learners need to ensure that their project timelines provide adequate time for multiple (e.g., 3-6) rounds of revision between the learners and mentor/co-investigators. Strongly consider meeting with the mentor to develop an outline before drafting a lengthy report or manuscript.

RESEARCH-IN-PROGRESS MEETINGS

Research-in-progress meetings are platforms for learners to provide updates on their projects and steps that have not yet been completed. These may occur within the institution or as a research-in-progress oral/poster presentation at a regional or national conference. These provide opportunities for learners to showcase their progress and preliminary results and discuss strategies to overcome potential barriers identified. The feedback received at these venues can shape the study's design and data analysis and attract new collaborators to the project.

REPORT, ANALYZE, AND IMPROVE

Quality assurance methods, like plan-do-check-act, can be applied to repetitive tasks within a project, such as data collection, data entry, screening, and enrollment. Frequent monitoring, especially early in project execution, can identify errors or inefficiencies that need to be addressed. For example, learners can analyze the first set of 10% to 20% of the study sample to look for unusual data. Reviewing and analyzing these unexpected data may help learners uncover strategies to improve the efficiency and accuracy of data collection tools.

Summary and Conclusions

This chapter identified the expertise, resources, and time needed to conduct practice-based research in pharmacy and focused on incorporating learners into project teams. Careful emphasis was placed on cultivating research experiences within existing pharmacy trainee learning experiences and identifying appropriate research mentors. One major obstacle to conducting practice-based research is the time and resources needed to have research learners onboard at the institution where the project takes place. This chapter describes strategies to minimize this administrative burden by sequencing longitudinal experiences at the same institution. Research learners can use this chapter's information to identify a capable practice-based research mentor to support complex and high-impact practice-based research in pharmacy.

Key Points and Advice

- A long-term mentor–mentee relationship can provide high-impact training opportunities and growth for a learner, and learners should proactively identify mentors early on during their formal training.
- Learners should not underestimate the amount of regulatory/HR onboarding and research credentialing that is needed by each health system where they will conduct practice-based research and should strategically identify those institutions early in the development of their research plans.
- High-quality, practice-based research in pharmacy may need up to one to three years to develop proposals into publications, and learners should initiate projects early to reach certain milestones prior to applying for postgraduate training and early career positions.
- Learners should leverage access to resources at their primary institution (e.g., university) and the institutions where the practice-based research will be conducted.
- Layered learning models provide learners with opportunities to support complex and high-impact practice-based research in pharmacy and to develop researcher, manager, and educator skills.

Chapter Review Questions

1. Describe research opportunities that exist within pharmacy learner programs using examples.
2. Discuss the benefits of longitudinal experiences and layered learning models in research training using examples.
3. Discuss how capabilities of research faculty/preceptors/sponsors using examples can impact research training for learners.
4. Describe resources that are available to research learners at training sites using examples.

Online Resources

- American Pharmacists Association. Conducting Research Projects. https://www.pharmacist.com/Practice/Practice-Resources/Research-Evidence/Conducting-Research-Projects
- American Society of Health-System Pharmacists. Research Resource Center. https://www.ashp.org/Pharmacy-Practice/Resource-Centers/Research-Resource-Center
- American College of Clinical Pharmacy Foundation. Investigator Development. https://www.accpfoundation.org/investigator/index.aspx

REFERENCES

1. American College of Clinical Pharmacy. The definition of clinical pharmacy. *Pharmacotherapy*. 2008;28(6):816-817.
2. Lee MW, Clay PG, Kennedy WK, et al. The essential research curriculum for doctor of pharmacy degree programs. *Pharmacotherapy*. 2010;30(9):966.
3. Deal EN, Stranges PM, Maxwell WD, et al. The importance of research and scholarly activity in pharmacy training. *Pharmacotherapy*. 2016;36(12):e200-e205.
4. American Council on Pharmaceutical Education. Accreditation Standards and Key Elements for the Professional Program in Pharmacy Leading to the Doctor of Pharmacy Degree "Standards 2016." 2015.
5. Lichvar AB, Smith Condeni M, Pierce DR. Preparing pharmacy trainees for a future in research and contributing to the medical literature. *JACCP*. 2021;4(1):71-80.
6. Fuji KT, Galt KA. Research skills training for the doctor of pharmacy in U.S. schools of pharmacy: a descriptive study. *Int J Pharm Pract*. 2009;17(2):115-121.
7. Slack MK, Martin J, Worede L, Islam S. A systematic review of extramural presentations and publications from pharmacy student research programs. *Am J Pharm Educ*. 2016;80(6):100.

8. Harirforoosh S, Stewart DW. A descriptive investigation of the impact of student research projects arising from elective research courses. *BMC Res Notes*. 2016;9:48.

9. Kao DJ, Hudmon KS, Corelli RL. Evaluation of a required senior research project in a doctor of pharmacy curriculum. *Am J Pharm Educ*. 2011;75(1):5.

10. Wuller CA. A capstone advanced pharmacy practice experience in research. *Am J Pharm Educ*. 2010;74(10):180.

11. Assemi M, Ibarra F, Mallios R, Corelli RL. Scholarly contributions of required senior research projects in a doctor of pharmacy curriculum. *Am J Pharm Educ*. 2015;79 (2):23.

12. American Society of Health-System Pharmacists. Required Competency Areas, Goals, and Objectives for Post-graduate Year One (PGY1) Pharmacy Residencies. 2015.

13. American Society of Health-System Pharmacists. Guidance Document for the ASHP Accreditation Standard for Postgraduate Year One (PGY1) Pharmacy Residency Programs. 2020.

14. American Society of Health-System Pharmacists. ASHP Accreditation Standard for Postgraduate Year Two (PGY2) Pharmacy Residency Programs. 2017.

15. Kwak N, Swan JT, Thompson-Moore N, Liebl MG. Validity and reliability of a systematic database search strategy to identify publications resulting from pharmacy residency research projects. *J Pharm Pract*. 2016;29(4):406-414.

16. Weathers T, Ercek K, Unni EJ. PGY1 resident research projects: publication rates, project completion policies, perceived values, and barriers. *Curr Pharm Teach Learn*. 2019;11(6):547-556.

17. Swan JT, Rizk E, Kwak N, Guastadisegni J, Thompson-Moore N, Liebl MG. Publication of pharmacy residency research: a 12-year cohort from an academic medical center. *J Pharm Pract*. 2021:8971900211021269.

18. Mueller EW, Bishop JR, Kanaan AO, Kiser TH, Phan H, Yang KY. Research fellowship programs as a pathway for training independent clinical pharmacy scientists. *Pharmacotherapy*. 2015;35(3):e13-e19.

19. Wiley TL, Rowe JM, Hammond DA. Making the most of advanced pharmacy practice experiences. *Am J Health-Syst Pharm*. 2017;74(10):648-650.

20. Bui LN, Pham VP, Shirkey BA, Swan JT. Effect of delirium motoric subtypes on administrative documentation of delirium in the surgical intensive care unit. *J Clin Monit Comput*. 2017;31(3):631-640.

21. Bui LN, Swan JT, Perez KK, et al. Impact of chlorhexidine bathing on antimicrobial utilization in surgical intensive care unit. *J Surg Res*. 2020;250:161-171.

22. Swan JT, Ashton CM, Bui LN, et al. Effect of chlorhexidine bathing every other day on prevention of hospital-acquired onfections in the surgical ICU: a single-center, randomized controlled trial. *Crit Care Med*. 2016;44(10):1822-1832.

23. Bui LN, Swan JT, Shirkey BA, Olsen RJ, Long SW, Graviss EA. Chlorhexidine bathing and *Clostridium difficile* infection in a surgical intensive care unit. *J Surg Res*. 2018;228:107-111.

24. Hughes CG, Mailloux PT, Devlin JW, et al. Dexmedetomidine or propofol for sedation in mechanically ventilated adults with sepsis. *N Engl J Med*. 2021;384(15):1424-1436.

25. Hwang GS, Rizk E, Bui LN, et al. Adherence to guideline recommendations for human rabies immune globulin patient selection, dosing, timing, and anatomical site of administration in rabies postexposure prophylaxis. *Hum Vaccin Immunother.* 2020;16(1): 51-60.

26. Lee R, Dahri K, Lau TTY, Shalansky S. Perceptions of hospital pharmacists concerning clinical research: a survey study. *Can J Hosp Pharm.* 2018;71(2):105-110.

27. The CITI Program. Published 2018. Accessed December 15, 2020. https://www.citiprogram.org/index.cfm?pageID=260

28. U.S. Department of Health & Human Services Office for Civil Rights. HIPAA for Professionals. Published 2017. Accessed Desember 15, 2020. https://www.hhs.gov/hipaa/for-professionals/index.html#

29. Occupational Safety and Health Administration (OSHA). Available from: www.OSHA.gov. Published 2020. Accessed December 15, 2020.

30. Chisholm-Burns MA, Vaillancourt AM, Shepherd M. *Pharmacy Management, Leadership, Marketing, and Finance (Book Only).* Burlington, MA: Jones & Bartlett Publishers; 2012.

31. American Society of Health-System Pharmacists. The consensus of the Pharmacy Practice Model Summit. *Am J Health Syst Pharm.* 2011;68(12):1148-1152.

32. Zellmer WA. Reflections on the key messages of the Pharmacy Practice Model Summit. *Am J Health Syst Pharm.* 2011;68(12):1153-1154.

33. American College of Clinical Pharmacy Research Affairs Committee, Fagan SC, Touchette D, et al. The state of science and research in clinical pharmacy. *Pharmacotherapy.* 2006;26(7):1027-1040.

34. American Society of Health-System Pharmacists. ASHP guidelines: minimum standard for pharmacies in hospitals. *Am J Health Syst Pharm.* 2013;70(18):1619-1630.

35. Giberson SYS, Lee MP. Improving Patient and Health System Outcomes through Advanced Pharmacy Practice. A Report to the U.S. Surgeon General. Office of the Chief Pharmacist US Public Health Service. 2011.

36. DesRoches C, Painter M, Jha A. Health information technology in the united states, 2015: transition to a post-hitech world. Cambridge, MA: Mathematica Policy Research [Google Scholar]. 2015.

37. Furukawa MF, Raghu T, Spaulding TJ, Vinze A. Adoption of health information technology for medication safety in US hospitals, 2006. *Health Aff.* 2008;27(3):865-875.

38. Centers for Medicare & Medicaid Services. Design and development of the Diagnosis Related Group (DRG). 2016.

39. World Health Organization (WHO). International Statistical Classification of Diseases and Related Health Problems (ICD). Published 2020. Accessed Decemeber 10, 2020. https://www.who.int/standards/classifications/classification-of-diseases

40. American Medical Association (AMA). CPT®. Published 2020. Accessed December 10, 2020. https://www.ama-assn.org/practice-management/cpt

41. Jetté N, Quan H, Hemmelgarn B, et al. The development, evolution, and modifications of ICD-10: challenges to the international comparability of morbidity data. *Med Care.* 2010;48(12):1105-1110.

42. United States Food and Drugs Administration (FDA). National Drug Code Directory. Published 2019. Accessed December 15, 2020. https://www.fda.gov/drugs/drug-approvals-and-databases/national-drug-code-directory

43. American Society of Health-System Pharmacists. AHFS Pharmacologic-Therapeutic Classification. Published 2020. Accessed December 10, 2020. https://www.ahfsdruginformation.com/ahfs-pharmacologic-therapeutic-classification/

44. National Library of Medicine (NLM). Unified Medical Language System® (UMLS®). Published 2020. Accessed December 15, 2020. https://www.nlm.nih.gov/research/umls/rxnorm/index.html

45. WHO Collaborating Centre for Drug Statistics Methodology. ATC/DDD Index 2021. Published 2020. Accessed December 15, 2020. https://www.whocc.no/atc_ddd_index/

46. Dowell D, Haegerich TM, Chou R. CDC Guideline for prescribing opioids for chronic pain—United States, 2016. *MMWR Recomm Rep.* 2016;65(1):1-49.

47. Berger MJ, Ettinger DS, Aston J, et al. NCCN Guidelines insights: antiemesis, version 2.2017. *J Natl Compr Canc Netw.* 2017;15(7):883-893.

48. Microsoft®. Microsoft 365. Published 2020. Accessed December 15, 2020. https://www.microsoft.com/en-us/microsoft-365

49. SurveyMonkey®. Surveys. Published 2020. Accessed December 10, 2020. https://www.surveymonkey.com/

50. Qualtrics®. Experience Management. Published 2020. Accessed December 15, 2020. https://www.qualtrics.com/experience-management/

51. Vanderbilt University. Research Electronic Data Capture (REDCap). Published 2020. Accessed December 10, 2020. project-redcap.org

52. Harris PA, Taylor R, Thielke R, Payne J, Gonzalez N, Conde JG. Research electronic data capture (REDCap)—a metadata-driven methodology and workflow process for providing translational research informatics support. *J Biomed Inform.* 2009;42(2):377-381.

53. Simpson SH, Johnson JA, Biggs C, et al. Practice-based research: lessons from community pharmacist participants. *Pharmacotherapy.* 2001;21(6):731–739.

54. Carr MB, Divine H, Hanna C, Freeman PR, Blumenschein K. Independent community pharmacist interest in participating in community pharmacy research networks. *J Am Pharm Assoc (2003).* 2011;51(6):727–733.

55. Awaisu A, Alsalimy N. Pharmacists' involvement in and attitudes toward pharmacy practice research: A systematic review of the literature. *Res Social Adm Pharm.* 2015;11(6):725–748.

56. American College of Clinical Pharmacy. Standards of practice for clinical pharmacists. *Pharmacotherapy.* 2014;34(8):794–797.

4

Chapter Four

Formulating Practice-Based Research Questions and Hypotheses

Marion K. Slack, PhD

Chapter Objectives

- Understand the structure, process, and outcomes of pharmacy practice
- Formulate practice-based research questions
- Identify sources of research questions in pharmacy practice
- Gather the literature to support the research question
- Understand the context to develop research hypotheses in pharmacy
- Understand scientific and practical considerations for the research question and hypotheses

Key Terminology

Structure, process, outcomes, research question, research hypothesis, population, intervention, comparison, outcome, timing, setting

Introduction

A research question can be defined as "an explicit query about a problem or issue that can be challenged, examined, and analyzed and that will yield useful new information."[1] The research question identifies the topic of the research query. Because it is the first step in the research process,[2] it has a critical role in the development of a research protocol. All parts of the protocol, including research design and methodology, connect to the research question either directly or indirectly. The research question sets the context for clinical- or laboratory-based research. The research question immediately identifies the topic of the study; that is, for instance, whether pain management or diabetes is being studied. It also identifies the experimental treatment being proposed, such as a new medication or a method to improve adherence. Finally, the research question identifies the aspect of the disease (outcome) that the treatment is expected to affect, for instance, glycosylated hemoglobin or the proportion of patients at goal.

Research forms the basis of evidence-based medicine. Evidence-based medicine uses the findings from research to improve the health and well-being of people. It also starts with a question to provide the context of patient care. Evidence-based medicine uses a process of (1) asking appropriate and answerable questions, (2) obtaining evidence from the results of studies, (3) assessing the study results to assure they are valid, and (4) applying the obtained evidence to patient care or practice. By asking appropriate questions in pharmacy practice and policy, the evidence can be obtained for optimal use of medications, pharmacist services, and pharmacy systems.[2]

The purpose of this chapter is to provide a framework for developing a precise research question with related hypotheses that can guide the development of a study protocol. First, the Population, Intervention, Comparison, and Outcome (PICO) framework[3] for developing a research question is introduced with each component described, and some examples of research questions are examined using the framework. Then we discuss sources that can assist with identifying practice-based research topics and identifying a mentor or project advisor. After a topic has been identified, literature relevant to the topic needs to be retrieved and reviewed. The literature review provides the information for refining and completing the research question by adding information on the timeline and study setting. The literature review also assists with writing the hypotheses. The research question and related hypotheses will be evaluated using the FINER criteria[4] applied in the context of student research projects. Finally, the relationship of the research question and the hypothesis to the study protocol is delineated. The goal of this chapter is to provide the information required for writing the research question and hypotheses that are part of a research protocol. The focus is on the primary research question; a similar process can be used for the secondary research questions.

PICO Components of the Research Question

PICO framework is often used in research to assure that all critical information required for designing a study is included in the research question or objectives and the hypotheses.[3,5,6] Each component of the research question with its definition and examples is shown in Table 4–1.[3] The first component is Population (P) and refers to the characteristics of patients with the health issue that the experimental treatment is thought to affect. For example, the experimental treatment may be thought to affect hemoglobin A1C levels of adults with diabetes; therefore, the population is adults with diabetes.

The second and third components, Intervention (I) and Comparison (C), represent the study groups or the primary independent variable of the study. The Intervention (I) represents the treatment or exposure thought to affect health status; it is the treatment/exposure that is being tested.[3] The intervention could be a medication, an exercise intervention, an educational intervention, or a new method of providing care, for example, Transition of Care (TOC) intervention. Because patients who receive the intervention may change even if the intervention did not affect health status, the outcomes of the group receiving the intervention are compared to the outcomes of a group of patients who did not receive the intervention. The presence of a comparison group provides reasonable confidence that the intervention and not some other factor was the cause of the change in health status. Comparison (C) in the PICO acronym represents the comparison.[3] The Comparison consists of patients who receive a placebo or usual care whose baseline characteristics, including clinical measures (e.g., A1C, BP), should not be statistically

TABLE 4–1. PICO COMPONENTS WITH EXAMPLES

Component	Definition	Examples
Population	Refers to the population studied. The population may be defined by disease state, demographic characteristics, or setting; designated as "P"	Adults with diabetes Women with chronic pain Clients of a community health center
Intervention	Refers to the experimental treatment or the topic being investigated. It could be a new treatment controlled by the investigator or it could be a treatment initiated outside the study; patients receiving the experimental treatment form the intervention group; designated as "I"	Medication Physical therapy Diet New management protocol Gender
Comparison	Refers to an alternate treatment or alternate condition; patients receiving the comparison form the control group. The comparison may or may not be controlled by the investigator. Designated as "C"	Placebo Usual exercise Usual diet Alternate treatment Care under old protocol
Outcome	Refers to the effect the intervention has on the patient, that is, the aspect of the disease or health that the intervention is expected to affect. Designated as "O"	Decreased blood pressure Decreased pain Absence of infection

Source: Data adapted from Turner 2014.[3]

different from the intervention group. Accordingly, the independent variable has two levels; the first level is the intervention (I) and the second level is the comparison, also called a control (C). Hence, an independent variable always has at least two levels, (I) and (C).

The fourth component of PICO is the Outcome (O). The Outcome is the health status dimension that the invention is thought to affect,[3] for example, A1C, sleep time, number of readmissions, or level of pain. The measure used to assess the outcome is known as the dependent variable; for instance, the number of readmissions in 30 days or the level of pain measured on an 11-point scale. After collecting data on the outcome, the investigator compares, for example, the mean response (e.g., A1C or Pain scale) for the intervention group to the control group. By conducting a statistical test, the investigator can determine if the intervention statistically increased, decreased, or did not affect the outcome compared to the comparison treatment (C).

Examples of research questions using the PICO format are shown in Table 4–2. The population, intervention, comparison, and outcomes are clearly identified. As can be seen, the populations vary, the interventions vary, the comparisons vary, and the outcomes vary, but each research question contains the four components. The first study is a classic clinical trial comparing the outcome (sleep time) for a group receiving medication (melatonin) to a group receiving a placebo.[7] The second study compares the use of a TOC intervention for decreasing readmissions to usual care.[8] Note that the TOC intervention is a change in patient care procedures that is being tested rather than medication. The third study does not involve an intervention. In contrast, the study compares two groups of patients based on a difference between the groups; in this example, the comparison groups are based on a demographic characteristic, gender, women versus men.[9] The outcome of interest is the level of pain. In the fourth example, patients using multidomain pain management strategies are compared to patients using only medications.[10] The outcome is the level of

TABLE 4–2. EXAMPLES OF RESEARCH QUESTIONS WRITTEN WITH PICO COMPONENTS

Example	Population	Intervention	Comparison	Outcome
1	In hospitalized older adults,	is melatonin more effective than	placebo	for increasing sleep time?
2	In hospitalized Medicare patients,	are TOC interventions more effective than	usual care	for preventing readmissions?
3	In community dwelling adults with chronic pain,	do women or	men	report higher levels of pain?
4	In community dwelling adults with chronic pain,	is use of multidomain pain management strategies compared to	use of only medications	associated with less disability?

TOC: Transition of Care
Source: Data adapted from Turner 2014.[3]

disability. The outcome of interest is measured for each group, then the groups are compared to determine if the outcomes are statistically different.

Framework for Pharmacy Practice Research

The goal of pharmacy practice research is to improve patient outcomes or health status. The Donabedian framework of structure, process, and outcome can provide the context for practice-based research.[11] The three components are shown in Table 4–3; they are generally depicted as progressing from structure to process to outcomes. Structure refers to the setting in which care is provided and includes material resources, personnel, and organizational structure. Process refers to the activities used by practitioners to provide care or used by patients to manage care. Outcome refers to the effect of care on the patient, including health status, quality of life, and other patient outcomes.[11] As shown in Table 4–3, a single topic, for example, the use of melatonin for sleep, could be studied from the perspective of structure, process, or outcome. The research question related to structure could involve insurance coverage

TABLE 4–3. STRUCTURE, PROCESS, AND OUTCOME COMPONENTS OF PHARMACY PRACTICE

Definition/Example	Structure	Process	Outcome
Definition	The setting in which care is provided, includes material resources, personnel, and organizational structure	Activities used by practitioners to provide care or used by patients to manage care	The effect of care on the patient including health status, QOL, and so on.
Example Question 1	Does insurance coverage for melatonin increase its use for sleep by older adults compared to no coverage?	What is older adults' level of knowledge of the use of melatonin for sleep?	In hospitalized older adults, is melatonin more effective than placebo for increasing sleep time?
Example Question 2	Does training personnel how to teach patients to self-monitor blood glucose increase patient satisfaction?	Is the accuracy of self-monitored blood glucose readings within acceptable limits?	How does the accuracy of self-monitored blood glucose influence treatment decisions made for women?
Example Question 3	Do refill limitations imposed by insurance compared to no limitations decrease adherence to metformin in older adults?	Do real-time reminders to refill metformin prescriptions vs. no reminder increase older adults' adherence?	How is adherence to metformin treatment related to HA1C levels in older adults?

Source: Data summarized from Donebedian, 1988.[11]

for melatonin, that is, does insurance coverage for melatonin increase older adults' use of melatonin? A question involving process could be assessing older adults' knowledge of the use of melatonin. The outcomes question could be a classic question of whether melatonin increases sleep time in older adults. A similar difference in research questions can be seen for self-monitoring blood glucose and adherence to metformin treatment. Further examples of research questions for each of the components, structure, process, and outcomes are described below. The example studies provided are for student projects.

Outcomes are probably the component most readily associated with pharmacy practice research because it is associated with improving health status. For pharmacy practice, the classic example would be a clinical trial to determine the effect of a new medication on disease, for example, the use of penicillin for infections. While students may not be involved in testing new medications, they could be involved in investigating the effects of pharmacy care on individual health status through such activities as pain management[9] or for populations, through activities such as immunization.[12] The studies could be conducted in either hospitals or community pharmacies. Both a study of melatonin for prevention of postoperative delirium in older adults[13] and a study of a TOC intervention was aimed at improving patient outcomes[14] in hospitalized patients. A study of the use of brentuximab vedotin in the management of non-Hodgkin lymphoma is another example of a study seeking to improve patient outcomes.[15]

Process refers to the activities used by practitioners to provide care (e.g., patient counseling) or used by patients to receive care (e.g., adherence to medication instructions). For example, one study assessed the impact of a real-time medication monitoring program on adherence to oral chemotherapy provided by a specialty pharmacy.[16] Another study examined the identification of drug therapy problems by pharmacists in community pharmacies through patient consultation.[17] A third study examined workflow changes in an outpatient hospital pharmacy.[18] A study comparing medication changes from comprehensive and noncomprehensive reviews also is an example of research into the process of providing pharmacy services.[19]

Structure refers to the setting in which care is provided and includes material resources (e.g., equipment), personnel (e.g., the contribution that pharmacists make to patient care or professional development), and organizational structure (e.g., methods of reimbursement). Studies of the electronic systems required to provide care are examples of research involving structure. One study examined the performance of drug-drug interaction software for personal digital assistants used to assist in providing pharmacy services.[20] Another example is a study on implementing a Health Information Exchange (HIE) at a county detention facility.[21] An additional example would be the comparison of the efficacy of two types of faxed medication interventions.[22] A study on preparing pharmacy graduates for interviews is an example of a study that contributes to professional development.[23] Research also can be conducted in other settings, including government, managed care, and professional organizations.

Sources of Research Questions in Pharmacy Practice

Sources of research questions in pharmacy practice include practitioners, faculty, reports of previous research, and a personal interest in developing a particular area of expertise. The sources of research questions are listed with the types of information available from each source in Table 4–4. Each source may be used by itself or in combination with other sources to identify a topic for a student research project.

Pharmacy practitioners or faculty often have practice issues that they would like to study but do not have time, so they may have suggestions. Another source of ideas is to review previous research. Scrolling through a journal in a specific area of interest could provide ideas on research topics. In addition, reviewing abstracts of research conducted by other students may be helpful. (See Online Resources) Previous research by the current faculty or former students can also be helpful. Another source of ideas is an interest in building expertise in a particular area. A particular interest in a specific area, for example, in the management of diabetes or the management of chronic pain, can serve as a source of ideas. By focusing on a specific area of practice, one could graduate with a specialty area in addition to the general pharmacy degree. A specialty focus also can differentiate applicants for specific pharmacy practice positions.

If a mentor or project advisor is not identified while identifying a research topic, then the next step is to find a mentor or project advisor. A research mentor is critical in learning

TABLE 4–4. SOURCES OF RESEARCH QUESTIONS WITH TYPE OF INFORMATION AVAILABLE

Source of Question	Type of Information Available
Practitioners	Relevance of research to practice; possibility of addressing issue of importance to the practice site
Faculty	Experience with conducting research; may have own research program with ideas for student research
Previous Research	Identify gaps in the literature; review discussion section of research reports as authors may suggest next steps in research on the topic
Previous Student Research	Identify the types of research that have been done via student research projects; reports may suggest next steps to research topic; also able to identify types of data collection procedures used in student research
Personal Interest	Can be sure that the topic is of interest to student
Theory	Identify new areas to research; identify novel approaches or topics

and applying the best practices of research. The best strategy for identifying an advisor if a topic has already been selected is to relate the topic to the specialty areas of faculty or practitioners. If the topic is pain management, then locate a possible advisor who works in that area by either checking their publication record or clinical expertise and checking with other faculty. When checking with a possible advisor and they say no, then be sure to ask them if they know someone else in their area who could be an advisor. Also, consider having co-advisors. Often one advisor will have expertise in the topic area, for example, diabetes, and the co-advisor will have expertise in research methods and statistics.

ROLE OF THEORY IN RESEARCH

Theory can provide guidance to the identification of a meaningful context for research as well as facilitate the identification of the research question. In addition, theory can provide interpretation for the data. To describe the role of theory, the biomedical paradigm is discussed, then the use of physical theories to guide research, and the addition of psychological and social theories that can increase the types of questions that can be asked related to patient care are described. In the biomedical paradigm, the overarching view of health and disease is that health and disease are the result of physical changes in the body. Theories in the biomedical paradigm involve physiological, pathological, and pharmacological mechanisms. The mind may be considered as separate from the physical body and not within the purview of medicine. However, there are efforts to incorporate social, psychological, and ecological factors as mediators of health and disease. Further development of theory related to social, psychological, and ecological factors and how they mediate health and disease can offer opportunities for research.[24]

As an example of the relationship between theory and research, consider the problem of chronic pain. Acute pain occurs when tissue has been physically damaged in some way. Pain lets the person know that damage has occurred, enabling the person to react to the threat. Typically, an acute injury will heal within three to six months. In contrast, chronic pain can occur without evidence of tissue damage and can occur for years. Management of pain is further complicated because pain is a subjective response that cannot be measured by any outside test, such as a blood test. Hence, a strictly biomedical perspective often fails to provide insight into the management of chronic pain. More recent efforts to improve pain management have resulted in the inclusion of psychological, social, and ecological factors into the management of chronic pain.[24] Several formulations of the biopsychosocial framework including pain as a disease, a multicomponent behavioral response to aversive stimuli, and a model based on learning theory are available.[25] For example, chronic pain without physical evidence of disease has been shown to be associated with negative life experiences such as abuse.[26] To address psychosocial factors, a bank of questionnaire items has been developed to assess the interference of pain in patients' lives, including items on the interference of pain with work, social activities, and so on.[27] Hence, the use of psychosocial theory can lead to new investigations that can improve patient care.

Review Relevant Research

The literature review has a specific role in developing a research protocol. The literature review provides the rationale for the research question and for the study design and methods delineated in the protocol. It shows that the research question and study design and methods are based on earlier work and not just someone's latest idea. This is particularly important when research involves human subjects as the latest idea that lacks a rationale could be harmful to patients. Therefore, a study protocol in pharmacy practice needs to be supported by a literature review. The discussion of the literature review below will focus on the literature related to the research question and hypotheses; however, the literature review also needs to include a rationale for the study design and methods proposed. Anyone reviewing the protocol should be able to identify the rationale for using specific treatment, for using a specific outcome measure, and for using a particular theoretical framework based on the literature review.

For the literature review, evaluate primary literature, that is, research reports of studies conducted in your area of interest. Research reports contain information, such as information on the research question, the intervention, the comparison, the outcomes measured, study design and methods, and the statistical analysis that are needed for writing a new protocol. If using theory, locate at least one study that reports research using the relevant theory. Other sources, such as textbooks, or guidelines will not have the specific information needed on the components of the protocol. However, textbooks and guidelines often cite primary research studies that may provide the needed information.

There are a number of strategies for identifying relevant literature. Probably the first step is to check with the project advisors. If they are conducting similar research, they can probably recommend a research report appropriate for review. Systematic reviews, with or without meta-analysis, on the topic, can identify research reports appropriate for review. Also, check the references in any relevant research reports already identified. Another strategy is to conduct a citation search of a previously identified research report. A citation search, using Scopus, Web of Science, or Google Scholar, will list all the studies that have cited the original report since it was published. Citation searches work best if the study report is at least four or five years old. General searches can also be conducted using keywords; their usefulness will depend on the area of study and searching skill. Consultation with a librarian can facilitate the search. Also, when conducting a general

TABLE 4–5. WORKSHEET FOR REVIEWING LITERATURE RELATED TO THE RESEARCH QUESTION

Citation[a]	Population	Intervention	Comparison	Outcome	Timeline	Study Design

[a]For citation, use first author's last name and date of publication.

search, be aware of the quality of the journal or source of the study. A safe rule of thumb is to use studies indexed in PubMed or the directory of open access journals (DOAJ).

To review the studies, use a worksheet such as that shown in Table 4–5. Reviews written for developing a protocol are not summaries of studies nor abstracts of study reports. The review is focused on the information that is needed for writing the protocol, which may or may not be contained in a summary or an abstract. For this part of the review, retrieve specific information on the target population, the intervention, the comparison, and the outcome related to formulating the research question. Also, collect additional information on the timing of the study and the study setting; the PICO framework is then expanded to the PICOTS framework, where T refers to the timeline and S refers to the study setting. The timeline refers to the length of time patients were followed after they received the initial dose of the intervention.

The number of studies needed for a review depends on the study and standards for student conducted studies. Typically, student research studies do not require the same type of comprehensive review required for a master's thesis or a dissertation. However, the number of studies should be adequate to provide the rationale for selecting a specific study population and appropriate study setting, forming the comparison group, and identifying the outcome as well as establishing a reasonable timeline for the study. One strategy would be to review four primary research reports (as required for student conducted research at the University of Arizona College of Pharmacy) then discuss the findings with an advisor/mentor to determine if more reviews are needed.

Refine the Research Question and Formulate the Hypothesis

Using the PICOTS framework, it is time to refine the original draft research question. The original draft research question provides information on the relevant components of the research study, including the population, intervention, comparison, and outcomes. The timing and study setting also need to be added to the research question if not already included. **Timing** for a research study indicates when the data were collected relative to the administration of the intervention or relative to the beginning of the study. The **study setting** is the site where the data were collected, such as a hospital or community pharmacy. Based on the literature review, an appropriate timeline and study setting can be identified. For the melatonin research question, the setting was already identified in the phrase, "In hospitalized older adults …," then by adding "after 14 days of therapy," the timeline for the study is described. The rewritten research question is shown in Table 4–6. The literature review on using TOCs to prevent readmissions indicated that the primary outcome of interest was the number of readmissions in the 30 days after discharge. Again, the study setting was already identified in the original research question when the patients were identified as "hospitalized." To complete the question, the 30-day time-frame is added in the phrase "for preventing 30-day readmissions?" In the third example comparing women and men on levels of pain, both the setting and the timeline need to be added. By adding the phrase "In community-dwelling adults with chronic pain …" at the beginning of the question and the phrase "at a single point in time?," both the setting and timeline are added. In a similar manner, in the fourth example, the phrases "In community-dwelling adults with chronic pain …" and "for at least six months …" explicitly identify the setting and the timeline.

The next step is to develop a hypothesis corresponding to the research question. A **research hypothesis** can be defined as a research question written in a form for statistical testing.[28] The hypothesis is one of the first steps in writing a protocol; the hypothesis and the protocol should be completed before any data are collected and analyzed. As discussed above, the research question provides information needed to write the protocol. The hypothesis provides the additional information needed for writing and interpreting the statistical analysis.[29,30] Theory can also assist with writing a hypothesis; for example, if a psychosocial theory is being used to study pain, then a hypothesis related to a psychosocial outcome, such as pain interference, can be used. The example research questions are shown with corresponding hypotheses in Table 4–6. Note the differences between the research question and the hypothesis. First, note that the research question is written in a format that indicates the investigators' rationale for the study; the investigator expects the experimental intervention to improve the health status of the patient, for example, to increase sleep time versus the comparison group. In contrast, the hypotheses are written as though the expectation is that the groups are not statistically different, that is, as a null hypothesis which is neutral with respect to outcome.[29] Also, note that the hypothesis specifically identifies the statistic being tested, for example, means or proportions. The statistic then indicates that a t-test could be used for testing for the difference in means and a Chi-square test for the difference in proportions (identified as rates in Example 4 in Table 4–6).

TABLE 4–6. PICOTS RESEARCH QUESTION AND CORRESPONDING HYPOTHESIS WITH IMPLICATIONS FOR STATISTICAL ANALYSIS

Example	Research Question with Hypothesis	Implications for Statistical Analysis
Example 1:		
Research Question **Hypothesis**	In hospitalized older adults, is melatonin more effective than placebo for increasing sleep time after 14 days of therapy? In hospitalized older adults, the mean sleep time for melatonin and placebo is not different.	The outcome variable is mean sleep time for the melatonin group compared to the placebo group indicating that a t-test could be used for the statistical test.
Example 2:		
Research Question **Hypothesis**	In hospitalized Medicare patients, are TOC interventions more effective than usual care for preventing 30-day readmissions? In hospitalized Medicare patients, the proportion of 30-day readmissions is not different in patients receiving TOC interventions and those receiving usual care.	The outcome variable is the proportion of readmissions for the TOC group compared to the usual care group indicating that a Chi-square test could be used for the statistical test.
Example 3:		
Research Question **Hypothesis**	In community dwelling adults with chronic pain, do women or men report higher levels of pain at a single point in time? In community dwelling adults with chronic pain, the mean pain levels reported by women and men are not different.	The outcome variable is mean pain level for women compared to men hence a t-test could be used for the statistical test.
Example 4:		
Research Question **Hypothesis**	In community dwelling adults with chronic pain, is use of multidomain pain management strategies for at least six months compared to use of only medications associated with less disability? In community dwelling adults with chronic pain, patients who use multidomain pain management strategies and patients using only medications experience rates of disability that are not different.	The outcome variable is number of patients with disability in the multidomain group compared to the medication only group, hence a Chi-square test for proportions could be used.

PICOTS: P=population; I=intervention; C=comparison; O=outcome; T=timeline, and S=setting; TOC: Transition of Care; t-test refers to a t-test for independent groups

Hypotheses do not have to be causal in nature. That is, the hypothesis does not have to propose that the intervention causes a change in the outcome. For example, a causal hypothesis would be "that melatonin affects sleep time … ." Causality is a function of research design, and it generally requires experimental research to evaluate a causal hypothesis. In contrast, one could also hypothesize that there are differences in the study groups or there exists a relationship between independent and dependent variables in nonexperimental research. For example, women experience different levels of pain than men. Both are hypotheses, but only the first is a causal hypothesis.[30]

When looking at the example hypotheses, note that the hypothesis is precise and that it can be measured. Precision and the ability to measure the outcome are related. The outcome to be measured must be identified precisely so that an appropriate measure can be identified. For example, the proportion of 30-day readmissions as an outcome is precise and can be measured by counting the number of patients who have been readmitted during the 30 days after discharge. A hypothesis that is precise and can be measured is considered a high-quality hypothesis.[31]

The research question and the hypothesis can also assist with the interpretation of study findings. Looking at the significance (p value) for the statistical test for the null hypothesis indicates if the statistic (i.e., means or proportions) are not different ($p > 0.05$) or if there is a difference greater than that expected from chance variation ($p < 0.05$). If the p-value is $p < 0.05$, then the research question can assist with interpretation of the difference. For example, in the melatonin study, the expectation is that melatonin will increase sleep time. If, for example, the melatonin mean sleep time is statistically greater than the mean placebo sleep time (i.e., $p < 0.05$), then the inference is that melatonin increases sleep time. If the mean sleep time for melatonin is statistically less than the mean for placebo ($p < 0.05$), then the inference is that melatonin decreases sleep time.

The melatonin example is based on a two-sided statistical test (e.g., t-test), that is, the objective is to determine whether the mean sleep time for melatonin is more or less than the mean sleep time for placebo. Both findings have implications for patient care. If sleep time is increased, then melatonin can be recommended to improve sleep. If sleep time is less, then the use of melatonin for sleep would be discouraged. Hence, as a rule of thumb, research with human subjects with implications for care should use a two-sided statistical test because knowing if an experimental treatment is ineffective is just as important as knowing if it is effective. In other areas of research, one-sided statistical tests may be used when the investigator is not concerned about using the information for patient care.

Evaluate the Research Question and Hypotheses

The FINER criteria have been developed to evaluate research questions and hypotheses. As shown in Table 4–7, the FINER criteria are: feasibility, interest of the topic, novelty, ethical considerations, and relevance.[4] However, when evaluating student projects,

TABLE 4–7. FINER CRITERIA, WITH STRATEGIES TO ADDRESS IN STUDENT RESEARCH

Criterion	Primary Concern	Strategies to Address
Feasibility	Limited time Limited resources Limited scientific expertise	Select types of studies that can be conducted with limited resources, e.g., nonexperimental studies using data already collected or using questionnaires; include a co-advisor with expertise in conducting research; restrict study scope
Interesting	Topic of the research should be interesting to the student Topic should be meaningful to the practice site or to the profession of pharmacy	Select study topics based on student interest, meaningful to the practice site, or the profession of pharmacy by addressing a practice or professional issue
Novel	Novelty	Conduct pilot studies in a new area; assure that the topic addresses a gap in the literature
Ethical	Use of human subjects in research	Work with study advisor and institutional review board
Relevant	Relevance to patient care, health policy, future research	Work with advisors who work in relevant areas

Source: Data from Hulley 2007.[4]

consideration should be given to the fact that it is student research, and the criteria should be modified as appropriate.

FEASIBLE

The proposed study should be feasible. Feasibility is an especially important issue for student research as students typically have a limited time frame and limited resources in which to conduct the study. One strategy to assure feasibility is to use nonexperimental study designs rather than experimental or interventional study designs. Nonexperimental study designs can use data that is already available from patient charts, databases, and published literature. Questionnaires are also a possibility if a specific population (e.g., patrons of a pharmacy) are accessible for the study. Generally, recruiting and consenting patients for an interventional study involves more time than is available for student projects. The same strategy of using data already collected also limits cost. In addition, most questionnaires and some educational interventions will have limited costs. Because time and costs are an issue, a timeline and study budget should always be developed so that feasibility can be assured. Another feasibility issue is the availability of research expertise; in cases where the primary advisor and the student have limited expertise, a co-advisor with research expertise could be added to the research team.

INTERESTING

It is particularly important for a research project to be interesting to the student who is conducting the research. One method to assure that the study is of interest is to identify how completing the study can assist in achieving other goals. For example, if one is interested in eventually working in management, then the study could involve a management issue. If one is interested in working in a specialized setting, for example, pain management, then the project could involve a pain management issue.

NOVEL

Novelty is another item that requires special consideration in the context of student research. The ideal in research is to conduct a study that investigates an issue in a new way or results in some type of new knowledge that can change patient care. Student research can be very useful for developing novel research ideas. Students can conduct pilot studies for developing methods to collect data, estimate sample size, or operationalization the intervention, which could be used for a larger study. Hence novelty should be considered in the context of the larger research program and previous work in the area.

ETHICAL

All student research proposals involving individual living humans must be reviewed to assure that the research is not harmful to the participants of the study. The Institutional Review Board (IRB) is usually the only entity that can determine if approval is needed; hence the best strategy is to always make an application to the IRB. Then if IRB approval is required for the presentation or publication of the study, documentation of IRB involvement is available.

RELEVANT

Relevance is primarily related to the application of the findings from the study to patient care and health policy or future research. Working with practitioners or practice sites that intend to use the study findings to improve patient care is one way to assure relevance.

PICOTS and Its Relationship with the Protocol

The research question using PICOTS provides key information for writing the study protocol. The relationship between the research question and hypotheses with sections of the

TABLE 4–8. **RESEARCH QUESTION AND HYPOTHESIS COMPONENTS WITH CORRESPONDING SECTIONS OF THE STUDY PROTOCOL**

Protocol Section	Research Question and Hypothesis Components	Protocol Sections
Introduction	Research question	Statement of the research question, typically as the last paragraph or sentence before the methods section.
Methods	(P) Population (S) Study setting	*Eligibility criteria*—A description of the criteria making a patient eligible for the study. Specify setting, demographic characteristics, and disease characteristics of the target population.
	Intervention (C) Comparison	*Intervention*—A description of the intervention and the comparison (i.e., the independent variable). For example, doses of medications, length of therapy, and so on for both the intervention and comparison treatment. If an alternate treatment is used, it should be described in some detail.
	(O) Outcome (T) Timeline	*Outcome measures*—Describe how the outcome will be measured, e.g., HgA1C, and time frame for the measurements, e.g., the HgA1C measured at six months after study entry.
	Specific statistic identified in the hypotheses (e.g., mean)	*Statistical analysis*—Describe the appropriate analysis for testing the identified statistic.

Note: There are other components to a protocol, only the components directly related to the research question and hypotheses are included. Typically, subheadings are used to denote these sections of the methods so that the key information related to the research question is easy to locate.

research protocol are shown in Table 4–8. In general, the research question and hypotheses identify the components specific to the proposed study, while the corresponding section in the protocol provides definitions and detail on how the component will be operationalized for the study. First of all, an appropriate research design should be identified for the objective. For example, if comparison groups based on random assignment are used, the research design could be specified as a randomized controlled trial. The Population component in the research question identifies the specific population and setting, for example, and the corresponding section in the protocol outlines the criteria for identifying a member of the target population (e.g., must be aged 18–80, with primary insomnia and sleep latency of at least 20 minutes) to be eligible for the study. In the methods section, the independent variable (I) is described. For example, patients in the melatonin group received 2 mg of PRM (prolonged-release melatonin) in the evening at bedtime for 21 weeks; patients in the comparison group received an identical placebo. The methods section also describes the outcome (dependent) variable. For example, the primary outcome measure was sleep latency recorded in a sleep diary by the patient every morning. Sleep latency was measured in minutes. Finally, the methods used to conduct the statistical analysis are described. For example, the mean latent sleep time between the PRM group and the placebo group was compared at 21 weeks using a t-test and an a priori alpha level of 0.05.

Given the importance of the terms used to designate the PICOTS components, it is best to carefully consider the words used to designate the components and be sure they accurately reflect the research question. The literature review can be helpful here as well; it can identify the terms currently being used for study components as well as increase the relevance of the proposed research to previous research in the area.

Summary and Conclusions

The research question has a critical role in designing the study and developing the study protocol. It sets the context of the research and provides the foundation for the development of the study protocol. The PICO acronym identifies the critical components of the research study, including the study population, the intervention, the comparison, and the outcome. This information can be used to guide the literature review, which in turn assists in identifying the timeline and the study design to expand the acronym to PICOTS. Identification of the timeline and study design then facilitate the development of the null hypothesis, which is needed for constructing the data analysis section in the protocol. Therefore, information in PICOTS provides the key information required for writing the protocol and connects directly and indirectly to other aspects of the protocol.

Understanding the structure, process, and outcome of pharmacy practice can guide pharmacy practice research. The research question should be constructed using the PICO components, including the population that the experimental treatment is expected to affect, the experimental intervention and the comparison group, and the health outcome that the experimental intervention is expected to affect. In general, the research question should delineate the goal of the research related to some type of change in health status. To formulate practice-based research questions, use a comprehensive framework that includes structure, process, and outcomes. A number of sources may be used to identify appropriate questions for investigation. Practitioners and college of pharmacy faculty may have care-related problems that need investigation. Reports of previous student research can also provide ideas for research studies. Research reports for completed studies frequently list suggested next steps in researching a specific topic in the discussion section, which may provide ideas for a new research project. Also, theories can provide ideas for testing new hypotheses as well.

Reviewing research related to the topic of interest provides information for identifying the outcome measures, methods for collecting data, and statistical analysis techniques that could be used in the new study. As a rule of thumb, a reader should not be surprised by any of the proposed methods, as the proposed methods should be clearly linked to the literature review. Hypotheses are developed from the research question to permit statistical testing. Hence, hypotheses require specific information related to the measurement of the outcome variable so that an appropriate statistical test can be identified. Throughout the process of stating the research question and hypotheses, actions need to be consistent with the requirements of scientific reasoning. Wording for the research question and hypotheses needs to be precise and consistent. Lack of precision and consistency will interfere with the ability to interpret the findings and make generalizations.

Key Points and Advice

- Research questions using PICOTS provide critical information for writing the hypotheses as well as sections of the research protocol; therefore, it is a good investment to spend time clarifying and refining the research question and hypotheses.
- Evaluation of the research question provides information essential to assuring that the study will provide meaningful evidence and that resources are available for the project.
- Identify a mentor and use structured worksheets to assist in writing the research question and hypotheses.
- Study protocols typically take time to write, particularly when working with a research team, so allow time for writing and for everyone involved to provide feedback.
- Remember that writing a research question, hypothesis, and protocol is an iterative process that typically requires discussion, revision, more discussion, and more revision.
- When working with a team, be careful with consistency in the protocol; each team member can write a section of the protocol, but then the sections need to be reviewed to assure consistency.
- If you are unsure of what to do next when writing the protocol, discuss the protocol with your advisor or another mentor. It is okay to say that you do not know what to do next.

Chapter Review Questions

1. Using the example PICOTS components provided below, compose a research question.
   a. Enoxaparin

b. Aspirin

c. Fewer blood clots

d. Hospitalized veterans having total knee arthroplasty

e. Within 30 days following surgery

2. Differentiate between the research question and the research hypothesis.

3. Identify three reasons for conducting a literature review.

4. For the example PICOTS hypothesis, identify the protocol section where the topic would be described and explain why you placed the topic there. Hypothesis: in (1) *patients receiving oral chemotherapy from a specialty pharmacy*, the (2) *mean medication possession ratio* is no different for (3) *real-time medication monitoring* and (4) *usual care* during (5) *one year of follow-up*.

5. Explain why the IRB should always be consulted when conducting research with living humans.

Online Resources

- Pharmacy Student Research Projects-University of Arizona. https://repository.arizona.edu/handle/10150/596334
- Pharmacy Student Research Projects—University of Utah available at: PharmD Projects—University of Utah. https://pharmacy.utah.edu/pharmdprojects/
- Resources available through the publisher, Elsevier. https://scientific-publishing.webshop.elsevier.com/research-process/finer-research-framework/
- Sage Research Methods (includes a wide variety of resources with a search function). https://methods.sagepub.com/

REFERENCES

1. Beitz JM. Writing the researchable question. *J Wound Ostomy Continence Nursing.* 2006;33(2):122-124.

2. Aparasu RR, Bentley JP. *Principles of Research Design and Drug Literature Evaluation.* New York, NY: McGraw Hill; 2020.

3. Turner M. PICO Framework and the Question Statement. Evidence-Based Practice in Health. 2014. Retrieved from University of Canberra website. Accessed November 11, 2020. https://canberra.libguides.com/evidence

4. Hulley SB, Cummings SR, Browner WS, et.al. *Designing Clinical Research.* 3rd ed. Philadelphia, PA: Lippincott Williams & Wilkins; 2007.

5. Aslam S, Emmanuel P. Formulating a researchable question: a critical step for facilitating good clinical research. *Indian J Sex Transm Dis AIDS.* 2010;31(1):47-50.

6. Richardson WS, Wilson MC, Nishikawa J, Hayward RS. The well-built clinical question: a key to evidence-based decisions. *ACP J Club*. 1995 Nov/Dec 1995;123(3):A12-A13.

7. Wade AG, Ford I, Crawford G, et al. Nightly treatment of primary insomnia with prolonged release melatonin for 6 months: a randomized placebo controlled trial on age and endogenous melatonin as predictors of efficacy and safety. *BMC Med*. 2010;8:51.

8. Arnold ME, Buys L, Fullas F. Impact of pharmacist intervention in conjunction with outpatient physician follow-up visits after hospital discharge on readmission rate. *Am J Health-Syst Pharm*. 2015;72:S36-S42.

9. Slack MK, Chavez R, Trinh D, Vergel de Dios D, Lee J. An observational study of pain self-management strategies and outcomes: does type of pain, age, or gender, matter? *Scand J Pain*. 2018 Oct 25;18(4):645-656. doi:10.1515/sjpain-2018-0070

10. Axon DR, Patel MJ, Martin JR, Slack MK. Use of multidomain management strategies by community dwelling adults with chronic pain: evidence from a systematic review. *Scand J Pain*. 2019;19(1):9-23. doi:10.1515/sjpain-2018-0306

11. Donabedian A. The quality of care: how can it be assessed. *JAMA*. 1988;260(12):1743-1748.

12. Baroy J, Chung D, Frisch R, Apgar D, Slack MK. The impact of pharmacist immunization programs on adult immunization rates: A systematic review and meta-analysis. *J Am Pharm A*. 2016;56:418-426.

13. Campbell AM, Axon DR, Martin JR, et. al. Melatonin for the prevention of postoperative delirium in older adults: a systematic review and meta-analysis. *BMC Geriatr*. 2019;19:272. doi:10.1186/s12877-019-1297-6

14. Rodrigues CR, Harrington AR, Murdock N, et. al. Effect of pharmacy-supported transition-of-care interventions on 30-day readmissions: a systematic review and meta-analysis. *Ann Pharmacother*. 2017;51(10):866-889. doi:10.1177/1060028017712725

15. Berger GK, McBride A, Lawson S. et al. Brentuximab vedotin for treatment of non-Hodgkin lymphomas: a systematic review. *Crit Rev Oncol Hematol*. 2017;109:42-50.

16. Mathews K, Cooley J, Russell K, Slack M. Impact of a specialty pharmacy-based oral chemotherapy adherence program on patient adherence. Accessed March 11, 2021. https://repository.arizona.edu/handle/10150/614015

17. Patel M, Campbell M, Mosleem M, Spriggle P, Warholak TL. Identifying drug therapy problems through patient consultation at community pharmacies: a quality improvement project. *J Patient Saf*. 2020;16(1):19-23. doi:10.1097/PTS.0000000000000228

18. Aguilar CP, Chau C, Giridharin N, Huh Y, Cooley J, Warholak TL. How to plan workflow changes: a practical quality improvement tool used in an outpatient hospital pharmacy. *J Pharm Pract*. 2013 Jun;26(3):214-219. doi:10.1177/0897190012451912

19. Buhl A, Augustine J, Taylor AM, Martin R, Warholak TL. Positive medication changes resulting from comprehensive and non-comprehensive medication reviews in a Medicare Part D program. *J Manag Care Pharm*. 2017;23(3):388-394.

20. Perkins NA, Murphy JE, Malone DC, Armstrong EP. Performance of drug-drug interaction software for personal digital assistants. *Ann Pharmacother*. 2006;40:850-855.

21. Hinchman A, Hodges S, Backus J, Warholak TL. Implementation of health information exchange (HIE) at the Pima County Adult Detention Complex (PCADC): lessons learned. *J Correct Health Care*. 2018;24(2):183-196.

22. Augustine J, Harrell T, Boesen K, Cerminara Z. *A comparison of the efficacy of two types of faxed medication interventions*. College of Pharmacy, The University of Arizona; 2014. https://repository.arizona.edu/handle/10150/614149

23. Powell AD, Yip S, Hillman J, Larson S, Cooley J, Davis LE. Preparing pharmacy graduates for interviews: a collaborative statewide mock interview session to improve confidence. *Curr Pharm Teach Learn*. 2015;7(5) 684-690. doi:10.1016/j.cptl.2015.06.009

24. Lima DD, Alves VLP, Turato ER. The phenomenological-existential comprehension of chronic pain: going beyond the standing healthcare models. *Philos Ethics Humanit Med*. 2014;9:2.

25. Quintner JL, Cohen ML, Buchanan D, et. al. Pain medicine and its models: helping or hindering? *Pain Med*. 2008;9(7):824-834.

26. Bullington J, Nordemar R, Nordemar K, Sjostrom-Flanagan C. Meaning out of chaos: a way to understand chronic pain. *Scand J Caring Sci*. 2003;17:325-331.

27. Amtmann D, Cook KF, Jensen MP, et al. Development of a PROMIS item bank to measure pain interference. *Pain*. 2010;150:173-182.

28. Farrugia P, Petrisor BA, Farrokhyar F, Bhandari M. Research questions, hypotheses, and objectives. *J Can Chir*. 2010;53(4):278-281.

29. Hoy WK. Analyzing the structure and substance of hypotheses. In: *Quantitative Research in Education: A Primer*. Thousand Oaks: SAGE Publications, Inc.; 2012. https://dx.doi.org/10.4135/9781452272061

30. Cheng GYT. A study of clinical questions posed by hospital clinicians. *J Med Libr Assoc*. 2004;92(4):445.

31. Behi R, Nolan M. Deduction: moving from the general to the specific. *B J Nurs*. 1995;4(6):341-344.

5

Chapter Five

Research Design and Methodology for Practice-Based Research

Margie E. Snyder, PharmD, MPH, FCCP, FAPhA and Molly A. Nichols, PharmD, MATS

Chapter Objectives

- Match research questions to appropriate research designs and methodologies commonly applied in practice-based research
- Identify the expertise needed to implement practice-based research
- Identify common pitfalls in planning for practice-based research
- Discuss practical considerations for practice-based research protocol development
- Apply theoretical frameworks to practice-based research protocol development
- Discuss important project management principles for practice-based research
- Discuss examples from published literature of student- and resident-led practice-based research

Key Terminology

Experimental designs, quasi-experimental designs, observational designs, quantitative methods, primary data collection, secondary data collection, qualitative methods, survey research, medical chart reviews, semi-structured interviews, focus groups, theoretical frameworks, project management

Introduction

Pharmacy students, residents, and fellows embarking on a research study for the first time often enter an initial meeting with a mentor with a study design and methodology in mind. For example, the junior researcher knows they want to pursue a descriptive, observational study. However, they begin planning for a survey due to their personal familiarity with surveys when their research question is better suited to be answered through qualitative interviews. It is important for researchers to pause and fully delineate their research question(s) and then proceed with matching these questions to appropriate study designs and methods. This will ensure the study is best designed to answer the research question(s) of interest. They need to further understand the practical considerations for planning the research because of limited time and resources. In addition, there are implications for appropriately applying theoretical frameworks from the literature to ensure a stronger overall study.

This chapter will describe important research designs and methodologies for learner-led research and common pitfalls in planning for practice-based research. Practice-based research is "research that is grounded in, informed by, and intended to improve practice."[1] This chapter provides practical advice for learners conducting research for the first time, and highlights examples from published literature of pharmacy students, residents, and other learner-led research. In addition, this chapter will enable readers to identify the expertise needed to successfully implement practice-based research and incorporate theoretical frameworks and important project management principles into the execution of their studies.

Common Study Designs

When considering both the study purpose and investigator orientation, study designs can be broadly categorized as experimental, quasi-experimental, or observational.[2] In experimental designs, the researcher is studying an intervention (e.g., drug, new pharmacy service) and randomizes groups to receipt of the intervention or not. Quasi-experimental designs also are used for studying an intervention; groups, however, are not randomized. In observational designs, researchers are studying what has occurred naturally (i.e., without researcher intervention or randomization). Given the resources and timelines needed for each design, students, residents, and fellows most often conduct quasi-experimental and observational research. These can include case, cross-sectional, and cohort studies. Therefore, these study designs, associated methodologies, and practical advice for their application will be the focus of the remaining sections of this chapter.

Common Study Methods

Both quantitative and qualitative methods are commonly used by learners. Quantitative methods are applied when the data to be analyzed are numerical. Quantitative methods use either primary (i.e., data collected for the specific study) or secondary (i.e., analysis of data collected for another reason) data collection. Qualitative methods are applied when the data to be analyzed are nonnumerical, typically text. Most commonly, learners conduct research using one of two common qualitative methods: one-on-one semi-structured interviews or focus groups.

Quantitative Methods

CONSIDERATIONS AND EXAMPLES OF APPROPRIATE RESEARCH QUESTIONS

Quantitative methods are the best match when a researcher asks questions such as, "how many...", "to what extent...", "what is the relationship between...", "what is the level of experience with...", or "what effect did..." Survey research is one example of a primary collection of self-report data methods that students, residents, and fellows often participate in. With regard to secondary data collection, learners often participate in medical chart reviews to answer practice-based research questions.[2] Therefore, survey and medical chart review methods will be the focus of this section. However, the guidance provided in this chapter can also be modified for other methods. Published examples of student, resident, and fellow projects the authors have mentored using these methods are summarized in Table 5–1.

SCIENTIFIC AND PRACTICE EXPERTISE FOR IMPLEMENTATION

Practice-based research is made possible by engaging a team with complementary expertise. Pharmacy students, residents, and fellows engaging in practice-based research are developing skills in both practice and research and will have varying levels of experience in each dependent on the stage of their training. Learners should help ensure that other team members involved in the design and execution of their project include both practitioners and researchers, as both bring valuable perspectives. During study conceptualization, practitioners can partner with researchers to formulate research questions that are clinically relevant and expected to help advance pharmacy practice. Practitioners should also be involved in the drafting and editing of survey items and chart abstraction

TABLE 5–1. PUBLISHED QUANTITATIVE EXAMPLES OF STUDENT, RESIDENT, AND FELLOW PROJECTS

Learner Type	Study Aims	Quantitative Method Used	Citation(s)
Student	To describe the experiences and opinions of pharmacists serving as site coordinators for the Medication Safety Research Network of Indiana (Rx-SafeNet)	Telephone Survey	Patel P, et al. *J Am Pharm Assoc.* 2015; 55:649-655
Student[a]	To describe primary nonadherence among subjects who opted-in to a bedside medication delivery (Meds-to-Beds) program at discharge compared to subjects who opted-out	Medical Chart Review	Damlos C. et al. *J Am Pharm Assoc.* 2019; 59: e39 [abstract] Myers J, et al. *J Am Pharm Assoc.* 2018; 57: e7 [abstract] Zillich AJ, et al. Evaluation of a "meds-to-beds" program on 30-day hospital readmissions. *J Am Coll Clin Pharm. 2019.* Published online ahead of print. doi:10.1002/jac5.1183
Resident	To: (1) characterize Indiana community-based pharmacist preceptors' knowledge and perceptions of medication-assisted treatment (MAT) for opioid use disorder (OUD) and (2) explore the desired resources, dispensing concerns, and preceptors' involvement in precepting students.	Internet Survey	Davenport ES, et al. *J Am Pharm Assoc.* 2020;60:S20-S28
Resident	To: (1) model the association between pharmacy technicians' attitudes and planned behaviors toward participating in medication therapy management (MTM) and MTM completion rates, (2) compare pharmacy technician and pharmacist attitudes and planned behaviors toward participating in MTM, and (3) identify respondent and pharmacy demographic factors associated with MTM completion rates	Telephone Survey[b]	Adeoye OA, et al. *J Am Pharm Assoc.* 2018;58:S7-S15

TABLE 5–1. PUBLISHED QUANTITATIVE EXAMPLES OF STUDENT, RESIDENT, AND FELLOW PROJECTS (*CONTINUED*)

Learner Type	Study Aims	Quantitative Method Used	Citation(s)
Fellow	To determine the use patterns of social media among graduating pharmacy students, characterize students' views and opinions of professionalism on popular social media sites, and compare responses about social media behavior among students seeking different types of employment	Internet Survey	Ness GL, et al. *Am J Pharm Educ* 2013;77:Article 146

[a]Damlos C. was a pharmacy student. Myers J. was a graduate student. Several abstracts/posters were produced from the same dataset collected via medical chart review. The main findings of the overarching study, which describes the methodology, are published in the Zillich et al. paper.

[b]Also included medical chart review component (i.e., modeled relationship between survey responses and medication therapy management completion rate and other pharmacy-level demographic data collected from respondents' pharmacies).

templates to ensure response options or data fields are complete and relevant to the practice setting. Moreover, at the point of dissemination, practitioners should review study findings and support researchers in the interpretation of findings and identification of key points for discussion, most pertinent to the clinical context. Researchers complement practitioners by ensuring a theoretical framework (discussed further in the section "Applying Theoretical Frameworks to Practice-Based Research") is applied to guide the research and bring critical methodological expertise. Researchers from disciplines outside of pharmacy (e.g., statistics, psychology, public health) should be consulted and invited to join the study team when needed.

PRAGMATIC CONSIDERATIONS

Resources Required

To successfully execute a survey study, a researcher needs various resources. First, a significant amount of time should be spent upfront to ensure the survey is well designed and mapped to the guiding theoretical framework, with response options appropriate for the audience. At this stage, the primary resource required is people—specifically, mentors and peers to assist in item development, pilot testing, and refinement. It is helpful to pilot test items first for content and then again for the timing to ensure the respondent burden won't be too great. Next, the researcher needs to consider the resources required for survey administration. This will partly depend on the format chosen for administration (e.g., mail, Internet, or telephone). For example, software packages exist for Internet-based survey administration, but the researcher must determine whether potential respondents have Internet access and how the URL for the survey will be provided (e.g., whether email addresses are known to the researcher or the URL will need to be sent in other formats, such as QR code in the mail) in order to determine if Internet-based administration is a good fit. If so, students and other new researchers should reach out to their institution's information technology team to determine whether the University has a subscription to a survey administration software program (e.g., SurveyMonkey, Qualtrics, REDCap) that can be used. If telephone administration is chosen, personnel will be needed to administer the survey and record data. Oftentimes, the resources available will inform what format for survey administration is taken. Financial resources for small incentives (e.g., gift cards) to encourage survey completion should also be considered. Finally, resources will be needed for data entry (when paper-based data collection is used), data cleaning, and analysis. These resources typically include trained personnel (e.g., statisticians) and software packages for data analysis (e.g., SPSS, R, SAS.) Statistical consulting services to assist with data management and analysis, as well as data analysis software packages, may be available through the researchers' institutions.

Some of the resources needed for a medical chart review are the same as those needed for surveys. For example, significant personnel resources are required to develop and pilot chart abstraction templates and to complete data collection and analysis. Software packages for recording (e.g., REDCap) and analyzing data are often used as well. One additional required resource is access to the medical charts themselves. The researchers will need to ensure that their study team includes individuals affiliated with the healthcare facility who can assist with navigating requirements for accessing medical charts for research purposes.

Timeframe

Pharmacy students, residents, and fellows typically have a rather short timeframe for getting a research study done during their training. Specifically, one year is a common timeline that learners, particularly residents, need to work within. Table 5–2 provides an example timeline for the survey and medical chart review studies to assist learners in planning accordingly and ensuring all-important study steps are considered. Creating a detailed timeline can help first-time researchers improve their likelihood of success in ultimately disseminating their work through abstracts and manuscripts.

Student Involvement, Roles, and Training Needs

Pharmacy students have many opportunities to get involved in practice-based research using quantitative methods. In some circumstances, students will be invited to take the lead on a project under the mentorship of faculty. For other projects, students might be asked to serve in a specific role, such as assisting with conducting a literature review, administering a survey, performing a medical chart review, or data cleaning and analysis. In both scenarios, it is critical that detailed training be provided. Learners leading projects

TABLE 5–2. EXAMPLE TIMELINE FOR A STUDENT, RESIDENT, OR FELLOW-LED SURVEY OR MEDICAL CHART REVIEW STUDY

July/August	September/October	November/December	January/February	March/April	May/June
• Identify mentor(s) • Draft research question(s) • Review theoretical frameworks to inform survey item/chart abstraction template development • Secure access to the medical charts (when applicable)	• Finalize research question(s) • Develop, pilot test, and finalize survey/chart abstraction instrument and data dictionary • Consult with statistician and finalize analysis plan and "skeleton" data tables • Submit IRB protocol • Draft introduction/methods sections of manuscript • Submit abstract and grant (residents, possibly others)	• Finalize logistics for survey administration/chart abstraction, depending on format chosen (e.g., build of electronic format, preparation of telephone number database, and so on) • Develop training materials and train personnel assisting with survey administration/chart abstraction • Present poster (some residents)	• Receive IRB approval • Administer survey/complete chart abstraction • Complete data collection and entry • Present poster (some residents)	• Data cleaning/analysis • Log any changes made to analysis plan and update draft methods section in manuscript • Present at residency conference (most residents)	• Draft results and fill in data tables and draft discussion/limitations • Submit manuscript to peer-reviewed journal

IRB, institutional review board

wherein more junior learners will be engaged should create clear learning objectives, associated training materials, and clear steps for assessing competence in the assigned task. Moreover, regular check-in meetings should be scheduled to address questions and take corrective action as needed. This level of communication between the study lead and learners is needed to ensure data integrity. Finally, students and other learners should be engaged early in direct conversations about their role(s) and how their work can best be reflected on their curriculum vitae. Project management will be further discussed in the section "Project Management and Helpful Tools."

Common Pitfalls and Lessons Learned

Planning ahead can help prevent many of the challenges that pharmacy students, residents, and fellows commonly encounter when conducting practice-based research using quantitative methods. Many checklists are available to help researchers ensure comprehensiveness in reporting the findings of different types of research studies; consulting these checklists in the planning stage is encouraged and can help ensure rigor and credibility in the research.

Examples of checklists for quantitative studies include:

- Good practice in the conduct and reporting of survey research[3]
- STROBE statement for observational research[4]
- PaCIR for pharmacist intervention studies[5]

Some challenges will likely still arise in practice-based research. Table 5–3 delineates some of the most common pitfalls experienced by new researchers, organized by each step in the project management process. Project management steps will be discussed in detail in the section "Project Management and Helpful Tools."

Qualitative Methods

CONSIDERATIONS AND EXAMPLES OF RESEARCH QUESTIONS

Qualitative methods are the best choice when a researcher asks questions such as, "why" or "how" something occurred. These methods provide rich insight into the lived experiences of individuals and allow researchers to explore attitudes and behaviors in depth. Most commonly, learners conduct research using one of two common qualitative methods: one-on-one semi-structured interviews or focus groups. **Semi-structured interviews** allow for in-depth probing of an individual's experience and are most appropriate when the research topic is considered sensitive or stigmatized (e.g., substance use

TABLE 5–3. COMMON PITFALLS ENCOUNTERED IN PRACTICE-BASED RESEARCH USING QUANTITATIVE METHODS

Project Management Step	Common Pitfalls	Tips for Success
• **Initiating**	• Inadequate focus; asking too many questions • Mismatch between questions and methods	• Learner-led projects should be simple to promote feasibility and likelihood for successful completion; try to narrow the scope to only one research question (see Chapter 4). • Be sure that method selection occurs after the research question is finalized.
• **Planning**	• Absent or inadequate statistical analysis plan and data dictionary • Inadequate application of theoretical framework • Insufficient training provided to team members	• Draft analysis plan and data dictionary (see Chapter 7) at the same time the IRB protocol is drafted, for review and editing by a data manager and/or statistician. • Mentors should help ensure that the theoretical framework is rigorously applied to all aspects of the study, including variable selection and plans for data collection and analysis. • Develop and deliver detailed training to all team members, tailored to their role on the study. Handouts, graphics, and slide decks can complement hands-on approaches (e.g., conducting a mock administration of a telephone survey).
• **Executing**	• Inadequate communication and learner oversight	• Students and other learners sometimes feel uncomfortable asking for help and believe they are sufficiently trained to complete tasks (e.g., data analysis) when oversight is needed. To prevent this, ongoing communication about assigned tasks and involvement of a statistician and senior mentors is needed to ensure data are analyzed and interpreted accurately.
• **Monitoring and controlling**	• Poor documentation of study changes	• Deviations from the analysis plan and any other changes made from the initial protocol should be documented in detail. A spreadsheet (e.g., created in Excel) can be a simple approach to this.

(Continued)

TABLE 5–3. COMMON PITFALLS ENCOUNTERED IN PRACTICE-BASED RESEARCH USING QUANTITATIVE METHODS (*CONTINUED*)

Project Management Step	Common Pitfalls	Tips for Success
• **Closing**	• Incomplete study close-out	• Learners should ensure that all steps outlined in the study protocol for appropriate study closure (e.g., secure data storage) are followed and/or communicate the status for assigned tasks to the PI once their role in the study ends. Creating a protocol checklist at the time of IRB approval and reviewing it throughout the study period can help ensure these steps are taken.

IRB, institutional review board; PI, principal investigator

disorder, sexually transmitted infections). Interviews are also preferred when convening participants for a single meeting wouldn't be practical (e.g., when the researcher wants to interview all of a pharmacy's staff about a new service being implemented).

On the contrary, focus groups are preferred when exploring group dynamics is relevant to the research question or when scheduling can leverage existing meeting times (e.g., dedicated lunch breaks or seminar time). When conducting focus groups, it is recommended that groups typically be homogenous (i.e., with people of similar background) and that at least two groups be held for each variable of interest.[6] For example, if the project is studying why some older adults choose to receive medication therapy management (MTM) while others do not, the researchers should consider conducting at least two groups each with: older males who received MTM, older males who did not receive MTM, older females who received MTM, and older females who did not receive MTM. Other variables (e.g., the complexity of their medication regimen) could also be considered and would increase the number of focus groups to conduct.

Because of their common use in learner-led research, semi-structured interviews and focus group methods will be the focus of this section. Published examples of student, resident, and fellow projects mentored by the authors using these methods are summarized in Table 5–4.

SCIENTIFIC AND PRACTICE EXPERTISE FOR IMPLEMENTATION

Just like for practice-based research projects using quantitative methods, complementary expertise is needed for projects using qualitative methods. Practitioners can assist

TABLE 5–4. PUBLISHED QUALITATIVE EXAMPLES OF STUDENT, RESIDENT, AND FELLOW PROJECTS

Learner Type	Study Aims	Qualitative Method Used	Citation
Student	To explore patient perceptions and the practical implication of using a brief nine-item scale to screen for medication-related problems in community pharmacies	Interviews, with patients	Kernodle AR, et al. *J Pharm Pract.* 2017;30:49-57
Student	To better understand perceived barriers and facilitators to providing medication therapy management (MTM) services by pharmacists who recently provided telephonic MTM services to home healthcare patients	Interviews, with pharmacists	Wellman BR, et al. *Consult Pharm.* 2015;30:163-174
Resident	To identify patient-perceived barriers to achieving A1C targets after receiving instruction in an accredited diabetes education program.	Interviews, with patients	Gildea CM, et al. *J Am Pharm Assoc.* 2017;57:S211-S216
Resident	To identify medical professionals' specific insights to implementing a transitions of care (TOC) clinic in a federally qualified health center (FQHC)	Focus groups, with medical clinic staff	Davis BT, et al. *J Am Pharm Assoc.* 2019;59:S12-S18
Fellow	To generate hypotheses for strategies contributing to community pharmacies' high performance on policy-relevant MTM quality measures	Interviews, with pharmacy staff	Adeoye-Olatunde OA, et al. *Res Social Adm Pharm.* 2021;17:1407-1419

learners and other researchers with the interpretation of coded transcripts. Researchers from other disciplines with expertise in qualitative methods (e.g., sociology, public health) are especially helpful additions to the team to assist in the development and refinement of interview and focus group guides and the logistics for data collection.

PRAGMATIC CONSIDERATIONS

Resources Required

When planning for interviews or focus groups, it is important to consider the numerous resources required. First, the researchers will need access to participants with experiences relevant for answering the research question(s). Sometimes, this is fairly obvious (e.g., studying service implementation and wanting to interview all participating staff) but often, this involves decisions. Participants should be selected carefully using purposive sampling approaches. Purposive sampling, in contrast with convenience sampling, means that potential participants are selected for a specific reason. Examples include homogeneous sampling, as mentioned above for focus groups, and "extreme" sampling, such as selecting the highest performers on a specific service.[6] Students, residents, and fellows should work with their mentors to delineate criteria that will be applied for selecting participants (e.g., age, stakeholder type, service performance level) and document the extent to which these criteria were met or not met in the final sample of participants. Thinking through these criteria also positions the team to consider the logistics for how eligible individuals will be located and invited to participate.

Interviews and focus groups can be conducted either in-person or remotely, via telephone or videoconferencing. If in-person, a quiet, private space is needed to help ensure confidentiality and sound quality if audio-recording. This might include patient consultation rooms, conference rooms, or even rooms in community spaces such as library study rooms. Telephone interviews are also convenient, and video-conferencing can work well for focus groups. In either case, if the conversation will be audio-recorded for transcription, a recording device will be needed and care taken to ensure data security. Again, personnel resources are also important to consider. For focus groups, separate moderator (i.e., the individual leading the discussion) and note-taker roles are ideal. This will enable the note taker to indicate the research subject identifier of different participants' statements, which is valuable during data analysis as it provides insight into the extent to which ideas are unique to one participant in the focus group or shared by many. People resources are also required to ensure sufficient pilot testing of interview and focus group guides and to conduct interviews and code/interpret data. Additionally, data transcription can be a time-intensive process. Professional transcriptionists can be used, but the service fees can be significant. The learner should work with the mentors to ensure that either resources exist for external transcription services or sufficient time and training is provided for internal transcription. Finally, while not required, qualitative data analysis software packages are helpful to support data management and coding, i.e., the process by which pieces of text are sorted and labeled to aid in interpretation. Bradley et al. provides a helpful taxonomy of the types of codes frequently used in qualitative data analysis.[7]

Timeframe

In Table 5–5, an example timeline is provided for a student, resident, or fellow-led interview or focus group study. In contrast to the timeline examples provided for quantitative research, a greater emphasis is placed on ensuring sufficient time for data analysis. This is due to the time requirements associated with the rigorous development and refinement of a codebook and transcript coding.

Student Involvement, Roles, and Training Needs

Pharmacy students can be successfully engaged in any part of a research project using qualitative methods. If not the project lead, students are often recruited to assist with

TABLE 5–5. EXAMPLE TIMELINE FOR A STUDENT, RESIDENT, OR FELLOW-LED INTERVIEW OR FOCUS GROUP STUDY

July/August	September/October	November/December	January/February	March/April	May/June
• Identify mentor(s)	• Finalize research question(s)	• Develop training materials and train personnel assisting with interviews/focus groups	• Continue conduct of interviews or focus groups	• Continue conduct of interviews or focus groups	• Complete data coding/interpretation and finalize audit trail
• Draft research question(s)	• Develop, pilot test, and finalize interview or focus group guide	• Receive IRB approval	• Continue data transcription and data coding/interpretation	• Continue data transcription and data coding/interpretation	• Draft results and fill in data tables and draft discussion/limitations
• Review theoretical frameworks to inform development of interview or focus group guide	• Draft analysis plans and consider initial deductive code development, using framework constructs	• Begin conduct of interviews or focus groups	• Maintain audit trail of codebook revisions	• Maintain audit trail of codebook revisions	• Submit manuscript to peer-reviewed journal
	• Draft "skeleton" data tables	• Begin data transcription and data coding/interpretation	• Present poster (some residents)	• Log any changes made to analysis plan and	
	• Submit IRB protocol	• Maintain audit trail of codebook revisions		• Update (if applicable) draft methods section in manuscript	
	• Draft introduction/methods sections of manuscript	• Present poster (some residents)		• Present at residency conference (most residents)	
	• Submit abstract and grant (residents, possibly others)				

IRB, institutional review board

conducting interviews and/or coding transcripts. Both are wonderful opportunities for students to gain exposure to qualitative methods; training, however, must be provided. Conducting a semi-structured interview is not easy and requires practice. Students should have the opportunity to conduct several mock interviews for feedback. Similarly, detailed training in data coding is necessary. Various workshops and short courses are available that can help mentors in providing students with this training. Students can start exploring these opportunities by asking their mentors about the training they've attended and by determining what workshops and/or short courses are offered locally. Internet searches are useful in identifying several external options as well.

Common Pitfalls and Lessons Learned

Many of the common pitfalls experienced in quantitative research can also occur in qualitative research. In Table 5–6, common pitfalls unique to qualitative research, and tips for success, are shared. These are focused on the first three steps in the project management process.

- Checklists also exist to help in planning for qualitative research. This is an example: COREQ checklist for interviews and focus groups.[8]

TABLE 5–6. **COMMON PITFALLS ENCOUNTERED IN PRACTICE-BASED RESEARCH USING QUALITATIVE METHODS**

Project Management Step	Common Pitfalls	Tips for Success
Initiating	• Unclear rationale for choosing interviews vs. focus groups	• The research topic, scheduling pragmatics, and resources required should be fully considered before choosing a specific qualitative method.
Planning	• Convenience vs. purposive sampling	• Developing clear sampling criteria up front can ensure that sampling is truly purposive.
	• Inadequate pilot testing/ training on qualitative data collection	• Plan for multiple rounds of pilot testing/mock interviewing to refine the interview/focus group guide and process in order to elicit detailed responses from participants.
Executing	• Insufficient resources for transcription	• Learners should discuss transcription needs with their mentors as soon as possible to ensure sufficient resources are available.
	• Not allocating enough time for data coding/ interpretation	• Qualitative data analysis is iterative and planning ahead for several months of data coding and interpretation is important to ensure the project can be completed on schedule.

Other Considerations in Practice-Based Research

DEVELOPMENT OF STUDY PROTOCOL OR PROPOSAL

All research involving human subjects must be approved by an institutional review board (IRB). However, most human subjects research led by learners falls either into exempt or expedited IRB review. In general, if the risk to participants in a study is not greater than the risks encountered in everyday life, the research will likely be exempt or expedited. It is important for researchers to look at the criteria for each and determine where the research fits best when submitting a protocol to IRB. This should involve a meeting between the learner and their mentor(s). It is important to note that receiving IRB approval can take a significant period of time. Often, a protocol will need to be revised and resubmitted before it gets officially approved. Remember, data collection cannot begin until IRB approval is received. At least one month should be budgeted to receive IRB approval.

FUNDING OPPORTUNITIES

Grants are an excellent resource for funding research activities. Grant funding may be utilized to support research assistants or statistical consultants for a project or to provide financial incentives for participants. Some grants may also be used for conference and travel expenses to share research findings through poster presentations. Allowable expenses for grant funding are specific to each grant and should be carefully reviewed when submitting an application. In addition to the practical advantages of research funding, developing grantsmanship skills is an excellent learning opportunity for any researcher, particularly learners. As a new investigator, pursuing small grants through local or national professional organizations is a great starting point for developing grantsmanship skills. Table 5–7 lists examples of small grant opportunities through national professional organizations (but note this is not a comprehensive list).

APPLYING THEORETICAL FRAMEWORKS TO PRACTICE-BASED RESEARCH

As mentioned previously, theoretical frameworks are excellent tools to use when crafting a research project. Theoretical frameworks are the structures that hold or support a theory of research study and explain why the research problem under study exists.[14,15] Applying frameworks can help ensure that all facets of the research question have been considered, and can serve as both a starting place and guide throughout the study design. For instance, if a researcher wants to answer a question about why patients behave a

TABLE 5–7. SMALL PHARMACY GRANT OPPORTUNITIES FOR STUDENTS, RESIDENTS, FELLOWS, AND NEW PRACTITIONERS

Organization	Grant Opportunity	Funding Amount	Eligible Applicants
College of Psychiatric and Neurologic Pharmacists Foundation[9]	Student Registration Grant Program	Conference-specific	Pharmacy students only
American Pharmacist Association Foundation[10]	Innovation in Immunization Practices Grant	$1,000	Pharmacy students, pharmacists only
College of Psychiatric and Neurologic Pharmacists Foundation[9]	Defining the Future Research Grant	$1,500	Pharmacy students, residents only
American Pharmacist Association Foundation[10]	Residents and Their Preceptors Incentive Grant	$1,000	Residents only
American Society of Health System Pharmacists Foundation[11]	Research Grant	$5,000	Residents only
Community Pharmacy Foundation (CPF) [12]	CPF Grant	Project-specific	Fellows, pharmacists only
American College of Clinical Pharmacy Foundation[13]	Futures Grant	$5,000-$40,000	Pharmacy students, residents, fellows, and junior investigators

certain way, using a theoretical framework about behavior can inform which questions to ask and shape the statistical analysis of results. It is important to "pull the thread through" when using theoretical frameworks and apply the framework throughout each step of the project from initial design to data analysis and write-up.

A vast number of theoretical frameworks exist, and highlighted below are a few common frameworks pertaining to behavior change. It is important to note that theoretical frameworks are not limited to specific types of methodologies; frameworks can be applied to both quantitative and qualitative research. The selection of a theoretical framework is driven by the question a researcher is trying to answer. In some cases, applying more than one framework may be appropriate to comprehensively answer the research question.

Examples of Behavior Change Frameworks[16,17]

The *Theory of Planned Behavior* (TPB), expanded from the Theory of Reasoned Action, attempts to predict intention to engage in certain behaviors by exploring an individual's: (1) attitudes toward the behavior, (2) subjective norms about the behavior, and (3) perceived control over the behavior.[16] The theory suggests that intent to perform a behavior increases with positive attitudes, affirmative subjective norms, and high perceived control, and that perceived control moderates the effect of attitudes and subjective norms.

The *Positive Deviance Approach* is based on observations of individuals or groups in a community whose behaviors deviate from their peers and allow for better problem-solving and outcomes.[17] This model asserts that, when resources and challenges remain the same in each community, differences in behavior influence positive or negative outcomes. Positive differences may be referred to as "best practices" and, once identified, can be promoted and disseminated within a community for sustained behavior change.

The *Social Cognitive Theory* (SCT), adapted from the Social Learning Theory, describes the reciprocal relationship between a person, a person's environment, and a person's behavior.[16] The SCT posits that people learn and perform behaviors based on both personal experiences and observed experiences from their environment. The SCT explores this relationship through six constructs: (1) reciprocal determinism, (2) behavioral capability, (3) observational learning, (4) reinforcements, (5) expectations, and (6) self-efficacy.

Examples from the Literature

Recall Adeoye-Olatunde et al.'s research from Table 5–4. Adeoye-Olatunde et al. applied two frameworks, the Positive Deviance Approach and the Chronic Care Model, to answer the question, "What strategies contribute to community pharmacies' high performance on MTM quality measures?" We will primarily highlight the use of the Positive Deviance Approach. The core research question focused on pharmacy performance, specifically positive performance, on MTM quality measures. The research team observed that pharmacy performance varied widely on MTM quality measures, with some pharmacies performing better than others. Using the Positive Deviance Approach, the team hypothesized that pharmacies with better scores on quality measures had better strategies, or best practices, compared to pharmacies with lower scores. The research team purposefully selected low-, moderate-, and high-performing pharmacy sites to interview staff members and attempt to characterize differences in staff behaviors between the sites. The research team utilized the Chronic Care Model to inform interview guides prior to interviewing pharmacy staff. Common themes from staff interviews resulted in the identification of eight strategies contributing to performance on MTM quality measures. After confirmation in future quantitative research, the positive contributing strategies identified in this project could be disseminated to all pharmacy practice sites to improve community performance.

PROJECT MANAGEMENT AND HELPFUL TOOLS

The lead investigator of a research project is primarily responsible for managing the research team. Good project management is essential to any team's success. **Project management** is defined as the application of knowledge, skills, tools, and techniques to meet project requirements, and its processes fall into one of five groups: (1) initiating, (2) planning, (3) executing, (4) monitoring and controlling, and (5) closing.[18] As a new investigator, the prospect of managing a team can feel overwhelming. Helpful tips for successfully leading research projects in each stage of the project management process are shared below.

Planning, Meeting Frequency, Time Management, and Study Documentation

Initiating: In the initiation phase, researchers will determine the main question the project will answer and conceptualize how to answer the question. The first three sections of this chapter explain in detail the factors to consider when selecting a research question and appropriate methodology in this stage of a research project.

Planning: Equally important to the conceptualization of a project is proper planning and time management to achieve the objectives. Taking care to plan ahead at the start of a research project for the entire project timeline will help the research team stay on track and not fall behind. When planning for projects, consider the following questions.

"Who Will Be on My Research Team?"

Reflect back on the scientific and practice expertise needed for quantitative and qualitative research projects. It is important to select team members with care and consider the strengths they will contribute to the team. Most new investigators will have at least one mentor for a project, typically serving in the PI role. New investigators may also have additional senior investigators serving as mentors on the project. Consider how peer or trainee investigators, such as students or residents, may contribute to the team.

"Who Will Be Responsible for What?"

Once the research team has been assembled, it is crucial to discuss the roles and responsibilities of each team member. As previously mentioned, the lead investigator will be responsible for project management in addition to other duties such as data collection. Data collection and other tasks may also be delegated to students or other learners. The PI and other senior mentors will be largely responsible for reviewing the work and providing input and suggestions for improvement. In addition to discussing roles on the project, it is best practice to determine upfront which members of the team will be authors of the research manuscript and in what order each name will appear. Utilizing CRediT (Contributor Roles Taxonomy)[19] can help guide the responsibility and authorship discussions.

"How Often Will My Research Team Meet?"

Regularly scheduled meetings will be essential in holding the team accountable for meeting project objectives on time. Find a consistent day and time that works best for everyone on the team and schedule recurring meetings in advance. In the beginning stages of the project, we recommend meeting once a week to ensure the team is moving at an appropriate pace. The meeting frequency may be reduced to every other week or once a month after the project is "off the ground," such as in Internet survey research, but this may not be appropriate in all circumstances. Remember, it is easier to cancel an unneeded meeting on the calendar than it is to schedule a needed meeting.

"How Long Will My Research Project Last?"

As mentioned previously, one year is a common timeline for learner-led research projects. Note the example timelines provided in Tables 5–2 and 5–5 and keep in mind that not all 12 months can be used for data collection. Around six months should be budgeted for project preparation (e.g., defining and refining the research question, designing project methods, training personnel, and so on) and submitting for IRB approval before starting to collect data. The remaining six months can be split roughly in half, three months for data collection and three months for data analysis and manuscript finalization. However, it is important to create timelines with flexibility in case something does not go as planned (which is likely!). Note that these suggested timelines are arbitrary and may need to be adjusted based on other deadlines, such as anticipated internal program launches or external presentation dates.

"What Is My Final Research Question?"

Now that the research team and project timeline are established, it is important to go back and refine the research question. Is it still feasible to answer the original question? Are there different methodologies that may be better suited to the timeline? It is critical to thoroughly review and revise project objectives and methodology prior to collecting data. Be careful not to underestimate how long revisions may take.

"Where Do I Want to Share My Work?"

The ultimate goal of most projects is to publish findings in a scientific journal. Take care to find a journal that best fits the purpose of the project to improve the odds of publication. Be on the lookout for calls for papers for special themed issues, such as the Residency Issue in the *Journal of the American Pharmacists Association (JAPhA)*. In addition to manuscripts, it is also important to consider sharing research through poster presentations at professional conferences, such as the American Society of Health System Pharmacists (ASHP) Midyear or the American Pharmacists Association (APhA) Annual meetings. Because deadlines for submitting abstracts occur months before these meetings take place, it is important to identify these opportunities at the start of the project timeline and budget ahead for deadlines.

"Will My Work Require Funding?"

It may be desirable to obtain funding for research projects, enabling the team to pay for statistical analysis or provide financial incentives to potential participants. As mentioned previously, there are small grant opportunities through national organizations in which to acquire funding for research projects. It is again important to identify these opportunities at the start of the project timeline and budget ahead for deadlines. Additionally, it is important to develop contingency plans in the event grant funding is not received.

Executing: Now that a detailed research plan has been determined, it is important to follow the schedule set for the team. Ensure each team member is aware of their assigned tasks as the project takes off. Consider tools that could aid in project execution, such as the online software Smartsheet for assigning tasks and tracking progress. Providing a central and accessible space for team members to access pertinent files, such as Dropbox, Box, or Google Drive platforms, allows for efficient documentation and editing. When choosing a file-sharing platform, ensure compliance with pertinent security considerations for the data shared. For instance, any patient-specific information should be stored in a secure platform to minimize potential Health Insurance Portability and Accountability Act (HIPAA) violations.

Monitoring and controlling: The lead researcher should check in on the team's progress at each recurring meeting and ensure that the work is submitted in a timely manner and with sufficient quality. Progress reports and decision documentation will help the project be successful. Adjust timelines as needed depending on the team's progress.

Closing: Once data collection, data analysis, and manuscript writing are finished, it is important to tie up any remaining loose ends. Ensure surveys, when applicable, are closed; all authors approve of the finished manuscript prior to submitting it for publication; and study closure activities occur as described in the IRB protocol.

Examples from the Literature

Two examples from the literature will be used to further illustrate project management concepts in practice-based research. Recall Davenport et al.'s Internet survey research from Table 5–1. Key aspects of project management for this quantitative research project are detailed below. First, look at the members of the research team and their roles and contributions to the project.

1. Elizabeth Davenport, PharmD, was a PGY-1 pharmacy resident at the time of the study. Her roles on the project were lead investigator and lead author. Dr. Davenport's project contributions included: *Conceptualization, Formal Analysis, Funding Acquisition, Investigation, Methodology, Project Administration, Visualization, Writing—Original Draft, and Writing—Review and Editing.*

2. Stephanie Arnett, PharmD, CDE, was an Adjunct Clinical Assistant Professor of Pharmacy Practice and Residency Program Director at the time of the study. Her roles on the project were co-investigator and co-author, and she served as research site mentor for Dr. Davenport. Dr. Arnett's project contributions included: *Conceptualization, Supervision, and Writing—Review and Editing.*

3. Molly Nichols, PharmD, was a fourth-year pharmacy student at the time of the study. Her roles on the project were co-investigator and co-author. Dr. Nichols' project contributions included: *Conceptualization, Data Curation, Investigation, Methodology, and Writing—Review and Editing.*

4. Monica Miller, PharmD, MS, was a Clinical Associate Professor of Pharmacy Practice at the time of the study. Her roles on the project were principal investigator and co-author, and she served as research faculty mentor for Dr. Davenport. Dr. Miller's project responsibilities included: *Conceptualization, Methodology, Supervision, and Writing—Review and Editing.*

The senior members of Dr. Davenport's team, Dr. Arnett and Dr. Miller, provided guidance from the outset of the project for research design, methodology, and objectives. They also provided supervision for project activities and edits for the manuscript materials. The junior members of the team, Dr. Davenport and Dr. Nichols, also had input in the design, methodology, and objectives, and were largely responsible for the creation of the survey instrument and data collection. While not an author on the research manuscript, a practice expert in substance use disorder participated in survey item pilot-testing to ensure appropriate content. Additionally, a statistician was consulted to ensure proper data reporting in descriptive statistics. Dr. Davenport scheduled biweekly meetings with her research team from August 2018 to January 2019, then monthly meetings thereafter. To facilitate project management, Dr. Davenport utilized a research training manual to outline team member expectations and Box to share files. Dr. Davenport's research manual is provided in Appendix 1. This manual was adapted from Dr. Stefanie Ferreri's student research training manual at UNC Eshelman School of Pharmacy.

Observe Dr. Davenport's project timeline below. Note the majority of the work took place in the planning stages of the project at the beginning of Dr. Davenport's residency year, most evidently in September and October:

July-August (2018): Drafted research questions and identified research mentors and co-investigators.

September-October (2018): Finalized survey questions, selected conceptual framework, drafted analysis plans, developed survey questions, drafted introduction and methods manuscript sections, submitted APhA Incentive Grant proposal, submitted APhA and ASHP poster abstracts.

November-December (2018): Pilot tested survey, revised survey questions, created the survey in the web-based platform, submitted IRB protocol, presented a poster at ASHP Midyear.

January-February (2019): Received IRB approval, recruited participants, began data collection.

March-April (2019): Ended data collection, presented a poster at APhA Annual, presented research at Great Lakes Pharmacy Residency Conference.

May-June (2019): Revised introduction and methods manuscript sections, drafted results, and discussion manuscript sections.

September (2019): Finalized and submitted manuscript to *JAPhA*.

November-December (2019): Revised and resubmitted manuscript to *JAPhA*.

February (2020): Manuscript published in *JAPhA*.

When asked about her experiences as a first-time lead investigator, Dr. Davenport noted, "Balancing research with other longitudinal residency experiences was difficult. I learned when to ask for help from my research team, and I asked for a lot of help. The most important task I completed was creating and establishing a timeline of expectations for what I needed from the different members of my research team. This provided me a framework to work from and work toward in order to keep the team and myself on track and able to finish my manuscript for submission to *JAPhA* by the end of my residency year."

Similarly, recall Adeoye-Olatunde et al.'s interview research from Table 5–4. Key aspects of project management for this qualitative research project are detailed below. First, look at the members of the research team and their roles and contributions to the project.

1. Omolola Adeoye-Olatunde, PharmD, MS, was a Community Practice Research Fellow at the time of the study. Her roles on the project were lead investigator and lead author. Dr. Adeoye-Olatunde's project contributions included: *Conceptualization, Methodology, Validation, Formal Analysis, Investigation, Resources, Data Curation, Writing—Original Draft, Writing—Review and Editing, Visualization, Project Administration, Funding Acquisition.*

2. Leslie Lake, PharmD was a community pharmacy site partner at the time of the study. Her roles on the project were co-investigator and co-author. Dr. Lake's project contributions included: *Formal Analysis, Investigation, Resources, Data Curation, Conceptualization, Methodology, Writing—Review and Editing.*

3. Celena Strohmier, PharmD, was a fourth-year pharmacy student at the time of the study. Her roles on the project were co-investigator and co-author. Dr. Strohmier's project contributions included: *Formal Analysis, Investigation, Resources, Data Curation, Writing—Review and Editing.*

4. Amanda Gourley, PharmD, was a fourth-year pharmacy student at the time of the study. Her roles on the project were co-investigator and co-author. Dr. Gourley's

project responsibilities included: *Formal Analysis, Resources, Data Curation, Writing—Review and Editing.*

5. Ashli Ray, PharmD, was a fourth-year pharmacy student at the time of the study. Her roles on the project were co-investigator and co-author. Dr. Ray's project responsibilities included: *Formal Analysis, Resources, Data Curation, Writing— Review and Editing.*

6. Alan Zillich, PharmD, FCCP, was a William S. Bucke Professor and Head of Pharmacy Practice at the time of the study. His roles on the project were co-investigator and co-author and served as a co-mentor for Dr. Adeoye-Olatunde. Dr. Zillich's project responsibilities included: *Conceptualization, Methodology, Writing—Review and Editing, Supervision.*

7. Margie E. Snyder, PharmD, MPH, FCCP, FAPhA was an Associate Professor of Pharmacy Practice at the time of the study. Her roles on the project were a principal investigator for the IRB protocol and co-author, and she served as Dr. Adeoye-Olatunde's fellowship program director and primary mentor on this project. Dr. Snyder's project responsibilities included: *Conceptualization, Methodology, Validation, Resources, Writing—Review and Editing, Visualization, Supervision, Project Administration, Funding Acquisition.*

As this was Dr. Adeoye-Olatunde's MS thesis, she spearheaded the study design, methodology, and objectives with input from the team's pharmacy partner (Dr. Lake) and thesis committee members (including Drs. Snyder [chair] and Zillich). They also provided supervision for project activities and edits for the manuscript materials. The PharmD student members of the team, Drs. Strohmier, Gourley and Ray, were instrumental to participant recruitment, qualitative data collection (i.e., semi-structured interviews), and analysis (e.g., creation of sub-codes, coding, thematic analysis). While not an author on the research manuscript, an expert in complex sampling methods assisted with extreme case site selection. Dr. Adeoye-Olatunde scheduled weekly to quarterly (depending on involvement and stage of research) meetings with research team members through the duration of the study. To facilitate project management, Dr. Adeoye-Olatunde also utilized a research training manual to outline team member expectations, as well as an institutional secured shared drive, Microsoft OneDrive, and FileLocker to share files with institutional and non-institutional team members.

Observe Dr. Adeoye-Olatunde's project timeline below. Note that in contrast to Dr. Davenport's one-year residency, Dr. Adeoye-Olatunde completed this project over a three-year fellowship.

March-May (2018): Drafted and submitted IRB protocol.

June-July (2018): Created list to draw sample from pharmacy locations, pilot-tested interview guide, began participant recruitment.

August-December (2018) and January (2019): Continued participant recruitment, began qualitative data collection.

February (2019): Ended data collection.

March-May (2019): Completed qualitative data analysis, pulled quantitative data, completed quantitative data analysis.

May-June (2019): Wrote thesis proposal.

July (2019): Defended and deposited thesis.

January (2020): Performed member-checking for study findings via participant advisory panel.

February-May (2020): Drafted manuscript.

June-September (2020): Revised manuscript and submitted to *RSAP.*

October (2020): Manuscript accepted and in press in *RSAP.*

Dr. Adeoye-Olatunde had one year of research experience when beginning this project. When asked about lessons learned over time as a new practitioner and researcher, Dr. Adeoye-Olatunde noted, "Never forget the 'practice' in practice-based research. As researchers, we tend to have our preferred timelines for various reasons; mine was wanting to defend my thesis in the spring. However, pharmacy practice is constantly evolving and can be very unpredictable, making it challenging for pharmacy partners to attend to research activities. When working with pharmacy partners, remain flexible, understanding, and appreciative, and anticipate changes to timelines. If you can do this, you will most likely still end up with a quality research product and maintain healthy collaborative relationships for the future."

Summary and Conclusions

Students, residents, and fellows have many opportunities to engage with faculty and other mentors on practice-based research. While often intimidating to new investigators, practice-based research can be very rewarding and many resources are available to help learners avoid common pitfalls. In this chapter, the study designs and methods most commonly used by students and residents were reviewed, and common pitfalls were summarized for each. Many examples from the literature were provided to highlight resources, project management tools, and learner roles for a variety of published learner-led practice-based research projects. Readers are encouraged to review these examples and advice provided throughout this chapter to help in planning ahead for the successful execution of their projects.

Key Points and Advice

- Research questions should be carefully delineated and matched to appropriate study designs and methods.
- Learners should take care to involve pertinent practitioners and scientific researchers to adequately address the research question.
- Applying one or more theoretical frameworks throughout a research project can help ensure all facets of the research question are considered to enhance study design.
- Good project management is essential to the success of any research project and avoids common pitfalls; care should be taken to carefully plan the timeline of the project from the beginning.

Chapter Review Questions

1. List at least three resources required for conducting a survey research project.
2. When would it be more appropriate to conduct focus groups as opposed to individual semi-structured interviews?
3. What checklist could be used to plan for reporting out on a pharmacist intervention study?
4. What is a theoretical framework and why should most projects apply one or more frameworks?
5. Name two grant opportunities available to pharmacy residents.
6. Which step in the project management process best sets research teams up for success?

Online Resources

- American Pharmacists Association. Conducting Research Projects. https://portal.pharmacist.com/node/1407400?is_sso_called=1
- American Society of Health-System Pharmacists: Essentials of Practice-Based Research for Pharmacists. https://elearning.ashp.org/products/5427/essentials-of-practice-based-research-for-pharmacists-not-for-ce
- Academy of Managed Care Pharmacy: Interpreting and Conducting Practice-Based Research: An Overview of Real-World Evidence. https://www.amcp.org/Resource-Center/real-world-evidence-research/interpreting-and-conducting-practice-based-research

REFERENCES

1. Westfall JM, Mold J, Fagnan L. *JAMA*. 2007 Jan 24;297(4):403-406.

2. Khanna R, Aparasu RR. Research design and methods. In: Rajender R. Aparasu John P. Bentleyeds. *Principles of Research Design and Drug Literature Evaluation*. 2nd ed. New York, NY: McGraw Hill; 2020.

3. Kelley K, Clark B, Brown V, Sitzia J. Good practice in the conduct and reporting of survey research. *Int J Qual Health Care*. 2003;15(3):261-266.

4. STROBE Statement: Checklist of items that should be included in reports of observational studies. Accessed December 18, 2020. https://www.strobe-statement.org/fileadmin/Strobe/uploads/checklists/STROBE_checklist_v4_combined.pdf

5. Clay PG, Burns AL, Isetts BJ, Hirsch JD, Kliethermes MA, Planas LG. PaCIR: a tool to enhance pharmacist patient care intervention reporting. *J Am Pharm Assoc*. 2019;59(5): P615-P623.

6. Ulin PR, Robinson ET, Tolley EE. *Qualitative Methods in Public Health: A Field Guide for Applied Research*. 1st ed. San Francisco, CA: Jossey-Bass; 2005.

7. Bradley EH, Curry LA, Devers KJ. Qualitative data analysis for health services research: developing taxonomy, themes, and theory. *Health Serv. Res*. 2007;42:1758-1772.

8. Tong A, Sainsbury P, Craig J. Consolidated criteria for reporting qualitative research (COREQ): a 32-item checklist for interviews and focus groups. *Int J Qual Health Care*. 2007;19(6):349-357.

9. College of Psychiatric and Neurologic Pharmacists Foundation: Grants. Accessed December 1, 2020. https://cpnpf.org/grants

10. American Pharmacists Association Foundation: Incentive Grants. Accessed December 1, 2020. https://www.aphafoundation.org/incentive-grants

11. American Society of Health System Pharmacists Foundation: Pharmacy Resident Research Grant. Accessed December 1, 2020. https://www.ashpfoundation.org/Grants-and-Awards/Research-Grants/Pharmacy-Resident-Research-Grant

12. Community Pharmacy Foundation. Accessed December 1, 2020. https://communitypharmacyfoundation.org/default.asp

13. American College of Clinical Pharmacy Foundation: Futures Grants. Accessed December 1, 2020. https://www.accpfoundation.org/futures/

14. Abend Gabriel. The meaning of theory. *Sociological Theory*. 2008 June;26:173-199.

15. Swanson Richard A. *Theory Building in Applied Disciplines*. San Francisco, CA: Berrett-Koehler Publishers; 2013.

16. Boston University School of Public Health: Behavioral Change Models. Accessed November 18, 2020. https://sphweb.bumc.bu.edu/otlt/mph-modules/sb/behavioralchangetheories/

17. Positive Deviance Collaborative. Accessed November 18, 2020. https://positivedeviance.org/

18. Project Management Institute: What Is Project Management? Accessed November 13, 2020. https://www.pmi.org/about/learn-about-pmi/what-is-project-management

19. CASRAI: CRediT – Contributor Roles Taxonomy. Accessed December 12, 2020. https://casrai.org/credit/

2018-2019 Research Training Manual

Elizabeth Davenport, PharmD, Walgreens/Purdue University
PGY-1 Community-Based Resident

1. Research Project Title:
Indiana community pharmacist preceptors' knowledge and perceptions of medication-assisted treatment.

2. Research Project Description:
The 38-item survey was developed using the *social cognitive theory* as conceptual framework which explains how people start and continue behaviors by emphasizing the relationship between people, their behavior, and their environments. Survey questions were adapted from previously published surveys with permission from study investigators. The study protocol was submitted to Purdue University Institutional Review Board, and data collection will begin upon approval. Study participants will include pharmacists who are at least 18 years of age or older, speak English, maintain an active Indiana pharmacist license, have been in their current community pharmacy practice setting for at least six consecutive months, and are active preceptors for Indiana based colleges of pharmacy. Experiential education directors at all Indiana colleges of pharmacy will recruit eligible participants, and an email invitation including the survey link will be sent to these individuals. Reminder emails will be sent every two weeks over a six-week period. Data collection will occur through a web-based survey tool. Survey questions will assess pharmacist knowledge, perceptions, and desired educational resources on MAT. To characterize the study population, participant demographics will be collected. Appropriate descriptive statistics will be used to describe preceptor knowledge, perceptions, and desired MAT resources. Regression analysis will be used to model the association between knowledge survey items, pharmacist demographics, and perceptions.

3. Research Participants and Roles:
Elizabeth Davenport, PharmD – Lead Investigator
Molly Nichols, P4 Pharmacy Student – Co-Investigator

Stephanie Arnett, PharmD, CDE – Co-Investigator, Site Mentor
Monica Miller, PharmD, MS – Principal Investigator, Academic Mentor

4. Tasks, Deliverables, and Experience to Be Gained for Student Research Experience:

TASK	PERSON(S) RESPONSIBLE	INTERNAL DEADLINE	ACTUAL DEADLINE
Review APhA Incentive grant proposal and provide feedback	All	Saturday 9/7	Grant submission deadline 11:59 PST Sunday 9/8
Review APhA *and* ASHP abstract draft and provide feedback	All	Friday 9/27	ASHP deadline Tuesday 10/1 APhA deadline Wednesday 10/2
CITI training: https:// www.citiprogram. org/?pageID=668 • Social Behavior Research: • Investigators and Key Personnel • Responsible Conduct of Research • Biomedical Research • Investigators and Key Personnel • Responsible Conduct of Research	All	Friday 10/25	All study investigators must complete training and survey items finalized prior to IRB submission
Review survey instrument, create and revise questions	Elizabeth and Molly	Wednesday 11/13	
Contact identified pharmacists for pilot testing of survey instrument	Molly	Friday 11/15 (Pilot testing to occur from 11/15 through 12/2)	
Review ASHP Midyear poster presentation and provide feedback	All	Monday 12/2	Print poster Thursday 12/5 Present poster 12/8 to 12/12
Review feedback from pilot testing and adapt survey instrument as necessary, finalize for IRB submission	All	Review Monday 12/2 to Friday 12/6 IRB submission Friday 1/5	
Input revised survey instrument into Qualtrics	Molly	Friday 12/6	

TASK	PERSON(S) RESPONSIBLE	INTERNAL DEADLINE	ACTUAL DEADLINE
Disseminate survey	Elizabeth	Pending IRB approval	
Review survey responses and troubleshoot identified issues	Molly	Ongoing throughout data collection (February-March)	
Review APhA Annual poster presentation and provide feedback	All	Friday 3/13	Print poster Wednesday 3/18 Present poster 3/20 to 3/23
Review incentive grant interim report and provide feedback	All	Friday 3/27	Grant report deadline Monday 3/30
Close survey instrument from further responses; organize and analyze data; participate in statistician meetings as necessary	Molly and Elizabeth	Close survey Tuesday 3/31 Data organization and analysis ongoing through April	
Review GLPRC PowerPoint presentation and provide feedback	All	Friday 4/17	GLPRC conference 4/23 to 4/26
Review incentive grant final report and provide feedback	All	Friday 6/12	Grant report deadline Monday 6/15
Review research manuscript and provide feedback	All	Ongoing through June	Manuscript to JAPhA Due 9/15

5. Authorship

Authorship implies responsibility and accountability for published work. Contributors who have made substantive intellectual contributions to a paper are given credit as authors. Contributors credited as authors understand their role in taking responsibility and being accountable for what is published.

Contributions meeting criteria of *co-authorship*:

1. Substantial contributions to the conception or design of the work; or the acquisition, analysis, or interpretation of data for the work;
2. Drafting the work or revising it critically for important intellectual content;
3. Final approval of version to be published; *AND*
4. Agreement to be accountable for all aspects of the work, ensuring that questions related to accuracy or integrity are appropriately investigated and resolved.

Contributions meeting criteria of *acknowledgment*:

* One or more, but not all, of the four criteria for authorship
* Acquisition of funding
* Technical or language editing or proofreading
* Clinical investigators
* Participating investigators

More information can be found at: http://www.icmje.org/recommendations/browse/roles-and-responsibilities/defining-the-role-of-authors-and-contributors.html

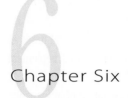

Chapter Six

Practice-Based Research and the Protection of Human Subjects

Mandy King, MS and John P. Bentley, RPh, PhD, FAPhA, FNAP

Chapter Objectives

- Understand the regulatory environment governing practice-based research
- Define human subjects research
- Describe the education and training requirements required for human subjects research
- Describe differences between exempt, expedited, and full board review procedures
- Discuss Institutional Review Board (IRB) procedures for research involving multiple institutions (IRB Reliance/Authorization Agreements)
- Describe the elements of informed consent and the procedures involved in the informed consent process
- Discuss IRB requirements after research has begun
- Describe best practices for learners in their interactions with IRBs
- Discuss important and unique elements of an IRB submission for practice-based research

Key Terminology

Adverse events, data use agreements (DUAs), exempt research, expedited review, full board review, human subject, human subjects research, informed consent, institutional review board (IRB), principal investigator (PI), protected health information (PHI), quality improvement, reliance/authorization agreement, research, unanticipated problems

Introduction

Institutions (such as universities and healthcare facilities) that receive federal funds to conduct research with human subjects must comply with regulations[1,2] that implement participant protections. This includes entering into a Federal Wide Assurance (FWA) to bind the institution to adherence to the regulatory text and registration of at least one Institutional Review Board (IRB) to review, approve, and monitor research with human subjects conducted by or for the institution. IRB review of proposed work with human participants is necessary to ensure researchers meet ethical, professional, and legal obligations and to allow the dissemination of results. Although the federal regulations for human research protections provide a detailed framework for IRB authority, function, and operation, they are the *minimum* requirements for assured institutions. As a result, institutions vary in how they assign IRB authority and define researcher expectations. Failure to follow institution-specific policies, procedures, and guidelines related to human subjects research can have consequences ranging from formal reprimand to retraction of publications.

There are many other laws, regulations, rules, and guidelines that may have an impact on the planning, conduct, and reporting of practice-based research. For example, Institutional Biosafety Committees (IBCs) oversee research involving pathogens, DNA, and/or human blood, other bodily fluids, or tissue.[3] Regulations from the Food and Drug Administration (FDA) may be applicable to certain practice-based research efforts.[2,4,5] In addition, there is significant oversight regarding integrity in the research process, focusing on research misconduct[6] as well as efforts to manage, reduce, or eliminate conflicts of interest.[7] These other mechanisms of oversight of the research process will not be discussed in this chapter, and pharmacy research learners are encouraged to have discussions with their mentors about these topics and seek input from individuals at their institutions to see what other regulations may apply depending on a learner's research project or situation.

This chapter is intended to provide a real-world guide for practice-based research involving human subjects. It is not meant to supplant standard training (as discussed later in the chapter), and therefore will not substantially duplicate the content of those curricula. After first providing a definition of what is meant by human subjects research, this chapter will next provide some general guidance and background about working with an IRB, followed by a discussion of important considerations when preparing your IRB submission. Additional IRB-related factors that learners may encounter after a research project starts are then presented. For each of these sections, helpful do's and don'ts based on the authors' experience are provided. The chapter concludes by considering additional matters that are specific to learner-led and learner-involved practice-based research projects in pharmacy settings.

Regulatory Definition of Human Subjects Research

The regulatory definitions of human subject and research are critical for an IRB to determine what (if any) review requirements to apply to a given project, as discussed in detail later in this chapter. For the specific purposes of IRB review, a **human subject** is "a living individual about whom an investigator (whether professional or student) conducting research (i) obtains information or biospecimens through intervention or interaction with the individual, and uses, studies, or analyzes the information or biospecimens; or (ii) obtains, uses, studies, analyzes, or generates identifiable private information or identifiable biospecimens" [45 CFR 46.102(e)(1)[8]]. According to federal regulations, **research** is defined as "a systematic investigation, including research development, testing, and evaluation, designed to develop or contribute to generalizable knowledge. Activities that meet this definition constitute research for purposes of this policy, whether or not they are conducted or supported under a program that is considered research for other purposes. For example, some demonstration and service programs may include research activities" [45 CFR 46.102(l)[8]]. It is important to note that the regulations explicitly exclude several activities from this definition, including public health surveillance activities. Thus, these activities are not deemed to be research according to these federal regulations. Combining these two definitions, and at the risk of sounding tautological, **human subjects research** is research that involves human subjects.

Working with Your IRB

The process of seeking IRB approval can seem intimidating and overwhelming, but research integrity and compliance staff at various institutions want to help researchers succeed. Their goals are to help researchers manage a seemingly complicated process so that they produce high-quality research while simultaneously protecting the rights and welfare of subjects involved with the research. The process is essential for the dissemination of results through publications and presentations, but it is also the right thing to do as part of an ethical approach to the conduct of research. This section will provide background on a number of IRB activities and functions. This basic background knowledge will help set the stage as learners begin to formulate the approach to their research and how they will seek any necessary approvals. The importance of establishing a good relationship, mandatory training and education, the categories of IRB review, and the basics of data use agreements (DUAs), as well as reliance/authorization agreements, are

TABLE 6–1. DO'S AND DON'TS WHEN WORKING WITH YOUR IRB

Do's	Don'ts
DO read and use the IRB's templates and guidance—most IRBs provide references, guidance, and template documents for researchers to use when drafting application materials. There can be local variations in requirements and expectations, so it is critical for you to use the materials provided by your IRB. Do read and follow instructions, and if something is not clear, then ask questions! Familiarity and utilization of these resources is a sure-fire path to a positive experience.	**DO NOT** think of the IRB as the enemy. They want you to ask questions along the way and want your research to succeed.
DO remember that every study is reviewed independently, and the process will not always mirror a previous experience for a similar study.	**DO NOT** rely on the IRB to tell you how to design your study (you have an advisor/mentor to guide you) or be your proofreader.
DO put forth effort when completing mandatory education and training. Do complete the training in a timely manner, well before your IRB submission. Education is a very important component of a comprehensive human research protection program. Be engaged with the material; efforts have been made to make sure that the offerings meet their stated purpose.	**DO NOT** forget about the participants' perspective. It is easy for researchers to view their work strictly through the lens of their goals and intent. Taking a step back and looking at things from the participants' point of view is critical.

all considered in the following sections. To set the stage, some do's, and don'ts when working with your IRB are described in Table 6–1.

ESTABLISHING A GOOD RELATIONSHIP

A good investigator–IRB relationship hinges on mutual respect for the other's perspective and responsibility in the protection of research participants. Given the tremendous workload of most IRBs (it is common for an IRB office to handle hundreds of new submissions in a given year), a common misconception among researchers is that the IRB functions like an assembly line of sorts. In reality, each research proposal represents a unique collaboration between the researcher and the IRB. Although it is common for IRB members to utilize standard operating procedures and checklists to review applications, the nuances of any given proposal will undoubtedly influence the feedback an investigator receives from the committee. In addition to the federal regulations that govern research with human participants, the IRB must consider the "local context" of the research under review. Any state or local laws, regulations, institutional policies, standards, or other local factors relevant to the research are all factors the committee weighs in its assessment of a proposal. In short, no two IRB reviews are created equal. Many frustrations can be avoided when investigators and IRB members approach new research proposals with that in mind.

MANDATORY TRAINING AND EDUCATION

Working with human research participants is a privilege. The scientific goals, individual health outcomes, and broader societal impacts of any given research project must be balanced with the risks, burdens, and equitable treatment of subjects. Current clinical and social practices have normalized these considerations to appear "common sense." Sadly, historical atrocities remind us this was not always the case. To ensure participant protections remain the ultimate priority for any research that requires human subjects, institutional and regulatory requirements for training and education must exist. In addition to fundamental ethical principles inherent to working with human subjects (such as those discussed in The Belmont Report[9] and The Nuremberg Code[10]) as well as the federal regulations,[1] educational requirements include topics such as protections of confidentiality, assessing risk, working with vulnerable populations, data security, and international research considerations. Many institutions rely on standardized training platforms, such as the Collaborative Institutional Training Initiative (CITI)[11] or the National Institutes of Health (NIH),[12] while others develop in-house programs to provide mandatory education. Even if you have previously completed training (at a different institution or as part of an academic curriculum), always verify what your institution's IRB requires and either complete it or confirm that your existing education is current and meets their criteria. Many IRBs require refresher training at regular intervals (three or four years). Delays in initiating data collection can be avoided by making sure training and education requirements have been met by all researchers.

CATEGORIES OF IRB REVIEW

It is worth reiterating that *the IRB is the appropriate body* to determine what, if any, regulatory requirements exist for any given research project. Not only does this protect the research participants, but it also protects the researchers and the institution. Dissemination of research results, whether as a presentation, thesis, dissertation, or peer-reviewed manuscript, will almost always require certification of IRB review. Regardless of the IRB's review category determination, failure to prospectively submit proposed research with human subjects to the IRB can have extreme consequences.

Not Human Subjects Research/Not Engaged

As previously discussed, the regulations governing human subjects research are driven by the definitions of "human subject" and "research." In practice-based research, it is not uncommon for a specific project to fail to meet one or both of the definitions and result in an IRB determination of "Not Human Subjects Research." For example, an IRB might regularly determine case studies (data from 1-3 subjects or even from a single clinic) are "Not Human Subjects Research" because the intention of the study and its results do not satisfy the requirement of "research" to contribute to generalizable knowledge. For the same reason, **quality improvement** initiatives or projects that use patient records to design and implement practices that improve patient care or serve clinical/practical/administrative purposes often fall in the "Not Human Subjects Research" category.[13] For a discussion of the key differences between quality improvement and research in the context of pharmacy-related research, see Phillips et al.[14] Some IRBs will issue guidance to communicate to their communities what they do or do not consider to be human subjects research. For example, at the University of Mississippi, the IRB has determined that the secondary analysis of certain preapproved public data files does not constitute human subjects research and therefore does not require IRB approval.[15]

Exempt

Exempt research includes certain types of "human subjects research" that meet specific requirements as per the federal regulations, also known as The Common Rule, and fall into one of several defined exemption categories. The label exempt research refers to the fact that such studies are exempt from additional IRB oversight and informed consent requirements.[16] The Common Rule was recently revised to expand the categories of exempt research, effectively reducing the administrative burden associated with a large body of research activities that involve human subjects. The Office for Human Research Protections (OHRP) with the U.S. Department of Health and Human Services (OHRP provides regulatory oversight of IRBs in the United States) provides useful decision charts[17] to help understand whether a study might be eligible for an exemption determination, and your IRB office will likely have specific guidance and procedures regarding the exempt review process. Turnaround times for exempt reviews are usually relatively quick.

The most common exempt categories for practice-based research fall into two categories (although a third category, research that only includes educational tests, survey procedures, interview procedures, or observation of public behavior meeting certain criteria, may be common in some settings): Category 3, or research that involves benign behavioral interventions and resultant data collected from adult participants, and Category 4, or research that involves secondary use of data. As defined in CFR 46.104,[16] benign behavioral interventions are "brief in duration, harmless, painless, not physically invasive, not likely to have a significant adverse lasting impact on the subjects, and the investigator has no reason to think the subjects will find the interventions offensive or embarrassing." Watching pharmacist-led presentations about medication compliance might be an example of a benign behavioral intervention. Secondary data refers to using data for research that was originally collected or will be collected for another purpose, such as patient records. It is important to note that there are restrictions on the exempt research when it involves minors, and no research involving prisoners is eligible for exempt determination.

Expedited

Nonexempt human subjects research is subject to the regulatory requirements set forth in the Common Rule. This means the IRB must determine the defined criteria for approval have been met, including all elements of informed consent. When nonexempt research involves no more than minimal risk activities, it may be eligible for expedited review. Minimal risk means that the likelihood of study activities causing harm, distress, or discomfort is no more than what is experienced in the study population's everyday life. Similar to exempt categories but not incorporated into the federal regulations, OHRP maintains a list of research activities that are eligible for expedited review.[18]

When an expedited review is determined to be suitable for proposed research activities, the IRB Chair or their designee conducts the review. It is common for IRBs to assign more than one reviewer to a protocol, and all reviewers must be voting members of the committee. Turnaround times for expedited review are typically longer than exempt determinations but faster than Full Board reviews.

The Dreaded Full Board

Studies that are not eligible for exempt determination or expedited review must be reviewed at a convened meeting of the Full Board (i.e., full board review). The Full Board is composed of at least five members, and some must meet defined roles. At least one member must be from a relevant scientific background, one must be from a nonscientific background, and one member must be otherwise unaffiliated with the institution. A nonscientific must be present at a convened meeting. When the Full Board convenes, a quorum of members must be present at all times during committee business. A quorum is a majority of voting members, or more than half. During a convened meeting, the Full Board will review all materials associated with the proposed research, and the investigator is often invited to attend the meeting to answer questions. The Full Board can approve, require modifications in order to approve, or disapprove the research. If minor revisions are needed, the committee can vote to allow expedited review in order to give final approval. If revisions are major (e.g., a required element of informed consent is missing), the revisions will go back in front of the Full Board.

Some institutions have more than one IRB. The schedule for convened meetings is usually disseminated, along with deadlines for receiving materials. Even the best-written submission that requires Full Board review will generally take some time to be approved, so early and consistent communication with the IRB Office is essential.

SPECIAL CONSIDERATIONS

Data Use Agreements

Data Use Agreements (DUAs) are commonly used contracts between parties that document the terms and conditions of transfer and use of nonpublic or otherwise restricted datasets. When a researcher proposes to use such human subjects data, such as existing human subjects research data, identifiable health information, or records from government agencies, as part of an IRB protocol, the institution (not the individual researcher) will negotiate and authorize the agreement. The administrative office with the authority to execute DUAs may vary across different institutions. The IRB Office will be able to direct you to the appropriate point of contact and provide guidance on their expectations for referring to the data source in your submission materials. An important consideration when planning research with data that may require a DUA is that completion of IRB review is often a required condition for data to be transferred.

Reliance/Authorization Agreements

When nonexempt human subjects research involves collaboration between investigators at two or more institutions, federal regulations allow (and in the case of federally funded research conducted in the United States, require) a single IRB to serve as the reviewing IRB for the study. This relationship is memorialized in a Reliance, or Authorization, Agreement that outlines the responsibilities of each institution for review, reporting, and recordkeeping. An authorized official at each institution is authorized to sign these agreements.

Reliance/authorization agreements are not used for exempt research. It is worth noting, however, that even if your collaborator's IRB has made an exempt determination for a research project you will be involved in, do not assume local IRB review is not required. While you may not need to submit a formal application or protocol, you should provide the protocol materials to your IRB to ensure they concur with the exempt determination.

When collaborators are not affiliated with an institution with an IRB and FWA, an IRB can elect to enter into an Individual Investigator Agreement (IIA). This agreement documents the responsibilities of the collaborator for the protection of human subjects and allows the institution to extend its FWA to them. An IIA is signed by the individual, the institution's investigator, and an authorized official for the institution.

Preparing Your IRB Submission

Once you and your mentor have developed your research questions and hypotheses and developed your research plan for conducting your project, it is time to prepare your IRB application materials (although in some situations, these are not necessarily ordered steps, and some activities when preparing the research plan may include IRB-related considerations). This section will provide additional background and guidance for preparing an IRB application. The initial discussion will focus on informed consent, and

TABLE 6–2. DO'S AND DON'TS WHEN PREPARING YOUR IRB SUBMISSION

Do's	Don'ts
DO make sure you use current application forms and templates. Experienced researchers often use previous applications to draft new ones. While this may seem like a time-saving strategy, if the IRB has updated their application forms and associated templates since previous projects were reviewed, you can end up wasting time by using an old version.	**DO NOT** hesitate to ask for a status update. Despite everyone's best efforts, missteps happen. Emails get missed or end up in junk folders. Files get misplaced. An advisor or colleague's desk may have a black hole where things go and are never seen again. Feel free to follow-up on your submission, at reasonable intervals (once a week, not four times a day).
DO communicate early and often with the IRB office. IRB Administrators can help familiarize you with procedures, give insight on current best practices and regulatory requirements, and provide sample materials or language to help you submit a complete application.	**DO NOT** use overly technical language and jargon in materials that will be provided to participants, such as information sheets and consent documents. The average reading comprehension level of an adult in the United States is eighth grade.
DO ask about realistic turnaround times and follow submission deadlines. The IRB and IRB Office understand that sometimes extenuating circumstances occur and will do their best to accommodate special requests, but "first come, first served" is the best rule of thumb.	

then a number of challenges and considerations related to the conduct of practice-based research will be presented. As with the previous section, Table 6–2 provides some do's and don'ts when preparing your IRB submission.

INFORMED CONSENT

Exempt Research

Again, research that is eligible for an exempt determination is not subject to the specific requirements of the federal regulations, such as required elements of informed consent. However, this does not exempt the ethical obligation of researchers to provide critical information related to the study and give potential participants an opportunity to voluntarily agree to complete the research activities. Often, this is accomplished using an abbreviated information sheet (or cover letter) that outlines the basics, such as the purpose of the study, description of study activities, risks, and benefits, costs and payments, confidentiality, right to withdraw, and a statement of consent. Signatures from participants are typically not required since exempt studies are often anonymous and/or very low risk and typically don't require researchers to collect data with identifiers. Therefore, implied consent statements are common in information sheets/cover letters. A statement that the study has been reviewed by an IRB and determined to be exempt is also standard.

Nonexempt Research

The majority of the IRB Office and IRB's efforts related to reviewing nonexempt research is devoted to the informed consent process and documents. **Informed consent** is the basic yet cornerstone element of ethical research involving human participants. When we say "informed consent" it is paramount to understand we are referring not just to a form that is read and signed, but a process by which potential participants give their voluntary consent to engage in research activities, having been fully informed of all the information necessary to make their decision.

Federal regulations [45 CFR 46.116(b)[19]] outline the required elements of informed consent. These include: the purpose of the research and its procedures, risks, benefits, alternatives, confidentiality of records and any exceptions thereof, compensation, contact information, the voluntary nature of participation and right to withdraw, and whether identifiable private information or biospecimens will be used for future studies. Certain research activities may require additional elements, when applicable or deemed appropriate by the IRB [45 CFR 46.116(c)[19]].

While the IRB's review of the informed consent process and document is done in the context of other application materials, a key tip for investigators is to remember the consent documents should be able to provide a stand-alone description of the research in order to facilitate a reasonable person's decision to engage in the activities (or not). There are many online guidance documents available regarding informed consent (e.g., see OHRP[20]), and most institutions have draft or sample consent documents for researchers to use as a template in preparing their submission. Using these templates saves considerable time and back-and-forth.

PRACTICE-BASED RESEARCH CHALLENGES

Waiver of Informed Consent and Waiver of Documentation of Informed Consent

The IRB has regulatory authority to waive some or all requirements of informed consent, as well as documentation (signature), for research that poses no more than minimal risk to participants. There are specific requirements the IRB must determine to be satisfied in order to approve a waiver, meaning simple convenience to the researcher is not a justification for a study design that eliminates the informed consent process.

Examples of research activities that may involve requests to waive some or all elements of consent include: studies that involve deception, studies that take place in educational settings, and secondary use of personally identifiable information (PII) or protected health information (PHI). Some researchers design recruitment and enrollment procedures to include an "opt-out" or "passive consent" methodology. From an IRB perspective, these methods are waivers of informed consent and must meet the regulatory criteria for their approval. Waivers of documentation of informed consent are common for research where the study would otherwise be anonymous (i.e., the participant's signature would be the only documentation linking them to the study) or when written consent wouldn't be required if the activities occurred in a context other than research.

In order for the IRB to grant a waiver, the investigator must demonstrate *all* of the following:

- The research presents no more than minimal risk to participants.
- The research could not practicably be conducted without the waiver.
- The waiver will not adversely impact the participants' rights or welfare.
- The participants will be provided information about their participation, where appropriate.

Patients as Subjects/Participants

In clinical practice settings, patients are often the most appropriate pool for potential participants in research studies. The dual role of provider and researcher can present unique challenges that thoughtful consideration, particularly when designing recruitment strategies. One of the basic ethical principles in human research protections is that of autonomy. Circumstances should not prevent a potential participant from making an informed, voluntary decision about whether to join a study. When the lead researcher is also a healthcare provider, an appearance of undue influence is possible. Your IRB should have guidance on current best practices to minimize or eliminate this concern. In general, patients recruited for research should be informed that their decision to participate (or not) will have no impact on their access to care or services. If possible, having a member of the research team that does not have an existing relationship with patients conduct recruitment and consent activities is highly recommended.

Additional Permissions

A common misconception among researchers that work with human subjects is that IRB approval is a golden ticket for blanket approval. While the IRB review process is likely to be the most time-consuming and comprehensive review required before research can begin, additional relevant permissions should be on your radar as you plan your research endeavors. In fact, the federal regulations (45 CFR 46.112[21]) state that research that an IRB has approved "may be subject to further appropriate review and approval or disapproval by the officials of the institution. However, these officials may not approve the research if it has not been approved by an IRB."

Within academic institutions, students will likely need input from their mentor/advisor/committee that oversees their research progress. It is also common for department chairs or other unit-level gatekeepers to review protocols prior to submission to the IRB. As an example of this, in their description of the development of a pharmacy resident research program, Baker et al. note that "although the residents complete all

IRB paperwork, the RRAB [residency research advisory board] reviews it before submission."[22] At many institutions, the IRB Office will have procedures in place to ensure those reviews are in place before it processes your submission materials.

Researchers proposing work that is conducted at outside institutions (e.g., schools, businesses, clinics) should seek permission from an authorized person to recruit, consent, or conduct activities at their site. Again, the IRB Office is likely to require documentation of this permission in order to move an application forward. The IRB may want the document to be read such that it is clear that the authorized representative has been provided sufficient information related to the study (e.g., the IRB application, surveys, consent form) to grant permission. Sometimes the IRB and the outside institution can seem to be in conflict when each wants the other to give approval before it finalizes its own. In these situations, the IRB may provide a letter of "conditional approval" to relay that the requirements for participant protections have been satisfied.

Working with Protected Health Information (HIPAA)

As a practice-based researcher, you should be well educated on the Health Insurance Portability and Accountability Act (HIPAA, Public Law 104-191[23]) and the HIPAA Privacy Rule (45 CFR 160 and 164[24]). HIPAA regulations are highly complex and require extensive oversight in the clinical setting. In the context of human research protections, there are a few key considerations to keep in mind when working with your IRB.

First and foremost, not all health information is subject to HIPAA. **Protected health information (PHI)** is health information created, received, or stored by a HIPAA-covered entity. HIPAA-covered entities include healthcare providers, health plans, and healthcare clearinghouses. So while patient records in a purely clinical setting are almost certainly PHI, health information disclosed solely for research use may not be.

In order to use PHI for research purposes, not only must an IRB review the proposed research under the federal regulations for research participant protections, but it must also consider the requirements of the Privacy Rule for obtaining written authorization from individuals. The term "authorization" should not be confused with "consent." The IRB can approve a consent process that incorporates authorization to release and use PHI, but the authorization is in addition to, not instead of, consent to participate in research activities.

For practice-based research, it is most common for researchers to require the use of existing PHI, for which obtaining prospective authorization would be impracticable. The Privacy Rule allows a Privacy Board to grant waivers of authorization under specific circumstances. At most academic institutions, the IRB will also serve as the Privacy Board, although university-affiliated healthcare settings may assign the role to a separate body. As repeated throughout this chapter, communicate early and often with your IRB Office to ensure you understand the process at your institution. The requirements for granting a waiver of authorization are outlined in 45 CFR 164.512(i)[25] and include: the use of disclosure of PHI presents no more than minimal risk to participants, the research could not be practicably conducted without the waiver, and the research could not be practicably conducted without access and use of the PHI. Further, before PHI can be obtained for research use, the covered entity must receive written documentation from the Privacy Board (IRB) that includes: a statement that the above criteria have been met, the specific PHI that may be released under the waiver, the date of approval, the method of review (must be expedited or full board), and a signature of the board's chairperson or authorized designee. This document is separate from a standard IRB approval/determination.

A common issue seen in the IRB review of HIPAA authorization waiver requests revolves around the specific PHI that may be released as part of the waiver. In practice-based research, the researcher often has access to all PHI at the covered entity. It is critical to understand that just because you have access to PHI by nature of your professional affiliation does not mean you are free to use it for research purposes. The reviewing board may only approve your access to the specific categories of PHI necessary to inform the research question. Additionally, you should not be the individual responsible for accessing the covered-entity systems in order to transfer the PHI for research use. A third party at the organization that has confirmed the waiver documentation satisfies HIPAA requirements should provide the data.

Working with Educational Records (FERPA)

Similar to HIPAA, student educational records are also subject to regulatory protections. The Family Educational Rights and Privacy Act (FERPA, 20 USC 1232g[26]) and its associated regulations (34 CFR 99[27]) provide parents of minor students or adult students the right to access and control the disclosure of PII from educational records.

When research involves access to educational records, FERPA requires authorization from the individual to access and use that data. Unlike human research protections and HIPAA regulations, there are very limited exceptions to the requirement to obtain prospective authorization for the use of identifiable data from educational records. A detailed discussion of the intersection of FERPA and the IRB is beyond the scope of this chapter; however, one key concept is important for practice-based researchers.

The U.S. Department of Education and the U.S. Department of Health and Human Services have released joint guidance on the application of HIPAA and FERPA to student health records.[28] In a nutshell, student medical records maintained at covered entities run by postsecondary institutions (i.e., student health clinics) are covered by FERPA, not HIPAA! In the same setting, nonstudent records are covered by HIPAA. This can pose significant difficulty for researchers to comply with the stricter FERPA requirements for authorization. If your research could involve health information from student records that would fall under FERPA, contact your IRB as early as possible to discuss the feasibility of your methods. The IRB may need to consult with multiple units at the institution to verify all regulatory requirements are met, and this could take significant time.

Conducting Research

Your interactions with the IRB do not end when you receive IRB approval for your research. Changes to your protocol may be necessary. You may need to add an investigator to help you collect data or analyze identifiable information. In some situations, you will be required to continue your communications with the IRB about your project (e.g., submitting progress reports or reporting unanticipated problems). These matters are described in the following sections. See Table 6–3 for some IRB-related do's and don'ts when conducting research.

AMENDMENTS AND MODIFICATIONS

IRB determinations/approvals are valid only for the research described and documented in the materials it has reviewed. If during the course of your research, you need to amend or modify any element of the study (even to add personnel), you must notify the IRB. For exempt research, this may be an informal process that involves an administrative verification that the modifications do not change eligibility for exemption. For nonexempt studies, this will require a formal review and approval process. If your study was approved via Full Board review, significant modifications would also require Full Board Review. As with the initial review process, always ask the IRB Office for reasonable expectations for turnaround time.

UNANTICIPATED PROBLEMS AND ADVERSE EVENTS

Researchers are responsible for informing the IRB promptly of any unanticipated problems or adverse events during the course of approved research activities. Unanticipated problems refer to any incident, experience, or outcome occurring during the course of

TABLE 6-3. **DO'S AND DON'TS RELATED TO IRBS WHEN CONDUCTING RESEARCH**

Do's	Don'ts
DO follow your approved protocol.	**DO NOT** assume the IRB is responsible for making sure you meet your deadlines.
DO stay in touch with the IRB Office, especially when you need to make changes or submit regular updates.	**DO NOT** miss deadlines when responding to requests made by the IRB (e.g., in the submission of a progress report).
DO use appropriate forms when needing to amend a protocol.	

research that is unexpected, related, or possibly related to the research and suggest the risk to participants is greater than was previously known or recognized. Adverse events refer to any unfavorable occurrence in a human participant, including any abnormal sign, symptom, or disease that is temporally associated with participation in the research, whether or not considered related to participation in the research. Your IRB Office will have specific procedures for when and how reports of unanticipated problems and/or adverse events must be handled. You should familiarize yourself with these requirements prior to beginning research.

PROGRESS REPORTS AND CLOSE-OUT

When the IRB issues its initial determination or approval for your research, they will communicate the continuing review interval and, if applicable, expiration date. Studies that require Full Board approval may not be approved for more than one year at a time. This means that the board must review and approve the work each year of the project's lifetime. Institutional procedures can vary widely in how progress reports and continuing reviews are handled for Expedited and Exempt studies. In general, researchers should expect to check in annually with the IRB to provide updates regarding project status. Additionally, researchers are responsible for informing the IRB that their study has concluded or will not be continuing. While most IRBs have systems in place to provide courtesy reminders about impending report deadlines and expiration dates, remember it is ultimately the investigator's responsibility to comply with these requirements. Conducting research even one day past the expiration date is serious noncompliance!

Other Practical Considerations for Learner-Led and Learner-Involved Projects

Some researchers have assessed the impact of a number of different barriers to the publication of pharmacy residency research projects. Feedback from residents and residency program directors suggests that while not the most significant barrier, difficulties obtaining IRB approval or compliance with other rules or regulations are perceived as a challenge by some.[29,30] Although all of the considerations, do's, and don'ts discussed previously in this chapter might help overcome this barrier, there are a few additional matters related to learner-led and learner-involved pharmacy research projects that merit additional discussion. Byerly[31] and Phillips et al.[14] provide reviews of IRB-related issues that are relevant to pharmacy research.

One matter to consider is who to designate as the principal investigator (PI) on an IRB submission. The PI is the lead investigator of a study, and in the IRB context, he or she is the person with overall responsibilities for the study,[32] meaning they will ultimately be responsible for all aspects of the research, including application submission, correspondence with the IRB, required reporting, and study closure. In some locations, learners (i.e., student pharmacists and trainees such as pharmacy residents) may not be eligible to serve as the PI on an IRB submission, while in other settings, learners are allowed to fulfill this role, but an advisor (such as a faculty member) must agree to monitor the research and supervise the learner's activities.[14] In the context of residency research, Barletta recommends that preceptors, not residents, should serve as the PI, especially because projects often continue after a resident's program is completed.[33] This is also useful advice when projects are learner-involved (e.g., a learner is assisting a faculty member with a faculty member's research project) rather than learner-led (e.g., an honor's thesis or another required research project) and also for research activities that are structured in a layered learning model. Serving as a PI on an IRB submission may be a valuable learning opportunity for those who plan to continue their development as a researcher.

Another consideration for learners is that they should be prepared for variability in review requirements in various settings in which they may be educated or trained. Recall that there is considerable latitude at the local level regarding IRB authority, functions, and operations. Thus, policies and procedures can be institution-specific. For example, Linden et al. documented meaningful variability in the review category as well as review time for the same protocol for an assessment of medical resident professionalism using a web-based survey conducted at 19 different sites (almost all university-affiliated).[34] Patel et al. observed similar findings in the conduct of a multisite, quality improvement study.[35]

Finally, learners are in potentially vulnerable positions because they are subordinate members in hierarchical relationships with their research advisors or mentors. This can be especially problematic when there are potential noncompliance issues with respect to human subjects research (or any broader situation regarding integrity in the research process). Learners should be aware of local resources within their institutions if ever confronted with research misconduct or human subjects research noncompliance. Institutional research integrity and compliance staff are potential sources of contact for more information. A trusted mentor or advisor could also be consulted, and many institutions have ombuds programs that may be able to provide assistance in such situations.[36]

Summary and Conclusions

Almost all practice-based research in pharmacy involves human subjects. Understanding the regulatory environment governing human subjects research is critical for all researchers, including pharmacy research learners. Although working with an IRB to submit application materials and manage the process of conducting human subjects research can seem overwhelming for learners (and even their mentors), many resources exist that serve as a real-world guide through the process. In addition, institutional research integrity and compliance staff are committed to helping researchers navigate the process and do the right thing. Learners should never be afraid to ask questions. Because there is considerable variability across institutions, it is imperative for pharmacy research learners to access, read, and follow local guidance and template documents. The entire human subjects research protections process is critical for the conduct of high-quality and ethical research. Attention to the little things is essential for complying with the requirements, but it is also extremely important to never lose sight of the perspective of those who elect to participate in our research. Their rights and welfare are worth protecting.

Key Points and Advice

- Familiarity and utilization of your IRB's templates and guidance is a sure-fire path to a positive experience.
- The IRB is not the enemy. Your IRB staff want you to ask questions, they want to help you navigate the process, and they want your research to succeed.
- Always remember the perspective of your participants. How would you want to be treated if you were a research subject?
- Be aware of and be prepared for variability within and between IRBs.
- Build IRB review time into your project timeline. While review times can vary, you can ask about turnaround times upon submission and request status updates during the review process.
- Follow your approved protocol and keep the IRB informed of any changes before you make them.

Chapter Review Questions

1. What is human subjects research?
2. Federal regulations for human research protections are the *minimum* requirements for assured institutions. What are the implications of this for the review, approval, and monitoring of research with human subjects in the United States?
3. What are the differences between exempt, expedited, and full board review procedures?

4. When would a Reliance (or Authorization) Agreement be needed in a pharmacy research setting?

5. What are some examples of research activities that may involve requests to waive some or all elements of consent?

Online Resources

- OHRP. https://www.hhs.gov/ohrp/index.html
- OHRP: Human Subject Regulations Decision Charts: 2018 Requirements. https://www.hhs.gov/ohrp/regulations-and-policy/decision-charts-2018/index.html
- OHRP: Exemptions (2018 Requirements). https://www.hhs.gov/ohrp/regulations-and-policy/regulations/45-cfr-46/common-rule-subpart-a-46104/index.html
- OHRP: Human Research Protection Training. https://www.hhs.gov/ohrp/education-and-outreach/online-education/human-research-protection-training/index.html
- The Collaborative Institutional Training Initiative (CITI Program). https://www.citiprogram.org/
- How to check reading comprehension level in a Word document. https://support.microsoft.com/en-us/office/get-your-document-s-readability-and-level-statistics-85b4969e-e80a-4777-8dd3-f7fc3c8b3fd2

REFERENCES

1. Office for Human Research Protections (OHRP). 45 CFR 46 (The 2018 Common Rule). Accessed August 26, 2021. https://www.hhs.gov/ohrp/regulations-and-policy/regulations/45-cfr-46/index.html

2. 21 CFR Part 56 – Institutional Review Boards. Accessed August 26, 2021. https://www.ecfr.gov/current/title-21/chapter-I/subchapter-A/part-56

3. National Institutes of Health. Institutional Biosafety Committees. Accessed September 13, 2021. https://osp.od.nih.gov/biotechnology/institutional-biosafety-committees/

4. 21 CFR Part 50 – Protection of Human Subjects. Accessed August 26, 2021. https://www.ecfr.gov/current/title-21/chapter-I/subchapter-A/part-50

5. 21 CFR Part 312 Subpart B – Investigational New Drug Application (IND). Accessed August 26, 2021. https://www.ecfr.gov/current/title-21/chapter-I/subchapter-D/part-312/subpart-B

6. Office of Research Integrity. Handling misconduct. Accessed September 13, 2021. https://ori.hhs.gov/handling-misconduct

7. Office of Research Integrity. Responsible Conduct Research: Conflicts of Interest. Accessed September 13, 2021. https://ori.hhs.gov/education/products/columbia_wbt/rcr_conflicts/introduction/index.html

8. Office for Human Research Protections (OHRP). 45 CFR 46.102. Accessed August 26, 2021. https://www.hhs.gov/ohrp/regulations-and-policy/regulations/45-cfr-46/revised-common-rule-regulatory-text/index.html#46.102

9. Office for Human Research Protections (OHRP). The Belmont Report. Published June 16, 2021. Accessed August 27, 2021. https://www.hhs.gov/ohrp/regulations-and-policy/belmont-report/index.html

10. National Institutes of Health. The Nuremberg Code. Accessed August 30, 2021. https://history.nih.gov/display/history/Nuremberg+Code

11. CITI Program. Research, Ethics, and Compliance Training. Accessed August 30, 2021. https://about.citiprogram.org/

12. National Institutes of Health. Training & Resources – Human Subjects. Accessed August 30, 2021. https://grants.nih.gov/policy/humansubjects/training-and-resources.htm

13. Office for Human Research Protections (OHRP). Quality Improvement Activities FAQs. Accessed August 30, 2021. https://www.hhs.gov/ohrp/regulations-and-policy/guidance/faq/quality-improvement-activities/index.html

14. Phillips MS, Abdelghany O, Johnston S, Rarus R, Austin-Szwak J, Kirkwood C. Navigating the institutional review board (IRB) process for pharmacy-related research. *Hosp Pharm*. 2017;52(2):105-116. doi:10.1310/hpj5202–105

15. The University of Mississippi. Guidance on Public Use Data Files. Accessed September 14, 2021. http://www.research.olemiss.edu/irb/guidance/public-data

16. Office for Human Research Protections (OHRP). 45 CFR 46.104. Accessed August 26, 2021. https://www.hhs.gov/ohrp/regulations-and-policy/regulations/45-cfr-46/revised-common-rule-regulatory-text/index.html#46.104

17. Office for Human Research Protections (OHRP). Human Subject Regulations Decision Charts: 2018 Requirements. Accessed August 26, 2021. https://www.hhs.gov/ohrp/regulations-and-policy/decision-charts-2018/index.html

18. Office for Human Research Protections (OHRP). Expedited Review: Categories of Research that may be Reviewed through an Expedited Review Procedure (1998). Accessed August 26, 2021. https://www.hhs.gov/ohrp/regulations-and-policy/guidance/categories-of-research-expedited-review-procedure-1998/index.html

19. Office for Human Research Protections (OHRP). 45 CFR 46.116. Accessed August 26, 2021. https://www.hhs.gov/ohrp/regulations-and-policy/regulations/45-cfr-46/revised-common-rule-regulatory-text/index.html#46.116

20. Office for Human Research Protections (OHRP). Informed Consent. Accessed August 31, 2021. https://www.hhs.gov/ohrp/regulations-and-policy/guidance/informed-consent/index.html

21. Office for Human Research Protections (OHRP). 45 CFR 46.112. Accessed August 26, 2021. https://www.hhs.gov/ohrp/regulations-and-policy/regulations/45-cfr-46/revised-common-rule-regulatory-text/index.html#46.112

22. Baker JW, Bean J, Benge C, McFarland MS. Designing a resident research program. *Am J Health Syst Pharm*. 2014;71(7):592-598. doi:10.2146/ajhp130318

23. Public Law 104 – 191 – Health Insurance Portability and Accountability Act of 1996. gov-info. Accessed August 30, 2021. https://www.govinfo.gov/app/details/PLAW-104publ191

24. The HIPAA Privacy Rule. Accessed August 30, 2021. https://www.hhs.gov/hipaa/for-professionals/privacy/index.html

25. 45 CFR 164.512(i) – Standard: Uses and Disclosures for Research Purposes. Accessed August 26, 2021. https://www.ecfr.gov/current/title-45/subtitle-A/subchapter-C/part-164/subpart-E/section-164.512#p-164.512(i)

26. 20 U.S.C. 1232g – Family Educational and Privacy Rights. Accessed August 30, 2021. https://www.govinfo.gov/app/details/USCODE-2011-title20/USCODE-2011-title20-chap31-subchapIII-part4-sec1232g

27. 34 CFR Part 99 – Family Educational Rights and Privacy. Accessed August 30, 2021. https://www.ecfr.gov/current/title-34/subtitle-A/part-99

28. Joint Guidance on the Application of FERPA and HIPAA to Student Health Records. Updated December 1, 2019. Accessed August 30, 2021. https://studentprivacy.ed.gov/resources/joint-guidance-application-ferpa-and-hipaa-student-health-records

29. Weathers T, Ercek K, Unni EJ. PGY1 resident research projects: publication rates, project completion policies, perceived values, and barriers. *Curr Pharm Teach Learn.* 2019;11(6):547-556. doi:10.1016/j.cptl.2019.02.017

30. Irwin AN, Olson KL, Joline BR, Witt DM, Patel RJ. Challenges to publishing pharmacy resident research projects from the perspectives of residency program directors and residents. *Pharm Pract.* 2013;11(3):166-172. doi:10.4321/s1886-36552013000300007

31. Byerly WG. Working with the institutional review board. *Am J Health Syst Pharm.* 2009;66(2):176-184. doi:10.2146/ajhp070066

32. Office for Human Research Protections (OHRP). Investigator Responsibilities FAQs. Accessed September 13, 2021. https://www.hhs.gov/ohrp/regulations-and-policy/guidance/faq/investigator-responsibilities/index.html

33. Barletta JF. Conducting a successful residency research project. *Am J Pharm Educ.* 2008;72(4):92. doi:10.5688/aj720492

34. Linden JA, Schneider JI, Cotter A, et al. Variability in institutional board review for a multisite assessment of resident professionalism. *J Empir Res Hum Res Ethics.* 2019;14(2):117-125. doi:10.1177/1556264619831895

35. Patel DI, Stevens KR, Puga F. Variations in institutional review board approval in the implementation of an improvement research study. *Nurs Res Pract.* 2013; Article ID 548591. doi:10.1155/2013/548591

36. International Ombudsman Association. What Is an Organizational Ombudsman? Accessed September 16, 2021. https://www.ombudsassociation.org/what-is-an-organizational-ombuds

Chapter Seven

Research Data Management and Statistical Analysis

Spencer E. Harpe PharmD, PhD, MPH, FAPhA and
John P. Bentley, RPh, PhD, FAPhA, FNAP

Chapter Objectives

- Discuss the resources needed for data management and statistical analysis for practice-based research in pharmacy
- Describe key concepts of effective data management
- Describe criteria for selecting statistical techniques for research
- Discuss considerations when selecting statistical software for research
- Identify characteristics of a successful statistical collaborator from the learner's perspective
- Describe best practices for learners while interacting with statisticians and data analysts

Key Terminology

Accessibility, bridger, data analysis plan, data archiving, data dictionary, data manipulation, data permanence, data preservation, data provenance, findability, interoperability, metadata, p-hacking, primary data, secondary data, research data repositories, reusability, sensitivity analyses

Introduction

It is critical for healthcare professionals,[1] including pharmacists,[2] to be literate in statistics. For PharmD students, this often translates into educational opportunities focused on knowledge and skills to read and understand the presentation of statistics in published articles. Statistical competence is needed to fully understand the results of research so that they can be translated into practice and the care of patients or populations. Courses in PharmD programs often attempt to use clinically relevant examples with a focus on why a particular statistical method was selected and how it answers a clinical question. However, learning to provide evidence-based patient care does not necessarily translate into having the knowledge and skills necessary to handle data management and statistical analysis tasks associated with the conduct of research. Not only are the statistical competencies needed for these activities different, but even for those focused on research applications, the degree of literacy required is not the same for every statistical competency, nor is the degree necessary the same for every pharmacy research learner. The implication of this is that student pharmacists and residents who wish to undertake research experiences need to dedicate structured time to expand their data management and statistics knowledge and skills, and this will likely be beyond what is learned in the standard, required PharmD curriculum. In addition, learners must be able to identify, learn from, communicate with, and collaborate with those who have relevant data management and analysis experience and expertise.

The intent of this chapter is to serve as an introductory resource for those wishing to expand their data management and statistical competencies necessary for the conduct of their own research. This chapter is not focused on what data to collect (that is described elsewhere in this book) but rather focuses on how to manage what data are being collected and how to support data analysis, interpretation, and dissemination. Although some discussion of selecting and implementing appropriate statistical methods will be provided, that is certainly not the primary aim of this chapter, as those reviews for pharmacy learners, practitioners, and researchers have been provided elsewhere.[3-7] General data management practices apply regardless of the analytical approach taken; thus, as a second focus, attention will be given to those practices. The third focus area of this chapter is how to efficiently and effectively work with others who have substantial expertise in the management and analysis of data. Successful research endeavors require alignment of the study objectives (or hypotheses), study design, sample size calculation, and planned (and executed) statistical analysis. This requires that researchers think with the end in mind, which may mean involving a statistician *prior* to conducting a study.

This chapter provides an overview of important considerations related to data management and statistical analysis when conducting pharmacy practice-based research.

First, general principles and recommendations about research data management are provided. This is followed by an overview of the data analysis process, including the development of data analysis plans and using statistical software. Then recommendations for learners to consider when collaborating with a statistician in the research process are presented. The chapter concludes with a brief discussion surrounding the future of statistics training in pharmacy education.

Managing Research Data

When conducting practice-based research, data come in many different varieties, from numbers in a spreadsheet from a survey to insurance claims data to biospecimens in a freezer to recordings of focus groups or interviews with patients. Collectively, these "research artifacts" are vital pieces of the research process and necessary for data analysis. Managing and protecting these data are key steps in the overall research process. Research data management plans may be required by certain funders, especially in relation to data sharing and transparency. For example, the U.S. National Institutes of Health (NIH) policy requires data generated from projects receiving at least $500,000 in NIH funding must submit a data management plan that includes how the data will be shared.[8] This policy has been revised, and beginning in 2023, it will apply to all NIH-funded research regardless of the level of funding.[9] Developing explicit data management plans is becoming a recommended best practice. The growth of the open science movement has also placed increased emphasis on sharing data to promote reproducible research.[10,11] Developing good habits related to research data management early in your training will certainly pay off later. Data management can be viewed from the perspective of the research data lifecycle. Many different versions of the data lifecycle have been described.[12-16] Figure 7–1 presents the general research data lifecycle being used to support the current discussion. The following sections describe the steps in this process.

PLANNING

A necessary first step before collecting any data is to develop a clear plan on what data are needed and how they might be obtained. The data needed for the project should flow directly from the previously developed research objective(s) or question(s), as described in Chapter 4. Remember to consider whether data need to be collected anew (aka, **primary data**) or whether you can use existing data (aka, **secondary data**). It is also important to consider the potential data collection approaches in order to obtain the best data for your particular project. For example, obtaining data through semi-structured

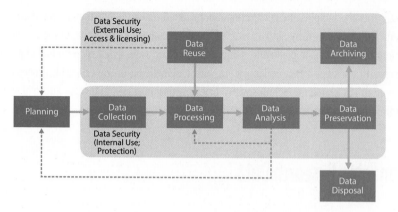

Figure 7–1. Research data lifecycle.
[Note: Solid lines represent the usual stepwise process. Dashed lines represent steps
that may be taken based on the findings or experience within a project.]

interviews with a smaller group of pharmacists may provide you with more appropriate data to answer your research question than to administer a survey to a large group of pharmacists in your region.

DATA COLLECTION

Once a plan for obtaining the necessary data has been developed, the next stage is data collection. This is the point at which the raw data are collected, recorded, or otherwise created. This may be through any variety of data collection mechanisms, such as administering questionnaires, performing blood tests, taking a biometric measurement (e.g., blood pressure or weight), or even recording an interview with a patient. Care must be taken at this stage to ensure that data collection procedures are clear and consistent for all involved in the process. Otherwise, the results of the subsequent use of the data may be adversely affected. Even if you are not directly involved in data collection or data creation, it is important to have some level of understanding of the data creation/collection process. This is particularly true when using secondary data. For example, data not originally created for research purposes, such as data from electronic health records (EHRs) or insurance claims data, are common data sources. It is important to understand the processes through which those data were initially created, the points in the data creation process that may be prone to error, and any specific biases that may be particularly relevant.[17,18]

When creating data files, there are a few decision points that must be made early in the process. Careful consideration of these can save substantial time, energy, and frustration for you and any statistician with whom you may be collaborating. When entering data, the best practice is to keep observations in the rows and variables in the columns

(A) Observations in the rows (recommended format)

Patient ID	Weight	Height	Age	Serum Creatinine	Sex
1	183	64	36	1.0	F
2	254	72	47	2.1	M
3	105	62	72	0.8	F
4	151	70	28	0.9	M

(B) Observations in the columns (do not use this format)

Variable	Patient 1	Patient 2	Patient 3	Patient 4
Weight	183	254	105	151
Height	64	72	62	70
Age	36	47	72	28
Serum Creatinine	1.0	2.1	0.8	0.9
Sex	F	M	F	M

Figure 7–2. Recommended and non-recommended layouts when preparing data files.

(Figure 7–2, Panel A). This is the standard format for statistical software and what a statistician will likely expect. Placing the observations in the columns and the variables in the rows (Figure 7–2, Panel B) is nonstandard and causes difficulty during data analysis. In keeping observations in the rows, you may wonder how to deal with multiple observations per subject (e.g., a lab value before and after the dose of a drug). There are two ways to approach this. One involves allowing multiple rows per subject (sometimes called a "long" data format). In this approach, there will be a row for each time point within the subject. If there are three-time points, then there will be three rows or observations for each subject. This requires the addition of a new time or period variable, as shown in Figure 7–3, Panel A. The other approach keeps one row per participant but repeating columns for each variable. This is sometimes called a "wide" data format. As shown in Figure 7–3, Panel B, "Pre" or "Post" are added to the variable names to denote the time period. We could just as easily have chosen to use a numerical suffix (e.g., Weight1 for PreWeight, Weight2 for PostWeight).

Another important consideration early in the data collection process is how you will maintain and manage your data. Usually, a simple spreadsheet will be sufficient. On occasion, the data may be complex and require multiple spreadsheets that need to be linked. For example, you may have one spreadsheet with patient demographics, a second with drug use information, and a third with laboratory values. As long as each spreadsheet has a consistent identifier for each patient, the various sources can be merged and combined as needed. For more complex or large data files, the use of database software may be necessary. The decision to use these more complex database approaches may require close consultation with a research mentor or information technology personnel. It is also important to remember that statistical

(A) Long data format (multiple rows per unique subject)

ID	Time	Weight	A1c	LDL
101	1	260	8.5	162
101	2	230	7.2	130
102	1	215	7.3	143
102	2	180	6.9	96
103	1	283	9.2	195
103	2	251	8.1	160

(B) Wide data format (one row per unique subject)

ID	PreWeight	PreA1c	PreLDL	PostWeight	PostA1c	PostLDL
101	260	8.5	162	230	7.2	130
102	215	7.3	143	180	6.9	96
103	283	9.2	195	251	8.1	160

Figure 7–3. Examples of long and wide data formats.

software may not be able to access data directly in certain databases, so early discussions with any collaborating statistician may also be necessary.

The creation of documentation to accompany the data is another extremely important issue to consider. This documentation, sometimes be referred to as a **data dictionary**, typically involves such information as a listing of the original variables in the dataset, the type of variable (e.g., character vs. numeric), and any coding used within the variable (e.g., for an insurance variable, 1 = Private, 2 = Public, 3 = None). This will be helpful as a reminder should you need to step away from the project and also to help others with whom you may share the data. The documentation may also include **metadata** that provides data about the actual data. This may include the number of observations, which is extremely helpful when importing data or merging multiple data sets; the number of variables in the dataset; the size of the data file in the computer's storage; and dates of creation and modification, which can help identify the most recent version of the file. It is extremely important to be consistent in your practices related to variable names, coding for data within variables, and filenames. For example, if you designate 1 for "Yes" and 0 for "No," then do this consistently for all variables where the data represent Yes/No entries. You may also decide to use certain terminology within the filename, such as including "WORKING" in those files that represent work in progress and "FINAL" for those ready for analysis. Taking time to develop your naming and coding practices prior to data entry, revising it regularly during data entry, and documenting any revisions will help you be consistent.

DATA PROCESSING

After collecting data, it is usually necessary to process those data to get them into a usable form ready for data analysis and interpretation. This may involve manual data entry (e.g., entering data from paper questionnaires) or the manipulation and cleaning of data collected through some automated extraction process (e.g., cleaning and merging data from various sources for a group of patients on anticoagulants). While there may still be a substantial amount of processing, there are notable efficiencies in obtaining data through automated extraction process (e.g., from EHRs or dispensing data) since you have data files that are ready to load into statistical software and potential errors from manual extraction and data (re)entry can be avoided. When using these automated extraction procedures to facilitate data processing, it is important to obtain readily usable files. For example, a PDF of a report of all serum creatinine values from patients receiving a certain antibiotic may be appropriate for completing clinical rounds, but it would not be ideal for research purposes. A file that contains the data in a readily usable form (e.g., a spreadsheet file or a comma- or tab-separated values file) would be ideal. Data processing may also be an important step when reusing previously collected data from your own projects or others.

Two key considerations during data processing deserve mention here. Data entry errors can sometimes be easy to identify by examining outliers (e.g., a weight of 100 kg for a study of infants or an intensive care unit length of stay greater than the total hospital length of stay). If the frequency of these potential errors is sufficiently low, the observations in question may be excluded from the analysis. If these are common, then it may require further investigation into the particular variables and perhaps a reconsideration of whether the research can proceed as initially planned. Missing data, especially patterns of missingness, are another consideration during data processing. In some situations, the data entry process used a certain code to denote missingness (e.g., 999 or 777). This should be specified in the data dictionary. These values are typically selected because they are implausible under normal circumstances. As an example, 888 may be used to indicate of a missing weight in a dataset where weight is measured in kilograms. Obviously, it is effectively impossible for a person to weigh 888 kilograms. Any observations with these entries would need to be handled specially during data analysis (e.g., telling the statistical software that 888 represents a missing value or manually converting these to missing values) or else they could skew the results. If you did not consult the data dictionary or if this were not included there, you would notice a spike at 888 when examining the distribution of that weight variable. Similar situations apply to categorical variables where certain codes are used, such as the previous example of insurance (1 = Private, 2 = Public, 3 = None). If you examined the frequency distribution of the insurance variable and noticed entries other than 1, 2, or 3, this might suggest an error in data entry, incomplete information in the data dictionary, or even an error when importing the data. This highlights the importance of examining descriptive statistics for all variables in the dataset.

Data manipulation is another important activity during the data processing step. Despite the potential negative connotations, this manipulation is a common and necessary part of data analysis. Data manipulation involves calculating new variables (e.g., calculating body mass index from weight and height), recoding existing variables (e.g., collapsing categories of an existing variable, such collapsing a variable measuring agreement from five categories into two like Strongly Agree/Agree vs. Neutral/Disagree/Strongly Disagree), or even merging different datasets.

With all of the changes that can occur during the data processing phase, keeping track of the different versions of your data files is extremely important. Generally speaking, it is best practice not to overwrite any file during the data processing stage. As mentioned earlier, you may want to use certain naming conventions to denote files where processing is being conducted from those that are final and ready for analysis. It may also be helpful to preserve periodic snapshots of your data files. Keeping these separate snapshots allows you to go back to a previous step of data manipulation without having to start over completely from the beginning. A simple approach is to include a date in the filename itself (e.g., DataFile-WORKING-2021-01-15). Merging requires some unique considerations since a date in the filename alone may not help. There are many different approaches to this snapshot approach during merging, ranging from including the variable names in the name of the data file to creating codes for each file (Merging-A for the first dataset Merging-AB after including dataset B, Merging-ABC after merging in dataset C, etc.). Consider discussing this with your research mentor, as they may have their own standard practices to recommend.

Finally, you may need to return to the data processing stage after you begin data analysis. For example, you may identify additional variables that need to be included in the analysis, but they were not previously cleaned. There could be alternate combinations or transformations of existing variables that are needed based on the results in the data analysis step. Another common occurrence is the need to conduct additional analysis based on peer reviewer comments after submitting a research manuscript to a journal for publication. This is why it is important to keep good notes and records during the data processing stage and be prepared to revisit that stage if needed.

DATA ANALYSIS

The next phase in the data lifecycle is data analysis. This involves using the processed and hopefully "clean" data for the prespecified data analyses to answer your research questions. The data analysis process is discussed in detail in a later section in this chapter.

DATA PRESERVATION

After data analysis, data preservation involves processes to ensure the data are available for as long as needed. For this discussion, preservation will be focused on maintaining research data to support the dissemination of your research findings, but there is substantial overlap with data archiving if the potential for data sharing exists. In its simplest form, data preservation may involve backing up your data. Remember the rule of three for backups: three copies on two different media with one backup located off-site. While it may be tempting to rely on keeping your data analysis files in some cloud storage platform as a form of backup, remember that backup files are not intended to be used actively. These should be separate files that you are not using for day-to-day research activities.

Backing up your data is just one part of data preservation. When you begin the process of disseminating your findings, you will need to take care to preserve your data in case you must revise your analysis based on feedback during presentations at professional meetings or peer review of any manuscripts. Some journals require data to be made available for reviewers. Most likely, there are also local policies at your institution specifying how long research data must be maintained (e.g., five years after final publication, ten years after the last subject completes the study). Similarly, funding agencies may place requirements on data retention and preservation. If you decide that you wish to make your data available for others to use, considerations about data preservation will lead to the data archiving stage.

Another way to think about data preservation is what happens to your data after you leave your current position or institution. Simply transferring your data files in your cloud storage account to your mentor or giving your mentor a USB drive or external hard drive with the research files is *not* data preservation. The focus should be on ensuring that all necessary documentation is available and associated with the data files to facilitate use by somebody not originally affiliated with the research project. Remember that the data collected at an institution generally belong to that institution, not the individual researcher. Local policies should describe whether and under what circumstances a researcher may take data with them if they leave the institution.

DATA DISPOSAL

Issues related to data disposal are an important part of the data lifecycle. Before considering disposing of or destroying your data, you should consider the potential implications of that. Will you want to reuse the data later? Would others benefit from access to the data? Just because you *can* dispose of or destroy your research data, you should ask yourself whether you *want* to do that. Data disposal can also apply to entire datasets. This typically happens when you are using secondary data obtained from another source, such as insurance claims data. The agreement covering the use of the data may specify when and how the data will be destroyed, deleted, or returned to the owner. In certain situations, you may be asked to sign documentation attesting to the disposal or destruction of the data. Data disposal or destruction may also apply to particular elements within your data. For example, participant identifiers may be retained until a certain period of time after data collection is finalized or after initial publication. One important consideration for data disposal plans is how that process will be managed if you share your data with others. This is why careful consideration must be given to what research data can be shared and under what circumstances.

DATA ARCHIVING

After you have analyzed the data and disseminated your findings, the story and life of your data are not finished. Those data may be reused by you for subsequent projects or by others. Making your data available may be a requirement of funding agencies. Also, scholarly journals are increasingly encouraging, and in some cases, even requiring that research data from publications be made available for others to use. This can generally be viewed as data archiving. Given the long-term nature of archiving, data permanence is a major consideration. Hard drives can fail. Cloud storage platforms will come and go. Data permanence considers how the preservation plan will account for data storage in perpetuity. Research data repositories, such as Dryad (https://www.datadryad.org), the Dataverse project (https://dataverse.org), Zenodo (https://zenodo.org), the Open Science Framework (https://osf.io), and Figshare (https://www.figshare.com), can facilitate long-term data archiving outside of an individual research group. These plat-forms are particularly useful for sharing since they provide mechanisms to improve the discoverability of your data by making metadata available to potential users and providing mechanisms to cite your data, thereby providing you with an additional form of scientific credit. The Registry of Research Data Repositories (http:///www.re3data.org) provides a way to search for available research repositories by general subject area and content type. This may be useful to identify a repository for your own data or to find data that you may want to use for a research project. When selecting a data repository, consider the sustain-ability plans of a potential repository since this can have serious implications for long-term archiving. In addition to data repositories, some journals allow you to publish your data as either a standalone publication or alongside your journal article as a supplemental file.

If you decide to archive your data for sharing and future reuse by others, remember to follow all appropriate regulations that may apply, such as those required by the Health Insurance Portability and Accountability Act (HIPAA). The FAIR principles (findable, accessible, interoperable, and reusable) have been proposed as a way to promote ethical, appropriate, and efficient sharing of data.[19,20] Although distinct, these four principles are interrelated. To illustrate these principles, we will consider a new restaurant opening in your city as an example.

The first principle is to ensure that data intended to be shared are findable (find-ability) or discoverable. In order for the new restaurant to be findable, it needs a unique physical address not shared with any other establishment. If you saw an advertisement for the new restaurant that simply said, "Visit us downtown," you would not be able to locate the restaurant. Shared data need to have a similar unique address. Since these files are often posted online, shared data need a persistent identifier since websites change over time. There are various approaches, but a common approach is to assign a digital object identifier (DOI) to data that are made available for reuse. Most data repositories can provide a DOI. Simply having a unique, persistent identifier is not sufficient. There needs to be a way for potential users to find the data. Turning to the restaurant example, this might involve creating a website to increase the chances that the restaurant could be found or discovered. This findability could be improved if the restaurant included important keywords about the restaurant in the website metadata to optimize indexing. This might include any variety of descriptors, such as the type of cuisine, the type of dining (e.g., casual vs. fine), or even price. Think of posting your data in a data repository as creating a webpage for your data that includes important information about the data and relevant keywords to facilitate searching.

The second principle is accessibility. In the restaurant example, you have found the restaurant's webpage and decided to try it for an upcoming meal. You know where it is and how to get there, but now you wonder if there are any important considerations when visiting the restaurant. Since the restaurant is downtown, parking may be an important consideration that could influence when you decide to visit. Promoting accessibility may be as simple as noting on the website that free parking is available or that they provide a discount for parking fees at a nearby parking garage. You may also wonder whether reservations are needed or required, if so, under what circumstances. This would be helpful to find on the restaurant's website. In the context of shared research data, potential users need to know how to access the data. This may include any special instructions or approval that may be required (e.g., data are shared after the data owner reviews the research plan of the researcher requesting the data). When posting your data in a research repository, on your own website, or mentioning the data are available within a journal article, it is important to clearly state any processes or restrictions on how the data can be accessed. This is particularly important if only certain variables are made available.

The third principle is interoperability, which refers to how the data (potentially) integrate with other data. Think about payment options the restaurant accepts. If the restaurant only accepts cash, but you never carry cash, then that could be a problem. You may also want to know if all major credit cards were accepted or only a few. This information would be important to know prior to visiting the restaurant to help you know whether the restaurant's payment approach was interoperable with, or integrated with, your own payment approaches. Similarly, you may expect information about food contents (allergens, gluten-free, lactose-free, etc.) and how allergen cross-contamination is managed by the kitchen on the menu. If you asked the server about these and were then provided with a binder containing a list of recipes and photocopies of the nutritional labels of the ingredients, you would likely leave the restaurant since that information was not in a format easy for you to process and use. From a data standpoint, reuse is promoted when data are provided in reasonably standard file formats (e.g., posting a comma-separated text file rather than the proprietary format of a statistical package). Interoperability also relates to the documentation provided with the data since that may contain important information about the original data collection processes, any initial data cleaning, and validation efforts, and variable coding explanations.

The final principle is that data should be reusable (reusability). This principle highlights the importance of clear and descriptive metadata. For the restaurant, simply having a website is not sufficient. The keywords mentioned earlier are extremely important. Assume that you visited the restaurant and found it to your liking. A few months later, you want to visit again, or maybe you are making a recommendation to a friend, but you cannot remember the name of the restaurant. All you remember is that it was a casual-dining restaurant serving Italian cuisine and was located downtown. Without the appropriate keywords on their website, you may not be able to easily find the restaurant again or "reuse" the restaurant. The same can be said of shared research data. Including descriptive metadata can facilitate others' finding your data. This is closely related to the findable principle. Another consideration for reusability is the importance of knowing how the data were originally created or collected, whether any prior manipulation or cleaning occurred, and whether they have been previously published. Collectively, these are referred to as data provenance. Back to the restaurant example, assume that your friend recommended a restaurant for you to try. You ask whether they have eaten at the restaurant. They have not, but received a recommendation from another friend. Before you eat at the new restaurant, you may ask your friend if the original recommender had tried the restaurant or if they have good taste (or at least similar taste) in food as your friend. This would help you determine where the recommendation came from (or its provenance) and if you wanted to act on it. A final consideration within this principle involves the way in which the data are licensed for reuse. While this is related to interoperability, this is also about legal considerations rather than technical interoperability. The data documentation should clearly describe what licenses or restrictions are placed on how the data are shared. For example, there may be license fees associated with obtaining the data, or there may be requirements that any data created based on the original data are made available under a similar license. There may also be expectations of having an original publication. It is also possible to cite the data themselves in subsequent publications if a DOI is assigned to the data.

DATA SECURITY

Regardless of whether individual identifiers are included, all research data are sensitive data. Data management plans should include efforts to promote data security, especially during the phases where there are individual identifiers present and when data are being shared or archived. From an internal use standpoint, data security primarily focuses on physical security and the protection of confidentiality of research subjects through data access restrictions. If identifiers or other protected information is part of the data, your project's ethical approval may require that only those individuals on the research protocol have access to the data. Even if not required as part of ethics approval, it is best practice to limit access to research data to those individuals directly involved with the research project. Keep in mind methods to secure access to your data, such as password protecting the data files or keeping files on a computer or server with access limited to authorized individuals. Managing access is important if you are required to provide an audit trail for regulatory purposes. Consulting with your local information technology department can be helpful in this area.

Data security also includes physical security, such as limiting access to computers where research data are stored or used. This does pose some logistical difficulties since laptop computers are commonly used, but this highlights the importance of keeping your computer password-protected and physically secured whenever possible. Removable storage media should be avoided except for backup purposes, and physical security of those should be ensured (e.g., kept in a locked filing cabinet). If you must keep your data on removable media, such as a USB flash drive, use password protection and consider encrypting the device.

When data are archived for potential reuse by others, data security takes a slightly different approach since data use is external to the original research team. Physical security (e.g., access to the physical servers) is still important, but this may be handled by the data repository. The focus on external use is access to the data (including specific data elements) and licensing. Completely de-identified data may be archived and made available for broad use. You may also make selected elements available only in certain situations after reviewing requests from another researcher. The variables available through limited access and the request approach should be fully disclosed when your data are archived to meet the previously mentioned FAIR principles. Most data repositories will ask for you to assign a license to your data, such as one of the Creative Commons licenses. The various repositories have additional guidance on the types of licenses available. The potential for data sharing should be described in your research project's ethics review application. You may also be asked to disclose the potential for research data sharing to research participants and sometimes provide ways for them to opt out of having their data shared.

Performing Statistical Analyses

Although the statistical analysis of data collected for a project occurs later in the research data lifecycle outlined in Figure 7–1, researchers should develop a data analysis plan early in the process. While a good practice in general, it will likely be a requirement for grant applications or formal projects, like a learner's honors thesis. A well-written data analysis plan will help researchers collect all needed data while also ensuring that all data collected are used. In addition, it facilitates communication between pharmacy research learners and their mentors and is essential for avoiding errors and misunderstandings in projects that involve multiple researchers. Different sections of the plan may also form the basis for abstracts, presentations, and manuscripts, facilitating the output of the research process. The following sections outline what is usually included in a data analysis plan, with some guidance on selecting appropriate statistical methods. Selecting and using statistical software also will be discussed. The focus in this section is on quantitative methods; for more information on the analysis of qualitative data, please see Chapter 15 or other sources.[21,22] In addition, this section is not intended to be comprehensive in nature but will provide some key considerations to guide the selection of appropriate statistical methods that are common in the pharmacy literature. Furthermore, an assumption is made that the reader is familiar with certain concepts (e.g., type of data, classification of variables, levels of measurement, independent vs. dependent variable, descriptive statistics, measures of association, hypothesis testing, confidence intervals, statistical significance vs. clinical significance, confounding, effect modification). The reader is referred to a number of references that elaborate on these foundational principles as applied to pharmacy research.[4-7, 23-29]

CREATING A DATA ANALYSIS PLAN

The contents of a data analysis plan may vary depending on the application and situation, but generally, the following are included[30,31]:

- A statement of the aims, research question(s), and/or hypotheses
- The source of the data to be analyzed
- A description of the study participants, including any inclusion and/or exclusion criteria
- Overview of the variables and study measures to be used in the analysis
- Steps in data management (e.g., data cleaning, outlier detection)
- Description of the statistical methods and software to be used
- Shells for planned tables and figures (these can then easily be populated after analysis)

Although some of these components are somewhat self-explanatory and others, such as data management, were described in detail earlier in this chapter, two components merit additional discussion. Regarding the study variables and study measures, this may include details if scoring is needed for any of the variables (e.g., how will a quality of life score be calculated based on a set of questions from a questionnaire, how will it be determined that someone has diabetes based on administrative claims data). If a continuous variable is going to be categorized (e.g., age in years categorized into two groups: under 65 years of age and 65 years of age or older), this should be stated in this section, including a justification as well as steps to be followed. When appropriate, researchers should state which variables are independent variables (exposure variables), dependent variables (outcome variables), or other covariates (like potential confounders, effect modifiers, and variables for subgroup analysis).

With respect to the description of the planned statistical methods, this is perhaps the most detailed part of the plan and may include descriptive statistics planned, tests or models proposed to address the research questions(s), methods to assess statistical assumptions and plans if there are violations, approaches for handling missing data, plans for assessing and addressing potential confounding, significance level for hypothesis testing, description of subgroup analyses, and a discussion of any **sensitivity analyses**[32,33] that are planned to assess the robustness of the study findings. Additional guidance on the selection of statistical methods will be provided in a subsequent section. Researchers should state what statistical software (and version number) they plan to use as well as the procedures and/or commands from that software.

In addition, although information about the size of the sample may be discussed in other sections of a research protocol, it is not uncommon for researchers to include information about sample size in their analysis plan (i.e., sample size estimation or justification) because such decisions are necessarily based on the study objective, study design, and planned statistical analysis as mentioned earlier in the chapter. A more detailed discussion of the principles of sample size calculation and related considerations is available elsewhere.[34]

Some tasks in a data analysis plan may be contingent on what is discovered during data analysis (e.g., variable transformation after assessment for assumption violations). It is also important to consider the responsibilities and capabilities of pharmacy research learners regarding the various components. Learners should be able to conduct many of the data management tasks, at least for small to moderate data sets based on primary data collection. When faced with data management tasks associated with a large administrative claims data set, most pharmacy research learners will require additional training and/or the guidance and support of an experienced researcher. Learners should also be able to run descriptive statistics for their projects and perhaps perform tests for differences and tests for an association but may need additional support before implementing multivariable or multivariate models. But even in these more complicated situations, learners must have an understanding of the data structure for their projects because it forms the basis for selecting the appropriate statistical procedure to use in a research project, a major part of the data analysis plan. At a minimum, learners should be able to specify whether their variables are categorical (i.e., discrete) or continuous and if appropriate, they should be able to classify their variables as independent or dependent.

SELECTING APPROPRIATE STATISTICAL METHODS AND TECHNIQUES

A number of authors have presented classification frameworks for statistical techniques, some more comprehensive than others, with some providing instruction regarding how the statistical method can be carried out in different software packages (e.g., see[4,35–40]). Such frameworks can be used to assist researchers in the selection of an appropriate statistical method and also to evaluate whether others have chosen wisely. The following questions provide important considerations for how to group together statistical methods:

1. What is the major research question to be addressed by the analysis?
2. How many and what type (i.e., continuous vs. categorical) of dependent variables are there?
3. How many and what type (i.e., continuous vs. categorical) of independent variables are there?
4. What role, if any, do "third variables" play in the proposed analysis? (e.g., confounders, effect modifiers, mediators)
5. Are correlated or clustered responses being analyzed (i.e., do we have "correlated data" or are our observations not independent)?
6. Other than independence (see previous questions), are any other standard assumptions violated?

There may be other considerations as well. For example, in the patient-reported outcomes literature, researchers sometimes use what are called latent variables in the analysis. Such variables are not observable in a dataset but may be operationalized through observed responses to a set of questions on a questionnaire or other measured variables. These variables may be used in analysis with techniques such as confirmatory factor analysis, structural equation modeling, and latent class analysis.[4] As another example, missing data can present a number of complications during data analysis. More detailed discussions relevant to pharmacy research are available elsewhere.[41–44] Given its complexity, this is an area where pharmacy research learners are encouraged to seek guidance from a statistician or an applied researcher with relevant experience and expertise.

Two common "broad" research questions commonly encountered by data analysts are to assess: (1) whether there are differences among groups and (2) the degree of relationship (or association) among variables. Table 7–1 outlines various tests for differences and association based on the nature of the dependent variable (i.e., continuous and normally distributed, continuous and not normally distributed, ordinal, or nominal), the number and nature (i.e., two groups or more than two groups) of the independent variables,

TABLE 7–1. TESTS FOR DIFFERENCES AND ASSOCIATIONS

Purpose of research (Type of statistics) →	Describe (Descriptive)	Identify Differences (Inferential)				Identify Associations (Inferential) (Also see regression chart in Table 7–2) *Nature of IV can vary for different measures*
		Categorical independent variables (IV or grouping variables)				
Number and types of groups →		Independent observations		Observations *not* independent (pairing, matching, repeating over time, observed multiply under different conditions)		Only looking at 2 variables (correlation as a descriptive tool)
Level/scale of measurement ↓		Comparing 2 groups (IV has 2 levels)	Comparing ≥3 groups[a] (Either 1 IV with ≥3 levels or 2 IVs with ≥2 levels)	Comparing 2 matched/paired groups or time points (or 2 treatments both administered to the same subjects)	Comparing ≥3 groups (≥3 timepoints within the same subject or 1 IV with ≥3 levels or 2 IVs where 1 is time-related)	
Level of Measurement of the Dependent Variable (DV) Continuous (Interval/Ratio) and normally distributed *or* "Long" ordinal (i.e., with ≥5 categories) and almost normally distributed	Mean and standard deviation (SD)	• Unpaired *t*-test	• One-way ANOVA (1 IV) • Two-way ANOVA (2 IVs) • *k*-way ANOVA (*k* IVs)	• Paired *t*-test	• Repeated measures ANOVA	• Pearson's *r* (product moment correlation)

(Continued)

159

TABLE 7–1. TESTS FOR DIFFERENCES AND ASSOCIATIONS (CONTINUED)

Continuous or "long" ordinal (≥5 categories) and not normally distributed	Median and interquartile range (IQR) or just the range	• Wilcoxon rank sum test • Mann-Whitney U test	• Kruskal–Wallis test (1 IV) • Multiple options (≥2 IVs)[b]	• Wilcoxon signed rank test	• Friedman's test	• Spearman's rho (ρ)
Discrete data (Nominal [e.g., dichotomous] or Ordinal with <5 categories, i.e., "short" ordinal)	Percentage or Frequency (For "short" ordinal, you may see Median/ IQR, but that is arguably pushing things a bit)	• Chi square • Fisher's exact test	• Chi square • Fisher's exact test	• McNemar's test	• Cochran's Q	• Chi square (can supplement with Phi, Cramer's V, Lambda, Gamma) • Fisher's exact test

[a]You can have more than three groups if you have either two or more independent variables examined simultaneously (e.g., cross-classification of treatment type and disease severity) or if you have one independent variable with more than two categories (e.g., disease severity measured as mild, moderate, or severe).

[b]There is some debate over this (i.e., what is the appropriate approach when trying to perform a non-parametric equivalent to two-way or k-way ANOVA). The Scheirer–Ray–Hare test is one option; others recommend Aligned Ranks Transformation ANOVA; yet others recommend the use of ordinal logistic regression (a type of generalized linear model, see Table 7–2, and is actually a generalization of the Wilcoxon rank sum, Mann–Whitney U, and Kruskal-Wallis tests).

and whether the observations can be considered independent or not. Information about a variety of regression methods that can be used to assess relationships (or associations) between a single continuous, categorical, or time-to-event dependent variable and one or more independent variables measured as continuous or categorical can be found in Table 7–2. It is important to note that the regression models discussed in Table 7–2 generalize many of the tests in Table 7–1, thus can be used for similar purposes under certain circumstances and can even extend the tests presented in Table 7–1 to more complex situations (e.g., the need to include additional variables to address potential confounding when testing for differences between groups).

There are a number of statistical methods beyond what is presented in Tables 7–1 and 7–2, but these tables present methods that are commonly used in the biomedical and pharmacy literature. If pharmacy research learners come across relevant literature that they would like to use to support the analysis for their projects and it seems complicated, they are encouraged to seek assistance or guidance from others with experience in those areas.

SELECTING AND USING STATISTICAL SOFTWARE

A multitude of options exists when it comes to statistical software packages. Although there are many differences between these packages, there are some similarities. As Grace-Martin observes, "the first one you learn is the hardest to learn ... So once you're learned one, it will be easier to learn the next one."[45] Some considerations in statistical software selection include interaction with the software (coding vs. graphical user interface vs. both), learning curve, cost, the familiarity of your mentor (and/or the statistician) with a given package, course requirement, and for those packages that are not freely available, site license availability at your college/school, university, or health-system. Historically, there were disciplinary norms (e.g., social sciences tended to use SPSS, manufacturing as well as the health and life sciences tended to SAS, economists and epidemiologists tended to use Stata), but this is less of an issue today. The need for handling different types of specialized issues (e.g., data from surveys that use complex sampling methods) may lead analysts to select a certain software package. Table 7–3 provides a comparison of selected statistical software packages based on the first three considerations stated earlier: interaction of the user with the program (menu-driven, programming/coding, or both), learning curve, and cost (for additional information, see also these references[45,46]). A few other observations based on the authors' experience are also provided in the table.

In addition to the packages outlined in Table 7–3, there are other specialized software packages that are used by some practice-based researchers. For example, Mplus is a latent variable modeling program that can do most of the regression methods mentioned in Table 7–2, but allows for additional capabilities by integrating the use of latent variables. As

TABLE 7–2. REGRESSION METHODS

	Nature of Dependent and Independent Variables	Assessment and Interpretable Quantity (IQ)	Mathematical Form
Observations are independent			
Linear (or ordinary least squares) regression	Dependent: Continuous Independent: Continuous or categorical	Model assessment: R-squared and residual analysis IQ: Regression coefficients (beta or β)	$Y_i = \beta_0 + \beta X_1 + \varepsilon_i$ or $E(Y) = \beta_0 + \beta X_1$
Logistic regression	Dependent: Categorical Independent: Continuous or categorical	Model assessment: Hosmer–Lemeshow test (goodness of fit) and sometimes ROC or C statistic (accurate prediction of outcomes) IQ: Odds ratio (OR) (comes from the exponentiated regression coefficient, that is, e^β)	$\ln\left[\dfrac{p(Y_i=1)}{1-p(Y_i=1)}\right] = \beta_0 + \beta X_1$ or $p(Y_i=1) = \dfrac{e^{\beta_0+\beta X_i}}{1+e^{\beta_0+\beta X_i}}$
Generalized linear model (GLM)	Dependent: Categorical or continuous Independent: Continuous or categorical	Model assessment: Depends on the type of model IQ: Similar to the above models in that the regression coefficient or exponentiated coefficients are used	Generally resembles $f(E(Y)) = \beta_0 + \beta X_1$ When using a GLM for analysis, you select a particular link (i.e., a function that relates the mean of the DV to the other side of the equal sign) and distribution (i.e., how the DV is assumed to be distributed)
Survival analysis, Cox proportional hazards regression, or Time-to-event analysis[a]	Dependent: Composed of two pieces—time (continuous) and outcome (categorical) Independent: Continuous or categorical	Model assessment: Goodness of fit and sometimes ROC/C statistic IQ: Hazard ratio (HR), rate ratio, or relative risk (comes from the exponentiated regression coefficient, that is, e^β)[b]	$h_i(t) = h_0(t)\, e^{\beta X_i}$ or $\ln h_i(t) = \ln h_0(t) + \beta X_1$

Observations are not independent			
Generalized linear mixed models (GLMM)	Dependent: Categorical or continuous Independent: Continuous or categorical; may be measured at different levels (e.g., patient vs. hospital; student vs. teacher)	Model assessment: Depends on the type of model IQ: Similar to the above models in that the regression coefficient or exponentiated coefficients are used; also there can be effects estimated at different levels in the same model (e.g., patient and hospital separately)	Resembles the GLM but includes additional terms for effects at "higher" levels

[a]There are variations in the actual statistical assumptions and approaches for these different techniques. We are keeping them as a general set since they are doing the same thing conceptually and interpretation is similar.
[b]Although there are differences between these three values, we will treat them all the same because, rightly or wrongly, most health sciences researchers tend to interpret them similarly.

TABLE 7–3. COMPARISON OF SELECTED STATISTICAL SOFTWARE PACKAGES

Name	Primary Interaction	Learning Curve	Cost[a]	Comments
Stata (https://www.stata.com)	Programming or Menu-driven	+ +	$$ (Annual or Perpetual License)	• Menu-driven approach provides full syntax associated with each analysis • Can produce high quality statistical graphics • User-written programs can be added to extend its capabilities • Commonly used in epidemiology and economics • Very active user community
SAS (https://www.sas.com)	Programming (some menu-driven options)	+ + +	$$$$ (Annual License)	• SAS Enterprise Guide provides menu-drive data analysis • SAS OnDemand for Academics provides cloud-based access and is free for students and educators • Commonly used in corporate environments
SPSS (https://www.spss.com)	Menu-driven (some programming options)	+	$$$$ (Annual License)	• Basic software extended with additional modules for specific uses (structural equation modeling, Bayesian analysis, decision analysis, etc.) • Certain statistical techniques may be part of add-on packages that require additional licenses • A number of extensions are freely available via the SPSS Predictive Analytics collection on GitHub; these can be accessed from the Extension Hub dialog when SPSS is opened • Commonly used in social sciences
R (https://www.r-project.org)	Programming	+ + +	Free and Open Source	• Statistical programming language • Coding approach provides extreme flexibility (if you can code it, you can do it) • Can produce high quality statistical graphics • Many thousands of specific-use programs (called packages) support a wide range of statistical analyses • Very active user community

Software	Interface		Cost	Features
R Commander (https://socialsciences.mcmaster.ca/jfox/Misc/Rcmdr)	Menu-driven or Programming	++	Free and Open Source	• R package that provides a graphical user interface for R • Menu-driven approach provides full syntax associated with each analysis • R Commander plug-ins provide menu-driven approaches for specific use cases (time series, evidence-based medicine, survival analysis, etc.)
Jamovi (https://www.jamovi.org)	Menu-driven	+	Free and Open Source	• Built on R and modeled after SPSS • Produces tables in APA format that can be copied into word-processing software • Optional modules allow more advanced or specific statistical analyses (psychometrics, meta-analysis, command-line programming, etc.)
JASP (https://jasp-stats.org)	Menu-driven	+	Free and Open Source	• Built on R and modeled after SPSS • Provides both frequentist and Bayesian approaches to common statistical analyses
JMP[a] (https://www.jmp.com)	Menu-driven (some programming options through scripts and SAS interface)	+	$$$ (Annual License)	• Provides many options for data visualization • Offers menu-driven access to various complex analytical approaches • Provides integration with SAS (both data and statistical procedures) • Includes special procedures for topics like design of experiments and statistical quality control analysis • "Pro" version offers additional advanced statistical techniques
GraphPad Prism[b] (https://www.graphpad.com/scientific-software/prism/)	Menu-driven	+	$$ (Annual or Perpetual License)	• General purpose statistical software • Many graphic options for results • Allows some level of automation (e.g., import and cleaning) without the need for coding • Links data, results tables, and graphs so that updating data can dynamically update results and graphs

(Continued)

TABLE 7–3. COMPARISON OF SELECTED STATISTICAL SOFTWARE PACKAGES (*CONTINUED*)

Name	Primary Interaction	Learning Curve	Cost[a]	Comments
Tableau[b] (https://www.tableau.com)	Menu-driven	++	$$$ (Annual License)	• Primarily focused on data visualization and the use of large datasets • Some basic analyses are available • Allows connection to R and Python for additional statistical analyses
Spreadsheets (Microsoft Excel, LibreOffice Calc, Apple Numbers, Google Sheets, etc.)	Varies	++	$$ (Annual or Perpetual License)	• Some options are free (LibreOffice Calc or Google Sheets) • There have been concerns with the accuracy of spreadsheet-based statistical analysis • Difficult to promote reproducible analysis and reporting • Add-on programs are available for some to provide menu-driven analysis
Python (https://www.python.org)	Programming	+++	Free and Open Source	• General purpose programming language; statistical analysis is performed using specific libraries (SciPy, NumPy, Pandas, etc.) • Popular in data science applications • Very active user community

[a]Discounts are often available for academic use; residents do not typically qualify for academic discounts, but discounts may be available for employees of non-profit organizations; when annual licenses are required, students may qualify for shorter-term licenses (e.g., a semester-long license) at a reduced price
[b]Not available for Unix/Linux

mentioned in the table, Microsoft Excel (and other spreadsheet programs) can be used for a number of data analysis-related activities. Examples of some basic spreadsheet functions and operators can be found in Table 7–4. Although spreadsheets can be used for more complicated analyses, most statisticians advise that other software packages be used for such analyses. In some situations, spreadsheets can provide inaccurate results and are not as well documented regarding statistical analysis when compared to other software packages. However, spreadsheets may be used for data entry, the manipulation of rows and columns prior to statistical analysis, and some basic descriptive analyses. There are also a number of online calculators and data analysis tools. Many of these tools can conduct analyses without the need for raw data (i.e., by providing means and standard deviations or frequency counts). For example, GraphPad provides an online utility to perform a t-test[47] and the VassarStat website can perform a chi-square test and a Fisher exact test.[48]

The wide availability of statistical software programs and online tools, oftentimes in a user-friendly format, may create some unintended consequences. Readers are cautioned to remember that just because you *can* perform some test or method within the software does not mean that you *should* perform it or that you know what all of the output actually means. There is such a thing as "knowing enough to be dangerous." For an interesting discussion of this problem in the context of structural equation modeling, a complicated statistical technique that also has somewhat user-friendly software programs as well as "easy-to-read" introductory textbooks, please see Steiger's aptly-named article, "Driving Fast in Reverse."[49] Steiger notes that direct guidance from someone with advanced statistical training and experience is often needed. Muthén makes a similar argument and states that "students should not be encouraged to *wing it* on their own and should be discouraged from seeking automated software solutions."[50] Statistical software has made relatively advanced techniques more widely available; that is not a bad thing. These advances in software do, however, require the user to understand the relationship between the question being asked and the analysis being performed, as well as any assumptions that accompany a particular statistical test or technique.

Working with a Statistician or Data Analyst

When working with a researcher or research group, the statistician[a] may serve a number of different roles. Kirk described five such roles: helper, leader, data-blesser, collaborator,

---

[a]The individual may not be labeled as a statistician or biostatistician, but rather may have training as a substantive researcher with significant methodological and statistical education and training. Thus, we will also use the term "data analyst."

TABLE 7–4. COMMON SPREADSHEET FUNCTIONS AND OPERATORS

Functions		

Functions always start with an equal sign. This tells Excel that there is a function for it to evaluate. The text in italics in parentheses are the required arguments for the function to work.

Function	Description	Example
=AVERAGE (*cell range*)	Calculates the average (or arithmetic mean) of a cell range	=AVERAGE (B2:B30)
=STDEV.S (*cell range*)	Calculates the sample standard deviation (i.e., the denominator is $n-1$) of a cell range	=STDEV.S (B2:B30)
=SUM (*cell range*)	Calculates the sum of a cell range (any missing or non-numeric values are ignored)	=SUM (B2:B30)
=MIN (*cell range*)	Returns the minimum (or smallest) value in a range	=MIN (B2:B30)
=MAX (*cell range*)	Returns the maximum (or largest) value in a range	=MAX (B2:B30)
=MEDIAN (*cell range*)	Returns the median value in a range	=MEDIAN (B2:B30)
=COUNT (*cell range*)	Counts the number of cells containing numeric values in a range	=COUNT (B2:B30)
=COUNTIF (*range, value*)	Counts the number of cells in a range that are equal to or contain a given value; if the value of interest is text, enclose it in double quotes)	=COUNTIF (B2:B30,1) =COUNTIF (B2:B30,"A")
=COUNTA (*cell range*)	Counts the number of cells that are *not* blank (regardless of their contents)	=COUNTA (B2:B30)
=COUNTBLANK (*cell range*)	Counts the number of cells that are blank	=COUNTBLANK (B2:B30)
=IF (*comparison to be performed, value if true, value if false*)	Performs a logical test (i.e., is the comparison statement true or false) and then returns the appropriate value. This is often done to return 0 or 1 (T/F;Y/N; etc.). If the true or false values are letters, enclose them in double quotes.	=IF (A2>B2,1,0) =IF (A2<>15,"T","F")

Mathematical Operators

Mathematical operators allow you to use Excel as a calculator. You can use them with individual numbers (3+2) or cell references (B2+C2). If you want Excel to perform the calculation, you must start with an equal sign (=) to tell Excel that a function follows. Otherwise, it will put exactly what you type into the cell as text.

Operator	Description	Example
+	Addition	=B2+C2
- (Hyphen)	Subtraction	=B2-C2

(Continued)

TABLE 7–4. COMMON SPREADSHEET FUNCTIONS AND OPERATORS (*CONTINUED*)

Functions		
* (asterisk, Shift 8)	Multiplication	=B2*C2
/	Division	=B2/C2
^ (caret, Shift 6)	Exponentiation	=B2^C2
ln(*cell reference*)	Natural log of a number	=ln(B2)
log10(*cell reference*)	Log (base 10) of a number	=log10(B2)
Parentheses ()	Spreadsheets follow standard order of operations, so watch your parentheses carefully. Parentheses are also helpful to clarify reading of functions. This helps when you share things with others.	=(A2+B2)^C2/D2

Logical Operators

Logical operators allow you to make comparisons between two or more quantities. This is usually done with numbers, but it can also be done with characters (e.g., =B2="Apple" asks Excel to tell you if the text in cell B2 is "Apple"). When comparing text, remember that case (upper or lower) matters and that there is a "natural" order based on the alphabet (using the locale set on your system). These operators are most useful with intermediate data manipulation steps or data quality checks. As with the mathematical operators, you must start with an equal sign to tell Excel to perform the actual comparison. Excel will evaluate the comparison and return "True" or "False" depending on what it finds.

Operator	Description	Example
>	Greater than	=B2>C2
>=	Greater than or equal to	=B2>=C2
<	Less than	=B2<C2
<=	Less than or equal to	=B2<=C2
=	Equal to	=B2=C2
<> (that is a less than sign followed immediately by a greater than sign)	Not equal to	=B2<>C2

Note: These are common functions and operators in MS Excel. These generally work in other spreadsheets, such as Google Sheets or LibreOffice Calc or Apple Numbers, but slight modifications may be required.

and teacher (see Table 7–5).[51] The first three roles represent the statistician having relatively little intellectual contributions to the overall research project; rather, the statistician is more of a technician or merely a second set of eyes. Having served in all of five roles, these chapter authors can speak to the personal and professional benefits of serving as true collaborators and teachers rather than merely providing technical support or passing input into a project.

It is important to emphasize what a statistician can do and what they cannot do in terms of research assistance. First and foremost, a statistician cannot tell you what your

TABLE 7–5. POTENTIAL ROLES OF A COLLABORATING STATISTICIAN

Role	Description
Helper	Low level of direct involvement in the research project beyond answering questions about statistics or performing data analysis
Leader	Assumes primary responsibility for all efforts to make sense of the data that has been collected; little effort in this area from the main researcher
Data-blesser	Performs little to no statistical analysis; primarily reviews statistical output or presentation of findings prepared by the primary researcher
Collaborator	Efforts to develop and conduct the research project are shared by the researcher and the statistician; ideally input from the statistician is made through all stages from research question development or refinement through final publication
Teacher	Builds off collaboration where the statistician helps the researcher learn more about statistics, data analysis, and how these can shape and be shaped by the research being conducted

Adapted from reference[51]: Kirk RE. Statistical consulting in a university: dealing with people and other challenges. Am Stat. 1991;45(1):28-34.

research question is or what it should be. While the statistician in a collaborator role can provide guidance on refining the research questions or developing the initial question when consulted from the very beginning of the project, statisticians may lack the disciplinary or content knowledge to know what is novel, important, or relevant in your area.[52] This is something that you must bring as the researcher. Similarly, the statistician cannot design the study for you. While they can provide important input on the relative advantages or disadvantages of various approaches, the study design needs to be linked to the research question. Statisticians can help with determining target sample sizes, but this requires information from you as the researcher, such as the expected differences or associations to be detected and an idea of the amount of variability in the quantities being measured.[34] In cases where general rules of thumb are used for sample size estimates,[53] statisticians can often provide insight into whether those general approaches hold true or if more in-depth approaches are required. A final example of what statisticians cannot do is to generate statistically significant findings from your data. Researchers may be tempted to send their data files to a statistician with a request to "make the data significant." This happens with surprising frequency and is a common source of frustration for many statisticians. The goal of any statistical analysis is not simply to find some statistically significant result. Instead, the goal is to use statistical tools to make sense of the available data in an attempt to answer a specific research question.[54] Asking a statistician to find something significant is at best inappropriate and at worst insulting even if it was not the intent. Be cognizant that statisticians, like pharmacists, have a set of professional ethics that guides their decision-making and behavior.[55] Requests for **p-hacking**[56] (i.e., trying multiple analytical approaches until one arrives at a desired or pleasing result, usually meaning one that is statistically significant; may also be called data-snooping, fishing, or significance-chasing) should not be made.

Ideally, the involvement of a statistician is pursued as early in the research process as possible.[52,57,58] While it is tempting to wait until you arrive at the point of data analysis or even the development of your data analysis plan, the statistician may have valuable insight into issues related to the research project in general. The type of input a statistician may have will look different depending on the stage of the research project. In the design stage, that is, anything before data collection has started, the statistician may offer insight into study design, the selection and measurement of important variables, and even focusing or clarifying the research question.[59] These efforts at clarifying the research question cannot be overemphasized. As John W. Tukey (of Honestly Significant Difference fame) said, "Far better an approximate answer to the right question, which is often vague, than an exact answer to the wrong question, which can always be made precise."[60] Once data have been collected, a statistician may be able to assist with performing the statistical analyses; however, the actual analysis plan should be developed prior to data collection. Keep in mind that statisticians may only be able to provide bad news if their first involvement is at this stage. If substantial problems are identified, there is little that can be done to change the study at this point beyond collecting new data on the topic or starting over from the beginning with a new question.[61] After the analysis is complete, especially if you conducted the analysis yourself, the statistician may be able to assist with interpreting the output of the statistical tests, presenting the results, and responding to reviewer comments if a manuscript has been submitted for publication.

Meeting with the statistician may seem anxiety-inducing, but it need not be. De Muth[62] provides guidance on how to prepare for your first meeting. Generally speaking, you should understand your research objective(s), be prepared to discuss the data that you plan to collect,[b] and have an idea of the differences or relationships you wish to assess based on your research objectives. It is a good idea to provide a brief overview or background of your research project to the statistician prior to the first meeting. This could be an abstract from your Institutional Review Board submission or a summary from a grant proposal if available. Providing key published articles also may be beneficial; this may include relevant articles in the content area or possibly other published research that reports the results of analyses of similar data. This overview will help orient the statistician to the project. Try to avoid a meeting without first providing background information to the statistician. This will make the meeting more efficient. The statistician may also have questions for you, such as other important variables (e.g., mediators, moderators, confounders) that may influence the differences or

---

[b] If you have any information on how certain measures you are using are scored, like a measurement scale for quality of life, it would be very helpful to share that information.

relationships you are trying to assess or information on previous results in the area that may be important for sample size estimation.

Remember that collaboration is built on open communication, so be clear and honest about expected contributions from each side during the meeting. As noted earlier, the statistician may have limited knowledge of the clinical conditions or the practice settings related to the research project. Similarly, you or your research mentor may have limited technical knowledge about the statistical approaches necessary for the project, which may have motivated you to seek statistical help in the first place. Rather than being perceived as limitations or drawbacks to the project, this collaboration can play to the strengths of the parties involved where content knowledge of you and your research mentor is complemented by the technical knowledge of the statistician. For insight into the training of applied statisticians regarding how they can be effective statistical collaborators, see Sharp, Griffith, and Higgs.[63]

One final important consideration when working with a statistician is how the statistician's efforts will be recognized.[64] In ideal situations where the statistician is involved throughout the research project, their services can be included in a grant proposal to provide financial support for the statistician's efforts.[65] This may not be the case for small grants often sought by trainees; however, this is certainly an expectation for larger grants from external sponsors like government agencies, nonprofit organizations, or the biopharmaceutical industry. Funding is not the only way to recognize the assistance of a statistician. When a statistician makes substantial contributions to the project and a manuscript is submitted for publication, the individual(s) providing statistical assistance should be included as an author if the criteria for authorship are met[64,65] (see also Chapter 24). When the statistician does not meet the criteria for authorship, their efforts should still be included as an acknowledgement in the paper. Unfortunately, this has not been applied consistently in the past.[66] Discussions surrounding funding, authorship, or other recognition should happen early in the collaboration process and be revisited as necessary over time. Expecting the statistician to provide any amount of effort without appropriate recognition in some form is inappropriate and could potentially be unethical. At the very least, failure to provide appropriate recognition may result in a lack of support from that statistician on future projects.

Best Practices for Learners Related to Statistical Collaboration

As with any form of collaboration, statistical collaboration is a bidirectional process involving active participation from all involved.[67] It is important to approach your interactions with the statistician as a collaborative effort rather than someone who is filling a technical or service provider role for you in the conduct of your research project. There are several key characteristics that make statistical collaboration successful for learners in particular. First, there should be a focus on learning and skills development. This is something that you may want as a learner. This should be conveyed to the collaborating statistician. Second, the collaboration should involve active support and guidance. This should come from both the collaborating statistician and your research mentor, especially if this is a different individual than the statistician. There should be regular and open communication between all parties involved. This may involve discussions of data collection and measurement processes, especially when the statistician is involved early in the research process. It could also involve discussion surrounding the development of a data analysis plan or assistance in interpreting the results of statistical analyses. Third, the collaboration should focus on the process, not just the product. The successful collaboration should involve more than the statistician simply sharing statistical output by email or providing a statistical analysis paragraph for a manuscript. A final characteristic is the availability and willingness of all involved parties to engage in the research process. This may be an important consideration to raise early in the collaboration. If you are seeking to learn and want close guidance in the process but the statistician cannot provide that, then you may need to consider seeking an alternate individual. The same can be said of your research mentor. This collaboration should result in a good research product while providing important educational benefits to you. This is why everybody must be committed to the collaboration—the statistician, the research mentor, and the learner.

Formal, consensus-derived best practices for statistical collaboration may not exist. Based on our experience as collaborating statisticians and research mentors, we can make some general recommendations for learners to consider during statistical collaboration. These include being clear on your desired learning outcomes early in the collaboration, being prepared to ask plenty of questions, not being afraid to make mistakes, and performing the work in tandem with the statistician. Table 7–6 provides these recommendations with brief discussions of the underlying motivation.

Future of Statistics Training in Pharmacy Education

Advanced and sophisticated statistical methods are becoming more and more common in practitioner-oriented journals.[68] In addition, practice-based research more frequently requires the use of complex analytical approaches to appropriately address research questions. In pharmacy education, the focus of the mastery of statistical competencies is often on preparing student pharmacists to be evidence consumers rather than evidence generators, and this is appropriate as an entry-level skill. Some elective experiences for

TABLE 7-6. RECOMMENDATIONS FOR LEARNERS DURING STATISTICAL COLLABORATION

Recommendation	Reasoning
Identify your desired learning outcome(s)	• In addition to obtaining statistical support, this should be a learning experience
	• Discuss what you hope to learn with your mentor and the statistician early in the process as this may influence the nature of the interactions
	• Wanting to learn to interpret statistical output vs. learning how to perform more complex data manipulation and analysis may require considerably different approaches and time commitments from the statistician
	• The desired outcome(s) can change, so be open and ready to revisit these as needed
Ask lots of questions	• Performing statistical analyses is both science and art
	• As with any process that comes with experience, the statistician may have internal thought processes that are not readily evident to you as a learner
	• Asking questions can help you learn about the analysis being performed and better understand the thought process of the statistician
Don't be afraid to make mistakes	• Decision making in statistical analysis does not often involve options that are completely "right" or "wrong"
	• Inappropriate or less than ideal decisions may result in undesirable or misleading conclusions
	• When collaborating with a statistician, you have an important source of support who can help identify and avoid any major mistakes
	• Making mistakes can be a useful means of learning, especially when discussing those mistakes with someone who has more experience, such as your statistician collaborator
Perform the work in tandem	• Learning data analysis is very much a hands-on process
	• Similar to your patient care training, you cannot learn these skills effectively by only watching somebody else perform the tasks
	• You may start by watching the statistician perform the analysis, but engaging in the work in tandem followed by comparison of the steps and outputs is extremely important

student pharmacists have provided additional learning opportunities with respect to statistical competencies needed for pharmacy research learners.[69] Postgraduate training can provide additional opportunities to enhance statistical competencies needed for pharmacy practice-based research.[c] However, statistical training for pharmacy residents

---

[c] Please note that the discussion contained in this section refers to PharmD education and training, rather than PhD programs in the pharmaceutical sciences. PhD programs usually have requirements for statistics education and training built into their curricula and the requirement of a doctoral dissertation usually requires a certain level of statistical competence or the involvement of such experts on a PhD student's dissertation committee.

is often limited, and residency program directors generally are not confident in the ability of residents to conduct their own statistical analyses for research projects.[70] Pharmacy residents themselves have been shown to have poor knowledge of biostatistics.[2]

All of this suggests that what is being taught in pharmacy education differs from what is actually needed by pharmacy research learners. There may be some success with structured residency research training programs with a greater focus on statistical knowledge and skills, but these activities require the availability of the necessary human resources (i.e., qualified experts to lead the training) and statistical software resources in addition to a willingness to dedicate time to such activities in an already busy resident training schedule.[70] Programs may be able to use local experts at their institutions to offer such training or even encourage online statistical training options.[70]

While these are all worthwhile approaches to consider, it is informative to consider two other questions that can help to advance this discussion: (1) What is the level of mastery needed for pharmacy research learners? (2) Are there people who can serve to help bridge the gap between advanced, sophisticated, specialized statistical knowledge/skills and that which is fundamental to the success of end-users, whether those be pharmacy evidence consumers or pharmacy evidence generators? Regarding the first question, Oster and Enders[1] describe a decade-long process undertaken to develop statistical competencies for medical research learners that can be used to guide curricular development, assessment, and improvement efforts. These competencies can serve as the basis for a similar exercise in pharmacy, but there may be a need for other competencies that may be more specific to pharmacy research learners, such as bioequivalence testing, the measurement of medication adherence, or the calculation and communication of risk concepts. But what is more relevant to this discussion is the explicit recognition by Oster and Enders that not every medical research learner is required to have the same level of competency in statistics. They state, "CTS [clinical and translational science] learners who intend to become independent principal investigators require more specialized training, while those intending to become informed consumers of the medical literature require more fundamental education."[1] They go on to state that, "our work has shown that learners who will be principal investigators require a higher level of understanding than those who will be coinvestigators."[1] The same arguments can be made regarding pharmacy research learners and also suggests the need for targeted approaches to statistical learning for this important group of people. But how should this be done, and who should be tasked with carrying this out?

That is where the second question asked earlier becomes relevant. Here again, it is helpful to look for guidance from our colleagues in other disciplines who have similarly struggled with related issues. In writing about the training of graduate students in educational psychology regarding sophisticated and advanced statistical methods, Muthén notes a lack of individuals "who can bridge the gap between the [statistical] theory provided and the intelligent use of these methods in practice."[50] Muthén calls these people **bridgers** and goes on to discuss the educational and training requirements for those who can serve as low-level and high-level bridgers between statistical theorists and users.[50] A similar case can be made for the need for bridgers in pharmacy. In some locations, there are "home-grown, pharmacy-educated" bridgers, while in other places, people seek assistance from those who are often outside of pharmacy (e.g., PhD-level or Master's-level biostatisticians in a School of Public Health). Such individuals are critical for advancing the statistical competencies of pharmacy research learners, whether for those interested in being evidence generators or better evidence consumers. Bridgers may be responsible for offering a structured training curriculum that enhances statistical competencies while also working with learners in the planning and execution of their research.

Some of these individuals already exist in pharmacy. For example, drug information specialists may serve as low-level bridgers (and maybe higher depending on the situation and their training). Substantive-area researchers with general research training and those who have emphasized methodological and statistical interests as part of their education and training may serve as low-level or high-level bridgers. In many schools/colleges of pharmacy, economic, social and administrative pharmacy (ESAP) faculty serve in these roles to varying degrees. Some ESAP faculty members may actually conduct methodological research, contributing new approaches to generate knowledge, especially in the area of pharmacoeconomics and, to a lesser extent, pharmacoepidemiology. There are even those in pharmacy who supplement their pharmacy education with statistics education and training and become PhD-level or Master's-level statisticians, biostatisticians, or psychometricians, although there are significantly fewer of these individuals. Within and across each of these categories of bridgers, you may find varying degrees of statistical competencies, with some having notable specialized skills and knowledge. Although bridgers do exist in pharmacy, the demand is certainly greater than the supply.

The two important takeaways of this discussion are that: (1) depending on the question, pharmacy research learners may not always need to seek a PhD-level biostatistician for advice and guidance, and (2) pharmacy as a profession should focus on the development of bridgers to overcome the challenges associated with limited functional statistical knowledge and abilities to appropriately use statistical analysis software in the education and training of pharmacy research learners. There is a need for educational paths for bridgers to develop their knowledge and skills, and there is also a need for viable career paths within health systems and educational institutions for such individuals. Having someone serve in multiple roles may be beneficial in some situations, but it may not be advantageous to fully realize the potential of a bridger with respect to enhancing the contributions of pharmacy research learners to the biomedical and pharmacy literature. Consideration should be given to paths to promotion, roles and responsibilities, and funding. Muthén[50] recommends a Master's degree in applied statistics (e.g., biostatistics) for high-level bridgers in educational psychology, and this seems appropriate for pharmacy as well. Perhaps pharmacy as a profession can encourage those with the capacity and interest to explore dual degrees during pharmacy residency programs.[71] Developing new programs within colleges/schools of pharmacy is possible but requires a clear vision for the required competencies to be achieved (both breadth and depth) as well as a critical mass of qualified faculty. Newsome et al. state that "statistical training should not be an afterthought in the residency process."[70] We wholeheartedly agree and extend the sentiment beyond the residency process to the entire pharmacy research infrastructure.

Summary and Conclusions

Data analysis is an important part of the research process. Managing and analyzing research data can be overwhelming for both learners and experienced researchers. Fortunately, there are many resources available to make this less stressful. Using the research data lifecycle can provide a useful guiding framework to approach research data management. Careful consideration of data needs and potential data use early in the research planning process can save time and frustration later. Involving a statistician can also make the data analysis process more efficient and effective. Learners at all levels can gain a great deal of experience and develop increased confidence in their own research skills by taking part in data analysis and data management.

Key Points and Advice

- Research data are a vital part of any research project, so they must be managed appropriately.
- Developing formal data management plans is becoming a recommended best practice.
- Data analysis plans are a key part of research and must be carefully developed prior to data collection.
- A wide variety of software is available to facilitate data analysis; consultation with research mentors or statisticians can help identify potential software to use for your project.
- Collaboration with statisticians can strengthen a research project, but they should be involved as early as possible in the research development process.

Chapter Review Questions

1. What are the various stages of the research data management lifecycle?
2. Briefly describe the FAIR principles as they relate to sharing research data.
3. Why is it important to develop a data analysis plan early in the research process?
4. What are the major components of a data analysis plan?
5. What are some major considerations when selecting a statistical analysis technique?
6. What are some major considerations when selecting statistical software?
7. Describe how the questions a statistician asks may change depending on the stage of the research process (e.g., from research development to data collection to data analysis to reporting or dissemination)?

Online Resources

- Registry of Research Data Repositories. https://www.re3data.org
- NIH Office of Science Policy: Scientific Data Management. https://osp.od.nih.gov/scientific-sharing/scientific-data-management/
- Data Documentation Initiative (DDI) Alliance. https://ddialliance.org/
- Data Management Plan (DMP) Tool. https://dmptool.org/
- SticiGui. https://www.stat.berkeley.edu/~stark/SticiGui/index.htm
- Statistical Consulting Services at the UCLA Institute for Digital Research and Education. https://stats.idre.ucla.edu/

REFERENCES

1. Oster RA, Enders FT. The importance of statistical competencies for medical research learners. *J Stat Educ.* 2018;26(2):137-142. doi:10.1080/10691898.2018.1484674
2. Bookstaver PB, Miller AD, Felder TM, Tice DL, Norris LB, Sutton SS. Assessing pharmacy residents' knowledge of biostatistics and research study design. *Ann Pharmacother.* 2012;46(7-8):991-999. doi:10.1345/aph.1Q772
3. Aparasu RR, Bentley JP, eds. *Principles of Research Design and Drug Literature Evaluation.* 2nd ed. New York: McGraw Hill Education; 2020.
4. Bentley JP. Statistical Analysis. In: Aparasu RR, ed. *Research Methods for Pharmaceutical Practice and Policy.* London: Pharmaceutical Press; 2011: 179-202.
5. Bentley JP. Biostatistics and pharmacoepidemiology. In: Yang Y, West-Strum D, eds. *Understanding Pharmacoepidemiology.* New York: McGraw Hill; 2011: 79-104.
6. DiCenzo R. *Clinical Pharmacist's Guide to Biostatistics and Literature Evaluation.* 2nd ed. Lenexa, KS: American College of Clinical Pharmacy; 2015.

7. Sutton SS, Cummings T. Chapter 71. Statistics. In: Sutton SS, ed. *McGraw Hill's NAPLEX® Review Guide*. 3rd ed. New York: McGraw-Hill Education; 2019.

8. NIH Data Sharing Policy and Implementation Guidance. National Institutes of Health. Updated November 3, 2020. Accessed February 15, 2021. https://grants.nih.gov/grants/policy/data_sharing/data_sharing_guidance.htm

9. Final NIH Policy for Data Management and Sharing. National Institutes of Health. Published October 29, 2020. Accessed February 15, 2021. https://grants.nih.gov/grants/guide/notice-files/NOT-OD-21-013.html

10. Fecher B, Friesike S. Open science: one term, five schools of thought. In: Bartling S, Friesike S, eds. *Opening Science*. Springer; 2014: 17-47.

11. McKiernan EC, Bourne PE, Brown CT, et al. How open science helps researchers succeed. *eLife*. 2016;5:e16800. doi:10.7554/eLife.16800

12. Higgins S. The DCC Curation Lifecycle Model. *International Journal of Digital Curation*. 2008;3(1):134-140. doi:10.2218/ijdc.v3i1.48

13. Ingram C. How and Why You Should Manage Your Research Data: A Guide for Researchers. Joint Information Systems Committee. Published January 7, 2016. Accessed February 24, 2021. https://www.jisc.ac.uk/guides/how-and-why-you-should-manage-your-research-data

14. Pennock M. Digital curation and the management of digital library cultural heritage resources. *The Local Studies Librarian*. 2006;25(2):3-7.

15. Strasser C, Cook R, Michener W, Budden A. Primer on Data Management: What You Always Wanted to Know (But Were Afraid to Ask). DataONE; 2012. https://old.dataone.org/sites/all/documents/DataONE_BP_Primer_020212.pdf

16. Surkis A, Read K. Research data management. *J Med Libr Assoc*. 2015;103(3):154-156. doi:10.3163/1536-5050.103.3.011

17. Harpe SE. Using secondary data sources for pharmacoepidemiology and outcomes research. *Pharmacotherapy*. 2009;29(2):138-153. doi:10.1592/phco.29.2.138

18. Schneeweiss S, Avorn J. A review of uses of health care utilization databases for epidemiologic research on therapeutics. *J Clin Epidemiol*. 2005;58(4):323-337. doi:10.1016/j.jclinepi.2004.10.012

19. Wilkinson MD, Dumontier M, Aalbersberg IJJ, et al. The FAIR Guiding Principles for scientific data management and stewardship. *Sci Data*. 2016;3:160018. doi:10.1038/sdata.2016.18

20. GO FAIR initiative. GO FAIR International Support and Coordination Office. Accessed February 15, 2021. https://www.go-fair.org/go-fair-initiative/

21. Austin Z, Sutton J. Qualitative research: getting started. *Can J Hosp Pharm*. 2014;67(6):436-440. doi:10.4212/cjhp.v67i6.1406

22. Sutton J, Austin Z. Qualitative research: data collection, analysis, and management. *Can J Hosp Pharm*. 2015;68(3):226-231. doi:10.4212/cjhp.v68i3.1456

23. Goodin A, Blumenschein K. Measurement and descriptive analysis. In: Aparasu RR, Bentley JP, eds. *Principles of Research Design and Drug Literature Evaluation*. 2nd ed. New York: McGraw Hill; 2020: 117-130.

24. Harpe SE. Interpretation and basic statistical concepts. In: Aparasu RR, Bentley JP, eds. *Principles of Research Design and Drug Literature Evaluation*. 2nd ed. New York: McGraw Hill; 2020: 87-101.

25. Slack MK. Bivariate analysis and comparing groups. In: Aparasu RR, Bentley JP, eds. *Principles of Research Design and Drug Literature Evaluation*. 2nd ed. New York: McGraw Hill; 2020: 103-115.

26. Friesner D, Bentley JP. Simple and multiple linear regression. In: Aparasu RR, Bentley JP, eds. *Principles of Research Design and Drug Literature Evaluation*. 2nd ed. New York: McGraw Hill; 2020: 75-85.

27. Bentley JP, Friesner D. Logistic regression and survival analysis. In: Aparasu RR, Bentley JP, eds. *Principles of Research Design and Drug Literature Evaluation*. 2nd ed. New York: McGraw Hill; 2020: 131-138.

28. Kauffman YS, Witt DM. Using biostatistics and analyzing quantitative data. In: Kauffman YS, Witt DM, eds. *The Essential Guide to Pharmacy Residency Research*. Bethesda, MD: American Society of Health-System Pharmacists; 2020: 75-90.

29. Kauffman YS, King J. Interpreting study findings. In: Kauffman YS, Witt DM, eds. *The Essential Guide to Pharmacy Residency Research*. Bethesda, MD: American Society of Health-System Pharmacists; 2020: 91-101.

30. Banks E, Paige E, Mather T. Developing a Quantitative Data Analysis Plan for Observational Studies. Australian National University College of Medicine, Biology & Environment. Updated November 25, 2013. Accessed September 1, 2021. https://rsph. anu.edu.au/files/Data_Analysis_Plan_Guide_20131125_0.pdf

31. Creating an Analysis Plan. Centers for Disease Control and Prevention (CDC). Published 2013. Accessed September 1, 2021. https://www.cdc.gov/globalhealth/healthprotection/ fetp/training_modules/9/creating-analysis-plan_pw_final_09242013.pdf

32. Thabane L, Mbuagbaw L, Zhang S, et al. A tutorial on sensitivity analyses in clinical trials: the what, why, when and how. *BMC Med Res Methodol*. 2013;13:92. doi:10.1186/1471-2288-13-92

33. de Souza RJ, Eisen RB, Perera S, et al. Best (but oft-forgotten) practices: sensitivity analyses in randomized controlled trials. *Am J Clin Nutr*. 2016;103(1):5-17. doi:10.3945/ ajcn.115.121848

34. Bentley JP. Sample size and power analysis. In: Aparasu RR, Bentley JP, eds. *Principles of Research Design and Drug Literature Evaluation*. 2nd ed. New York: McGraw Hill; 2020: 139-150.

35. Hair JF, Black WC, Babin BJ, Anderson RE. *Multivariate Data Analysis*. 8th ed. Andover, Hampshire, United Kingdom: Cengage Learning; 2019.

36. Simpson SH. Creating a data analysis plan: what to consider when choosing statistics for a study. *Can J Hosp Pharm*. 2015;68(4):311-317. doi:10.4212/cjhp.v68i4.1471

37. Tabachnick BG, Fidell LS. *Using Multivariate Statistics*. 7th ed. New York: Pearson Education; 2019.

38. White SE. *Basic & Clinical Biostatistics*. 5th ed. New York: McGraw Hill Education; 2020.

39. Quantitative Analysis Guide: Choose Statistical Test for 1 Dependent Variable. NYU Data Services. Accessed August 30, 2021. https://guides.nyu.edu/quant/choose_test_1DV

40. Choosing the Correct Statistical Test in SAS, Stata, SPSS and R. UCLA: Statistical Consulting Group. Accessed August 30, 2021. https://stats.idre.ucla.edu/other/mult-pkg/whatstat/

41. Bounthavong M, Watanabe JH, Sullivan KM. Approach to addressing missing data for electronic medical records and pharmacy claims data research. *Pharmacotherapy*. 2015;35(4):380-387. doi:10.1002/phar.1569

42. Mirzaei A, Carter SR, Patanwala AE, Schneider CR. Missing data in surveys: key concepts, approaches, and applications. *Res Social Adm Pharm*. 2022;18(2)2308-2316. doi:10.1016/j.sapharm.2021.03.009

43. Narayan SW, Yu Ho K, Penm J, et al. Missing data reporting in clinical pharmacy research. *Am J Health Syst Pharm*. 2019;76(24):2048-2052. doi:10.1093/ajhp/zxz245

44. Zhang N. Methodological progress note: handling missing data in clinical research. *J Hosp Med*. 2020;14(4):237-239. doi:10.12788/jhm.3330

45. Grace-Martin K. SPSS, SAS, R, Stata, JMP? Choosing a Statistical Software Package or Two. The Analysis Factor. Accessed September 6, 2021. https://www.theanalysisfactor.com/choosing-statistical-software/

46. Quantitative Analysis Guide: Which Statistical Software to Use? NYU Data Services. Accessed September 6, 2021. https://guides.nyu.edu/quant/statsoft

47. t Test Calculator. GraphPad. Accessed September 7, 2021. https://www.graphpad.com/quickcalcs/ttest1/?format=SD

48. For a 2x2 Contingency Table. VassarStats. Accessed September 7, 2021. http://vassarstats.net/tab2x2.html

49. Steiger JH. Driving fast in reverse. *J Am Stat Assoc*. 2001;96(453):331-338. doi:10.1198/016214501750332893

50. Muthén B. Teaching students of educational psychology new sophisticated statistical techniques. In: Wittrock MC, Farley F, eds. *The Future of Educational Psychology*. Hillsdale, NJ: Lawrence Erlbaum Associates; 1989: 181-189.

51. Kirk RE. Statistical consulting in a university: dealing with people and other challenges. *Am Stat*. 1991;45(1):28. doi:10.2307/2685235

52. Hall M, Richardson T, Berry JG, Ambroggio L, Shah SS, Roberts KB. Collaborating with a statistician: bringing a clinical perspective to statistics. *Hosp Pediatr*. 2016;6(12):750-752. doi:10.1542/hpeds.2016-0054

53. Van Belle G. *Statistical Rules of Thumb*. 2nd ed. Wiley; 2008.

54. Abelson RP. *Statistics as Principled Argument*. L. Erlbaum Associates; 1995.

55. Ethical Guidelines for Statistical Practice. American Statistical Association. Published April 14, 2018. Accessed August 26, 2021. https://www.amstat.org/asa/files/pdfs/EthicalGuidelines.pdf

56. Head ML, Holman L, Lanfear R, Kahn AT, Jennions MD. The extent and consequences of p-hacking in science. *PLoS Biol*. 2015;13(3). doi:10.1371/journal.pbio.1002106

57. Li L. Collaboration with Biostatisticians: Why, How, When, and Where. American Society for Cell Biology. Published December 18, 2018. Accessed February 24, 2021. https:// www.ascb.org/careers/collaboration-with-biostatisticians-why-how-when-and-where/

58. Li Z, Wang X, Barnhart HX, Wang Y. Working with statisticians in clinical research. *Stroke.* 2018;49(11):e311-e313. doi:10.1161/STROKEAHA.118.022266

59. Hand DJ. Deconstructing statistical questions. *J R Stat Soc Ser A Stat Soc.* 1994;157(3):317-356. doi:10.2307/2983526

60. Tukey JW. The future of data analysis. *Ann Math Statist.* 1962;33(1):1-67. doi:10.1214/aoms/1177704711

61. Carley S, Lecky F. Statistical consideration for research. *Emerg Med J.* 2003;20(3):258-262. doi:10.1136/emj.20.3.258

62. De Muth JE. Preparing for the first meeting with a statistician. *Am J Health Syst Pharm.* 2008;65(24):2358-2366. doi:10.2146/ajhp070007

63. Sharp JL, Griffith EH, Higgs MD. Setting the stage: Statistical collaboration videos for training the next generation of applied statisticians. *Journal of Statistics and Data Science Education.* 2021:1-11. doi:10.1080/26939169.2021.1934202

64. Perkins SM, Bacchetti P, Davey CS, et al. Best practices for biostatistical consultation and collaboration in academic health centers. *Am Stat.* 2016;70(2):187-194. doi:10.1080/00031305.2015.1077727

65. Parker RA, Berman NG. Criteria for authorship for statisticians in medical papers. *Stat Med.* 1998;17(20):2289-2299. doi:10.1002/(sici)1097-0258(19981030)17:20<2289::aid-sim931>3.0.co;2-l

66. Altman DG, Goodman SN, Schroter S. How statistical expertise is used in medical research. *JAMA.* 2002;287(21):2817-2820. doi:10.1001/jama.287.21.2817

67. Moses L, Louis TA. Statistical consulting in clinical research: the two-way street. *Stat Med.* 1984;3(1):1-5. doi:10.1002/sim.4780030102

68. Arnold LD, Braganza M, Salih R, Colditz GA. Statistical trends in the *Journal of the American Medical Association* and implications for training across the continuum of medical education. *PLoS ONE.* 2013;8(10). doi:10.1371/journal.pone.0077301

69. Lichvar AB, Smith Condeni M, Pierce DR. Preparing pharmacy trainees for a future in research and contributing to the medical literature. *J Am Coll Clin Pharm.* 2021;4:71-80. doi:10.1002/jac5.1320

70. Newsome C, Ryan K, Bakhireva L, Sarangarm P. Breadth of statistical training among pharmacy residency programs across the United States. *Hosp Pharm.* 2017;53(2):101-106. doi:10.1177/0018578717746416

71. Shannon SB, Bradley-Baker LR, Truong H. Pharmacy residencies and dual degrees as complementary or competitive advanced training opportunities. *Am J Pharm Educ.* 2012;76(8)145. doi: https://doi.org/10.5688/ajpe768145

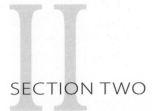

SECTION TWO

CONDUCTING PRACTICE-BASED RESEARCH

Chapter Eight

Case Reports and Case Series in Pharmacy

Katie E. Barber, PharmD and Jamie L. Wagner, PharmD, BCPS

Chapter Objectives

- Define case reports and case series in pharmacy settings
- Discuss various sources for case reports and case series in pharmacy settings
- Identity common research questions in case reports and case series
- Understand the practical and technical considerations for case reports and case series
- Discuss the strategies for harnessing the expertise needed for conducting case reports and case series
- Describe an example of learner-involved case reports or case series project
- Understand the dissemination framework for case reports and case series

Key Terminology

Case reports, case series

Introduction

Case reports and case series are used primarily to convey unique or interesting clinical scenarios that help the medical community identify new diseases, recognize rare disease manifestations, utilize new diagnostic approaches, discover the pathophysiology of a disease process, detect new side effects of medications, or prescribe alternative therapeutic treatments.[1] These studies can help identify observations that would normally be missed or overlooked in larger clinical trials. The Food and Drug Administration encourages reporting of these observations to aid in documenting post-marketing experiences using the FDA *MedWatch* Portal.[2] Therefore, case reports and case series should be educational and provide useful, practical, and easy-to-follow instructions for others to accurately identify the scenario described.

The use of case reports and case studies in pharmacy literature is abundant. A simple search in Pubmed/MEDLINE with the terms "case report" or "case series" and "pharmacy" returns over 150,000 articles published in peer-reviewed journals. Unfortunately, case reports and case series are not always highly valued based on their low level in the research design hierarchy.[3,4] However, Murad et al. described an adapted hierarchy that suggests the divide between study design types is not as strict and can vary based on the information and bias contained within the report.[4] This chapter will provide a guide to understanding common research questions in case reports and case series within pharmacy practice, sources for case reports and case series, practical and technical considerations, expertise needed, and examples of learner-led reports.

Case Reports and Case Series

A case report or case series is a clinical synopsis regarding an individual patient or patients, which includes signs, symptoms, laboratory values, imaging, diagnosis, treatment, clinical outcome, and, if applicable, long-term follow-up.[5] Specifically, **case reports** contain information about a single patient in a unique scenario, whereas a **case series** describe more than one patient with similar treatment or diagnoses.[6,7] Case reports can be categorized into three different types of reports, namely diagnostic, treatment, or educational.[8] Of these, the most common are case reports that describe the management of a patient, including their treatment and outcomes in significant depth. Educational case reports often include a review of the literature, whereas diagnostic case reports focus on rare or difficult to diagnose diseases that seldom have treatment modalities. These reports generally consist of a case or scenario not already reported in the literature. Additionally, these kinds of reports are usually accompanied by a review of literature, including any other similar case reports. The main purpose of case reports is to educate providers about patients with unusual problems.[9] It is not to make claims, far-reaching conclusions, or prove anything.[8] Despite that these are typically shorter in length, standard technical writing expectations that apply to other forms of medical writing also apply to case reports/case series.

Before writing a case report or case series, authors should determine the following items:[10]

What am I going to report?
Why am I going to report this?
How should I report this?

The methodology for composing a case report or case series begins with a thorough literature evaluation to determine if the case report/case series is truly novel. Next, authors need to determine if they wish to write a retrospective or a prospective case report/case series.[8] Retrospective studies are more common and are often easiest for beginning authors. Prospective designs require significantly more planning ahead of time in order to ensure that the study process continues to progress appropriately. Most prospective case reports/case series are pharmacokinetic centric case reports that evaluate the pharmacokinetics of a drug that requires patient samples, or alternatively, they assess new management options. Once the literature has been assessed, and the timing of the study selected, accessing patient data in the medical record is the next step. Novice case report/case series authors often struggle with the next step, which is determining relevant information for the specific case report or series. As a rule of thumb, only the laboratory values, imaging, and treatment pertinent to the specific event/diagnosis should be included. The final step is formalizing this distilled information and writing it into a concise case report/case series. Authors should rely on using the CARE guidelines to help guide the format of the case report/case series, thus ensuring the essential information is included prior to submitting it for publication.[11] The CARE guidelines help authors to reduce the risk of bias in their reporting, increase the transparency of the information presented, and provide clues as to what worked for which patients under which circumstances.[11]

The biggest difference between case reports versus case series is the level of detail in the presentation section of the manuscript. While a case report presents information on one patient, a case series can vary with a range of up to 20 patients. Typically, in a case series, less information is provided for each case, with the amount of data provided dependent upon the total number of patients included. Additionally, to keep within word limitations of the journal, details on the case series patients often are included in a table as well. The information of the table typically describes the intervention, outcome, and other applicable information pending the disease state or agents utilized. Journals often have specific author instructions for the various types of literature, but the general format for case reports is fairly consistent regardless of the journal (Table 8–1).[6] Below, we will discuss specific considerations for each section of a case report/case series.

TABLE 8–1. RECOMMENDATIONS FOR INCLUDED MATERIAL IN CASE REPORTS AND CASE SERIES

Abstract

  a. Introduction and objective

  b. Case report/case series (briefly)

  c. Discussion

  d. Conclusion

Introduction (<3 paragraphs)

  a. Describe the subject matter: background information, definitions.

  b. Describe the strategy of the literature review and provide search terms.

  c. Justify the merit of the case report/case series by using the literature review.

  d. State the purpose of the case report/case series.

  e. Introduce the patient case(s) to the reader.

Patient Case(s) Presentation (in chronological order)

  a. Describe the case(s) in narrative form.

  b. Provide patient demographics (avoiding patient identifiers).

  c. Describe the chief complaint.

  d. List the present illness, medical/family/social/dietary history, and allergy history. Include the name of the drug and the date/type of allergic reaction.

  e. List and verify the medication history, including prior to admission and throughout the reporting period. Include pertinent herbals, vaccines, depot injections, nonprescription medications, and indications for all. List each drug's name, strength, dosage form, route, and dates of administration. List any adverse drug reaction history and the dates of the reaction.

  f. Provide renal and hepatic organ function data in order to determine the appropriateness of medication dosing regimens.

  g. Provide pertinent serum drug levels and include the time of each level taken and relationship to the given dose.

  h. Provide pertinent findings on physical examination.

  i. Provide pertinent laboratory values that support the case.

  j. Provide the reference range for laboratory values that are not widely known or established.

  k. List the completed diagnostic procedures that are pertinent and support the case; paraphrase the pertinent results of the procedures.

  l. Provide photographs of histopathology, roentgenograms, electrocardiograms, skin manifestations, or anatomy as related to the case.

  m. Obtain permission from the patient to use the patient's photographs.

  n. Ensure that the presentation provides sufficient detail to establish the case's validity.

Discussion and Conclusion

  a. Compare and contrast the nuances of the report with the literature review through explaining or justifying the similarities and differences.

  b. List the limitations of the report and describe their relevance.

  c. Confirm the accuracy of the report by establishing a temporal and causal relationship (see Naranjo Scale).

  d. Summarize the main take-home points of the report while also justifying its uniqueness.

  e. Draw evidence-based recommendations and justified conclusions.

  f. Describe how the information learned applies to practice.

  g. List opportunities for future research.

ABSTRACT CONSIDERATIONS

An abstract of a case report may be required by some journals, but this should only be a brief synopsis of what is to come in the full case. Typically, this type of abstract should include the rationale for why the case or information is unique and valuable, a brief synopsis of the case to be reported, and a summary with or without needed future directions.

INTRODUCTION

This portion of a case report should be kept to a minimum. This is in part because little data should exist on the topic, but also because these reports often have word count restrictions. This section should generally be a simple introduction into what the disease state or therapeutic agent that was involved. In addition, addressing the gap in published literature is appropriate. The end of the introduction should lead logically into the patient case.

CASE PRESENTATION

The goal of this section is to provide details from the initial case presentation and describe pertinent details of what happens to the patient over their course of admission. This section should follow the flow of the patient from hospital admission to discharge or death. If the patient was from an outpatient setting, a thorough history preceding the index event should also be provided. The case description should begin with the initial patient presentation, including initial physical examination, laboratory, imaging, and other findings before proceeding to the patient's clinical progression. Patient clinical progress should also include chronological updates on the aforementioned values, as well as pertinent medication therapy updates. The reader should be able to understand why certain procedures were performed and medications administered. For certain disease states, the inclusion of pictures is often beneficial. However, if pictures are included, it is imperative to protect the confidentiality of the patient by not showing patient identifiers, i.e., blurring the face, including eyes, tattoos or scars, would be needed. Additionally, many journals require written patient consent before allowing authors to include pictures.

DISCUSSION

The discussion should contain two key elements. First, if there are similar case reports, they should be described briefly and compared. Second, the authors should provide further explanation to describe why certain decisions were made in the patient case. The discussion should conclude with recommendations on what readers should do or now take into consideration as a result of this novel case report or case series. All case reports should include references throughout the discussion; however, the list should be relatively small compared to other types of published literature.

Common Research Questions in Case Reports and Case Series

As opposed to many chapters in this text, case reports and case series often focus on noticing unique clinical cases rather than developing formal research questions. Prospective case reports are the exception, as mentioned previously, and commonly involve noticing gaps in pharmacokinetic drug data in special populations or common use scenarios which may be useful to improving understanding or developing best practices for medication use. It is likely more helpful for readers to identify research questions that have been answered to more accurately place case series and case reports in the literature.

Many research questions can be answered through case reports and case series. Examples include offering new insights into disease pathogenesis, describing unusual clinical features or mechanisms of a disease that add to previously known information, describing improved procedures which may result in more formal research, reporting unusual drug interactions, and describing patient adverse reactions to care.[8] One of the most common types of research questions answered by these publications is the off-label use of medications. Given inherent limitations to the drug approval process, many agents are utilized for a variety of off-label indications once they are available to use in practice. For example, ceftaroline fosamil was originally FDA approved for the treatment of acute bacterial skin/skin structure infections.[12,13] Shortly after becoming available for use, clinicians began utilizing this agent for the treatment of bloodstream infections. Subsequently, several case series were published regarding the use of ceftaroline fosamil for the treatment of bloodstream infections.[14–17]

Other common questions answered by case reports or case series include special populations, pharmacokinetics, and atypical disease states. Special population case reports exist because, while inclusion and exclusion criteria for clinical trials are extensive, not all patients meet the criteria outlined by clinical studies. Some commonly excluded patient populations include obese patients, patients on hemodialysis, immunocompromised patients, pediatric patients, burn patients, and patients with cystic fibrosis.[18–22] Case reports become a valuable source of data to inform practice in these excluded populations and can be even more valuable and specific with combinations of excluded patients, for example pediatric patients with burns.[21] Direct-acting oral anticoagulants (DOACs) provide a great example, as when these drugs first became available, several excluded populations are either not routinely recommended DOAC treatment or offered adjusted therapy due to limited clinical trial data, i.e., patients with body mass index >40 kg/m^2 or 120 kg.[23] However, on account of published case studies expanding evidence in excluded patients, there is now data regarding the use of DOACs in obese patients,[24] immunocompromised patients,[25-27] and hemodialysis patients, which has led to larger clinical studies.[24-32] Pharmacokinetic case reports by contrast typically assess the penetration of drugs into hard-to-reach places, including the central nervous system or the bones in order to improve clinical decision making.[33-35] Lastly, case reports or case series reports often describe atypical disease states or disease presentations that are rarely observed, including patient/patients treated appropriately but who have atypical responses, including lack of improvement/failure or adverse events that have not been previously reported.[36-38] Table 8–2 offers a list of additional reasons and published examples for consideration when publishing a case report/case series.

TABLE 8–2. REASONS TO CONSIDER SUBMITTING A CASE REPORT/SERIES FOR PUBLICATION AND SUPPORTING EXAMPLES

Reason[9]	Published Example
Unusual etiology, setting, or diagnosis of a disorder	A case report of peritoneal tuberculosis: a challenging diagnosis. *Case Rep Infect Dis.* 2018;2018:4970836
Mistakes in healthcare	Overlooked guide wire: a multicomplicated Swiss Cheese Model example. Analysis of a case and review of the literature. *Acta Clin Belg.* 2020;75(3):193-199
Unreproducible information	Robust planning for a patient treated in decubitus position with proton pencil beam scanning radiotherapy. *Cureus.* 2017;9(9):e1706
Hypothesis generating and confirmation that stimulates further research	Ebola virus transmission initiated by relapse of systemic Ebola virus disease. *N Engl J Med.* 2021;384:1240-1247
Insight into disease pathogenesis	Case report: re-emerging significance of surgical embolectomy in pulmonary embolism. *Ann Med Surg (Lond).* 2018;39:26-28
Unusual clinical features	Neurobrucellosis: a case report with an unusual presentation. *Recent Pat Antiinfect Drug Discov.* 2020;epub ahead of print. doi:10.2174/15748 91X15999200917153454
Improved procedures	Minimally invasive endoscopic maxillary sinus lifting and immediate implant placement: a case report. *World J Clin Cases.* 2019;7(10):1234-1241
Drug interactions	Significant drug interaction between voriconazole and dexamethasone: a case report. *J Oncol Pharm Pract.* 2019;25(5):1239-1242
Rare adverse reactions	Case report: Albendazole associated psychosis. *Ment Health Clin.* 2019; 9(6):397-400

Practical and Technical Considerations for Case Reports and Case Series

There are several considerations that must be taken into account when writing case reports or case series. The first is determining if institutional review board (IRB) approval is needed. For IRB submissions, Collaborative Institutional Training Initiative (CITI) Program coursework will likely need to be completed (https://about.citiprogram.org/en/homepage/). Certification through the CITI Program ensures that researchers are trained to conduct research ethically and safely. Once the case report/series is approved or deemed exempt by the IRB, exploration through the patient or patients' charts can begin seeking to determine which information will be added to the report. The second consideration is the time that it will take to prepare and write the manuscript. As most case reports/case series are retrospective in nature, substantial background research must take place to ensure that the case report/case series is new and additive to the already published literature. Authors should anticipate spending approximately one to four hours researching existing literature, with another four to eight hours reading through the literature to determine which could be useful in the Introduction section versus the Discussion section of the manuscript. Ideally, in the Introduction, the authors need to frame how this case will contribute to the literature, otherwise known as "framing the gap." Some ways to achieve this include stating how big of a problem this case report/case series topic is (e.g., incidence, number of previously reported cases, and so on), how has this topic been handled previously, and how this case report/case series can expand on what is already known.

In determining which patient-specific information is pertinent to include in the Case Presentation section, authors should provide sufficient detail so that readers can easily follow the clinical course and repeat the same protocol. The case information should also be presented in chronological order to allow readers the ability to come to their own conclusions about the case's validity. It is imperative that verified sources of data are used to describe the case (e.g., visual analog pain scale, vital signs, laboratory values, imaging) as these enhance the manuscript's reliability. Authors are discouraged from including inferences on the patient case in this section. If reporting an unusual reaction, many author guidelines require the reporting of the Naranjo score.[39] This scoring system helps to determine the probability of the treatment in question being related to the reaction experienced by the patient. Given that case reports and case series are often descriptive in nature, there are usually no statistics needed.

Once all the objective case information is detailed, the Discussion section is used to explain the case in the context of existing literature, provide opinions, and expound on new information and/or applicability to clinical practice. When comparing the current case to existing literature, authors should preferentially highlight any differences to help emphasize the uniqueness of the case report/case series. Additionally, the authors should seek to prove the objectivity of their case assessment by demonstrating knowledge of the problem, including an appropriate evaluation of the case and literature supporting it.

Writing the case report should be guided by the CARE guidelines, as well as the selected journal's "Instructions for Authors". CARE-Writer (https://care-writer.com/) may help organize and format the information needed to abide by the CARE guidelines. Most journals have a word limit for case reports/case series, ranging from 500 to 2,000 words, with an average of 1,000 words. It is imperative that the CARE guidelines are followed while adhering to the word limit of the journal; therefore, first writing down all the pertinent information before cutting the manuscript to fit the word count is advised for beginners. Additionally, a research mentor can help cut down on the word count once all the information is compiled into a cohesive manuscript.

Additional considerations for publication include publication costs and other resources needed. Many journals require authors to pay publication costs upon acceptance. These can range from hundreds to thousands of dollars, depending on the journal. Publication costs are typically readily available on each journal's website. If not, in the submission process, it will be explicitly stated, and the submitter will have to agree to the costs if accepted for publication. Some journals may offer a deferral of publication costs if the authors can prove financial hardship (e.g., student-led) in paying for the submission. Lastly, resources, including personnel, may be needed for some case reports or case series. For example, some case reports include additional laboratory evaluations, such as drug concentrations or microbiological culture information.[40] This may require staff support in nursing or the microbiology or clinical laboratory, as well as supplies needed. A research mentor will be able to help guide the author through the process, as well as the CARE guidelines once the author is prepared to compile all the information into a cohesive submission.

When publishing a case series or case report, it is helpful to frame these manuscripts considering commonly noted advantages and disadvantages of this research. Some advantages to case reports and case series include inciting inquiry into a new research area, providing stronger evidence (case series), their simplistic observational methodology, educational information provided from findings, typically a quick process from identification to publication, and capturing of rare manifestations.[41] Disadvantages cited for these types of studies include their uncontrolled design, the inherent difficulty in comparing cases, limited external validity, selection bias, and missing follow-up.[41] Using these advantages and disadvantages can help researchers decide if they want to pursue a case report/case study and also may help in creating a better manuscript for submission.

Expertise Needed for Conducting Case Reports and Case Series

While no specific upfront expertise is required to start a case report or case series, it is imperative that researchers become affluent in the subject matter. Specifically, it is essential that researchers have an in-depth understanding of the disease state and pharmacologic agents discussed in the report or series. An extensive background literature search strategy must also be employed to identify any other available data. If other articles exist, authors must ensure the novelty or uniqueness portrayed in their case, or it will likely result in wasted effort and rejection after submission. Ideally, seeking out someone with expertise in diagnostic or therapeutic subject matter helps in deciding on the novelty and ultimately the ability of the case to be published. If the case meets the novelty requirement, it is logical for this expert to then take a senior role in conducting the case report or case series. This expert could be anyone in the medical profession, including nurses, pharmacists, prescribers, or clinical laboratory specialists (e.g., pathologists, technicians). While statisticians may be useful in other types of clinical studies, statistical analyses are rarely performed in case studies or series, so that expertise is not needed.

Exemplars of Learner-Involved Published Case Reports or Case Series

Case reports/case series are ideal scholarship opportunities for pharmacy students and other trainees. They are an excellent way to help develop analytical skills and enhance curiosity for scientific inquiry. Publishing a case report or case series is a great way to easily and quickly produce scholarship and gain experience in scientific writing. The following is an example of a learner-involved case series published out of the University of Mississippi School of Pharmacy.

A third professional year student expressed interest in performing research to a senior pharmacy faculty member, a research idea to examine the use of ceftriaxone in treating methicillin-susceptible *Staphylococcus aureus* (MSSA) bacteremia was proposed. The use of ceftriaxone to treat MSSA was relatively uncommon; in fact, this drug was usually not even considered by most professionals in the standard bacteremia treatment course of MSSA. However, at this institution, physicians had recently started to prescribe ceftriaxone in an effort to help facilitate early patient discharge from the hospital, as ceftriaxone is a once-daily drug. After identifying a potentially novel topic, the student performed a thorough literature search to confirm the novelty of this approach and to identify further pertinent information for the Introduction section. Based on this review, and discussions with appropriate experts, multiple gaps that could be addressed with this research were found, including a limited number of patients receiving treatment with ceftriaxone, a paucity of data surrounding the efficacy and safety of this drug when treating MSSA bacteremia, and limited data on if this treatment facilitated early hospital discharge. These three criteria are examples of framing the gap and adhere to suggested criteria for publishable case reports and case series.[6] Based on these findings, the decision was made to pursue a case series instead of a case report due to the larger number of patient cases available at the institution that had received this treatment regimen for the specified indication.

After deciding to pursue a case series, the next step was to decide which patient-specific data needed to be collected. The student was responsible for reading the literature to determine what data elements would be necessary to collect on each patient, getting documentation for IRB submission, and proceeded to collect data on 15 patients with MSSA bacteremia treated with ceftriaxone. The data were presented as a poster at the Infectious Diseases Society of America Annual Meeting in 2016 and received significant attention. Upon returning from the conference, the student was offered the chance to begin developing a case series to submit for publication. A target journal was identified, and author guidelines for submitting a case series, as well as the CARE guidelines, were followed. The case series was officially published in 2017 in the Journal of Pharmacology and Pharmacotherapeutics.[42] Spurred by this case series, several subsequent larger studies were conducted and published to help guide providers in utilizing ceftriaxone to treat MSSA bacteremia,[43,44] including a randomized controlled trial.[45]

Dissemination Considerations and Frameworks

While publishing case reports and case series might seem easy and straightforward, there are a variety of guidelines (i.e., CARE) that authors should use to reduce the risk of bias, increase transparency, and provide early guidance on what works, in whom, and under which circumstances.[6,11,46,47] Case reports and case series typically are formatted with three to four main sections: introduction, patient presentation, and the discussion with/ without conclusion. Some key concepts to make sure to discuss in the patient presentation section include de-identified patient demographics, chief complaint, past medical/ family/social history, medication history, allergy status and reactions, diagnostic procedures and findings, therapeutic interventions, and any follow-up or outcomes assessed. Strict attention must be paid to the timing of the case(s) presented, as well as the smallest

TABLE 8–3. "THINK. CHECK. SUBMIT." CHECKLIST

Do you or your colleagues know the journal?
- Have you read any articles in the journal before?
- Is it easy to discover the latest papers in the journal?
Can you easily identify and contact the publisher?
- Is the publisher name clearly displayed on the journal website?
- Can you contact the publisher by telephone, email, and post?
Is the journal clear about the type of peer review it uses?
- Does the journal site explain what these fees are for and when they will be charged?
Do you recognize the editorial board?
- Have you heard of the editorial board members?
- Do members of the editorial board mention the journal on their own websites?
Is the publisher a member of a recognized industry initiative?
- Do they belong to the COPE?
- If the journal is open access, is it listed in the DOAJ?
- If the journal is open access, does the publisher belong to the OASPA?
- Is the publisher a member of another trade association?

details (e.g., drug dose, formulation, and route). Additionally, the formatting of the case report or case series is very dependent upon the author guidelines for the target journal. A great tool to start investigating available journals is using J.A.N.E. (Journal / Author Name Estimator; https://jane.biosemantics.org/). This tool provides suggestions for possible journals to consider publishing based upon keywords typed into the suggestion box. While this is a great place to start, another method includes the "Think. Check. Submit." method (Table 8–3).[7] This checklist relies upon knowing more about the journal, either through colleagues, the publisher, the editorial board, or what organizations the journal belongs to. Knowing the publisher can be crucial in determining if the journal is reputable. The Committee on Publication Ethics (COPE) provides guidelines for publishers to abide by to sustain the current publication methods (https://publicationethics.org/guidance/Guidelines). The Open Access Scholarly Publishing Association (OASPA) is an organization that works to encourage and enable Open Access as the primary modality for publishing scholarly output (https://oaspa.org). If a journal claims to be Open Access, there should be no charge for publishing, and they should be found on the Directory of Open Access Journals (DOAJ) website (https://doaj.org).

Since 2010, there has been a stark increase in peer-reviewed journals that will exclusively publish case reports and case series.[7,48] Many journals with higher impact factors are no longer accepting case reports or case series; however, many pharmacy-specific journals still are (e.g., Journal of the American College of Clinical Pharmacy, Pharmacotherapy, Annals of Pharmacotherapy, and so on). You can visit the journal's website and examine the

"Author Guidelines" to determine if they accept these types of submissions. If they do not specify, authors can always contact the journal editor to confirm.

Summary and Conclusions

Case reports and case series provide an opportunity to enhance the medical literature through reporting of new diseases, rare disease manifestations, new diagnostic approaches, new side effects of medications, or alternative therapeutic treatments. It is imperative to ensure that all pertinent data is reported within the report/series and that IRB approval is obtained prior to publication if needed. There are many journals that accept case reports and case series, either as part of all their submissions or as the only submissions accepted. These manuscripts are a great way for students to learn more about a disease state and gain a quick publication in peer-reviewed journals.

Key Points and Advice

- Case reports and case series are a great learning experience for students' first introduction to scientific publishing.
- Knowledge of the published literature and/or utilizing a mentor are keys to identifying criteria for publishable case reports and case series.
- Sufficient clinical details, i.e., signs/symptoms, medication doses/routes, and so on, are key when drafting the case report or case series.
- Many pharmacy-related journals will accept case reports and case series, especially if the publication has the potential to spur further scientific exploration.
- J.A.N.E. and "Think. Check. Submit." are great ways to identify possible target journals to submit a case report or case series.

Chapter Review Questions

1. What are some common research areas that case reports and case series often target?
2. What are some limitations of case reports and case series?
3. What are some ways to identify an appropriate target journal when publishing a case report or case series?

4. What kinds of information should be included within the case report and case series?

5. Who are experts that can be recruited to help formulate the case report or case series to ensure all pertinent information is included?

Online Resources

- CARE-writer. https://care-writer.com/
- Scientific Writing in Health and Medicine. https://www.swihm.com/
- Naranjo Adverse Drug Reaction Probability Scale worksheet. https://www.ncbi.nlm.nih.gov/books/NBK548069/bin/Naranjoassessment.pdf

REFERENCES

1. Sun Z. Tips for writing a case report for the novice author. *J Med Rad Sci.* 2013;60(3):108-113.

2. U.S. Food and Drug Administration. MedWatch Online Voluntary Reporting Form. Accessed December 17, 2020. https://www.accessdata.fda.gov/scripts/medwatch/index.cfm

3. Murad MH, Asi N, Alsawas M, Alahdab F. New evidence pyramid. *BMJ Evid Based Med.* 2016;21(4):125-127.

4. Sayre JW, Toklu HZ, Ye F, Mazza J, Yale S. Case reports, case series – from clinical practice to evidence-based medicine in graduate medical education. *Cureus.* 2017;9(8):e1546.

5. Guidelines to writing a clinical case report. *Heart Views.* 2017;18(3):104-105.

6. Cohen H. How to write a patient case report. *Am J Health-Syst Pharm.* 2006;63(19):1888-1892.

7. Rison RA, Shepphird JK, Kidd MR. How to choose the best journal for your case report. *J Med Case Rep.* 2017;11:198.

8. Green BN, Johnson CD. How to write a case report for publication. *J Chirop Med.* 2006;2(5):72-82.

9. Peat J, Elliott E, Baur L, Keena V. *Scientific writing, easy when you know how.* London: BMJ Books; 2006: 176-178.

10. Wildsmith JAW. How to write a case report. In: Hall GM, ed. *How to Write a Paper.* 3rd ed. London: BMJ Books; 2006: 85-91.

11. CARE Group. CARE case report guidelines. 2014. Accessed December 17, 2020. https://www.care-statement.org/

12. Corey GR, Wilcox MH, Talbot GH, et al. CANVAS 1: the first phase III, randomized, double-blind study evaluating ceftaroline fosamil for the treatment of patients with complicated skin and skin structure infections. *J Antimicrob Chemother.* 2010;65(Suppl 4):iv41-iv51.

13. Wilcox MH, Corey GR, Talbot GH, et al. CANVAS 2: the second phase III, randomized, double-blind study evaluating ceftaroline fosamil for the treatment of patients with

complicated skin and skin structure infections. *J Antimicrob Chemother.* 2010;65(Suppl 4):iv53-iv65.

14. Jongsma K, Jason J, Heidari A. Ceftaroline in the treatment of concomitant methicillin-resistant and daptomycin-non-susceptible *Staphylococcus aureus* infective endocarditis and osteomyelitis: case report. *J Antimicrob Chemother.* 2013;68(6):1444-1445.

15. Ho TT, Cadena J, Childs LM, Gonzalez-Velez M, Lewis JS. Methicillin-resistant *Staphylococcus aureus* bacteraemia and endocarditis treated with ceftaroline salvage therapy. *J Antimicrob Chemother.* 2012;67(5):1267-1270.

16. Lin JC, Aung G, Thomas A, Jahng M, Johns S, Fierer J. The use of ceftaroline foasmil in methicillin-resistant *Staphylococcus aureus* endocarditis and deep-seated MRSA infections: a retrospective case series of 10 patients. *J Infect Chemother.* 2013;19(1):42-49.

17. Polenakovik HM, Pleiman CM. Ceftaroline for methicillin-resistant *Staphylococcus aureus* bacteraemia: case series and review of the literature. *Int J Antimicrob Agents.* 2013;42(5):450-455.

18. Niño-Taravilla C, Espinosa-Vielma YP, Otaola-Arca H, Poli-Harlowe C, Tapia LI, Ortiz-Fritz P. Pediatric inflammatory multisystem syndrome temporally associated with SARS-CoV-2 treated with tocilizumab. *Pediatr Rep.* 2020;12(3):142-148.

19. Zhang L, Borish L, Smith A, Somerville L, Albon D. Use of mepolizumab in adult patients with cystic fibrosis and an eosinophilic phenotype: case series. *Allergy Asthma Clin Immunol.* 2020;16:3.

20. Law N, Logan C, Yung G, et al. Successful adjunctive use of bacteriophage therapy for treatment of multidrug-resistant *Pseudomonas aeruginosa* infection in a cystic fibrosis patient. *Infection.* 2019;47(4):665-668.

21. Streetz VN, Patatanian LK. Intravenous enoxaparin in pediatric burn patients: a case series. *J Pediatr Pharmacol Ther.* 2019;24(5):456-461.

22. Gragnani A, Müller BR, Oliveira AF, Ferreira LM. Burns and epilepsy—review and case report. *Burns.* 2015;41(2):e15-:e18.

23. Martin K, Beyer-Westendorf J, Davidson BL, et al. Use of direct oral anticoagulants in obese patients: guidance from the SSC of the ISTH. *J Thromb Haemost.* 2016;14(6):1308-1313.

24. Jennings ST, Manh KNP, Bita J. Morbidly obese patient on rivaroxaban presents with recurrent upper extremity deep vein thrombosis: a case report. *J Pharm Pract.* 2020;33(5):712-719.

25. Jóźwik A, Lisik W, Czerwiński J, Kosieradzki M. Simultaneous pancreas-kidney transplantation in a patient with heparin-induced thrombocytopenia on dabigatran therapy. *Ann Transplant.* 2018;23:232-235.

26. Yamamura K, Beppu T, Kinoshita K, et al. Hepatocellular carcinoma with extensive cancer-associated thrombosis successfully treated with liver resection and direct oral anticoagulant: a case report. *Anticancer Research.* 2020;40(11):6465-6471.

27. Nakao S, Masuda T, Sakamoto S, et al. Cerebral embolism during edoxaban administration for venous thromboembolism in a patient with lung adenocarcinoma: a case report. *Medicine (Baltimore).* 2019;98(12):e14821.

28. Kalani C, Awudi E, Alexander T, Udeani G, Surani S. Evaluation of the efficacy of direct oral anticoagulants (DOACs) in comparison to warfarin in morbidly obese patients. *Hosp Pract.* 2019;47(4):181-185.

29. Netley J, Howard K, Wilson W. Effects of body mass index on the safety and effectiveness of direct oral anticoagulants: a retrospective review. *J Thromb Thrombolysis.* 2019;48(3):359-365.

30. Agnelli G, Becattini C, Meyer G, et al. Apixaban for the treatment of venous thromboembolism associated with cancer. *N Engl J Med.* 2020;382;1599-1607.

31. Farge D, Frere C. Recent advances in the treatment and prevention of venous thromboembolism in cancer patients: role of the direct oral anticoagulants and their unique challenges. *F1000Research.* 2019;8(F1000 Faculty Rev):974.

32. Kufel WD, Zayac AS, Lehmann DF, Miller CD. Clinical application and pharmacodynamic monitoring of apixaban in a patient with end-stage renal disease requiring chronic hemodialysis. *Pharmacother.* 2016;36(11):e166-e171.

33. Kullar R, Chin JN, Edwards DJ, Parker D, Coplin WM, Rybak MJ. Pharmacokinetics of single-dose daptomycin in patients with suspected or confirmed neurological infections. *Antimicrob Agents Chemother.* 2011;55(7):3505-3509.

34. Rhoney DH, Tam VH, Parker DJr, McKinnon PS, Coplin WM. Disposition of cefepime in the central nervous system of patients with external ventricular drains. *Pharmacother.* 2003;23(3):310-314.

35. Grillon A, Argemi X, Gaudias J, et al. Bone penetration of daptomycin in diabetic patients with bacterial foot infections. *Int J Infect Dis.* 2019;85:127-131.

36. Knoll BM, Hellmann M, Kotton CN. Vancomycin-resistant *Enterococcus faecium* meningitis in adults: case series and review of the literature. *Scand J Infect Dis.* 2013;45(2):131-139.

37. Rac H, Bojikian KD, Lucar J, Barber KE. Successful treatment of necrotizing fasciitis and streptococcal toxic shock syndrome with the addition of linezolid. *Case Rep Infect Dis.* 2017;2017:5720708.

38. Barber KE, Albrecht S, Stover KR. Persistent cryptococcal meningitis treated with antiretroviral therapy and alternative antifungals. *J Pharmacol Pharmacother.* 2019;10(1):35-37.

39. Naranjo CA, Busto U, Sellers EM, et al. A method for estimating the probability of adverse drug reactions. *Clin Pharacol Ther.* 1981;30(2):239-245.

40. Barber KE, Rybak MJ, Sakoulas G. Vancomycin plus ceftaroline shows potent in vitro synergy and was successfully utilized to clear persistent daptomycin-non-susceptible MRSA bacteraemia. *J Antimicrob Chemother.* 2015;70(1):311-313.

41. Ballentine C. "Sulfanilamide Disaster". FDA Consumer 1981. Accessed December 12, 2020. https://www.fda.gov/files/about%20fda/published/The-Sulfanilamide-Disaster.pdf

42. Lowe RA, Barber KE, Wagner JL, Bell-Harlan AM, Stover KR. Ceftriaxone for the treatment of methicillin-susceptible *Staphylococcus aureus* bacteremia: a case series. *J Pharmacol Pharmacother.* 2017;8(3):140-144.

43. Kamfose MM, Muriithi FG, Knight T, Lasserson D, Hayward G. Intravenous ceftriaxone versus multiple dosing regimes of intravenous anti-staphylococcal antibiotics for methicillin-susceptible *Staphylococcus aureus* (MSSA): a systematic review. *Antibiotics (Basel).* 2020;9(2):39.

44. Carr DR, Stiefel U, Bonomo RA, Burant CJ, Sims SV. A comparison of cefazolin versus ceftriaxone for the treatment of methicillin-susceptible *Staphylococcus aureus* bacteremia in a tertiary care VA medical center. *Open Forum Infect Dis.* 2018;5(5):ofy089.

45. ClinicalTrials.gov [Internet]. Bethesda (MD). National Library of Medicine (US). February 29, 2000. Identifier NCT04141787, Ceftriaxone as Home IV for Staph Infections; 2019 Oct 28 [cited 2020 Dec 18]; [about 4 screens]. https://clinicaltrials.gov/ct2/show/NCT04141787

46. Gagnier JJ, Kienle G, Altman DG, et al. The CARE guidelines: consensus-based clinical case report guideline development. *J Diet Suppl*. 2013;10(4):381-390.

47. Carey TS, Boden SD. A critical guide to case series reports. *SPINE*. 2003;28(15):1631-1634.

48. Akers KG. New journals for publishing medical case reports. *J Med Libr Assoc*. 2016; 104(2):146-149.

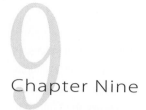

Chapter Nine

Intervention Research in Pharmacy Settings

Divya A. Varkey, PharmD, MS and
Elisabeth M. Wang, PharmD, BCCP

Chapter Objectives

- Define intervention research in pharmacy settings
- Discuss various types of interventions that can be evaluated in pharmacy settings
- Identify common research questions in intervention research in pharmacy settings
- Understand the practical considerations for intervention research in pharmacy settings
- Understand the technical considerations for intervention research in pharmacy settings
- Discuss the strategies for harnessing the expertise needed for conducting intervention research in pharmacy settings
- Describe an example of a learner-involved intervention research project in a pharmacy setting
- Understand the dissemination framework for intervention research in pharmacy settings

Key Terminology

Intervention research, medication use process, treatment fidelity, delivery arrangements, financial arrangements, governance arrangements, implementation strategy, problem theory, program theory

Introduction

Intervention research is defined as the study of systematic changes within processes and can be conducted in a wide variety of pharmacy practice settings.[1] Interventions are often used to implement a change in practice and subsequent research is conducted to determine the impact of this change. A change in practice can range from interventions that influence the use of a single medication for a specific patient population to the institution-wide implementation of a new electronic health record (EHR). Similarly, the outcomes evaluated can range broadly, from disease and health-related outcomes like the achievement of goal blood pressure to institution-wide outcomes including operational (i.e., efficient delivery of medications) and financial (medication control and supply expenses) impacts.

Pharmacy personnel, like medication and process experts, play an integral role in identifying and conducting intervention research throughout the continuum of patient care. Through intervention research, pharmacists can positively impact patient care on a larger scale—whether at a pharmacy department level, institution-wide, or even across the profession by identifying needed changes to improve health outcomes, demonstrate value, and expand patient services. One example of a positive impact on patient care is demonstrated when data analysis confirms that the development and/or modification of treatment protocols improves compliance with treatment guidelines. Intervention research not only allows members of the research team to become more adept at research but also provides an opportunity for both personal and professional development. The opportunity to communicate the results of intervention research with a variety of stakeholders, learn practice and administrative nuances within the institution, and utilize expertise gained to continue to move patient care forward are rewarding in many ways. The purpose of this type of research is to implement a change in pharmacy practice and subsequently determine the impact of this change. This chapter can serve as a guide to the development and execution of a student- or resident-led interventional research project and will discuss various interventions as examples. Specifically, this chapter will review the components of interventional research, including identification of a research question, research considerations, and the presentation of research results.

Common Research Areas

Intervention research offers the opportunity to improve all parts of the medication use process.[2] The *medication use process* consists of the following steps: *Prescribing,*

Transcribing, Dispensing, Administration, and *Monitoring.*[3] Each step can be broken down into detailed processes that involve a variety of healthcare workers across the spectrum of care to ensure safe and optimal patient outcomes. Pharmacists and pharmacy technicians are most commonly responsible for the steps noted as *Transcribing* and *Dispensing.* Significant opportunities for intervention research can be found within these steps. However, the impact of pharmacists and the opportunity for intervention research span the full medication use process, even when pharmacy personnel is not the primary driver.

The *Prescribing* step refers to the decision-making process for selecting appropriate therapy once a diagnosis is determined. In this step, specific prescriptions are prescribed for a patient based on the assessment and diagnosis. This is driven by the patient's healthcare professional with prescribing authority—most often, the physician. Pharmacists consistently impact this step by serving as the medication expert and providing recommendations for appropriate therapy regarding specific medications, dose, route, timing, contraindications, and many other factors. Pharmacists commonly lead interventions focused on modifying prescribing patterns. Examples of this type of intervention research include evaluating the impact of targeted medication education to prescribers for a commonly misprescribed drug, assessing formulary compliance after implementing automatic conversions (brand to generic, antibiotic double checks, IV to PO switches), or measuring guideline compliance after implementation of standardized prescribing forms.[4-6] Intervention research in the prescribing step often involves studying the change of prescribing patterns after specific interventions are implemented to improve patient outcomes (e.g., compliance for prescribing all guideline required medications at discharge for patients after an acute myocardial infarction) or financial impact (e.g., assessment of cost savings due to implementation of prescribing restrictions for intravenous acetaminophen).[7,8]

Once the medication order has been prescribed, the *transcribing* step involves the review of medication orders, ensuring the order is safe and optimal for the patient.[9] Pharmacy settings utilize various software platforms to process medication orders. Integrated software platforms, such as an EHR or e-prescribing, allow for the prescribing and transcribing step to be done electronically through a "verification" process. If the order is received physically (via fax or paper prescription), it involves manually entering information into a pharmacy system. Pharmacists use this step to review the appropriateness of the prescription (term used in community settings) or order (term used in hospital settings). In addition to assessing the same factors considered in the prescribing step, pharmacists determine the appropriate method for preparation and dispensing during the transcribing step. Considerations range from correct diluent and volume for compounded medications to the quantity to be dispensed based on the dose prescribed and the number of days supplies required. Appropriate transcription can be defined as accurately interpreting what is prescribed once deemed safe and optimal.[9] Interventions focused on creating safety and quality in transcribing prescriptions are common intervention research projects, including examples like evaluating the effectiveness of safety alerts or tall man lettering on transcription.

The output of transcription drives the *dispensing* step. This involves the process of physically preparing the medication for the patient and ensuring items such as the drug, dose, and instructions are accurate.[9] Medication preparation involves a wide range of systems dependent on several factors, including common examples listed below:

- *Setting*: outpatient or inpatient
- *Route of administration*: intravenous, oral, topical, rectal
- *Product availability*: Sterile or nonsterile compounding, bulk or unit dose
- *Timing and quantity of dose(s) required*: Emergent or routine, appropriate days' supply
- *Storage requirements*: Secured, temperature-related

Operational considerations in this step provide a multitude of opportunities for intervention in both the community and inpatient settings aimed at improving the medication dispensing process and, ultimately, patient care. For example, in a community pharmacy setting, the dispensing step may include the use of automated dispensing machines, and an intervention research project may evaluate if these dispensing machines reduce misfilled prescriptions (i.e., the appropriate medication is ready for the correct patient to pick up or be delivered). Similarly, in the inpatient pharmacy setting, an intervention project in this step may evaluate the impact of different medication delivery schedules on medication availability to nursing personnel. Other examples of dispensing interventions range from the implementation of a new technician and pharmacist workflow, implementation of dispensing technology (e.g., medication carousels or robotics), or integration of medication synchronization. The goal of many interventions within this step, regardless of the setting, is an accurate and efficient use of pharmacy resources to ensure the timely availability of the correct medication for the patient.[9]

The primary resource involved in the *administration* step is human resources within the larger healthcare environment. The administration step involves the patient actually receiving/taking the medication. Therefore, in the community setting, the patient or caregiver is responsible; however, this step is often dependent on nursing personnel in the hospital or nursing home. Intervention research opportunities in this step involve ensuring those responsible for administration correctly administer the medication and understand all safety precautions (i.e., the five patient rights: [1] patient; [2] drug; [3] dose; [4] route; and [5] time).[6] Intervention research in this step may include studying the impact of patient counseling on medication adherence or appropriate medication administration such as insulin administration; or evaluating compliance with safe handling precautions for hazardous medications such as chemotherapy or timely administration of time-sensitive medications.[10–12]

The final step of the medication use process is *monitoring*; the frequency of monitoring is variable but will involve checking parameters such as lab values to confirm medication safety and efficacy. Monitoring will be less frequent for chronic disease management as compared to a critically ill patient where monitoring may be continuous. Interventions in this step may involve ensuring that the correct parameters are checked at the appropriate time. Outcomes for several interventions made throughout the medication use process are often reflected in the data that is contained in the monitoring step. Metrics from this step allow for the determination of intervention effects and to identify areas to target in future intervention research.

Common Interventions in Pharmacy Practice

There are a variety of interventions to consider when starting a project that can be classified into various groups. In 2015, the **Effective Practice and Organisation of Care (EPOC)** group developed four domains to categorize types of health system interventions. These four domains include: delivery arrangements, financial arrangements, governance arrangements, and implementation strategy. Subcategories within these larger domains further describe intervention types and help with classification (Table 9–1).[13]

Delivery arrangements are defined as changes in who delivers healthcare and how, when, or where healthcare is organized and/or delivered. An example of this type of intervention is a comparison of the accuracy of medication reconciliations completed by nurses versus pharmacists. *Financial arrangements* assess changes in how reimbursement is collected, how services are purchased, overarching insurance plans, and financial incentivization. An example of a financial arrangement research project is the evaluation of medication refill rates in patients who receive vouchers versus patients who pay out-of-pocket for medication. *Governance arrangements* are interventions that impact the way power is carried out—such as enforcing employee participation or accountability. An example of this may be a change in the process of recertification of a healthcare professional. *Implementation strategies* are interventions that lead to changes in the healthcare system, healthcare professional behavior, or utilization of services by patients. Providing nursing education about a new medication process would be implementation strategy intervention research.

Steps in Intervention Research

Intervention research is differentiated from other types of research by its focus on the *design* and *development* of the interventions. The design component incorporates the

TABLE 9–1. EFFECTIVE PRACTICE AND ORGANIZATION OF CARE (EPOC) TAXONOMY OF HEALTHCARE SYSTEMS INTERVENTIONS

Intervention Type	Definition	Intervention Subcategories
Delivery Arrangements	Changes in how, when, and where healthcare is organized and delivered, and who delivers healthcare	How and when care is delivered Where care is provided and changes to the healthcare environment Who provides care and how the healthcare workforce is managed Coordination of healthcare and management of care processes Information and communication technology
Financial Arrangements	Changes in how funds are collected, insurance schemes, how services are purchased, and the use of targeted financial incentives or disincentives	Collection of funds Insurance schemes Mechanisms for the payment of health services Targeted financial incentives for health professionals and healthcare organizations
Governance Arrangements	Rules or processes that affect the way in which powers are exercised, particularly with regard to authority, accountability, openness, participation, and coherence	Authority and accountability for health policies Authority and accountability for organizations Authority and accountability for commercial products Authority and accountability for health professionals
Implementation Strategies	Interventions designed to bring about changes in healthcare organizations, the behavior of healthcare professionals or the use of health services by healthcare recipients	Interventions targeted at healthcare organizations Interventions targeted at healthcare workers Interventions targeted at specific types of practice, conditions, or settings

concepts of problem and program theory. **Problem theory** identifies potential risk factors. **Program theory** describes how an intervention is connected to the results that lead to the observed impact. To design an intervention, it is critical to incorporate previously published research and knowledge with the strategies or protocol of the research project. Careful design decreases the likelihood of implementation failures.[1]

The development of interventions has been described as a six-phase process (problem analysis and project planning; information gathering and synthesis; design of the intervention; early development and pilot testing; experimental evaluation and advance development; and dissemination).[1] Another process of intervention research development outlines three stages: (1) developing the first draft and testing it for feasibility, (2) expanding the draft to provide guidance on implementation and training, and (3) refining a tested protocol for use in diverse settings.[14] Ultimately, the development of interventional research occurs over the course of multiple studies—from less-controlled to more controlled evaluations of the intervention.

Systematic approaches to intervention development are important, especially with regard to ensuring treatment fidelity. Treatment fidelity is a combination of treatment integrity (how closely the implemented treatment is to what was intended) and treatment differentiation (how treatments differed from each other and if it was as intended).[15] For example, in a study where the intervention was to implement a new nursing-driven protocol and compare it to an already established protocol, if the new protocol was not implemented as intended, it would be difficult to assess a finding of no difference between the groups. The intervention not being carried out as designed limits the ability to display effectiveness. To avoid issues like this, researchers should clearly outline treatment definitions, appropriately train implementers, have clearly outlined treatment manuals, and provide ongoing supervision to ensure fidelity.

In 2008, the Medical Research Council (MRC) developed a stepwise system to develop an intervention. Step 1 is the development of the intervention, followed by Step 2, which includes assessing intervention feasibility through piloting. Steps 3 and 4 include evaluation of the effectiveness of interventions and implementation through monitoring, surveillance, and dissemination of knowledge. Figure 9–1 illustrates the MRC framework described.

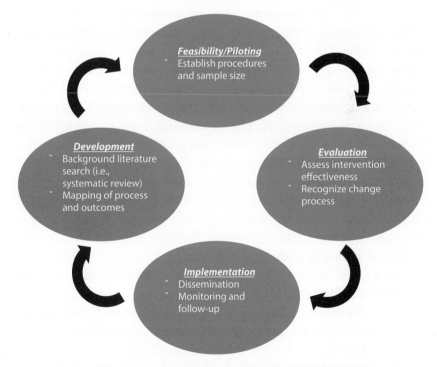

Figure 9–1. Medical Research Council framework for the intervention development.

While developing an intervention (steps outlined above) is key, the overall steps of the intervention research process beyond development are equally critical. Fraser et al. highlight five steps of the intervention research process: (1) develop problem and program theories; (2) specify program structures and processes; (3) refine and confirm in efficacy tests; (4) test effectiveness in practice settings; (5) disseminate program findings and materials.[1] To effectively design and develop an intervention, it is crucial to recruit research partners who (1) have expertise in the nuances of the setting being evaluated and (2) have the ability within the organization to effectively help implement the intervention. Depending on the research project, this may lead to a variety of experts on the team to help mold the project and ensure the processes and implementation strategies are well-defined.

Practical Considerations when Designing an Interventional Research Project

Interventional research ideas can arise from a variety of different perspectives, including clinical conundrums within patient care, operational considerations, or a continuous quality improvement project. Defining PICOTS (population, intervention, comparison group, outcomes, timeline, and setting) can help orient the research team at the beginning of the project to the purpose of the research project. From there, it is helpful to develop a study protocol or a document that would allow others to replicate the study. The American Society of Health-System Pharmacists provides guidance to approach writing a study protocol.[16] When a research question is posed, a natural follow-up is to delve into the current body of literature. The platform used to assess current literature will depend on the research question posed. Examples of potential options include PubMed, EMBASE, and the Institute for Healthcare Improvement (a database housing research about quality improvement). A background literature search allows for the increased familiarity of the topic and to assess research gaps where a research project would add to the literature and/or enhance processes within the institution. Thorough background research is a key step to inform and develop a valid research question.

Next, the scope of the research project should be established, and goals clearly described. Goals will be defined by the changes in the outcome that is expected due to the intervention. This leads to the development of specific study objectives. Goals and study objectives determine timeline planning, application for funding, and stakeholder involvement. Stakeholders may include a wide variety of people within the pharmacy department (preceptor, practitioner, administrator, pharmacy technician), the institution (physicians, nurses, executive leadership), or even colleagues across multiple institutions. Identifying key personnel with interest in the project's outcomes ensure that the research team is comprehensive and equipped to appropriately design the study.

Specific deadlines should be established to ensure the timely completion of subsections and the overall research project. This is especially important when working on a fixed schedule—such as a one-year residency project. Another planning step is to determine the implementation of processes needed for the collection and evaluation of data. Data collection can be gathered in a variety of ways that include: data extraction from an EHR, survey administration using online platforms such as REDCap or Qualtrics, or manual data collection, i.e. paper survey, chart reviews, and so on. REDCap and Qualtrics are web-based applications that allow users to build online surveys and collect data through online databases. Of note, REDCap is compliant with Health Insurance Portability and Accountability Act regulations and is becoming a preferred electronic survey modality among hospital systems. During the planning phase, researchers should also create a document to record data points to allow data to be easily shared between research team members and also allow for critical evaluation of which data points are necessary to evaluate the predefined project outcomes. Figure 9–2 is an example data collection sheet one could use for manually extracting information from patient profiles. Often, the data collection sheet will evolve and change throughout the course of a project. Pilot testing the datasheet with a handful of patient charts may be helpful to refine the sheet and determine if additional data points should be included or possibly excluded from the original draft. The goal of the datasheet is to create a standardized form that is thorough, efficient, and allows for appropriate data collection necessary for analysis.

Institutional infrastructure, such as the Information Technology (IT) department or pertinent institution committees, should be considered when planning. IT can play a key role in helping to gather data and is integral in implementation if the intervention research involves EHR changes such as revising clinical decision-making software or implementing a new prescription order set in the EHR. A clear understanding of the scope and roles of IT within the institution, including their specific capabilities applicable to intervention research, can greatly enhance the planning, implementation, and analysis of a project.

Investigators also need to include time for a project to go through the Institutional Review Board and any other approvals that may be required depending on the scope and intent of the intervention. Examples of other committee approvals include the Pharmacy and Therapeutics (P&T) Committee, specialty specific committees (e.g., Critical Care Committee, Anticoagulation committee, and so on), legal review, and any administrative committees within the institution (e.g., executive committee with nursing, pharmacy, medicine administrators). These various panels can provide valuable feedback and

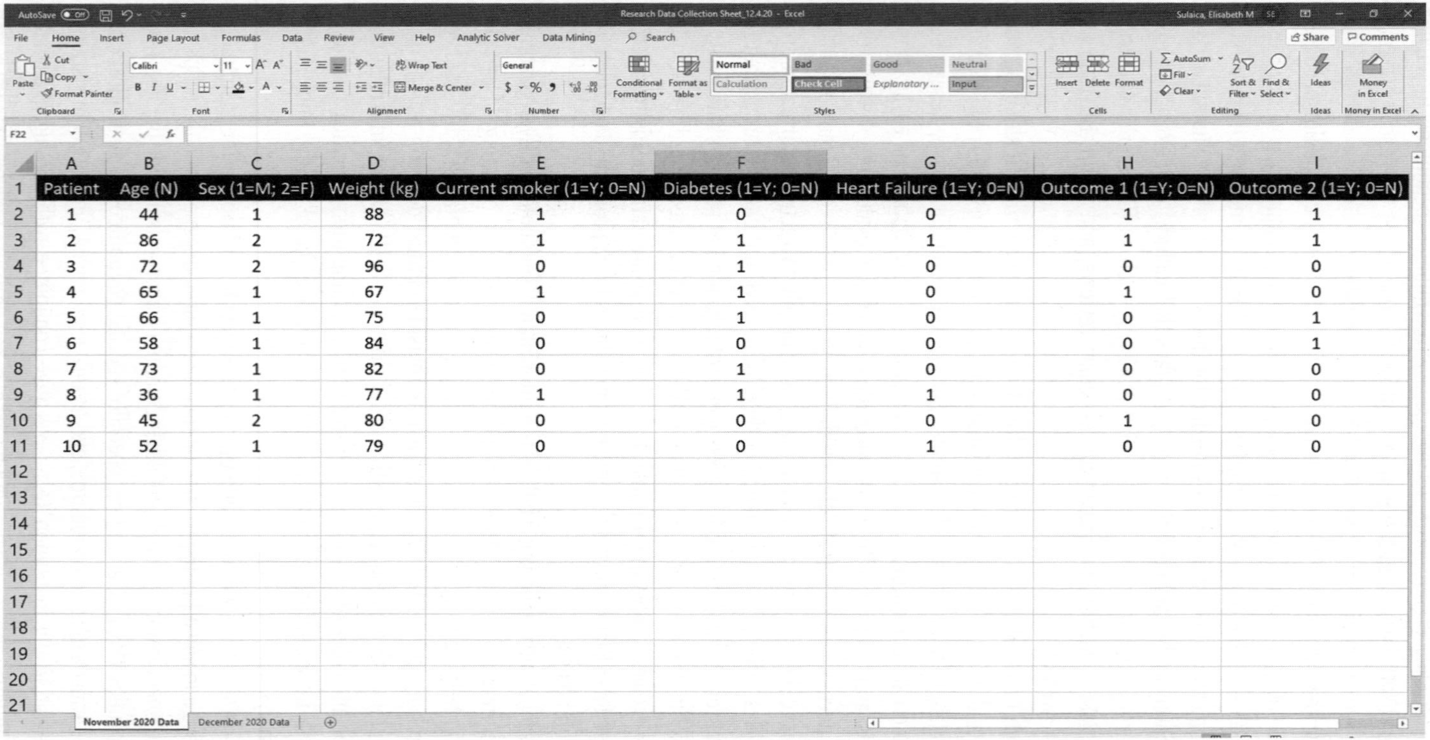

Patient	Age (N)	Sex (1=M; 2=F)	Weight (kg)	Current smoker (1=Y; 0=N)	Diabetes (1=Y; 0=N)	Heart Failure (1=Y; 0=N)	Outcome 1 (1=Y; 0=N)	Outcome 2 (1=Y; 0=N)
1	44	1	88	1	0	0	1	1
2	86	2	72	1	1	1	1	1
3	72	2	96	0	1	0	0	0
4	65	1	67	1	1	0	1	0
5	66	1	75	0	1	0	0	1
6	58	1	84	0	0	0	0	1
7	73	1	82	0	1	0	0	0
8	36	1	77	1	0	1	0	0
9	45	2	80	0	0	0	1	0
10	52	1	79	0	0	1	0	0

Figure 9–2. Example of data collection sheet.

perspective to improve and tailor research projects. Funding is another consideration investigators should consider when starting a project. Funding for intervention research may be used to hire a statistician, order supplies, hire a research assistant, or pay for other ancillary costs that may arise. Obtaining funding often will require completing an application and/or a grant submission. Organizations such as the American College of Clinical Pharmacy and the American Society of Health-System Pharmacists have research grants available for trainees to apply for. Institutions often have an individualized process for internal submission and approval for projects seeking funding that must be completed before applying to the funding organization. This internal review and approval can take time and require additional planning along with a complete understanding of the project needs.

Technical Considerations when Designing an Interventional Research Project

Study design considerations should be assessed when posing the study question and outlining the study protocol. Interventional research is usually prospective and involves implementing an intervention to cause a change. The intervention research can be experimental if there is randomization leading to randomized trials. The intervention research can also be observational studies if there is no randomization. For example, a study question may lend itself to be observational in nature rather than a randomized trial if the research question does not require randomization of an intervention but instead documentation of intervention exposure and subsequent outcome.

Randomized controlled trials (RCT) are the most commonly recognized type of intervention research project. They are considered one of the strongest research designs within the hierarchy of scientific evidence. Randomization will ensure that both groups are similar, and the quality of an RCT increases with the incorporation of methodologies such as blinding and allocation concealment. Alternatively, nonrandomized or observational studies involve patients who are not randomized to treatment arms. In these studies, participants may be assigned to groups based on factors such as convenience, interest among patients and providers, ability to follow-up or pay, or other factors. The observational study designs for intervention research include cohort study, pre- and post-observational study, and time-series analyses. These designs are often used by learners when there is limited time and resources to implement RCT. Compared to RCTs, observational studies are considered a weaker form of evidence and are more susceptible to selection bias as differences between groups could impact the results of the trial. Also, observational studies require strong statistical approaches to control for observed and unobserved biases.

How to Navigate an Intervention Research Project

Navigating the intervention research process can be challenging; time management, project management, and communication skills are required for successful completion. A common issue encountered by novice researchers is setting appropriate expectations and managing time effectively in order to accomplish research goals within the required time frame. This becomes particularly challenging given that most research projects are longitudinal and will be completed while simultaneously fulfilling day-to-day responsibilities, such as patient care tasks, meetings, or other routine obligations. Strategies may include setting deadlines for subsections and holding oneself accountable to those deadlines, understanding realistic time frames to complete work, and being intentional in scheduling time to complete the work. Honing time management strategies allows for efficient and effective work with improved accuracy. Along with time management skills, project management skills are essential in intervention research. Project management skills refer to the ability to distill the overarching project into logical steps and define how the work will be accomplished within a period of time. Early identification of and working through barriers is another aspect of project management. The value of timely and effective communication with all stakeholders throughout the process cannot be overstated. Appropriate verbal and written communication methods to all project team members are the best way to maintain support, keep the team informed, and ensure successful outcomes.

It is important to outline the roles, responsibilities, and expectations of each member of the team to understand the communication pathways. Project team members will include a primary investigator or project lead, stakeholders, and potentially support personnel. The primary investigator or project lead will be responsible for the majority of research, but decisions will be informed by input from all project team members. Mentors and experts within the area will be considered stakeholders. Their input and expertise will guide the progress throughout the project and they should be consulted routinely. Setting routine meetings or "check-ins" ahead of time should be considered. In the initial phases, a mentor or expert within the area can help evaluate if an interventional research project would be a worthwhile investment of time. Additionally, guidance and mentorship for grant submission by an experienced member of the research team may be helpful. Support personnel may include IT resources that provide necessary data and/or create the specific intervention. Another example may be other learners that support the data collection process. Overall, finding key team members and leveraging their expertise can ensure the project is successful.

Exemplars of Learner-Involved Intervention Research

Intervention research can be conducted across a wide range of healthcare settings; commonly identified areas are community pharmacy, ambulatory, and acute care settings. Across all settings, the needs of the organization will drive the focus of the intervention. Organizational needs are prioritized by ensuring safe and optimal care efficiently while maintaining responsible financial considerations. Organizations are guided by regulatory and accrediting agencies such as Centers for Medicare and Medicaid (CMS), the Joint Commission, Drug Enforcement and Administration, Occupational Safety and Health Administration, state boards of pharmacy, among others that outline best practices to optimize healthcare and requirements to maintain licensure. These agencies define quality indicators and financial incentives that often provide the foundation for identifying needed interventions.

A research example within community pharmacy may include assessing the effects of patient counseling on the access to and understanding of medications. In this example, the intervention is the act of counseling, and the outcome is the improvement in access to and/or understanding of the medication.[17] An additional example is demonstrating the value of the prescription drug monitoring program (PDMP), an electronic database that provides essential information regarding all controlled substance prescriptions with regard to opioid stewardship. The intervention would be the use of the PDMP, and the outcome would be the effects on opioid stewardship.[18] In this example, the intervention (e.g., use of PDMP) occurs in the transcription step of the medication use process and would be considered an implementation strategy. Within the transcription step, pharmacists utilize information to assess the validity and appropriateness of all prescriptions. The ability to evaluate the impact of the pharmacists' use of the PDMP (*intervention*) is studied through data collected from surveys completed by pharmacists (*research methodology*) to demonstrate a change in the number of prescriptions verified (*outcome*), thus reducing the opportunity for prescription drug misuse (*positive impact*).[18] For this example, practical considerations would include creating a research team with experts, gaining an understanding of the opioid epidemic and contributing factors via a thorough background literature search, understanding of PDMP data, and how pharmacists utilize that data to form a research question. Additional considerations include survey development (what data should be collected to answer the question; what software should be used), survey dissemination plan (how and to who), and how best to analyze the information within a specified timeline.

Intervention research in ambulatory care can include assessing the impact of pharmacist-provided care for chronic disease states such as diabetes and hypertension.[19] The intervention in these studies is often the additional patient care provided by the pharmacist, and the outcome is a change in the disease state metric such as achievement of goal blood pressure and hemoglobin A1c or glycemic control for diabetes.[20] This specific example would be characterized as delivery arrangements as it compares three versions of pharmacist-led counseling that occur throughout the administration and monitoring steps of the medication use process. The ability to compare three versions of pharmacist-led counseling (*intervention*) is studied through comparing changes in insulin persistence, hemoglobin A1c, and healthcare utilization for each group (*research methodology*) to determine the most effective pharmacist-led counseling (*outcome*), thus allowing pharmacists to efficiently and effectively utilize their time and knowledge to optimize health outcomes (*positive impact*). Another example would be pharmacist involvement to improve prescribing of evidence-based medicine.[21] Active pharmacist involvement in this scenario would be considered the intervention, and increased adherence to therapeutic guidelines recommendations is the outcome.

The concept of medication reconciliation in which a healthcare provider compares lists of medications when there is a change in the level of care (i.e., admission, transfer from acute care to critical care or discharge) is an example of intervention research within inpatient care. As guided by CMS, performing medication reconciliation ensures safe and quality care by identifying potential duplication of or omission of therapy. As such, to maintain accreditation, organizations are required to provide this service. However, organizations must determine how to best utilize limited resources to optimally reconcile medications. Interventions categorized as delivery arrangements may focus on identifying who performs this service (e.g., nurse, pharmacist, pharmacy technician, or student) and which patients are prioritized (high-risk patients, patients with multiple transitions of care). Therefore, medication reconciliation interventions may be process-focused with the goal of increasing the efficiency of providing this service.[22] Alternatively, influencing clinical decision support within EHRs, including reducing the number of alerts displayed to prescribers and measuring the perceived effectiveness, is another example of inpatient intervention research.[23]

Throughout the continuum of care, there are numerous opportunities to conduct intervention research. This, in conjunction with the ever-evolving nature of healthcare, allows for meaningful pharmacy personnel and trainee involvement in this area. These examples are just a few of countless opportunities to assess the impact of pharmacists within healthcare.

Dissemination Framework for Intervention Research

Results of an intervention research project can be presented at professional conferences through abstract and poster presentations, infographics via professional social media accounts, and PowerPoint presentations. Findings will likely also be presented to key internal stakeholders—such as hospital administration or hospital committees. All facets of the intervention, such as the stages and fidelity of implementing the intervention, should be incorporated into the presentation. These stakeholders will help to assess the effectiveness of the intervention to determine if it should be more widely implemented throughout the institution, permanently implemented, or not at all.

A common concern about disseminating information is the inconsistency in describing the development, reporting, and evaluation of intervention research projects. This makes it difficult to interpret and/or replicate results. Specific details of the intervention—from design to implementation and results—should be clearly reported when presenting results. There are multiple guidelines that provide criteria for conducting and reporting interventional research projects, such as the Consolidated Standards of Reporting Trials (CONSORT) and the Criteria for Reporting the Development and Evaluation of Complex Interventions in healthcare (CReDECI2).[24,25]

The CONSORT statement was developed to improve the consistency of reporting of randomized controlled trials. This document highlights sections including title and abstract, introduction, methods, results, and discussion. Within the methods section, a granular description of the intervention should be reported to allow for replication. The CReDECI2 guideline is intended to provide direction on the process of intervention research and is divided into three stages—development, feasibility, and piloting, and evaluation. There are 13 items described in the guideline that calls for an extensive description of the intervention. Items include describing the theory behind the intervention, the intervention components, and the interaction between components. Description of the comparator, delivery of the intervention, tools, and fidelity should also be reported. In contrast to the CONSORT statement, CReDECI2 was not developed for a specific type of study design and can be applied to interventional research in any healthcare setting.

These guidance documents should be consulted for best practices in the dissemination of methods, protocols, and findings in intervention research. This allows for systematic reporting and ensures that the interventional research project is able to be replicated.

Summary and Conclusions

Pharmacy personnel plays a key role in intervention research, and their involvement can lead to a large impact on patient care. Practice-based research can be conducted within any of the medication use process steps, which include: *Prescribing, Transcribing, Dispensing, Administration,* and *Monitoring.* Pharmacists, pharmacy technicians, and pharmacy learners are the primary drivers in the *Transcribing* and *Dispensing* steps resulting in a significant opportunity for intervention research, but there is an opportunity for collaboration with other healthcare providers for research focused within any of the medication use steps. There are many factors to consider when initiating an intervention research project, and these include: conducting background research, setting research goals, identifying stakeholders, setting a timeline for each step of the project, planning data collection strategies, applying for funding (if needed), and navigating institution-specific infrastructure. Planning, in conjunction with time management and effective communication, is paramount for executing the project. Balancing day-to-day tasks with a longitudinal research project can be challenging but is more attainable when appropriate deadlines are set and subsequently met.

Intervention research can be conducted across the spectrum of healthcare, including within the community, ambulatory, and acute care settings. Similarly, results obtained from these settings are able to be disseminated to target audiences over a wide variety of platforms—from live presentations to published manuscripts. Overall, this enables researchers to reach a larger audience and have a wider opportunity to affect the practice. Intervention research requires dedication and focus, but with appropriate planning, time management, and communication, pharmacy personnel has the opportunity to broadly impact patient care over a wide variety of settings.

Key Points and Advice

- Intervention research is designed to measure the impact of interventions within a process.
- Intervention research questions can be developed within all steps of the medication use process and in all healthcare settings.
- There are many factors to consider when initiating an intervention research project, and these include components such as: conducting background research, setting research goals, identifying stakeholders, setting a timeline for each step of the project, planning data collection strategies, applying for funding (if needed), and navigating institution-specific infrastructure.
- The development of interventional research occurs over the course of multiple studies—from less-controlled to more controlled evaluations of the intervention.

Chapter Review Questions

1. What is the purpose of intervention research?

2. Discuss example intervention research opportunities within the steps of the medication use process and provide the outcomes evaluated.
3. Describe the value of background research for an intervention research project.
4. Why is it essential to define stakeholders?
5. What factors should be considered when planning data collection?

Online Resources

- American Pharmacists Association Research & Evidence Practice Resources. https://www.pharmacist.com/Practice/Practice-Resources/Research-Evidence
- American Society of Health-System Pharmacists Research Resource Center. https://www.ashp.org/pharmacy-practice/resource-centers/research-resource-center?loginret urnUrl=SSOCheckOnly
- Consolidated Standards of Reporting Trials (CONSORT) Resources. http://www.consort-statement.org/

REFERENCES

1. Fraser MW, Galinsky MJ. Steps in intervention research: designing and developing social programs. *Res Soc Work Pract.* 2010;20(5):459-466. doi:10.1177/1049731509358424
2. Vest JR, Kern LM, Abramson E, Ancker JS, Kaushal R, HITEC Investigators. Effect of a state-based incentive programme on the use of electronic health records. *J Eval Clin Pract.* 2014;20(5):657-663. doi:10.1111/jep.12195
3. United States Pharmacopeial Convention. General Chapter 1006: Physical environments that promote safe medication use. Accessed December 21, 2020. https://www.uspnf.com/sites/default/files/usp_pdf/EN/USPNF/c1066.pdf
4. Budiman T, Snodgrass K, Komatsu Chang A. Evaluation of pharmacist medication education and post-discharge follow-up in reducing readmissions in patients with ST-Segment Elevation Myocardial Infarction (STEMI). *Ann Pharmacother.* 2016;50(2):118-124. doi:10.1177/1060028015620425
5. Karel LI, Delisle DR, Anagnostis EA, Wordell CJ. Implementation of a formulary management process. *Am J Health-Syst Pharm AJHP Off J Am Soc Health-Syst Pharm.* 2017;74(16):1245-1252. doi:10.2146/ajhp160193
6. Sano HS, Waddell JA, Solimando DA, Doulaveris P, Myhand R. Study of the effect of standardized chemotherapy order forms on prescribing errors and anti-emetic cost. *J Oncol Pharm Pract Off Publ Int Soc Oncol Pharm Pract.* 2005;11(1):21-30. doi:10.1191/10781552 05jp149oa
7. Shanbhag D, Graham ID, Harlos K, et al. Effectiveness of implementation interventions in improving physician adherence to guideline recommendations in heart failure: a systematic review. *BMJ Open.* 2018;8(3):e017765. doi:10.1136/bmjopen-2017-017765

8. Vincent WR, Huiras P, Empfield J, et al. Controlling postoperative use of i.v. acetaminophen at an academic medical center. *Am J Health-Syst Pharm AJHP Off J Am Soc Health-Syst Pharm.* 2018;75(8):548-555. doi:10.2146/ajhp170054

9. Billstein-Leber M, Carrillo CJD, Cassano AT, Moline K, Robertson JJ. ASHP Guidelines on preventing medication errors in hospitals. *Am J Health-Syst Pharm AJHP Off J Am Soc Health-Syst Pharm.* 2018;75(19):1493-1517. doi:10.2146/ajhp170811

10. Palacio A, Garay D, Langer B, Taylor J, Wood BA, Tamariz L. Motivational interviewing improves medication adherence: a systematic review and meta-analysis. *J Gen Intern Med.* 2016;31(8):929-940. doi:10.1007/s11606-016-3685-3

11. Truong TH, Nguyen TT, Armor BL, Farley JR. Errors in the Administration Technique of Insulin Pen Devices: A Result of Insufficient Education. *Diabetes Ther Res Treat Educ Diabetes Relat Disord.* 2017;8(2):221-226. doi:10.1007/s13300-017-0242-y

12. Guillemette A, Langlois H, Voisine M, et al. Impact and appreciation of two methods aiming at reducing hazardous drug environmental contamination: the centralization of the priming of IV tubing in the pharmacy and use of a closed-system transfer device. *J Oncol Pharm Pract Off Publ Int Soc Oncol Pharm Pract.* 2014;20(6):426-432. doi:10.1177/1078155213517127

13. Effective Practice and Organisation of Care (EPOC). EPOC Taxonomy. Published online July 15, 2021. doi:10.5281/zenodo.5105851

14. Onken LS, Blaine JD, Battjes RJ. Behavioral therapy research: a conceptualization of a process. In: Henggeler SW, Santos AB (eds.), *Innovative Approaches for Difficult-to-Treat Populations.* American Psychiatric Association; 1997:477-485.

15. Moncher FJ, Prinz RJ. Treatment fidelity in outcome studies. *Clin Psychol Rev.* 1991;11(3):247-266. doi:10.1016/0272-7358(91)90103-2

16. Kauffman YS, Billups SJ. *Developing the Research Idea.* ASHP; 2020. Accessed August 13, 2021. https://publications.ashp.org/view/book/9781585285617/ch01.xml

17. Milosavljevic A, Aspden T, Harrison J. Community pharmacist-led interventions and their impact on patients' medication adherence and other health outcomes: a systematic review. *Int J Pharm Pract.* 2018;26(5):387-397. doi:10.1111/ijpp.12462

18. Norwood CW, Wright ER. Integration of prescription drug monitoring programs (PDMP) in pharmacy practice: improving clinical decision-making and supporting a pharmacist's professional judgment. *Res Soc Adm Pharm RSAP.* 2016;12(2):257-266. doi:10.1016/j.sapharm.2015.05.008

19. Elnaem MH, Rosley NFF, Alhifany AA, Elrggal ME, Cheema E. Impact of pharmacist-led interventions on medication adherence and clinical outcomes in patients with hypertension and hyperlipidemia: a scoping review of published literature. *J Multidiscip Healthc.* 2020;13:635-645. doi:10.2147/JMDH.S257273

20. Lauffenburger JC, Lewey J, Jan S, et al. Effectiveness of targeted insulin-adherence interventions for glycemic control using predictive analytics among patients with type 2 diabetes: a randomized clinical trial. *JAMA Netw Open.* 2019;2(3):e190657. doi:10.1001/jamanetworkopen.2019.0657

21. Burns KW, Johnson KM, Pham SN, Egwuatu NE, Dumkow LE. Implementing outpatient antimicrobial stewardship in a primary care office through ambulatory care pharmacist-led audit and feedback. *J Am Pharm Assoc JAPhA*. 2020;60(6):e246-e251. doi:10.1016/j.japh.2020.08.003

22. Audurier Y, Roubille C, Manna F, et al. Development and validation of a score to assess risk of medication errors detected during medication reconciliation process at admission in internal medicine unit: SCOREM study. *Int J Clin Pract*. Published online August 8, 2020;75(2):e13663. doi:10.1111/ijcp.13663

23. Bhakta SB, Colavecchia AC, Haines L, Varkey D, Garey KW. A systematic approach to optimize electronic health record medication alerts in a health system. *Am J Health-Syst Pharm AJHP Off J Am Soc Health-Syst Pharm*. 2019;76(8):530-536. doi:10.1093/ajhp/zxz012

24. Schulz KF, Altman DG, Moher D, the CONSORT Group. CONSORT 2010 statement: updated guidelines for reporting parallel group randomised trials. *BMC Medicine*. 2010;8(1):18. doi:10.1186/1741-7015-8-18

25. Möhler R, Köpke S, Meyer G. Criteria for reporting the development and evaluation of complex interventions in healthcare: revised guideline (CReDECI 2). *Trials*. 2015;16(1):204. doi:10.1186/s13063-015-0709-y

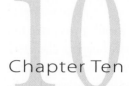

Chapter Ten

Implementation Science in Pharmacy Settings

Douglas Thornton, PhD, PharmD

Chapter Objectives

1. Define implementation science in pharmacy settings
2. Identity common research questions in implementation science
3. Discuss various research implementation models
4. Understand common research designs in implementation science
5. Understand the practical and technical considerations for implementation science
6. Discuss the strategies for harnessing the expertise needed for conducting implementation science projects
7. Describe an example of a learner-involved implementation science project in a pharmacy setting
8. Understand the dissemination framework for implementation science in pharmacy settings

Key Terminology

Implementation science, health services research, implementation models, logic model, dissemination research

Introduction

A "chasm" exists between scientific knowledge, which helps identify patient care that could potentially be given, and the actual care that patients receive.[1] Implementation science is one emerging field of study that can help close the gap between basic science and fully realized evidence-based practice. Implementation science, as defined by the National Institutes of Health, is "the study of methods to promote the adoption and integration of evidence-based practices, interventions, and policies into routine healthcare and public health settings to improve the impact on population health."[2] This discipline can be used to generalize research findings, sustain evidence-based practices over time, and even de-implement harmful or unnecessary practices. As implementation science is a new and developing field that incorporates many scientific and patient care disciplines, there can be some overlap in terminology. For the purposes of this chapter, the terminology used will be implementation science, which is used by United Kingdom's Medical Research Council and the World Health Organization (WHO). Other names include the broader field of Dissemination and Implementation (D&I) research which is used by Veterans Administration's Quality Enhancement Research Initiative and Patient Centered Outcomes Research Institute (PCORI), among others, and Knowledge Translation which is used by the Canadian Institutes for Health Research. All of these fields overlap in that they focus on methods to promote the incorporation of scientific findings and evidence-based practices into "real world" healthcare policy and practices.

In this chapter, the reader will be provided a more detailed history of implementation science, including a review of methods that are used in this discipline. The chapter will also go through an example project and discuss how dissemination relates to implementation science. Finally, this chapter will dive into best practices for reporting on implementation science projects. While this chapter is certainly not enough to make a pharmacist or pharmacy student an implementation science expert, it can build an appetite for more learning and point the reader in the direction of additional resources on the topic.

Value of Implementation Science in Pharmacy

One of the known problems with the healthcare system is that it takes nearly two decades to turn a small fraction of research into a benefit for patient care.[3] This research gap shows that many routine practices do not produce any of the positive outcomes that were identified through clinical research or basic science. Evolving pharmacy practice and the inclusion of pharmacists throughout the healthcare system have helped to close this gap with key interventions, including medication therapy management (MTM), immunization, and aiding in transitions of care. For pharmacy practice to continue to grow and the profession to remain a central pillar of the modern healthcare system, pharmacists need to prove their value beyond traditional roles. Implementation science is a field ready for pharmacists to show their professional abilities to incorporate evidence-based practices, improve quality, reduce or control costs, and maximize value for patients as well as the healthcare system.

The two key dimensions of implementation science are research and practice. Pharmacists are excellently trained healthcare providers who can work in complex practice sites and do their best to avoid error-prone processes that are rampant in the modern healthcare system. However, pharmacists tend to work in only one of these two silos. Evidence-based practices designed by and for pharmacists are needed to propel the profession into the future. Additionally, training in implementation science, specifically on how to bridge the research and practice dimensions, is critical. Pharmacists will need to learn what intervention components are, how to effectively implement and sustain them, and who to turn to for help in this process.

Pharmacists have been involved with quality improvement for decades, so one might wonder why there needs to be such an emphasis on a relatively new discipline. Implementation science and quality improvement are often confused because they share some similarities—primarily to improve patient care. However, these two practices are not the same and are often at odds due to their distinct methodologies and effect on the healthcare system.[4] Quality improvement is an iterative practice whereby the processes within an organization are reviewed, evaluated, improved, and ultimately optimized to improve patient outcomes. The practices within an organization that are being "improved" are certainly not all evidence-based. This is the key distinction. Implementation science, on the other hand, is based on theory and an underlying evidence-based practice. As evidence-based practices have been emphasized and promulgated by clinicians and policymakers, there was an understanding that a systematic process was necessary to improve their uptake. Implementation science is the process of integrating evidence-based practice into a real-world clinical setting and evaluating if the intended effects remain the same.

Implementation Science: History and the Need

HISTORY OF IMPLEMENTATION SCIENCE

Turning research into clinical practice is a time-consuming and difficult process. The goal of generating a body of research to be able to consider a clinical practice to read evidence-based practice is to be able to have other clinicians repeat it. As primary evidence is generated and spread throughout research and practice communities, new clinicians and practice sites seek to adopt these research findings. Implementation science is the study of this adoption process that dives into what happens before, during, and after the adoption of a new evidence-based practice within a specific practice site. A large portion of implementation science projects are performed to establish if the evidence-based practice will still have the intended effect when applied to "real world" practice conditions.[5]

While the methods have solidified around implementation science, especially over the previous 2 decades, the study of how new ideas get spread through populations of potential adopters is not new. The discipline of communication studies has described the diffusion of innovations since the early 1960s, and the origins of that theory go back even further.[6] New practices and policies are adopted in pharmacy settings nearly every day. The study of the adoption of these new practices is the focus of this chapter: implementation science. The practice site is the location where the implementation of new practices takes place, and an implementer is a person who is changing their practice by adopting innovation or new research. Finally, sustainability, or how to support the long-term upkeep of a new practice, is an important part of implementation science.

The initial diffusion of the innovation must start somewhere by being communicated through members of a social system over time. The best way to stimulate this diffusion process is through trusted, informal thought leaders. Another name for this type of person is a clinician "champion" who advocates for innovation and helps with the uptake of the new practice through word-of-mouth communication and social modeling. In the healthcare setting, new practices, knowledge, and the use of technology can culminate in providing evidence-based medicine to use a wide range of information to improve clinical decision-making and patient care. Evidence-based medicine emphasizes the role of new information over an individual's clinical experiences, but both are necessary to inform clinical decision-making.[7] This process can also be applied to public health, where the desire for valid and generalizable evidence to inform decisions has been labeled as evidence-based public health.[8] The variety of these domains show how implementation science can positively impact patients and society by improving decision-making in healthcare and public health.

NEED FOR IMPLEMENTATION SCIENCE AS PART OF HEALTH SERVICES RESEARCH

Simply put, **health services research** (HSR) is the study of how people access healthcare, pay for it, and what results they receive. According to the Agency for Healthcare Research and Quality (AHRQ), HSR is a "multidisciplinary field of scientific investigation that studies how social factors, financing systems, organizational structures and processes, health technologies, and personal behaviors affect access to healthcare, the quality and cost of healthcare, and ultimately, our health and well-being." The goals of this field of research are to provide the evidence needed to make healthcare more affordable, safe, effective, equitable, and patient-centered.[9] As you have learned from earlier in this chapter, the next step after evidence generation is adoption by other clinicians and practices. This puts implementation science at the core of health services research since it is the critical mechanism for spreading replicable evidence-based practices to various providers.

DIFFERENCES IN IMPLEMENTATION SCIENCE AND CLINICAL INTERVENTION RESEARCH

Primary evidence generation, often in the form of clinical intervention research, must precede implementation science. Clinical trials and other intervention research focus on the efficacy of the intervention. These findings will be the benchmark for which implementation science will seek to replicate as the evidence-based practices are spread to practice sites other than where the initial clinical research took place. Both clinical research and implementation science emphasize the need to have high fidelity of the intervention and typically have the same clinical outcomes the research is seeking to measure. Having high intervention fidelity means that the intervention is delivered the same way it was described in the study protocol, and lack of fidelity is a threat to internal study validity.

There are differences between clinical and implementation research. The first difference is in the population being studied. In clinical research, the emphasis is on the patient, whereas in implementation science, all parties involved with delivering and receiving the evidence-based practice are important study participants (e.g., pharmacists, doctors, patients). Next, the setting in which the research takes place moves away from academic medical centers where the most clinical research is performed to other clinical settings where the intervention will be delivered (e.g., critical access hospitals, rural health clinics, community pharmacies). Lastly, in implementation science, the availability of research support can be much different and will be highly dependent on the facility where the implementation is taking place. These differences highlight why implementation science is so critical to closing the quality chasm in healthcare.

Another way to look at the relationship between intervention research and implementation science is through the lens of translational research. Translational research is the process of moving basic science discoveries to clinical practice quickly and efficiently and can be described as being a five-step process commonly denoted as "T0" through "T4." As seen in Figure 10–1, the first three steps involve non-human basic science, including genomic association studies (T0), basic science through early human testing (T1), and establishing effectiveness in human populations (T2). The next step, T3, is all about implementation science and how to maintain the positive effects established in previous translational steps. To complete the process, T4 focuses on outcomes and population effectiveness.[10]

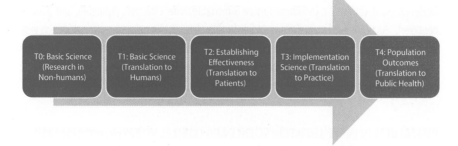

| T0: Basic Science (Research in Non-humans) | T1: Basic Science (Translation to Humans) | T2: Establishing Effectiveness (Translation to Patients) | T3: Implementation Science (Translation to Practice) | T4: Population Outcomes (Translation to Public Health) |

Figure 10–1. Translational research continuum.

Common Implementation Science Research Questions in Pharmacy

IMPLEMENTATION SCIENCE IN DIFFERENT PHARMACY SETTINGS

In 2017, one of the leading figures in implementation science, Geoffrey Curran, wrote an editorial describing how pharmacy practice could be advanced by embracing implementation science.[11] The editorial was part of a special issue on implementation science. The majority of the implementation science described focused on interventions in the community pharmacy setting. These interventions included value-based payment models for primary care services,[12] incentive strategies to improve MTM implementation,[13] and appropriate thromboprophylaxis use in hospitalized patients.[14] Beyond these specific studies, the editorial expanded on what pharmacy practice could gain from moving away from just showing effectiveness to a pharmacy intervention toward understanding and systematically testing the best ways to support implementation and sustainability of the interventions. Ultimately, there was a call to action for more robust study designs to advance evidence-based practices for pharmacists and improve the quality and effectiveness of interventions performed by the profession.

Research starts by identifying a research problem, often by asking a question, then the study performed aims to answer that question. In implementation science, the research questions are focused more on how an intervention can be best performed, what are the barriers and facilitators to performing an evidence-based practice in a "real world" setting, how can practice settings affect intervention success, and what are techniques to de-implement inappropriate (non-evidence based) practices. Example implementation science research questions are provided in Table 10–1. One suggestion for how to form implementation science research questions stems from a government implementation workshop which recommends relating the question to a challenge related to one of the following.[15]

TABLE 10-1. EXAMPLE IMPLEMENTATION SCIENCE RESEARCH QUESTIONS

Pharmacy Practice Setting	Research Questions
Community Pharmacy	What are the most effective techniques to keep a patient adherent to their chronic disease medication?
	How do the contextual factors of the community pharmacy workspace influence patient care practices?
	What is the best way to de-implement pharmacy practices that are no longer effective?
Hospital/Acute Care	What is the fastest way to reliably deliver first dose antibiotics to patients with sepsis?
	What are the determinants of hospital readmission when patients are discharged after an acute myocardial infarction?
	What pharmacy services can be provided during non-peak shifts?
Ambulatory Care	How can we ensure patients return to the clinic for their mammography?
	What is the best way to deliver a comprehensive medication review?
	What is the best reimbursement strategy to provide pharmacy services within the clinical setting?

- Scaling Up: Adoption of evidence-based practice at a new practice location while accounting for implementation issues that arise
- Sustainability: Building a process by which an evidence-based practice can remain in place and adapt when needed to maintain the desired long-term outcomes
- Replication: Similar to "scaling up" but by organizations not involved with the initial implementation of the evidence-based practice
- Program Integration: Focuses on how specific evidence-based practices can be packaged and delivered within practice sites
- Equitability: Assuring that the implementation of the evidence-based process would remain consistent across different types of practice settings, including those that serve different patients (e.g., low-income, racial/ethnic minorities, different languages)
- Real-World Effectiveness: In the context of implementation science, this focuses on unintended consequences, cost-effectiveness, and whether the evidence-based practice has the intended public health impact.

Technical Considerations for Implementation Science

COMMON STUDY DESIGNS IN IMPLEMENTATION SCIENCE

The wide range of study designs that are used in implementation science can be roughly broken into three categories: randomized controlled trials including hybrid designs, quasi-experimental designs, and mixed methods that include qualitative designs.[16] Other nonexperimental research can be performed as part of an implementation science project (e.g., patient or provider satisfaction assessed cross-sectionally), but for the most part, the main design should fit into one of these groups.

First, randomized controlled trials are experimental research designs where participants are randomly assigned to an intervention or control group. While randomized controlled trials are critical to establishing efficacy, they can have some limitations when used to establish an evidence-based practice at a new practice site. Variations of randomized clinical trials include cluster randomized controlled trials,[17] stepped-wedge designs,[18] and hybrid designs.[19] Hybrid designs are particularly powerful and informative because they focus on assessing both the clinical effectiveness and implementation at the same time. However, they can be difficult and require extensive expertise and planning.

Quasi-experimental designs are studies that are used to estimate the causal impact of an intervention without the use of random assignment and are the second category of study designs used in implementation science. This type of study is particularly helpful when the randomization is either ethically impossible or logistically infeasible. Since one of the goals of implementation science is to assess the process of adopting an evidence-based practice in a new setting, oftentimes, quasi-experimental designs are used. Commonly used studies in this category include interrupted time series,[20] regression discontinuity,[21] and pragmatic clinical trials. Pragmatic clinical trials, also known as practical clinical trials, are a relatively new concept that places importance on external validity by sacrificing some internal validity. The defining characteristics of this type of quasi-experimental design are: (1) selecting two or more clinically relevant interventions to compare, (2) include a diverse sample of study participants that represent clinical practice, (3) recruit participants from real practices with minimal exclusion criteria, and (4) collect data on a wider range of health or patient report outcomes.[22]

The final broad category of study designs used in implementation science is mixed methods. Mixed methods research is characterized by combining qualitative and quantitative components. Qualitative research is the in-depth study of human phenomena within their natural setting (e.g., pharmacists working in a pharmacy, patients receiving care in an ambulatory clinic) used to better examine the "why" of the research question being studied. Quantitative research is the process of collecting, grouping, and analyzing numerical data. These two research methods can be combined by: (1) collecting and analyzing both types of data in response to research questions and hypotheses, (2) integrating the two types of data and the results, (3) organizing data collection procedures into specific research designs, and (4) framing the data collection within the theory.[23] A mixed methods study design can be particularly helpful to describe a patient's point of view; however, the process of combining the data collection and analysis requires additional methodological expertise.

DEFINE IMPLEMENTATION THEORIES, FRAMEWORKS, AND MODELS

Although theories, frameworks, and models are often discussed together in the implementation science literature, they are quite different.[24] A theory is the most unique in this group as it is testable and can help predict and evaluate specific factors that affect an outcome. Ideally, a theory would be able to provide an explanation of how different concepts relate to one another, ultimately leading to an outcome of interest. Implementation frameworks and implementation models, however, describe relationships between different concepts but do not attempt to explain them. A framework lays out the concepts and how they relate, but they do not provide explanations- the "why." Models can be thought of as being in between both theories and frameworks. They do try to distill an idea or process, like a theory, but as a framework, they are only descriptive rather than explanatory and testable.[25] Still, in implementation science, with all its complexity, frameworks, and models offer tremendous benefits in terms of planning, organization, and communication.

SELECTING AND ADAPTING A MODEL FOR YOUR RESEARCH

For this chapter, the focus will be on one popular way of organizing the numerous theories, frameworks, and models. A narrative review was published that made an attempt to make sense of theories, frameworks, and models in implementation science by grouping them by their intended use. The three approaches for applying theory in implementation science are: (1) describing and/or guiding the process of translating research into practice, (2) understanding and/or explaining what influences implementation outcomes, and (3) evaluating implementation.[25]

The first approach focuses entirely on process models, which help specify steps in the process of turning research into practice. Process models can provide more practical guidance to help plan for and engage in implementation activities. Popular examples of process models include the Canadian Institutes of Health Research Model of Knowledge Translation,[26] the Knowledge to Action Framework,[27] and the Ottawa Model.[28]

The next approach to applying theory in implementation science focuses on understanding influences on implementation outcomes. This category can be broken down into three groups based on the origins of the theories or frameworks: Determinant frameworks, classic theories, and implementation theories. Determinant frameworks help specify facilitators and barriers that affect implementation outcomes with the overall goal of measuring their relationship. Examples of these include the Theoretical Domains Framework,[29] the Consolidated Framework for Implementation Research,[30] and the Promoting Action on Research Implementation in Health Services Framework.[31] Classic theories originated in other disciplines but have been used in implementation science to help provide context or understanding to aspects of this type of research. Examples of classic theories are numerous and cover broad topics, including decision making, social cognitive theories, and other organizational theories. The third subgroup in this approach is the implementation theories which have been specifically developed for implementation science to provide a better understanding of this discipline. Examples of these are Capacity-Opportunities-Motivation-Behavior[32] and Implementation Climate.[33]

The third and final approach is evaluating implementation, where evaluation frameworks are used. Evaluation frameworks are specifically designed to identify aspects of implementation projects that can be evaluated to determine a successful intervention. Popular examples of evaluation frameworks include RE-AIM[34] and PRECEDE-PROCEED.[35]

Practical Considerations

Logic models are graphical depictions of how a program, project, or research study will work and how elements interact.[36] They have been used for decades for program evaluation to communicate more effectively with various stakeholders about the "what" and "how" of proposed projects. Logic models can be useful in the planning, organization, implementation, and evaluation stages of a large project, especially when diverse groups of clinicians and researchers with different backgrounds are involved. National funders, including the AHRQ, National Institutes of Health, and PCORI, require or strongly recommend the use of a basic version of a logic model.[37]

Many different disciplines, including public health, policy analysis, and implementation science, use logic models, so they do not always all have the same types of information. This chapter will focus on the Implementation Research Logic Model (IRLM).[36] The IRLM was created based on the specific needs of implementation science projects, the discipline's unique terminology, and the diversity of frameworks, theories, and models used. A printable and fillable version of the IRLM is available online, and an example is reproduced in Figure 10–2.[36] This "standard" version of the IRLM does not include a section on the evidence-based practice being implemented because, for most practical projects, the practice will be established prior to the implementation project.

The IRLM is broken down into four categories: Determinants, Implementation Strategies, Mechanisms, and Outcomes.[36,38] Determinants, also known as barriers and facilitators, are factors that help or hurt the implementation of evidence-based practice. Implementation strategies are how specific aspects of the current clinical practice are being supported, changed, or intervened on to support the adoption of the evidence-based practice. Mechanisms of action are how an implementation strategy has its desired effect. For example, a causal process could be the use of fidelity monitoring strategies among pharmacists performing MTM activities to assure the evidence-based practice is

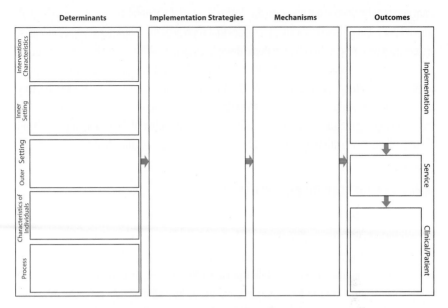

Figure 10–2. Implementation Research Logic Model (IRLM) Standard Form.[36]

being carried out the same way every time, which would lead to increased fidelity of delivery and sustainability. Finally, outcomes are the effects of specific actions taken to implement evidence-based practice and can be indicators of the implementation process itself, outcomes of the practice, or clinical outcomes. The key, however, is linking which implementation strategies are theoretically affecting which outcomes and through what mechanisms. Laying out a logic model in this way will improve the reproducibility of the implementation science project.[36]

Starting Implementation Science Projects in Pharmacy

FINDING RESEARCH TEAM MEMBERS

Every research project needs a good team, and this is especially true for something as potentially complex as an implementation science project. Since this book is written with pharmacy trainees in mind, identifying a mentor with both clinical practice and research experience is important. Since there is not a huge number of practicing pharmacists that can fill both of these roles simultaneously, an experienced mentor should be sought in each area of expertise. After identifying a mentor (or mentors), or if you will be the principal investigator, the team needs to be fleshed out based on the desired project. In general, the team should be multidisciplinary and diverse to include members that represent the following groups: clinicians, project manager, researcher(s) in multiple disciplines as needed based on the research question (public health, statistics, social science, etc.), community members, and a stakeholder advisory committee.[39] As you see, there are a large number of specialties needed to carry out an implementation science project, so finding the right clinical and research mentors are critical. Outlining the roles and responsibilities for each member of the research team ahead of time will improve communication and help with recruiting team members.

COMMUNICATING WITH THE RESEARCH TEAM

As a pharmacist in training, whether that be a pharmacy student, intern, resident, or fellow, you will have to wear many different hats. As you plan and carry out an implementation science research project, besides being a clinician and aspiring researcher, you will need to be an excellent communicator and use skills from the field of project management. First, you will be the main point of contact for the project and make sure all meetings run smoothly. This can be easily overlooked, but you will oversee making sure meetings are scheduled, calendar invites are sent out, agendas are made (and followed), and notes are taken to record progress. Keeping track of all components of a complex implementation science research project can be daunting, so familiarizing yourself with the tools available in the Microsoft Office Suite and online apps like "Trello" will be critical to your success in your trainee role. Sloppy project management is an easy way for you to get side-tracked, deadlines to be forgotten about, and ultimately for the project to fall behind schedule. When you are working on an academic schedule, like most trainees are, a few days or weeks can mean a project does not get completed. Project management is the process of organizing a project, including setting goals and deliverables for a specific project. Communicating effectively with your team is important, but it can be especially prudent to communicate clearly with administrators when given the opportunity. They can help your project by identifying and acquiring the necessary resources (e.g., financial support, personnel, goodwill). By communicating the goals, significance, and potential outcomes of the research project to your "higher-ups," you will have a much better chance at success.

Dissemination Models

DEFINE DISSEMINATION RESEARCH

Dissemination and implementation are complementary and often used in combination yet are distinct from one another. As discussed in this chapter, implementation science is the process of integrating evidence-based practices into clinical practice. An antiquated and narrow view of dissemination relies on the submission of research findings in peer-reviewed journals or through presentations at research conferences. These methods of dissemination limit the number and types of stakeholders who are able to learn about the research findings being shared. Journal paywalls and lack of targeted messaging make these passive dissemination processes part of the reason the chasm exists between research and clinical practice.

Modern dissemination research is the active process for identifying target audiences and tailoring communication to them.[5,40] These communication strategies are designed to engage stakeholders, increase awareness and understanding of the evidence gained through implementation science and advocate for its use in policy, practice sites, and among individual clinicians or patients. This definition of dissemination has components of external validity and scaling up in that researchers seek to have replicable findings across different settings and conditions. To do this, potential adopters can be sought out systematically with the end goal of effectively spreading an innovative practice across various disciplines.[5]

COMBINING DISSEMINATION AND IMPLEMENTATION MODELS

Understanding that there is a wide variety of stakeholders involved in patient-centered research, the PCORI commissioned a D&I Framework.[40] Implementation science begins after the dissemination process successfully spreads an innovative process with new potential adopters. The framework calls for plans for dissemination and implementation to begin before the study findings are complete. If the studies that form the body of literature that support the evidence-based practices plan for dissemination and implementation from the outset, the entire translational process will speed up. Ultimately, patients and researchers both benefit from this more rigorous planning.

Reporting Guidelines for Implementation Research

NEED FOR STANDARDIZED REPORTING

As discussed throughout this chapter, implementation science is a relatively new and growing discipline. As terminologies grow and adapt to the science being performed, researchers performing the studies and stakeholders that want to use the study findings both have a difficult time keeping track of and interpreting the research. This can be due to inconsistently labeled implementation science studies and poorly described implementation strategies undertaken as part of the research. In 2013, there was a call to action for more rigorous reporting of implementation science studies, specifically in the naming, defining, and operationalizing implementation strategies used.[41] The goal of standardized reporting is the increase in the reproducibility of the research being performed.

STANDARDS FOR REPORTING IMPLEMENTATION STUDIES (StaRI) STATEMENT

Years after this call to action, in 2017, the Standards for Reporting Implementation Studies (StaRI) Statement was published.[42] The goal of this statement was to have guidelines in place to promote a more transparent and accurate report of implementation science studies. Similar to the PRISMA checklist for systematic reviews or the STROBE statement for observational research, StaRI is a checklist of 27 items that is discussed as part of a manuscript or research report that will improve the reporting of the research. There are seven sections in the StaRI checklist that closely follow the sections of a manuscript and include: (1) Title and Abstract, (2) Introduction, (3) Methods: Description, (4) Methods: Evaluation, (5) Results, (6) Discussion, and (7) General statements. Each of the items in the checklist is listed as pertaining to either the implementation strategy and/or the intervention itself. If the StaRI checklist is reviewed during project planning and diligently followed during manuscript writing, the research team will save a lot of time and potential headaches.

Exemplar of an Implementation Project in a Pharmacy Setting

INTRODUCTION TO RESEARCH PROJECT

With the United States surpassing 93,000 drug overdose deaths in 2020, opioid stewardship has been a clinical thrust of many inpatient and outpatient practice settings. The goal of opioid stewardship is to improve, monitor, and evaluate the use of opioids in these settings. In this example, the pharmacy resident will be implementing an intervention in an acute care hospital with the goal of reducing long-term opioid use among patients who have been treated for a cardiac condition that required surgery.

RESEARCH QUESTION

How do prescriber training and a reduction in the default opioid prescribing limits of the electronic medical record–based ordering system change the use of outpatient opioid medications at the time of discharge as well as three and six months post-discharge?

STUDY DESIGN

Since pain management prescriptions, including opioids, can be assessed as multiple observations, over time, for a number of consecutive points before and after an intervention, an interrupted time series design (ITSD) can be used. ITSD is a quasi-experimental design that can be used to estimate the causal impact of the opioid stewardship intervention without requiring random assignment. Specific details about this study design as well as other alternatives can be found in the companion book *Principles of Research Design and Drug Literature Evaluation.*[43]

SETTING

An acute care hospital that performs cardiac surgeries including coronary artery bypass grafts, heart valve replacement, insertion of pacemakers or ventricular assist devices, and heart transplants

TEAM

As a resident, you will need to focus on what local resources are available. Start with your residency director (if you were a student, start with your preceptor), as they should have the best understanding of who is able and willing to fill roles you will need on your research team. Now that your immediate mentor is in place, it is important to think about the project idea and ask yourself a few questions from Table 10–2.

TABLE 10–2. QUESTIONS TO HELP FIND TEAM MEMBERS

Category of Need	Questions to Determine Need	Team Research Role
Diffusion of Intervention	Who are the "champions" or thought leaders at the institution that would help drive the project forward?	Clinical Champion
Data Collection and Analysis	Do you need help with chart reviews or gathering data?	Other residents, Research Fellows, APPE Students
	What data is needed, and who has access to it?	Information Technology, Quality Management Team, Informatics Team
	Do you need statistical support?	Statistician, Clinical Research Manager, Academic faculty
Administration	Do you need funding?	Director of Pharmacy, Vice President that the pharmacy department reports to

LOGIC MODEL

An abbreviated logic model is provided in Figure 10–3, which lists the key components of the IRLM (Determinants, Implementation Strategies, Mechanisms, and Outcomes) for this project. Completing the logic model will help you walk through the entire project and help plan the implementation. Having a complete (or mostly complete) logic model will make conversations with other members of the research team much easier because they can see where they fit in the implementation project.

IMPLEMENTATION MODEL

This example implementation science project is based on the RE-AIM framework that is an evaluation framework and one of the easiest to start with for a first-time implementation science researcher. RE-AIM is an efficient framework for planning and evaluating clinical implementation projects[44] and focuses on five elements that are also reflected in the logic model:

1. Reach: Number or proportion of individuals eligible to participate in a new intervention
2. Effectiveness: Impact of the invention on the eligible population
3. Adoption: Number or proportion of individuals that participate in the implementation
4. Implementation: How well the evidence-based practice was followed by different groups of adopters
5. Maintenance: How well the intervention can be sustained after the research study is over

DATA COLLECTION

Data collection will be informed mostly by four key components: (1) your research question (including previous research), (2) your research team, (3) the key outcomes identified and listed in your logic model, and (4) resources available. First, you will need to review the literature to identify the gap in the research. By reviewing the literature, you will also familiarize yourself with common outcomes being measured in studies published in high-impact journals. You and your team can then strive to collect data on the same outcomes and in the same manner as done in those studies. Next, your research team will help you interpret the findings of the literature review and potentially fill in any "blind spots" you may have missed. Third, by this point, you will have drafted out your logic model, so a preliminary list of outcomes and how they

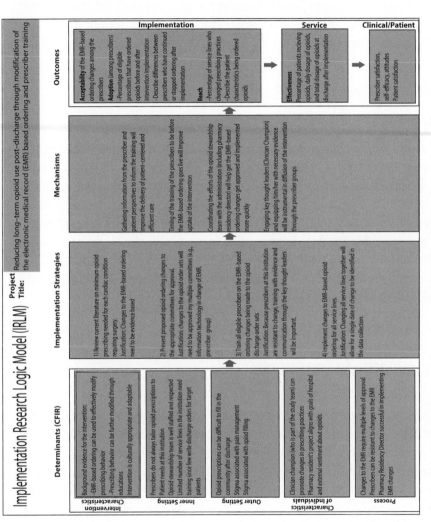

Figure 10–3. Filled in Implementation Research Logic Model (IRLM) Standard Form for example of implementation science project.

fit into your chosen framework will be available for you and your research team (see examples in the Outcomes section of the logic model). Finally, data collection for any project will be limited in some ways by the resources you have at your disposal. The biggest resource you have as a trainee is time, so planning how and when data will be collected will determine the types of data collection procedures you undertake. In addition to time, other costs to consider are personnel costs (for chart reviews), printing costs (for surveys), and transcription costs (for interviews). If you have a statistician on the team, they can also let you know if you need any data management programs to help you record data for them to help analyze.

ADAPT

Adaption will be required by any new adopter as each clinical practice site is unique. As you and your team collect data on this implementation project, it will be necessary to consider who the next adopters will be and make the information as transferrable as possible. Can you offer suggestions for how the implementation process could be changed based on barriers you and your team faced? If so, recording and providing specific information about how to adapt to these barriers will be immensely beneficial to the new adopters. This type of information is great to add to a discussion section of a research publication or presentation—no one wants to reinvent the wheel or guess what your research team did, especially in implementation science.

Summary and Conclusions

Well-designed implementation science research projects can improve the speed at which evidence-based practices translate from clinical research to patient care. Accelerating this process will help close the quality chasm that exists and keeps patients from receiving high-quality, evidence-based care. An implementation science project can take many forms, use different research designs, follow one of a variety of different frameworks, but it will always take a team of researchers and good communication. You have been provided with both technical and practical considerations for carrying out an implementation science research project. Also, this chapter provides an example logic model, one of the most critical pieces of planning and evaluating and implementation science project. As a pharmacy trainee, you will now be armed with enough information to talk to your academic mentor or workplace advisor about undertaking an implementation science project.

Key Points and Advice

- Pharmacists can benefit from a better understanding of what implementation science is and how it affects their practice sites.
- Before starting an implementation science project, find one or two mentors that can guide you through the clinical and research aspects of the research project.
- Dissemination and implementation go hand in hand and are both parts of the translational research continuum.
- Logic models will help guide many parts of an implementation science research project and should be completed at the onset of a new project.
- The StaRI Checklist should be used whenever findings from an implementation science project are shared as part of a research report or manuscript.

Chapter Review Questions

1. How does implementation science differ from quality improvement?
2. How can you choose when theory, model, or framework to use for your implementation science project?
3. How can a logic model improve an implementation science project?
4. What are the benefits of a substantial dissemination strategy?
5. Why is it important to provide standardization for reporting of implementation studies? What types of information are necessary to report?

Online Resources

- University of Washington's Implementation Science Resource Hub. https://impsciuw.org/
- United States Department of Veteran's Affairs Quality Enhancement Research Initiative (QUERI) Center for Evaluation and Implementation Resources (CEIR). https://www.queri.research.va.gov/ceir/resources.cfm
- National Institutes of Health Fogarty International Center Toolkit for Implementation Science Methodologies and Frameworks. https://www.fic.nih.gov/About/center-global-health-studies/neuroscience-implementation-toolkit/Pages/methodologies-frameworks.aspx
- Standards for Reporting Implementation Studies (StaRI) Checklist. https://www.equator-network.org/reporting-guidelines/stari-statement/
- Dissemination and Implementation Models in Health Research and Practice. https://dissemination-implementation.org/

REFERENCES

1. Insititute of Medicine. *Crossing the Quality Chasm: A New Health System for the 21st Century.* Washington, DC: National Academies Press; 2001.

2. National Cancer Institute. Implementation Science. Published 2021. Accessed 21 March, 2021. https://cancercontrol.cancer.gov/is

3. Morris ZS, Wooding S, Grant J. The answer is 17 years, what is the question: understanding time lags in translational research. *J R Soc Med.* 2011;104(12):510-520.

4. Koczwara B, Stover AM, Davies L, et al. Harnessing the synergy between improvement science and implementation science in cancer: a call to action. *J Oncol Pract.* 2018;14(6):335-340.

5. *Dissemination and Implementation Research in Health: Translating Science to Practice.* 2nd ed. England: Oxford University Press; 2017.

6. Rogers EM. *Diffusion of Innovations.* 5th ed. New York: Free Press; 2003.

7. Sackett DL, Rosenberg WM, Gray JA, Haynes RB, Richardson WS. Evidence based medicine: what it is and what it isn't. *BMJ.* 1996;312(7023):71-72.

8. Brownson RC, Fielding JE, Maylahn CM. Evidence-based public health: a fundamental concept for public health practice. *Annu Rev Public Health.* 2009;30:175-201.

9. Agency for Healthcare Research and Quality. *An Organizational Guide to Building Health Services Research Capacity: Introduction.* Agency for Healthcare Research and Quality. Published 2014. Accessed January 15, 2021. https://www.ahrq.gov/funding/training-grants/hsrguide/hsrguide-main-page.html

10. Fort DG, Herr TM, Shaw PL, Gutzman KE, Starren JB. Mapping the evolving definitions of translational research. *J Clin Transl Sci.* 2017;1(1):60-66.

11. Curran GM, Shoemaker SJ. Advancing pharmacy practice through implementation science. *Res Social Adm Pharm.* 2017;13(5):889-891.

12. Smith MA. Implementing primary care pharmacist services: Go upstream in the world of value-based payment models. *Res Social Adm Pharm.* 2017;13(5):892-895.

13. Stafford R, Thomas J, Payakachat N, et al. Using an array of implementation strategies to improve success rates of pharmacist-initiated medication therapy management services in community pharmacies. *Res Social Adm Pharm.* 2017;13(5):938-946.

14. Diamantouros A, Kiss A, Papastavros T, David U, Zwarenstein M, Geerts WH. The TOronto ThromboProphylaxis Patient Safety Initiative (TOPPS): A cluster randomised trial. *Res Social Adm Pharm.* 2017;13(5):997-1003.

15. Evaluation M. Fundamentals of Implementaion Research. US Agency for International Development. Published 2012. Accessed March 15, 2021. https://www.measureevaluation.org/resources/publications/ms-12-55

16. University of Washington. Overview of Study Designs in Implementation Science. University of Washington. Published 2021. Accessed January 3, 2021. https://impsciuw.org/implementation-science/research/designing-is-research/

17. Hemming K, Eldridge S, Forbes G, Weijer C, Taljaard M. How to design efficient cluster randomised trials. *BMJ.* 2017;358.

18. Hemming K, Lilford R, Girling AJ. Stepped-wedge cluster randomised controlled trials: a generic framework including parallel and multiple-level designs. *Stat Med.* 2015;34(2):181-196.

19. Curran GM, Bauer M, Mittman B, Pyne JM, Stetler C. Effectiveness-implementation hybrid designs: combining elements of clinical effectiveness and implementation research to enhance public health impact. *Med Care.* 2012;50(3):217-226.

20. Bernal JL, Cummins S, Gasparrini A. Interrupted time series regression for the evaluation of public health interventions: a tutorial. *Int J Epidemiol.* 2017;46(1):348-355.

21. Maciejewski ML, Basu A. Regression discontinuity design. *JAMA.* 2020;324(4):381-382.

22. Tunis SR, Stryer DB, Clancy CM. Practical clinical trials: increasing the value of clinical research for decision making in clinical and health policy. *JAMA.* 2003;290(12):1624-1632.

23. Creswell JW, Plano-Clark VL. *Designing and Conducting Mixed Methods Research.* 3rd ed. Los Angeles, CA: SAGE Publications, Inc; 2017.

24. University of Washington. Pick a Theory, Model, or Framework. Published 2021. Accessed March 19, 2021. https://impsciuw.org/implementation-science/research/frameworks/

25. Nilsen P. Making sense of implementation theories, models and frameworks. *Implement. Sci.* 2015;10:53.

26. Canadian Institutes of Health Research. Knowledge Translation at CIHR. Published 2016. Accessed January 5, 2021. https://cihr-irsc.gc.ca/e/29418.html

27. Wilson KM, Brady TJ, Lesesne C, Translation NWGo. An organizing framework for translation in public health: the Knowledge to Action Framework. *Prev Chronic Dis.* 2011;8(2):A46.

28. Graham ID, Logan J. Innovations in knowledge transfer and continuity of care. *Can J Nurs Res.* 2004;36(2):89-103.

29. Atkins L, Francis J, Islam R, et al. A guide to using the Theoretical Domains Framework of behaviour change to investigate implementation problems. *Implement Sci.* 2017;12(1):77.

30. Damschroder LJ, Aron DC, Keith RE, Kirsh SR, Alexander JA, Lowery JC. Fostering implementation of health services research findings into practice: a consolidated framework for advancing implementation science. *Implement Sci.* 2009;4:50.

31. Kitson A, Harvey G, McCormack B. Enabling the implementation of evidence based practice: a conceptual framework. *Qual Health Care.* 1998;7(3):149-158.

32. Michie S, van Stralen MM, West R. The behaviour change wheel: a new method for characterising and designing behaviour change interventions. *Implement Sci.* 2011;6:42.

33. May C, Finch T. Implementing, embedding, and integrating practices: an outline of normalization process theory. *Sociology.* 2009;43(3).

34. Glasgow RE, Vogt TM, Boles SM. Evaluating the public health impact of health promotion interventions: the RE-AIM framework. *Am J Public Health.* 1999;89(9):1322-1327.

35. Green L, Kreuter M. *Health Program Planning: An Educational and Ecological Approach.* 4th ed. New York: McGraw-Hill Humanities/Social Sciences/Languages; 2004.

36. Smith JD, Li DH, Rafferty MR. The Implementation Research Logic Model: a method for planning, executing, reporting, and synthesizing implementation projects. *Implement Sci.* 2020;15(1):84.

37. Funnell SC, Rogers PJ. *Purposeful Program Theory: Effective Use of Theories of Change and Logic Models.* 1st ed. Jossey-Bass; 2011.

38. Proctor E, Silmere H, Raghavan R, et al. Outcomes for implementation research: conceptual distinctions, measurement challenges, and research agenda. *Adm Policy Ment Health.* 2011;38(2):65-76.

39. World Health Organization. *Implementation Research Toolkit: Workbook.* 2014.

40. Esposito D, Heeringa J, Bradley K, Croake S, Kimmey L. PCORI Dissemination and Implementation Framework. Patient-Centered Outcomes Research Institute. Published 2015. Accessed January 15, 2021. https://www.pcori.org/sites/default/files/PCORI-DI-Framework-February-2015.pdf

41. Proctor EK, Powell BJ, McMillen JC. Implementation strategies: recommendations for specifying and reporting. *Implement Sci.* 2013;8:139.

42. Pinnock H, Barwick M, Carpenter CR, et al. Standards for Reporting Implementation Studies (StaRI) Statement. *BMJ.* 2017;356:i6795.

43. Aparasu RR, Bentley JP. *Principles of research design and drug literature evaluation.* 2nd ed. New York: McGraw-Hill; 2020.

44. Kwan BM, McGinnes HL, Ory MG, Estabrooks PA, Waxmonsky JA, Glasgow RE. RE-AIM in the real world: use of the RE-AIM framework for program planning and evaluation in clinical and community settings. *Front Public Health.* 2019;7:345.

Chapter Eleven

Survey Research in Pharmacy Settings

Anandi V. Law, BPharm, MS, PhD, FAPhA and Sun Lee, PharmD

Chapter Objectives

- Define survey research in pharmacy settings
- Identify common research questions that can be addressed with survey research in pharmacy settings
- Understand the practical and technical considerations for conducting survey research in pharmacy settings
- Describe the advantages and disadvantages of developing a new survey or adopting an existing survey (or existing measurement scales) for research in pharmacy settings
- Discuss the strategies for harnessing the expertise needed for conducting survey research in pharmacy settings
- Describe an example of a learner-involved survey research project in a pharmacy setting
- Understand the dissemination framework for survey research in pharmacy settings

Key Terminology

Branching, coverage error, deliberate sampling, in-person surveys, Internet (web-based) surveys, mail surveys, measurement error, mixed mode surveys, nonresponse error, random sampling, response rate, sample, sampling error, sampling frame, target population, telephone surveys, survey research

Introduction

Survey research is a method used to gather information by asking a relevant group of people questions on a specific topic.[1] The survey method is essential when addressing topics such as opinions or individuals' self-reports about knowledge, attitudes, perceptions, and behaviors. Surveys have become a commonly used research tool in healthcare in general and pharmacy in particular. For example, a review of the literature published in 2017 revealed that 52% of all original research articles in high-impact medical education journals used survey research methods.[2] In pharmacy, the use of survey research methods can be found in student-, resident-, practitioner-, and researcher-led projects from diverse pharmacy practice settings including health-systems, ambulatory care, community, pharmaceutical industry, managed care organizations, regulatory agencies, and academia.

Despite their common use and the wide availability of tools to support their use, conducting a survey research project is not easy and involves many considerations. The purpose of this chapter is to provide practical guidance to develop, administer, and report survey research. It begins by defining and discussing the steps in the process of conducting a survey research project and describing various research questions in pharmacy settings that can be addressed with survey research. A number of practical and technical considerations for conducting survey research in pharmacy settings are outlined, including a discussion of the trade-offs between developing a new survey tool versus using or adapting existing surveys or measures. Finally, an example of a learner-involved project involving the use of survey research in a pharmacy setting is described to demonstrate the application of the various considerations involved in the process. This chapter can help learners who are planning to develop a survey, administer new or existing surveys to conduct research, and/or assess the quality of a research article employing survey methods.

Steps in Survey Research

Alreck and Settle outline six major steps in the survey research process: (1) specifying information needs, (2) sampling design, (3) instrumentation, (4) data collection, (5) data processing, and (6) report generation.[3] These steps correspond with the basic steps of the scientific research process that have been described in other sections of this book. For example, specifying information needs is another way to describe "posing a research question and hypothesis." Sampling design and instrumentation are key elements of the research plan when conducting survey research as they specify the sample to be selected and the survey instrument to administer. The researcher's information needs (i.e., research questions) often dictate subsequent steps in the process. The next two sections explore different types of research questions in pharmacy settings that can be addressed with survey research, along with some practical and technical considerations that can be used to support decisions regarding the research plan and the collection of data from a survey study.

Research Questions that Can Be Addressed with Survey Research

Survey research has been applied to answer a wide assortment of research questions in pharmacy settings. These research questions may be: (1) exploratory (i.e., addressing questions to explore or gain insight on a topic), (2) descriptive (i.e., addressing questions of "who," "what," "when," and "where"); or (3) analytic (i.e., addressing questions of "why" and "how" about the relationships between variables/constructs). Depending on the type of research, the research question can be formulated to examine independent (exposure or perception) and dependent variables (outcomes or behaviors) and their relationships.

Surveys can be used to measure important outcomes in any prospective research project, including experiments/clinical trials and nonexperimental research. For example, Chapter 12 describes how patient-reported outcome measures (which are collected from patients using survey research methods) are used in clinical trials or intervention studies. Surveys have also been used to collect feedback from patients, providers, or others in the evaluation of programs and services (e.g., measures of patient satisfaction). Surveys can also be used in nonexperimental/observational research. While many think of surveys being collected in a cross-sectional manner, it is certainly possible to collect data in a longitudinal manner via survey research methods for cohort studies. Table 11–1 provides several examples of studies that have used surveys in pharmacy research in each of these categories.

A clearly defined research question is an essential step in implementing survey research. As described in Chapter 4, a well-defined research question should contain information about the population (or patient situation or problem of interest), intervention (or exposure or patient perceptions), comparator (if relevant), outcome, timing, and setting using the PICOTS model.[10,11] When using PICOTS, the outcome can be measured using survey research. Examples of two research questions that are addressed using survey methods along with the elements from the PICOTS framework are provided in Table 11–2.

TABLE 11–1. EXAMPLES OF RESEARCH QUESTIONS FROM THE PHARMACY LITERATURE ADDRESSED WITH SURVEY RESEARCH

General Category of Research	Authors	Research Question / Study Objective	Study Findings
		Example	
Descriptive and exploratory studies	Xiong et al.[4]	To evaluate the perspectives and perceived barriers that pharmacy personnel have in providing pharmacist-prescribed tobacco cessation services in the community pharmacy setting	About 92.4% of pharmacists who responded to the survey agreed that community pharmacists should provide tobacco cessation service, and 54.4% reported that "lack of time during normal workflow to deliver tobacco cessation service" was the biggest barrier to implement a tobacco cessation service in community pharmacy.
Survey development and validation studies	Livet et al.[5]	To develop and validate the Implementation Outcomes Questionnaire (IOQ), which assesses the implementation of medication optimization services, starting with Comprehensive Medication Management (CMM)	The results supported the reliability and validity of the 40-item IOQ to assess the implementation of medication optimization in domains related to service adoption, acceptability, feasibility, appropriateness, penetration, and sustainability.
Association studies and theory-driven/ theory-testing studies	Burstein et al.[6]	To evaluate pharmacist attitudes regarding recommending pharmacy-based naloxone	The findings suggested that working in a pharmacy that had a standing order or collaborative practice agreement to allow pharmacists to dispense naloxone without a physician's prescription was associated with a positive attitude toward opioid overdose prevention and public health prevention.
Patient and provider feedback/ evaluation of programs and services	Kelly et al.[7]	To capture the opinions of family physicians and community pharmacists in Newfoundland and Labrador (NL) regarding collaborative practice	A survey of Canadian family medicine physicians and pharmacists revealed that both groups agree that collaborative practice can positively affect patient outcomes. Both groups identified reimbursement models and insufficient time in the clinic as barriers to facilitate collaborative practice between the two professions.
Longitudinal studies that use surveys (e.g., to evaluate change)	Lee et al.[8]	To assess the effectiveness of an educational intervention to improve prescription label understanding	The findings suggest that the focused education on the prescription label at the community pharmacy helps improve prescription label understanding and observed action to fill the pillbox correctly following the prescription label instruction.

(Continued)

TABLE 11–1. EXAMPLES OF RESEARCH QUESTIONS FROM THE PHARMACY LITERATURE ADDRESSED WITH SURVEY RESEARCH (CONTINUED)

General Category of Research	Authors	Research Question / Study Objective	Study Findings
		Example	
Educational research	Crawford et al.[9]	To examine students' self-perceptions at different stages in a pharmacy curriculum of competence related to serving culturally diverse patients and to compare self-reported competence of a student cohort near the beginning and end of the degree program	There were differences in cross-sectional perceptions of knowledge, skills, and comfort in multicultural clinical encounters, which were highest for students in the P4 (fourth professional) year. Longitudinal analysis of the same cohort of students in P1 (first professional) and P4 years found a similar pattern, where perceptions of cultural competence improved in terms of knowledge, skills, and clinical encounters comfort.

TABLE 11–2. EXAMPLES OF LITERATURE-BASED SURVEY RESEARCH QUESTIONS ALONG WITH THE ELEMENTS FROM THE PICOTS FRAMEWORK

Research Question	PICOTS Study Elements
What is the change in first-year student pharmacists' competence and perceptions regarding pharmacogenomics before and after experiencing an interactive learning method?[12]	Population: First-year student pharmacists Intervention: Lecture, discussion, and patient care laboratory training on the topic of pharmacogenomics Comparison: None but a repeated measure of the same sample's pre-post survey results Outcome: 27-item survey on attitude toward the use of pharmacogenomics Timing: Before the intervention (pre-survey) and after the intervention (post-survey) Setting: Distribution of the survey done using Qualtrics in a classroom setting
What is the impact of a blended learning program related to the preconception, pregnancy, and lactation topics on community pharmacists?[13]	Population: Community pharmacists Intervention: e-learning and on-site training program Comparison: None but a repeated measure of the sample's pre-post survey results Outcome: Survey to capture self-reported barriers and competence (14 items), knowledge about preconception, pregnancy, and lactation (11 items) Timing: Pre-survey was administered before participating in the program, and post-survey was administered three-six months after participating in the program. Setting: Community pharmacy setting

Technical and Practical Considerations for Survey Research

SAMPLING DESIGN AND THE SAMPLE

Sample vs. Population

Selecting a subset of the population (i.e., a sample) is important to adequately answer a specific research question. In pharmacy-related research, surveys may be administered to the general public, patients with certain health conditions, patients from a specific clinic or pharmacy, members enrolled in a health plan, healthcare practitioners, administrators, and students and residents in a health professional program. Administering a survey to all potential respondents or to the entire general public is impractical because of the size and accessibility of the population and/or the difficulty and cost in identifying all possible respondents. For these reasons, survey researchers often select samples. When selecting sources of survey respondents, it is important to first define and determine a target population, or the subset of people who researchers intend to draw conclusions about as part of their survey research project, before deciding on sampling techniques. This process helps the investigator to formulate a well-defined PICOTS question by defining the Patient (P). Other questions to ask when defining the target population include: "who is the optimal sample?," "where will the sample be drawn from?," "what kind of sampling technique is feasible to implement?," and "how many respondents need to complete the survey?." Knowledge of the target population is essential for selecting a sampling frame or a list of persons in the target population from which a sample is drawn (note that in some situations, a good sampling frame may not exist).

Finding Respondents

There are several ways to find potential respondent pools. When administering the survey in-person, surveyors can utilize waiting areas in outpatient clinics and pharmacies. Before collecting survey data using such an approach, it is important to receive Institutional Review Board (IRB) approval regarding the use of the waiting area. IRBs will often ask for written documentation of permission from an authorized individual (e.g., the clinic or pharmacy manager) to collect data at outside institutions (see Chapter 6 for more details). When administering the survey telephonically, researchers may be able to use records of telephone numbers housed in information systems maintained by hospitals, clinics, pharmacies, or insurance companies. Certainly, IRB approval, along with permission from these outside institutions, is required to access such information. Internet or web-based survey distribution has enabled a number of flexible options for reaching a wide range of respondent pools. Using appropriate approvals and permissions, the email addresses of those in the target population can be obtained. As another example, when conducting a survey of practicing pharmacists, researchers may be able to gain access to potential respondents via an email list acquired from state boards of pharmacy or by sending an email through a state pharmacy association.

Some survey researchers have even posted a link to a survey at a website or in an online forum that is often visited by members of the target population. If using this approach, it is important to include screening questions at the beginning of the survey to ensure respondents are members of the target population and to implement methods to avoid receiving duplicate responses from the same individual. Another way to distribute a web-based survey is by working with paid vendors who maintain and facilitate access to panels of respondents, such as patients with certain medical conditions or healthcare professionals within a specific discipline. Examples of such vendors include Amazon Mechanical Turk, Qualtrics Mailer, and Upwork.[14,15]

Sampling Techniques

Sample selection can be random or deliberate. Random sampling, also known as a probability sampling design, is implemented when everyone in the target population has an equal (or at least known) chance of being selected to be included in the study. Deliberate sampling, also known as a nonprobability sampling design (convenience sampling, quota sampling, and purposive sampling are examples of nonprobability sampling designs), is implemented when investigators cannot estimate the chance of a given individual being included in the study.[16] There are a number of other sampling design options that are beyond the scope of this chapter (e.g., stratified sampling, cluster sampling). Readers are referred to a number of sources[3,17,18] that discuss these topics in greater detail, and learners should consult with their mentors or perhaps a biostatistician when constructing a sampling design.

The use of an appropriate sampling technique is important in order to answer the original research question and objectives. Survey designs in healthcare often use nonprobability sampling because the research is usually focused on a specific sub-population for which it may be difficult to find a well-defined list (e.g., patients with a certain condition or pharmacists with experience delivering a certain service). The potential to generalize information gathered from survey respondents to a target population depends on the size of the sample and the extent to which respondents are similar to nonrespondents. It is challenging to determine whether there are differences in survey responses between respondents and nonrespondents. Therefore, an appropriate sampling technique is needed to achieve a high response rate (please see later section on possible errors in survey research) that addresses the generalizability of the study findings.

Sample Size Considerations

An appropriate sample size is key for analysis and to make inferences from the results. Several factors should be considered when determining the sample size needed for a survey research project.[3,17,18] These include[18]: (1) the heterogeneity of the population being studied, (2) the level of precision desired when estimating results from a survey study, (3) the type of sampling design being used, (4) the number of subgroup breakdowns one is interested in (i.e., the number of different distinct categories of interest that one wishes to divide the sample into to look for differences in responses to certain survey questions), and (5) the analysis planned for the survey data based on the research question. Regarding these last two considerations, it is important to consider the statistical methods that will be used to analyze survey data (which is based on the aim of the study and the primary outcome(s) of interest) prior to the collection of any data.

One simple rule of thumb is to use about 5 to 10 participants for each survey item. Some literature supports the use of a minimum of 30 participants to have a meaningful analysis using the tests that are based on the Central Limit Theorem. Other literature considers a range of 200 to 300 participants (or even much higher) to be an appropriate sample size. Keep in mind that this is the actual number of respondents needed; the number of potential respondents one needs to contact may be much higher depending on the expected response rate to the survey. There are a number of tools and resources available for determining needed sample size, and depending on their situation, learners may need to seek advice from a biostatistician when making decisions about sample size.

INSTRUMENTATION

Developing a New Survey vs. Using or Adapting an Existing Survey

Investigators can choose to develop a new survey or use an existing survey to answer the study objective(s) based on the availability of the survey tools. Each approach has its pros and cons, as listed in Table 11–3, which also illustrates the purposes of using a new survey or an existing survey. Please keep in mind that it may be possible for a survey to include some measurement scales that have already been developed (e.g., a generic health-related quality of life measure or a self-reported measure of medication adherence) while also including measures that are newly developed for a particular study. Investigators often spend considerable time searching the literature to determine whether there are existing measurement scales that are suitable to address their research questions. In addition, many disciplines have repositories of developed measures that are specific to those fields, and investigators are encouraged to review these resources. For example, the online resources section at the end of this chapter provides a link to the HealthMeasures website (also known as the Person-Centered Assessment Resource), which provides details about hundreds of measures that can be used to assess physical, mental, and social health, symptoms, well-being and life satisfaction, as well as sensory, motor, and cognitive function. These measures include the PROMIS (Patient-Reported Outcomes Measurement Information System) toolset, which can be used to assess multiple domains of health in adults and children (for more information about PROMIS, please see Chapter 12).

TABLE 11-3. PURPOSE, ADVANTAGES, AND DISADVANTAGES OF DEVELOPING A NEW SURVEY OR ADOPTING AN EXISTING SURVEY

Category	Purpose	Advantages	Disadvantages
Developing a new survey	A lack of an existing survey to answer the research question of interest	Original contribution to the literature	Time and effort to develop a new survey; may not always fit into the time frame for a student/resident project
		Customizable to answer the study objective	
	Limited reliability and validity evidence with the existing survey		Need to validate reliability and validity of the new survey
	Existing survey does not include questions that will answer the study objective		Run the risk of developing a survey with low reliability and validity, resulting in the need to modify the survey to answer the study objective
Using or adapting an existing survey	Existing body of literature supports the use of the validated survey to answer a specific question	Save time and efforts in survey development and validation	May not be customizable to answer the study objective
		Confidence in using the validated survey to capture a specific domain and theme to answer the study objective	As a good practice, should contact the original authors to ask for permission to use the existing survey; this process may take time
		Easy to compare with the results of the existing research (e.g., PHQ-2 of a specific population can be compared with the general U.S. population through the existing survey result)	

Considerations for the development of a new survey can be found in a simplified seven-step process outlined in Table 11–4. Some of the steps described in Table 11–4 also pertain to research conducted with an existing survey (e.g., cover letters, pilot testing, reliability, and validity testing).

It is important to note that data collected from survey research projects designed and conducted by others are often made publicly available for use by researchers as secondary data. These include national population surveys such as the Medical Expenditure Panel Survey (MEPS) and the National Survey on Drug Use and Health (NSDUH), as well as surveys of providers such as the National Ambulatory Medical Care Survey (NAMCS). For more information on these types of secondary data sources, which often use complex sampling methods, please refer to Chapter 14 where links to online resources for many of these national population surveys and provider surveys are available. In addition, a

TABLE 11–4. SEVEN-STEP PROCESS OF DEVELOPING A NEW SURVEY

Steps	Practical and Technical Considerations
1. Item generation	This is a brainstorming step to consider and include all potential items to capture ideas and concepts. The goal is to identify domains, categories, and themes to help answer the research objective. A thorough literature review is necessary, which may reveal theoretical frameworks that can be utilized to set up the survey tool. Best practices include an initial qualitative approach using focus-group or interview sessions with potential respondents and experts to generate items. Item generation should continue until no new ideas emerge. The Delphi process can be used at this step.
2. Item reduction	Once all relevant ideas and concepts are captured in a list of items, the investigator reviews the list and reduces the items into a manageable form. Some have recommended that a survey should include less than 25 items and no more than five items per each domain;[19] however, the length of a survey is dependent on the research objective(s). Item reduction can also continue following pilot studies.
3. Question stem	Each question should target a single domain, construct, or category. Question stem should be composed of less than 20 words, using a nonjudgmental and unbiased tone. Avoid using absolute terms such as always, never, or none. Avoid using complex terminology and abbreviations.
4. Response formatting	Responses can use open-ended or closed-ended formatting. Closed-ended response formatting includes binary (yes or no), nominal, ordinal, interval, and ratio measurement. One of the common closed-ended response methods to capture the varying degree of response level is the Likert scale. Use of published textbooks[3,20–22] to choose the appropriate scale is recommended during the response formatting stage. Finally, it is important to be mindful of the reverse-coding based on the positive and negative question stems and how it is captured through the response formatting.
5. Handout including cover letter and survey questions	A cover letter for a survey describes the study objective(s) and reasons for being selected as a potential respondent. In many cases, it serves to provide the necessary consent information as required by an IRB. This letter should be concise and easy to understand. Providing contact information for any questions related to the study could instill trust in potential respondents, possibly resulting in an improved response rate. Depending on the methods to distribute and administer the survey, the survey questions can be represented in a paper or web-based format.
6. Pilot testing	Pilot testing can be conducted by administering the survey to a small group of potential respondents and content experts. The respondents and experts could provide information related to flow, readability, redundancy, confusing and poorly worded questions, and time to complete the survey. Following the pilot testing, investigators could decide to add, edit, or remove any questions.
7. Reliability and validity (i.e., psychometric validation)	At this stage of gathering results from the pilot testing, it is important to work with a biostatistician or researchers with expertise in psychometric validation. There are several tests that can be run to test for the reliability and validity of the survey or measurement scales contained within a survey. Internal consistency reliability can be assessed using a statistical method (i.e., Cronbach's coefficient alpha). Additional reliability tests such as test-retest and inter-rater reliability tests can be performed, if appropriate. If the pilot testing was done with a sample size greater than five respondents per item, factor analysis could be run to further investigate the revision and removal of the domain. Methods to capture the validity of the survey to answer the research question include the face, content, construct, and criterion validity. For more information, please see these references.[22–24]

valuable source for publicly available survey data related to the social, behavioral, and health sciences is the Inter-university Consortium for Political and Social Research (ICPSR) housed at the University of Michigan (https://www.icpsr.umich.edu/web/pages/).

Basic Principles of Question Writing

When planning to develop a new survey, it is important to carefully consider and plan the research question(s) based on the PICOTS model. Researchers could also use theoretical models or conceptual frameworks as the foundation for developing the survey. It is useful to involve content experts in the field, colleagues, and members of the target population to identify essential themes and domains to answer the research question(s). Researchers may decide to use qualitative methods such as conducting focus groups or in-depth interviews with potential respondents in the early stages of survey development to provide guidance.

Once the appropriate themes are identified, questions should be formulated and written in a clear and concise manner. Readers are referred to Dillman and colleagues for a detailed treatise on survey item writing.[17] The use of all capital letters (i.e., "all caps") should be avoided, and the questions should be numbered clearly. Questions that contain double negatives and ambiguous items should be avoided. Double-barreled questions should be avoided, which means that it is important to include one target item per one question. For example, a question about "how satisfied were you with the pharmacist interaction and with the pharmacy waiting time?" should be divided into two separate questions "how satisfied were you with the pharmacist interaction?" and "how satisfied were you with the pharmacy waiting time?". When asking sensitive questions, it is important to disclose the purpose of the study as clearly as possible at the front of the survey. In addition, steps to ensure respondents' anonymity should be taken and explained to potential respondents. Some IRBs may require additional disclosures and provision of additional information depending on the nature of the sensitive questions.

New investigators sometimes struggle with how and when to ask questions to gather information about respondents' demographic information (e.g., sex, gender, age, race, ethnicity, income, education level, employment status, marital status, insurance status, practice setting [for surveys of pharmacists and other practitioners]). Researchers should always consider how much demographic information needs to be collected and what they intend to do with the information. An excessive number of demographic questions may create a burden for respondents, possibly leading to lower response rates or failures to complete the survey. Experienced researchers sometimes add these questions to the end of the survey rather than the beginning in order to gather relevant information in the event the respondent decides not to respond to all demographic questions. Researchers are encouraged to explore the wording of demographic questions in sources such as the

American Community Survey (ACS) conducted by the U.S. Census Bureau (https://www.census.gov/programs-surveys/acs) or one of the many national population surveys conducted by various government agencies.

Other best practices include the formulation of a clear cover letter explaining the duration of the survey, the purpose of the survey, and possible benefits and risks associated with completing the survey. Additional details can be found in Table 11–4.

DATA COLLECTION METHODS

Common survey data collection methods include in-person interviews (i.e., face-to-face interviews), telephone interviews, mail data collection, and Internet (web-based) distribution platforms such as SurveyMonkey, Qualtrics, REDCap, and Google forms. In-person surveys involve a two-way interaction between the researcher and the respondent. The response rate is often high, but it is time-consuming and costly compared to other methods. Telephone surveys, similar to face-to-face interviews, allow for two-way interactions between the researcher and the respondent. They are quicker and cheaper to administer, but can be seen as intrusive and refusals to participate are generally more prevalent compared to in-person surveys. For a number of reasons, this approach as a stand-alone method of conducting surveys has decreased over the past 20 years.[17]

Sending printed questionnaires via the mail (i.e., mail surveys) does not allow two-way interactions between the researcher and the respondent; thus, it is important for instructions to be very clear.[3] Such an approach is fairly quick to administer, but concerns for low response rates need to be addressed by offering incentives to respond and by contacting a larger number of individuals to account for attrition and receive a desired number of respondents. Postage for initial survey distribution and for respondents to mail in their replies, as well as printing costs, also need to be taken into consideration.

Web-based survey administration (i.e., Internet or web-based surveys) has become a more prevalent method among survey researchers due to its relatively low cost and ease of administration and speed of data gathering. A key advantage of the web-based survey method is that responses are automatically captured in electronic form that can then be conveniently used for data analysis. In addition, branching (i.e., questions or sections of a questionnaire that are contingent on responses to previous questions) is much easier to implement with a web-based survey than a printed survey. There are also potential challenges to overcome with web-based surveys. For example, respondents may choose to complete a survey on different devices (i.e., desktops, laptops, tablets, or mobile devices), and the survey may not always appear the same on these devices. Researchers are encouraged to use tools from web-based survey distribution platforms to evaluate the appearance of different devices and to pretest their surveys on different devices. Low response rates are also an important concern to address. There are now several ways to communicate electronically, and some people may not regularly check all of their electronic forms of communication, which means that a standard approach to contact potential respondents (e.g., only using email) may not be very effective in some situations. Junk email filters may also be a challenge in reaching potential respondents. Similar to mail surveys, offering incentives may be necessary to achieve reasonable response rates with web-based surveys.

It is also possible to combine these survey data collection methods, leading to what is known as **mixed mode surveys**. This approach can include offering individuals more than one way to complete a survey. It may also be used to expand the sampling frame given that researchers may only have one type of contact information (i.e., postal mailing address, phone number, email address) available for potential respondents. Researchers may also decide to use one mode as the primary data collection approach and then switch to another mode in an attempt to collect additional responses, perhaps from more difficult-to-reach respondents. A mixed mode approach may also include sending a prenotification letter to potential survey respondents by mail prior to emailing a link to a web-based survey or texting reminders to individuals about responding to an email or web-based survey. For more information on mixed mode survey data collection, see Dillman, Smyth, and Christian.[17]

DATA ANALYSIS AND REPORTING

The purpose of data analysis is to summarize the collected data to answer the research question(s). For any survey project, researchers should spend time developing a data analysis plan prior to fielding their survey. It is important to consider the research question(s) and study endpoint(s) when choosing appropriate data analysis methods. In addition, the data analysis plan should include information about how to handle missing or incomplete data. There are a number of available resources to guide researchers in the selection of appropriate data analysis methods. Some of these resources are described in Chapter 7; in addition, this chapter provides advice about how to collaborate with statisticians.

Two considerations in the analysis of survey data deserve brief discussion: (1) the analysis of data from Likert and other close-ended rating scales, and (2) the analysis of data from open-ended questions. With respect to the former, Harpe describes the appropriate use of parametric and nonparametric analytical methods when analyzing rating scale data that are often generated from surveys.[25] Although there is still controversy surrounding the handling of such data, Harpe provides some useful recommendations. For example, data from summated (or aggregated) rating scales generally can be treated as continuous, as can data from individual rating items that use a numerical response format with at least five categories.[25] Nonparametric approaches or categorical data analysis methods should be considered for data from individual rating items that use numerical response formats with four or fewer categories or that use nonnumerical response formats.[25] Regarding the analysis of data from open-ended questions, many novice researchers assume that such analyses are simple and easy, when in practice, they can be quite challenging. One approach to the analysis of such data is to use qualitative research methods, such as content or thematic analysis (for more information, see Chapter 15).

POSSIBLE ERRORS IN SURVEY RESEARCH

According to Dillman and colleagues, errors that may occur when conducting survey research can be categorized into four types.[17] These errors include coverage error, sampling error, nonresponse error, and measurement error. Although it is not possible to completely eliminate all forms of these errors when conducting a survey project, researchers are encouraged to think about ways to minimize these errors in all stages of the survey research process because they can lead to inaccurate survey results (i.e., biased estimates during data analysis). In this section, definitions of each type of error and suggestions to minimize such errors are reviewed.

Coverage error is caused by a failure to accurately represent (or cover) the population of interest (the target population) in the list that will be used to generate the sample (the sampling frame). If those who are excluded from the sampling frame are different from those that are included in terms of what is being estimated by the survey, coverage error can be introduced. Survey researchers must define the target population for their study *and* make sure that the sampling frame used to draw their sample is as complete as possible. Researchers should also think critically about who might have been excluded from receiving the survey in the first place and how they might differ from those who are contacted. Sampling error is simply unavoidable whenever a sample is used to make inferences about a population. If everyone in the population (i.e., a census) completed a survey, there would be no sampling error. Thus, it is an error that results when surveying a sample of the population rather than everyone. It is fairly easily quantified and is commonly reported in survey findings as $+/-3\%$ (or something similar). Researchers have the ability to control the amount of sampling error; larger samples are associated with less sampling error. How much sampling error one is willing to tolerate can be used to help determine the appropriate sample size for a survey project.

Nonresponse error occurs when those in the sample who do not respond to the survey (i.e., nonrespondents) are different from those who do (i.e., respondents) in ways that are important to the topic of the survey. One important consideration that may serve as a warning regarding the presence of nonresponse error is a low response rate to a survey. The response rate is calculated as the number of returned and completed surveys divided by the number of eligible respondents in the sample. Thus, it is the proportion of individuals in the sample who completed the survey. There are a variety of approaches for increasing response rates to a survey, including:[17] (1) writing well-crafted cover letters that provide a convincing rationale for people to participate; (2) employing multiple contacts and follow-up requests (i.e., reminders) targeted to nonrespondents; (3) offering incentives for participation; (4) using several modes or switching survey modes; and (5) considering the length, appearance, and difficulty of the survey (i.e., take efforts to minimize response burden). It is important to keep in mind that a low response rate does not mean that nonresponse error definitely is present. Furthermore, although higher response rates do reduce the probability of nonresponse error, a high response rate does not guarantee the absence of nonresponse error. One must ask whether respondents are systematically different than nonrespondents on important survey questions to evaluate for nonresponse error. Some researchers will send abbreviated surveys to a random sample of nonrespondents in an attempt to evaluate differences between likely nonrespondents and those who responded to the full survey.

Measurement error refers to inaccurate or imprecise answers to survey questions and may be due to interviewers, data processors, survey questions, and respondents. When an in-person survey is the data collection mode, poorly trained interviewers may make mistakes such as "leading" (either consciously or unconsciously) respondents to respond in certain ways. When data processors are inputting survey responses into analyzable form, it is important to follow the predefined data input (coding) plan. Poorly designed coding plans may lead to measurement errors when a respondent's answer is not what is represented in a dataset. Poorly written survey questions (e.g., vague questions, double-barreled questions, questions with considerable jargon, leading questions) can introduce measurement error.[3] Finally, respondents may be unwilling or unable to provide accurate answers for a variety of reasons. Proper training and significant attention to question writing practices as well as pretesting are critical for minimizing measurement error.

Harnessing the Expertise Needed for Conducting Survey Research

When conducting a survey project, researchers may need to collaborate with or involve a number of different kinds of experts. For those analyzing publicly available survey data as secondary data, experts with experience using the specific dataset as well as those with knowledge of analyzing data acquired through complex sampling methods may be needed. When fielding one's own survey, there are a number of people who might be sought out for their expertise. Clinicians who work in settings relevant to the research question(s), as well as patients or other potential respondents, might be able to serve as content experts for question writing as well as pilot testing. Psychometricians, methodologists, or statisticians might be able to provide guidance about sampling designs, sample size calculations, analysis plans, as well as validity and reliability testing. Learners are encouraged to identify the expertise needed as well as potential experts by talking with their mentors. Examination of publications by researchers and faculty at their local institutions might also help identify those with the needed expertise. Many schools/colleges of pharmacy have economic, social, and administrative pharmacy (ESAP) faculty with specific training and education in survey research as well as scale development.

Other Considerations for Learner-Involved Survey Research Projects in Pharmacy Settings

Other important aspects for learners to consider when planning to conduct survey research projects in the pharmacy setting include establishing a timeline for survey development, administration, analysis, and dissemination, in addition to receiving any necessary approvals. Depending on a number of factors, the project may require financial support. Table 11–5 illustrates considerations related to setting a timeline, funding, and IRB review.

Dissemination of Survey Research

Because survey research can be used to help address a variety of questions, many scientific and professional conferences, as well as peer-reviewed journals, accept presentations, abstracts, and articles that utilize survey research methods. Examples of survey-based research in the biomedical literature, including research conducted in pharmacy settings, are readily available. Table 11–1 provides examples of published articles that have used surveys in pharmacy research across a number of different topics. As another example, a review of medical education journals revealed that 52% of original research articles were published using survey studies.[2] There are abundant opportunities available to publish survey research in peer-reviewed journals.

Prior to submitting a manuscript to a journal for the dissemination of their survey research findings, researchers are encouraged to review the Guide for Authors of their target journal. Some journals, such as the *Journal of the American Pharmacists Association*,

TABLE 11-5. PRACTICAL CONSIDERATIONS FOR LEARNERS WHEN CONDUCTING A SURVEY RESEARCH PROJECT

Considerations	Descriptions
Timeline	The timeline depends on the goals, objectives, administration methods, and sample size of the survey. On average, a survey study can take anywhere from a couple of months upwards, from beginning to end.
Funding	Like any other research, funding opportunities are available to conduct survey research from governmental and private entities. For example, resources for survey research may be available from the Agency for Healthcare Research and Quality (AHRQ), the National Opinion Research Center (NORC), the Association of Academic Survey Research Organization (AASRO), and the American Association for Public Opinion Research (AAPOR). The American Foundation for Pharmaceutical Education's (AFPE) Gateway to Research Scholarship program is designed to help student pharmacists participate in a faculty-mentored research project in the pharmaceutical sciences and may include research-related expenses for projects using survey research methods. Learners' own institutions also may have small grant programs to support learner-involved research projects. The secured funds can be used to provide incentives to survey respondents, pay to access panels of respondents through vendors (e.g., MTurk), and cover fees for the license to use any copyrighted measurement scales.
Institutional Review Board (IRB)	Survey research is generally eligible for exempt or expedited review unless otherwise indicated by an institution's IRB. Be sure to allocate one-three months to receive IRB approval in the research timeline. Multi-institution projects may require a signed collaboration agreement by the research collaborators unless otherwise indicated by the respective institution.
Other Best Practices	Review SURGE (non-web-based), CHERRIES (web-based), and/or CROSS guidelines regarding designing and reporting of survey studies; these guidelines also serve as useful quality assessment tools. When a learner is leading a survey research project, it is important to update the research team members at each stage of the project.

provide specific instructions to authors who are submitting an article that uses surveys or questionnaires.[26] Journals also require or strongly recommend that authors consult and follow reporting guidelines in the preparation of manuscripts. Such guidelines are useful for ensuring complete and transparent reporting, which is critical in order for the results of survey research to provide meaningful information for clinicians and researchers. Researchers have proposed guidelines for best practices to ensure that a standard reporting procedure is being adopted by authors of manuscripts that report survey research. While a gold standard has not been established, a recent review by Turk and colleagues provides suggestions on standardizing a reporting procedure for authors.[27] These authors assessed the quality of reporting of survey studies by examining 100 web-based and 100 non-web-based survey studies in reference to the two guidelines available at the time of the examination. The SUrvey Reporting GuidelinE (SURGE)[28] tool was used to assess the quality of reporting of non-web-based surveys (i.e., in-person, mail, telephone, and mixed method), and the Checklist for Reporting Results of Internet E-Surveys (CHERRIES)[29] guideline was used to assess quality reporting of web-based surveys.

Some of the key components of the SURGE tool include, description of: (1) the survey itself (including the provision of evidence of validity and reliability), (2) sample selection (including discussion of sampling frame as well as sample size calculation or justification), (3) survey administration (e.g., mode, incentives), (4) analysis (analysis to fulfill objectives, calculation of response rate, assessment for nonresponse error, and handling of missing data), (5) strengths and limitations of the study, and (6) ethical considerations (e.g., IRB approval, consent, funding). There is significant overlap between the CHERRIES checklist and the SURGE tool, with notable differences being related to a greater focus on the assessment of quality practices associated with surveys that are web-based. For example, CHERRIES has checklist items related to the following: (1) the use of randomization of items and adaptive questioning, (2) the number of questions per page, (3) implementation of completeness checks, (4) whether respondents were allowed to change responses, (5) the status of the survey as open vs. closed, and (6) the use of methods to prevent multiple entries from same people.

The findings from Turk and colleagues suggest that there was under-reporting of many of the elements of both the SURGE and CHERRIES guidelines, suggesting significant room for improvement.[27] Recently (in 2021), another guideline was published that addresses the reporting of both web- and non-web-based surveys, the Consensus-Based Checklist for Reporting of Survey Studies (the CROSS guideline).[30] The CROSS guideline was made available to provide an evidence-based, universal checklist that can be used to improve the quality of reporting of survey studies.

A standard reporting tool such as SURGE, CHERRIES, or CROSS must be reviewed by authors, researchers, clinicians, and learners so as to become familiar with the necessary components for the quality dissemination of a survey study. Students and resident learners can also examine these reporting guidelines when evaluating articles that use survey research methods while preparing to lead a journal club discussion. This practice also helps learners recognize the requirements for a scientific article to be considered quality literature. Clinicians and pharmacists can use the reporting guidelines to map the necessary steps in designing surveys to answer clinical questions. Educators and researchers with expertise in psychometric validation can use the guidelines to advise practitioners and learners on how to conduct survey research.

Exemplar of a Learner-Involved Survey Research Project

The following example illustrates a survey research project that involved several pharmacy learners. This description starts from an idea and research question development and includes survey development, sample definition, the IRB process, data collection, analysis, and dissemination. The team consisted of one clinical pharmacist (chapter author Sun Lee) and three third-year student pharmacists (P3s). The project involved the conduct of a cross-sectional survey regarding the self-management of blood pressure and mental health during the SARS-CoV-2 pandemic (COVID-19). The clinical pharmacist has a faculty appointment through a pharmacy school and works at a physician group clinic as an ambulatory care pharmacist. Table 11–6 illustrates the progression of the survey-based research that was performed while dealing with certain restrictions associated with the COVID-19 pandemic.

TABLE 11–6. ILLUSTRATION OF A SURVEY RESEARCH PROCESS AND ITS TIMELINE

Timeline	Process	Description
2 weeks	Defining a research question	Three third-year pharmacy students were enrolled in an independent research elective with the clinical pharmacist (principal investigator, PI). The research project had to be changed due to the COVID-19 pandemic research restrictions barring researchers from face-to-face interactions at the clinic. Therefore, the PI discussed a new research opportunity with the students related to assessing self-management of blood pressure and mental health during the SARS-CoV-2 pandemic period (COVID-19). Following the PICOTS model, the team defined the research question as "In patients with hypertension diagnosis, what is the psychological impact of COVID-19 on self-management of blood pressure at home?". To answer the question, a decision was made to implement a cross-sectional descriptive study design.
4 weeks	Survey development	Due to the original nature of the research, the research team was unable to locate an existing survey related to pandemic-induced self-management of blood pressure and mental health. Therefore, the team developed the survey by conducting a literature search related to the self-management of blood pressure control. The team consulted a psychometrician, other clinical pharmacists, and patients to conduct face and content validity.
2 weeks	IRB submission and approval	The project received IRB approval under expedited review due to the nature of the project being a survey method. It is important to allot two weeks to three months for the IRB review and approval process.
2 weeks	Setting up a survey distribution method	Upon IRB approval, the PI communicated with the Medical Director at the clinic to gather information about how to distribute the survey using the clinic list-serv. The team used REDCap to house the survey. Other online survey tools such as Qualtrics were considered.
2 weeks	Survey distribution	A link to the survey on REDCap was embedded into an email and sent to approximately 7,000 patients. The estimated budget spent was 700 dollars (10 cents per email to generate and send out an email with an embedded link x 7,000 potential patients receiving the email). The survey was open for two weeks. The budget and available resources at the clinic limited the number of times that the team could send out the email. To improve the response rate, it would have been possible to send second and third emails as reminders.

(Continued)

TABLE 11–6. ILLUSTRATION OF A SURVEY RESEARCH PROCESS AND ITS TIMELINE (CONTINUED)

Timeline	Process	Description
4 weeks	Data analysis	The team exported the collected data from REDCap to an SPSS-compatible file format. The student learners led the analysis with close supervision and feedback from the PI. Individual responses were screened for completion, and any survey that was stopped prematurely before completing 100% was eliminated from the data analysis. The team used SPSS to perform data analysis. The response rate was calculated, and the demographic information of the sample was compared with the target population (i.e., patients diagnosed with hypertension enrolled in the clinic). The team consulted a psychometrician to perform reliability and validity tests. The survey included two domains with 17 items, requiring at least 85 patients to run the psychometric tests (i.e., five respondents per each item). The reliability and validity tests mentioned in step 7 of Table 11–4 were performed. Additional analyses included examining the relationship between behavior on self-management of home blood pressure monitoring and financial concerns based on answers to the 17-item survey.
2+ weeks	Dissemination	The team submitted an abstract and presented a poster at a national pharmacy conference.[31] The PI reviewed and provided feedback on the abstract drafted by the students, and this process took about two weeks. The team spent about four weeks to develop the poster that was used to be presented at the conference.

There were several elements that helped the PI to effectively advise and manage the three students while leading this survey-based research project. The most important factor was guiding the learners with respect to the purpose and objective of the project. This step was achieved through sharing articles related to survey-based research on similar disease topics and clinic settings. Setting early expectations related to time commitments was very helpful. Instead of receiving monetary compensation for their time, students received a pass/fail credit as part of the research elective course in the third year curriculum. Students were physically present in the student office to work on the project for two hours each week. Once every two weeks, the team met to discuss the progress of the project, and this structured time commitment expectation helped the team to be productive throughout the research cycle.

Summary and Conclusions

The use of survey research methods in healthcare is very prevalent, and this approach to research can be used to address many different questions in pharmacy. However, limited time is spent in the pharmacy curriculum reviewing guidelines for good practices with respect to research in general and survey research in particular. In this chapter, we have defined survey research and reviewed practical and technical considerations to conduct survey research in pharmacy settings. Such research can be conducted using preexisting validated tools, or new measures can be developed following a planned scale validation process, a process that can be time-consuming and may not always fit into the time frame for a student or resident project. As illustrated via an example, there are opportunities for learners to be involved in survey research projects, and we have highlighted practical steps and timeline considerations from idea generation to the dissemination of the findings. Finally, helpful checklists are available to guide researchers concerning key elements to include for reporting purposes, as well as for assessing the quality of published literature that reports the results of survey research.

Key Points and Advice

- It is important to formulate a well-defined PICOTS question when conducting survey research. This step will help define selecting a target population, choosing a sampling method, and determining the use of a new or existing survey.
- If student learners are involved in the survey research project, it is critical to set an early expectation regarding time and effort commitment, as well as the research objective and purpose.
- Survey research can be conducted using a preexisting validated tool to collect data, or a new scale can be developed following the planned scale validation process.
- It is strongly recommended that learners refer to SURGE, CHERRIES, and CROSS guidelines prior to designing the survey research plan; these guidelines can help researchers develop a checklist of items that are important to improve the quality and structure of a survey research project.

Chapter Review Questions

1. List two to three challenges related to designing a new survey compared to adopting an existing survey in survey research.
2. Discuss the purpose of having a cover letter attached to the survey during the survey dissemination and data collection stage of the survey research.
3. Select any published article using a survey research design, and restate the research question based on the PICOTS model.

4. Discuss the purpose of the three survey research guidelines (i.e., SURGE, CHER-RIES, CROSS) discussed in this chapter.

Online Resources

- Enhancing the QUAlity and Transparency Of health Research. https://www.equator-network.org/reporting-guidelines/
- HealthMeasures. https://www.healthmeasures.net/index.php
- The Association of Academic Survey Research Organization. https://www.aasro.org/
- American Association for Public Opinion Research. https://www.aapor.org/
- Qualtrics: How to write great survey questions (and avoid common mistakes). https://www.qualtrics.com/blog/writing-survey-questions/
- Qualtrics: Survey data analysis: Best practices, helpful tips, and our favorite tools. https://www.qualtrics.com/experience-management/research/analysis-reporting/

REFERENCES

1. Groves RM, Fowler FJ, Couper MP, Lepkowski JM, Singer E, Tourangeau R. *Survey Methodology.* 2nd ed. Wiley; July 2009.
2. Phillips AW, Friedman BT, Utrankar A, Ta AQ, Reddy ST, Durning SJ. Surveys of health professions trainees: prevalence, response rates, and predictive factors to guide research-ers. *Acad Med.* 2017;92(2):222-228.
3. Alreck PL, Settle RB. *The Survey Research Handbook.* 3rd ed. Boston: McGraw-Hill/Irwin; 2004.
4. Xiong S, Willis R, Lalama J, Farinha T, Hamper J. Perspectives and perceived barriers to pharmacist-prescribed tobacco cessation services in the community pharmacy setting. *J Am Pharm Assoc.* 2021;61(4):S39-S48.
5. Livet M, Blanchard C, Richard C, et al. Measuring implementation of medication optimiza-tion services: development and validation of an implementation outcomes questionnaire. *Res Soc Adm Pharm.* 2021;17(9):1623-1630.
6. Burstein D, Baird J, Bratberg J, et al. Pharmacist attitudes toward pharmacy-based nalox-one: a cross-sectional survey study. *J Am Pharm Assoc.* 2020;60(2):304-310.
7. Kelly DV, Bishop L, Young S, Hawboldt J, Phillips L, Keough TM. Pharmacist and physi-cian views on collaborative practice: findings from the community pharmaceutical care project. *Can Pharm J CPJ.* 2013;146(4):218.
8. Lee S, Khare MM, Olson HR, Chen AMH, Law AV. The TEACH trial: tailored education to assist label comprehension and health literacy. *Res Soc Adm Pharm.* 2018;14(9):839-845.
9. Crawford SY, Awé C, Tawk RH, Pickard AS. A cross-sectional and longitudinal study of pharmacy student perceptions of readiness to serve diverse populations. *Am J Pharm Educ.* 2016;80(4).

10. Guyatt G, Rennie D, Evidence-Based Medicine Working Group, American Medical Association. *Users' Guides to the Medical Literature: A Manual for Evidence-Based Clinical Practice.* AMA Press; 2002.

11. Agency for Healthcare Research and Quality. Effective Health Care Program. Developing a Protocol for Observational Comparative Effectiveness Research: A User's Guide. Accessed August 11, 2021. https://effectivehealthcare.ahrq.gov/products/observational-cer-protocol/research

12. Assem M, Broeckel U, MacKinnon GE. Personal DNA Testing increases pharmacy students' confidence and competence in pharmacogenomics. *Am J Pharm Educ.* 2021;85(4):281-287.

13. Ceulemans M, Liekens S, Van Calsteren K, Allegaert K, Foulon V. Impact of a blended learning program on community pharmacists' barriers, knowledge, and counseling practice with regard to preconception, pregnancy and lactation. *Res Social Adm Pharm.* 2021;17(7):1242-1249.

14. Amazon Mechanical Turk. Accessed August 11, 2021. https://www.mturk.com/

15. Qualtrics Online Panels. Accessed August 11, 2021. https://www.qualtrics.com/support/survey-platform/sp-administration/brand-customization-services/purchase-respondents/

16. Daniel J. *Sampling Essentials: Practical Guidelines for Making Sampling Choices.* SAGE Publications; 2014.

17. Dillman DA, Smyth JD, Christian LM. *Internet, Phone, Mail, and Mixed-Mode Surveys: The Tailored Design Method.* 4th ed. Hoboken, NJ: John Wiley & Sons; 2014.

18. Singleton R, Straits BC. *Approaches to Social Research.* 6th ed. New York: Oxford University Press; 2018.

19. Burns KE, Duffett M, Kho ME, et al. A guide for the design and conduct of self-administered surveys of clinicians. *CMAJ.* 2008;179(3):245-252.

20. Bourque LB, Fielder EP. Format of the questionnaire. In: *How to Conduct Self-Administered and Mail Surveys.* 2nd ed. Thousand Oaks, CA: SAGE Publications, Inc.; 2003:96-141.

21. Johnson RL, Morgan GB. *Survey Scales: A Guide to Development, Analysis, and Reporting.* Guilford Publications; August 2016.

22. DeVellis RF. *Scale Development: Theory and Applications.* 4th ed. SAGE Publications; April 2016.

23. Streiner DL, Norman GR, Cairney J. *Health Measurement Scales: A Practical Guide to their Development and Use.* 5th ed. Oxford University Press; November 2014.

24. Boateng GO, Neilands TB, Frongillo EA, Melgar-Quiñonez HR, Young SL. Best practices for developing and validating scales for health, social, and behavioral research: a primer. *Front Public Heal.* 2018;6:149.

25. Harpe SE. How to analyze Likert and other rating scale data. *Curr Pharm Teach Learn.* 2015;7(6):836-850.

26. *Journal of the American Pharmacists Association.* Guide for Authors. Elsevier. Accessed August 11, 2021. https://www.elsevier.com/journals/journal-of-the-american-pharmacists-association/1544-3191/guide-for-authors

27. Turk T, Elhady MT, Rashed S, et al. Quality of reporting web-based and non-web-based survey studies: What authors, reviewers and consumers should consider. *PLoS One.* 2018;13(6).

28. Bennett C, Khangura S, Brehaut JC, Graham ID, Moher D, Potter BK, Grimshaw JM. Reporting guidelines for survey research: an analysis of published guidance and reporting practices. *PLoS Med.* 2010;8(8):e1001069.

29. Eysenbach G. Improving the quality of Web surveys: the Checklist for Reporting Results of Internet E-Surveys (CHERRIES) [published correction appears in doi:10.2196/jmir.2042]. *J Med Internet Res.* 2004;6(3):e34. Published 2004 Sep 29.

30. Sharma A, Minh Duc NT, Luu Lam Thang T, et al. A Consensus-Based Checklist for Reporting of Survey Studies (CROSS). *J Gen Intern Med.* 2021;36(10):3179-3187.

31. Edwards AL, Helms M, Suszynsky T, Lee S, Hwang A. SARS-CoV-2 pandemic and home blood pressure management among patients with hypertension. Poster Abstracts. Academy of Managed Care Pharmacy Virtual 2021. *JMCP.* 2021;27(Suppl 4-a). https://www.jmcp.org/doi/abs/10.18553/jmcp.2021.27.4-a.s1

Chapter Twelve

Patient-Reported Outcomes Research in Pharmacy

Nalin Payakachat, BPharm, MSc, PhD and Amy M. Franks, PharmD

Chapter Objectives

- Define patient-reported outcomes (PROs) and the importance of PRO research in healthcare and pharmacy settings
- Explain psychometric properties of PRO measures and their importance in PRO research
- Describe various sources of PROs that can be evaluated in pharmacy settings
- Identify common research questions that can be addressed with PRO research in pharmacy settings
- Describe the practical and technical considerations for PRO research in pharmacy settings
- Discuss the strategies for harnessing the expertise needed for conducting PRO research in pharmacy settings
- Provide an example of a learner-involved PRO research project in a pharmacy setting
- Discuss the dissemination framework for PRO research in pharmacy settings

Key Terminology

Activities of daily living (ADLs), disease-specific PROMs, generic PROMs, health-related quality of life (HRQoL), instrumental activities of daily living (IADLs), patient-reported outcomes (PROs), patient-reported experience, patient satisfaction, psychometric properties, quality of life (QoL), internal consistency reliability, test-retest reliability, responsiveness, content validity, construct validity, criterion validity, well-being

Introduction

"Patient-reported outcomes (PROs)" is an umbrella term that refers to *"any self-reported health information obtained directly from patients, without interpretation by a clinician or anyone else."*[1] PROs do not include biomarkers (e.g., A1c, blood pressure, bone mineral density, genetic tests), which are objective measures of medical signs (as opposed to symptoms reported by the patient) of disease or the effects of treatment.[2] Self-reported health information includes state of disease severity (e.g., symptoms or a change from a previous symptom measure) and the effect of medical intervention on one or more concepts of health (e.g., physical or mental functioning to measure the severity of a disease condition). The Institute of Medicine (2001) included patient-centered care (PCC) as one of the six essential aims of the healthcare system.[3] Since then, PCC has been recognized as a measure of the quality of care. Because PRO research captures a unique and crucial health perspective that only the patient knows, it has grown exponentially in the past two decades, and PROs have become the primary outcomes used in PCC. To date, PROs have several wide-reaching applications, including patient-centered therapeutic decisions, performance measures of value-based care, health technology assessment, drug development, and research in disease progression. Additionally, PROs can be used in clinical trials to support regulatory approval for obtaining a labeling claim, defined as any treatment benefit mentioned in the Food and Drug Administration (FDA) product label (i.e., package insert).[1,4]

Advances in information technology present unprecedented opportunities for capturing and integrating PROs into electronic health records (EHRs) with less human labor.[5] The integration of PROs into EHRs can also enable PRO data aggregation across medical centers and allow researchers to collect large PRO datasets over time. These datasets can be used for studying the impact of diseases in diverse populations (i.e., real-world evidence studies). With improved informatics, various PROs now can be efficiently sorted to identify the most meaningful data to assist in decision making in clinical settings, thus incorporating PRO data into routine clinical practice. In addition, electronic PRO measures also have the potential to be integrated into patient registries to address questions regarding treatment choices and effectiveness that are unaddressed by traditional clinical trials. PRO research can ultimately drive changes in healthcare delivery, improve healthcare quality, and inform evidence-based practice and patient-centered care.[6,7]

The purpose of this chapter is to present a basic overview of PROs, including taxonomy, measures, data collection, scoring and analysis, interpretation, and dissemination. This chapter covers practical and technical considerations when conducting PRO research in healthcare and in pharmacy settings. Lastly, this chapter provides examples of PRO research to enhance understanding of the importance of PROs and to equip young investigators for conducting future PRO research in pharmacy.

Patient-Reported Outcomes and their Measures

SOURCES OF PROs

The most proper and desired source of PROs should be the patient. However, when self-reports are not possible to be collected reliably or validly, observer-reports (so-called observer-reported outcomes—ObsROs) are the alternative. ObsROs can be used instead of PROs when patients cannot report for themselves (e.g., infants, toddlers, individuals who are cognitively impaired).[1] The importance for ObsROs is that the information should be reported by the primary caregiver who cares for the patient in the patient's daily life, such as a parent of the sick child or a caregiver of the cognitively impaired individual. *Importantly, PROs and ObsROs should be collected using valid instruments that are purposefully developed to capture intended concepts or perspectives of health.* Thus, no single set of PRO measures (PROMs) currently in use can be considered a gold standard. Thousands of valid PROMs exist, and new instruments are continuously being developed. It is crucial for researchers to carefully select PROMs to collect the PRO data that best serve their study's objectives.

PROs: TAXONOMY

To better understand PROs and PROMs, it is important to first review the taxonomy of concepts for which PROMs are typically used to capture. Clinicians and researchers should not underestimate the importance of clearly recognizing and carefully defining the concepts they desire to measure to help ensure the selection of appropriate PROMs for projects or clinical work. Table 12–1 summarizes concepts and examples of PROMs taxonomically.

Symptoms and Severity

Symptoms and severity of disease are the most common forms of PROs. They are reports of physical and psychological effects that are not directly observable or measurable; therefore, they are only known by the patient. A symptom is typically reported as a negative, uncomfortable feeling resulting from disease. Symptoms, such as pain, fatigue, and nausea, and their severity are of common interest in both research and clinical settings. A combination of the presence and severity of symptoms (so-called symptom burden) are best assessed using PROMs.[20] This symptom burden captures symptoms, their severity, and the impact experienced with a specific disease, and it is useful for monitoring changes from interventions or treatments.

Disability and Functional Status: ADLs and IADLs

Functional status refers to an individual's ability to perform both basic activities of daily living (ADLs), and more advanced instrumental activities of daily living (IADLs).[21,22]

TABLE 12–1. TAXONOMY AND EXAMPLES

Concept	Description	Examples of Concepts	Examples of PRO Instruments
Symptoms	Reports of physical and psychological symptoms that are not directly observable or measurable	Pain Pain interference	Brief Pain Inventory[8] Numeric Rating Scale (NRS-11)[9]
Severity	Frequency and intensity of symptoms	Pain intensity	
Disability and functional status	Decline or impaired ability to perform both basic activities of daily living (ADLs) and more advanced instrumental activities of daily living (IADLs)	ADLs, IADLs	Katz ADL index[10] IADL Scale by Lawton and Brody[11]
Quality of life	An individual's perception of their position in life in the context of the culture in which they live and in relation to their goals, expectations, standards, and concerns	General quality of life in adults	WHOQOL-BREF[12]
Health-related quality of life	A reflection of the impact of disease and treatment on disability and daily functioning	General health-related quality of life in adults	SF-36[13] EQ-5D-5L[14]
Well-being	Individual's positive evaluations of their lives	Life satisfaction	The Satisfaction with Life Scale[15,16]
Patient-reported experience	Patients' views of their experience while receiving care	Treatment burden Healthcare experience	Patient Experience with Treatment and Self-management (PETS)[17] Assessment of Healthcare Providers and Systems (CAHPS)[18]
Patient satisfaction	Patient's considerations of whether their healthcare expectations were met	Patient satisfaction	Patient Satisfaction Questionnaire Short Form (PSQ-18)[19]

ADLs include basic physical activities (e.g., walking, climbing stairs), cognitive activities (e.g., focusing attention, communicating), and routine ADLs (e.g., eating, bathing, dressing, toileting). IADLs refer to more complex activities necessary to live independently in society as well as to participate in life situations (e.g., school, play [in children], household chores, medication-taking). Decline or impairment in functioning and the subsequent loss of ADLs/IADLs are increasingly being used to measure disability, which happens when an individual's ability to carry out such activities or performance is compromised because of a health condition, injury, or aging.

QoL and HRQoL

First and foremost, researchers need to distinguish the difference between the two concepts of quality of life (QoL) and health-related quality of life (HRQoL). The World Health Organization (WHO) defines QoL as *"An individual's perception of their position in life in the context of the culture in which they live and in relation to their goals, expectations, standards, and concerns."*[23] This definition, however, is a broad construct that is influenced by many factors, including social context and culture where people live. HRQoL, on the other hand, is *"generally considered to reflect the impact of disease and treatment on disability and daily functioning; it has also been considered to reflect the impact of perceived health on an individual's ability to live a fulfilling life."*[24] It is important to correctly differentiate between these two concepts because a measure of QoL is unlikely to be a measure of HRQoL. In fact, HRQoL is only a small subset of QoL.

Well-being

Another important term that needs attention is well-being. The term "well-being" is defined as *"peoples' positive evaluations of their lives, and includes positive emotion, engagement, satisfaction."*[25] Well-being should include measures of cognitive and affective aspects that people perceive of their lives and should capture global judgments of life satisfaction and feelings ranging from depression to joy. Therefore, it has a significant overlap with QoL and HRQoL concepts. Moreover, because different studies assess different domains of well-being in different ways, it is often difficult to know what exact concepts are being measured. As a result, researchers should clearly specify which "well-being" is being measured (e.g., subjective well-being, psychological well-being)[26] in their projects.

Patient-Reported Experience

Patient-reported experience is a patient's view of their *experience* while receiving care rather than the *outcomes* of healthcare provided.[27] In fact, patients are the best source of information assessing which aspects of healthcare matter to them the most.[28] Therefore, they are able to provide essential feedback on the quality and experiences of the care they receive. This information can be used as an indicator of the quality of patient care and the impact of the care process on the patient's direct experience. For example, the clarity of communication and timeliness of care received can be important indicators of patient care.[29] It is important to note that patient-reported experience is different than patient satisfaction, although they are often used interchangeably.[30] Patient satisfaction reflects a patient's evaluation about whether their expectations in a healthcare encounter were met. Therefore, it is possible that two people who receive the exact same care can give different satisfaction ratings because of differing expectations.

VALUE OF PRO RESEARCH IN PHARMACY SETTINGS

PROs are important to all areas of patient care. This is especially important to pharmacists because pharmacists provide direct patient care in many diverse settings (e.g., acute care, ambulatory care, community pharmacy, health-system settings). As pharmacists continue to advance their impact on patient care and increase their visibility as important members of the healthcare team, it is valuable to embrace PRO research as a mechanism to learn from patients and document pharmacist impact.

PRO research has been a part of pharmacy research for several decades. For example, patient satisfaction and patient-reported experience are commonly used as performance measures for medication therapy management (MTM) programs and patient care services outcomes in community pharmacy settings.[31,32] Another example is using PROs in medication adherence research.[33] Medication nonadherence is a significant problem, and pharmacists are in unique positions to help maximize medication adherence, given their accessibility and frequency in which they interact with patients.[34–36] HRQoL can be used, along with clinical outcomes, for medication adherence research[37,38] that is often conducted in both community and clinical pharmacy settings. Another example is an ongoing funded pharmacy research project that implements the PatientToc™, a mobile application for PRO collection, health screening, and patient monitoring, in community pharmacies.[33] Importantly, pharmacists are able to immediately use these data to inform their counseling during routine visits. Additionally, pharmacists who collect PRO data and report PROs during the provision of MTM or other clinical services also improve patient experience and engagement.[39] In the inpatient and ambulatory care settings, a pharmacist may assess the severity of symptoms using the PRO-based New York Heart Association (NYHA) functional classification[40] in a patient with heart failure. This measure is frequently used for clinical assessment but could also be used in research projects to assess the impact of medication therapy interventions. With these PRO data, pharmacists can assess care on an individual level as well as retrospectively review entire cohorts of patients. PROs serve as a meaningful outcome in pharmacy research.

Steps in PRO Research

As described in other chapters of this section of the book, the scientific research process has a basic set of steps that are common to all areas of inquiry: (1) pose a research question and hypothesis, (2) develop and implement a research plan, (3) perform data collection and analysis, and (4) prepare a research report.[41] For PRO research, each of these steps involves a number of different considerations (see Figure 12-1

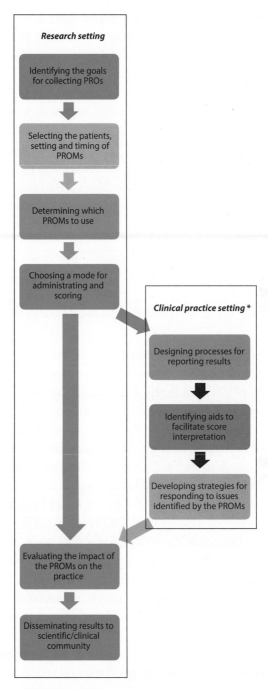

Figure 12–1. Step-by-step guidance on conducting PRO research, adapted from the ISOQOL's User's Guide for Implementing Patient-reported Outcomes Assessment in Clinical Practice.[61] *These three steps are additional steps when conducting PRO research in clinical practice settings.*

for further information). For example, the research question being asked has significant implications for the selection of a PROM. In addition, PROMs can be used to represent important variables in a variety of study designs, including randomized controlled trials, observational studies, cross-sectional studies, or longitudinal studies. Furthermore, while many PRO studies are conducted as primary research, a number of PROMs are included in secondary data sources, such as national population surveys. Moreover, there are a number of considerations involved in the scoring of PRO measures that have implications for data analysis and interpretation of findings. Researchers are strongly encouraged to use the available literature to guide the decision-making process in each of these steps. Types of PRO research questions, as well as a number of practical and technical considerations that can be used to support decisions regarding the steps in the conduct of PRO research, are covered in the subsequent two sections.

Common Research Questions Addressed with PRO Research

PROs are the outcomes when framing clinical research questions using the PICOTS (patient, intervention, comparison, outcome, and time) framework, as discussed in Chapter 4. Evaluating PROs is not merely an aspirational objective for delivering better healthcare; it is now one of the key outcomes of clinical practice as it provides crucial information about patients' responses to treatments and reflects how well healthcare processes/services are received. However, PRO research should include outcomes that patients notice and care about, such as functions, symptoms, or HRQoL.[42] PROs, if used as primary or secondary outcomes, should be clearly specified in the research protocol. A systematic review of randomized controlled trials that used PROs from 1989 to 2016 classified research questions addressed with PRO research into three categories: process of care (i.e., how PROs could improve a process of care), health outcomes (i.e., how treatments/intervention could improve PROs), and satisfaction with healthcare (i.e., how patients were satisfied with healthcare).[43] In observational research, PROs can also be used to evaluate variations across demographic groups, regions, and diseases. Table 12–2 provides other examples of PRO research conducted in medical settings, including pharmacy.

Given time, resources, and other constraints, it may not be possible for pharmacy learners to lead a project to address all of the questions stated in Table 12–2. For example, the article by Basch et al.[58] would be very challenging for a student pharmacist or pharmacy resident to undertake as a capstone or standalone research project as part of their professional training.

TABLE 12–2. EXAMPLES OF RESEARCH QUESTIONS ADDRESSED WITH PRO RESEARCH

Research Question	Authors	Study Objective	Examples Study Design, Country	PRO Measures Used
Whether PROs vary across demographics and disease	Oldsberg et al. (2019)[44]	Explore geographical variations in patient-reported outcomes in total hip arthroplasty and determine to what extent potential geographical variations are explained by patient-related and socioeconomic variables	A nationwide observational registry study, Sweden	• EQ-5D-3L[45] • Pain Visual Analogue Scale (VAS) • Satisfaction VAS
	Riazi et al. (2003)[46]	Examine the relative impact of two chronic neurological disorders; multiple sclerosis, and Parkinson's disease	A cross-sectional mailed survey study, U.K.	• SF-36[13]
PROs across treatments	Cohen et al. (2013)[47]	Determine whether the Individual Burden of Illness Index for Depression (IBI-D) would be as useful in evaluating the full impact of treatment	The STAR*D (Sequenced Treatment Alternatives to Relieve Depression) study (a series of sequenced, randomized treatment trial, U.S.)	• IBI-D[48]
	Lewis et al. (2019)[49]	Investigate the clinical effectiveness of sertraline in patients in primary care with depressive symptoms ranging from mild to severe and tested the role of severity and duration in treatment response	A pragmatic, multicenter, double-blind, placebo-controlled randomized trial, U.K.	• Patient Health Questionnaire, nine-item (PHQ-9)[50] • Beck Depression Inventory (BDI-II)[51] • Generalized Anxiety Disorder Assessment seven-item version (GAD-7)[52] • SF-12[53] • EQ-5D-5L[14]
Intervention effects on PROs	Al-Jumah & Qureshi (2012)[34]	Evaluate different types of pharmacist interventions used to enhance patients' adherence to antidepressant medication	A systematic review	• Patient satisfaction

(Continued)

TABLE 12–2. EXAMPLES OF RESEARCH QUESTIONS ADDRESSED WITH PRO RESEARCH (*CONTINUED*)

Research Question	Authors	Study Objective	Examples Study Design, Country	PRO Measures Used
	Moczygemba et al. (2010)[54]	Measure patient satisfaction with a pharmacist-provided telephone MTM program	A nonexperimental and cross-sectional survey study, U.S.	• Patient satisfaction
	Germain et al. (2007)[55]	Explore the effects of a very brief intervention for post-traumatic stress disorder (PTSD)–related nightmares and insomnia in victims of violent crimes with PTSD	A prospective, open-label design study, U.S.	• Pittsburgh Sleep Quality Index (PSQI)[56]
Using PROs in patient care	Lavallee et al. (2016)[57]	Examine the opportunities for using patient-reported outcomes to enhance care delivery and outcomes as healthcare information needs and technology platforms change	Review, U.S.	• Not applicable
	Basch et al. (2016)[58]	Test whether the systematic web-based collection of patient-reported symptoms during chemotherapy treatment, with automated alerts to clinicians for severe or worsening symptoms, improves HRQoL as well as survival, quality-adjusted survival, ER use, and hospitalization	A randomized, controlled trial, U.S.	• EQ-5D-5L[14]
	Wohlfahrt et al. (2020)[59]	Evaluate provider perspectives and experiences on the use of PROs in heart failure (HF) as a foundation for developing recommendations for implementing PROs in HF care	A multicenter qualitative study of diverse providers to describe the barriers and facilitators of routine PROs use in HF clinics, U.S.	• Not applicable

Practical and Technical Considerations in PRO Research

PROs can be used in many settings, including clinical trials, clinical practice, real-world evidence studies, patient registries, and regulatory approvals. PROs become essential data when there are no objective clinical outcomes to monitor the progress of disease conditions or to measure treatment benefits. This section provides practical and technical considerations when conducting PRO research.

SELECTING A PRO MEASURE

Conducting PRO research is not much different from other clinical studies in regard to research planning. However, a somewhat unique distinction of PRO research is selecting appropriate PROMs to serve the goals of the study and interpret PRO data in a meaningful way. For example, the SPIRIT (Standard Protocol Items: Recommendations for Intervention Trials) PRO extension recommends 16 PRO-specific items that should be addressed and included in clinical trial protocols when PROs are primary or key secondary outcomes.[60] The FDA advises researchers to first determine whether existing PROMs are adequate to address and measure the concepts of interest or whether they could be modified to serve the study's objective before developing a new PROM.[1] This is important because the development of a new PROM requires additional work and can be very time-consuming. If a new PROM is developed, it must first be validated to establish its psychometric properties in the target population prior to its use in a study. Please consult the FDA PRO Guidance to Industry for more details on developing a new PROM and the validation process.[1]

Figure 12–1 summarizes step-by-step guidance on conducting PRO research, adapted from the "User's Guide for Implementing Patient-reported Outcomes Assessment in Clinical Practice" published by the International Society for Quality of Life Research (ISOQOL).[61] The first step is to identify research goals and objectives for collecting PROs. In this step, researchers should have a clear idea of what PRO concepts are needed for the study. Next, researchers will need to specify the target population (e.g., age, sex, disease condition) to be studied. Once these two steps are specified, researchers can review and identify potential PROMs for measuring those concepts in the target population. Important considerations for choosing PROMs are discussed in the following subsections.

Type of PROMs

PROMs are categorized into generic and disease-specific measures. Generic PROMs are not specific to any disease conditions and can be used in the general population as well as patient populations. Examples of generic PROMs for measuring HRQoL are the

SF-36[13] and the EQ-5D-5L.[14] Generic PROMs generally cover multidimensional concepts or domains related to many areas of life. As a result, they enable score comparison in relation to population norms and between different disease conditions. Generic PROMs may also be developed for a specific age group (e.g., Pediatric Quality of Life [PedsQL] instrument[62]) or concept (e.g., Patient Satisfaction Questionnaire Short-Form [PSQ-18][19]). However, an important shortcoming of generic PROMs is that they may not cover relevant concepts that are specific to a disease condition. Therefore, they may be less sensitive to changes within those specific domains of the disease.

Disease-specific PROMs, on the other hand, are developed specifically for particular disease conditions. Such measures may be broadly defined, such as the Functional Assessment of Cancer Therapy (FACT)[63] instrument and the Asthma Quality of Life Questionnaire (AQLQ)[64] for measuring HRQoL in adult cancer patients and adult asthma patients, respectively. Broad disease-specific PROMs often have bolt-on scales to specifically apply to different forms of a disease (e.g., FACT-B—Breast cancer module[65]) or treatments (e.g., FACT-BMT—Bone Marrow Transplantation[66]). As disease-specific PROMs are tailored to topics relevant to a given condition, they are likely to be more sensitive to changes within those disease conditions compared to generic PROMs. However, a shortcoming of disease-specific PROMs is that they may fail to capture general aspects that may be affected by treatments, such as adverse effects.

Psychometric Properties of PROMs

Psychometric properties refer to the quality characteristics of a measurement tool and provide information on how the measure is constructed and how well it works to capture the desired concept. As measurement tools, it is essential that PROMs have good psychometric properties to measure concepts that are relevant to and established in the target population. These properties include validity, reliability, and responsiveness (ability to detect change). Findings from valid PROMs can then be used for clinical decision making, interpreting treatment benefits, or determining the impact of a disease condition on an individual's or population's health. Table 12–3 summarizes psychometric properties and approaches/statistical methods used to evaluate the properties.[1]

Administrative Burden

When selecting PROMs for research and clinical practice, researchers should be mindful of the patient's expected time to complete PROMs. A minimum number of PROMs should be selected to capture the most relevant outcomes and concepts. The frequency of follow-up data collection should be appropriate with how the disease condition is monitored. Basch et al. recommended limiting PRO data collection to be within 20 minutes at baseline and 10 to 15 minutes at follow-up time points.[67] As a general rule, a shorter PROM set is better to optimize response rates and obtain completed PROMs.

TABLE 12–3. A SUMMARY OF PSYCHOMETRIC PROPERTIES OF PROMS

Psychometric Properties	Definition	Approach/Statistical Methods to Evaluate the Properties
Validity	Accuracy	
Content validity	The extent to which the PROM captures the concepts intended to measure	The desired contents that derive the items of the PROM should come from patients and then be examined by a group of experts.
Criterion validity	The extent of the relationship between the PROM and the criterion	Correlation coefficients
Construct validity	The extent to which a particular PROM relates to other measures (convergent and divergent) consistent with theoretically derived concepts	Factor analysis to examine the construct of multi-item PROMs as well as their convergent and divergent validity
		Correlation coefficients
Reliability	Reproducibility	
Internal consistency reliability	The extent to which items are homogenous in relation to the same concept or domain	Cronbach's alpha (>0.7 is desirable)
Test-retest reliability	The stability of a PROM	Intraclass correlation coefficient (>0.7 is desirable)
Responsiveness	The ability to measure a meaningful or clinically important change	Cohen's effect size

Copyright/Licensing to Use PROMs

One of the important considerations when selecting PROMs is whether a PROM is subject to copyright and must be licensed for use. Unauthorized use of certain PROMs can lead to claims of copyright infringement, which may cost thousands of dollars to resolve. Some cases may also lead to publication retraction similar to when the Morisky Medication Adherence Scale (MMAS-8) was used without permission.[68,69] Researchers should also be aware *not* to modify a PROM without permission from the developer.

PRO DATA COLLECTION METHODS

PROMs can be administered as self-report (preferred), interviewer-administered (either via phone or in-person), or observer-report (from the primary caregiver of the patient). The administration and format of PROMs should be determined ahead of time and taken into consideration.[61] The traditional format of PROMs is a paper-and-pencil format that requires someone to collect and enter the data into an electronic platform for data analysis. Electronic PROMs have been introduced in the past two decades and have been increasingly popular in recent years. They can be administered via web-based or mobile applications and also be incorporated into EHRs. An example of a validated PROM that is available in both paper-and-pencil and electronic formats is the PROMIS (Patient-Reported Outcomes Measurement Information System) toolset.[70,71] The PROMIS toolset offers many generic and disease-specific PROMs that are also available in a psychometrically-robust computer adaptive testing system, compatible with an EHR enterprise like the Epic system. The integration of PROMs in EHRs facilitates meaningful use of PRO data in clinical practice[72] and real-world evidence studies.[73]

PRO SCORING AND ANALYSIS

Two of the important considerations in conducting PRO research are scoring and interpretation of a PROM. These steps should be done according to the developer manual for the PROM. Researchers should *never* assume how to score PRO data from a PROM. Due diligence is required to ensure the scoring manual or the original literature on the development of the PROM is reviewed and applied in a manner consistent with its intention. Deviating from the scoring manual may lead to misinterpretation of PRO data and PROM and can result in inappropriate clinical decisions for interventions.[68] Researchers may also check the availability of automated scoring services for some PROMs such as the PROMIS toolset (https://www.assessmentcenter.net/ac_scoringservice) and the SF12v2 (https://www.qualitymetric.com/scientific-consulting/scoring-interpretation/). In some cases, researchers can submit raw data via a web-based application or a downloadable program to generate PRO scores. Other scoring tools are provided when the PROM is incorporated into a data collection tool, like REDCap (https://www.healthmeasures.net/implement-healthmeasures/administration-platforms/redcap). One advantage of using these scoring services is that most have some advanced capability of handling missing PRO data (i.e., item-level missingness).

Analysis of PRO data should follow a set of best statistical practices, described by the International Council on Harmonization (ICH)[74] and the Setting International Standards in Analyzing Patient-Reported Outcomes and Quality of Life (SISAQOL)[75] that are broadly applicable for clinical studies and PRO research. When dealing with multiple PRO endpoints or multiple PRO domains, researchers need to properly handle multiplicity problems to control Type I errors. Please consult with a biostatistician and follow the recommendations from the ICH's E9 Guidance for Industry on Statistical Principles[74] and SISAQOL[75] to deal with multiplicity.

Another important issue in PRO research and analysis is missing data. Missing data often occur in clinical studies, including PRO research. Researchers should have a thorough plan to minimize missing data (see the PCORI Methodology Standards[42] and SISAQOL[75]) and be familiar with appropriate methods (see the ICH's E9[74]) to address them.

EXPERTISE NEEDED

For conducting PRO research, researchers may consider collaborating with, or at least consulting, the following experts:

- *Patients* are not only the target population but also can help review research questions, select relevant PROs that are important to them, and consult whether PRO data collection and mode of administration are appropriate.
- *Clinicians,* who are specialized in disease conditions being studied, can provide their expertise to help shape PRO concepts, along with patients.
- *PRO researchers* can help review research questions, research design, and methodology.
- *Psychometricians* can help select appropriate PROMs for the study's objectives, conduct psychometric properties evaluation, if needed, and PRO scoring and interpretation.
- *Information technologists* can assist researchers in building PROMs in electronic format for use in EHRs and also can help extract PRO data for analysis.
- *Statisticians* can assist with data analysis and maybe a necessary resource when dealing with missing data or other complicated issues that may arise before or during statistical analysis.

Other Considerations for Learner-Involved PRO Research Projects in Pharmacy Settings

PRO research is one of many types of research conducted in pharmacy settings. It is also a type of research in which learners (e.g., student pharmacists, pharmacy residents) can have the opportunity to be involved in many of the steps of PRO research from the beginning to the end. They can participate in setting a study's goal and writing a study's objectives. They may also be involved directly in the data collection by assisting with patient interviews or indirectly by educating patients or clinical staff on the administration of PROMs. Although they may not be able to design the study independently, it is a great learning experience to participate in conversations with the research team on how to design and launch a PRO research study.

Through these conversations, learners can be more involved in drafting, finalizing, and submitting a PRO research protocol for institutional approvals. PRO research, like other clinical studies, needs approval from the institutional review board to ensure that the proposed study follows the ethical standard for research when it involves human subjects. All researchers, including learners involved in the research project, must have the proper training to conduct research studies involving human subjects. Please see the Collaborative Institutional Training Initiative program[76] for training courses for researchers.

Another important consideration for PRO research is a study's timeline. Learners need to be realistic about what can be done in the available timeframe of their research experience. For example, pharmacy residents typically have one year to complete their research projects. Therefore, they need to carefully select what PROs can be collected and how often for follow-up PRO data collection. A general rule for a one-year study timeline is to limit data collection to a total of a six-month period to allow time for data analysis, reporting, and dissemination of results.

Lastly, researchers may need resources to conduct PRO research. In addition to the National Institutes of Health funding, the Patient-Centered Outcomes Research Institute (PCORI), a private nonprofit institution, has provided hundreds of millions of dollars to fund patient-centered studies, including PRO research, since 2012. Many professional organizations (e.g., American Association of Colleges of Pharmacy, American College of Clinical Pharmacy, American Heart Association) also offer research funding for PRO research. Specific funding available to students, such as that from the American Foundation for Pharmaceutical Education (AFPE) Gateway to Research Award, can also be used to support the student's effort in PRO research. Researchers and learners may consider applying for internal funding within their institutions if the project does not require significant resources. Funding can then be used, for example, to support study personnel time and effort to conduct a study, compensate study subjects for their time completing PROMs, pay for study materials needed for the study (including licensing fees for PROMs if necessary), and travel to present study results.

Dissemination of PRO Research

Similar to other clinical research, many scientific conferences and peer-reviewed clinical journals accept PRO research work. There are also journals specific to PRO, such as the *Journal of Patient-Reported Outcomes*. In addition, there are several journals dedicated to the dissemination of research in specific areas within the realm of PRO, such as the fields of quality of life and health-related quality of life (e.g., *Quality of Life Research, Health and Quality of Life Outcomes*). For journal outlets, researchers should carefully review the aims and scope of a journal to help decide whether the journal is an appropriate target to disseminate their research findings. Once the decision is made for the target journal, the journal's guidelines for authors should be reviewed for what is required for the manuscript, such as the manuscript's structure (abstract, components of the main text, and word limit), reporting standard, and references used.

Researchers should also consult PRO reporting guidelines designed to enhance the quality and transparency in the reporting of PRO research. One such example is the Consolidated Standards of Reporting Trials PRO (CONSORT PRO) extension,[77] which was developed using the methodology proposed by the Enhancing the Quality and Transparency of Health Research (EQUATOR) Network. Although the CONSORT PRO extension is oriented toward reporting PRO data from clinical trials, it provides useful guidance for PRO reporting in general. Some of the key components of the checklist specific to PRO research include:

- Identify PROs as primary or secondary outcomes in the abstract.
- State the PRO hypothesis and identify relevant PRO domains, if applicable, in the introduction.
- Specify psychometric properties of PROMs used, how PRO data are collected, administration mode, and format of PROMs in the methods.
- Provide a clear statistical approach to deal with missing data in the statistical analysis.
- Discuss PRO-specific limitations as well as implications for clinical practice and generalizability of the results in the discussion.

Exemplars of Learner-Involved PRO Research

The authors have been fortunate to have worked with several student pharmacists, graduate students, and pharmacy residents to conduct PRO research. This section provides examples based on the authors' experience of PRO research that involved learners. The first example was a randomized-controlled study conducted among pregnant women receiving care at two women's clinics at one U.S. medical center.[78] This study evaluated if a Tdap vaccine information statement (VIS) affected overall perception, vaccination intention, and components of a health behavior model associated with Tdap vaccination rates. The two participating student pharmacists learned how to develop a PRO research protocol and design survey questions to collect PROs (i.e., attitudes and perceptions toward Tdap) and assisted with data collection, PRO interpretation, and reporting. Under supervision, they conducted a literature search to review existing vaccine studies (e.g., flu vaccination, Tdap) in pregnant women and gathered information about their attitudes and whether there were existing PROMs that could be used in the current study. The student pharmacists also consulted with clinical pharmacists and other clinicians to inform the development of the PRO questionnaire. They helped prepare the paper-based survey, recruited patients into the study, and administered the survey. Moreover, they were closely involved with PRO interpretation during weekly meetings and assisted in drafting the first manuscript. One of the two student pharmacists also helped draft a second manuscript[79] that focused on maternal knowledge of pertussis and Tdap vaccine and the use of a Tdap VIS to improve that knowledge.

The second example is a cross-sectional, observational survey study that explored the attitudes of the Arkansas community toward medical cannabis (MC) regulation and the role of pharmacists in dispensing MC and examined whether participants' demographics and characteristics were associated with these attitudes.[80] The student pharmacist teamed with graduate students in Masters and PhD programs to score the PROs (i.e., low health risk using the Comprehensive Marijuana Motive Questionnaire[81]), conduct preliminary data analysis, and draft and revise the manuscript. In each project, the students practiced reviewing relevant literature to develop the research plan, which included identifying pre-existing, validated PROMs. Importantly, they considered the applicability of these PROMs in the specific clinical and patient contexts of their projects. The authors encouraged the students to independently consider the PRO results and how these data may be interpreted to improve patient care and education. The student pharmacists who participated in both PRO research projects were funded by a summer research fellowship offered by the authors' college of pharmacy.

From our experience, student pharmacists appreciate the opportunity to learn about and participate in PRO research. Before these research experiences, they are sometimes unaware of PRO research and have more familiarity with bench-based basic research as the "typical" research endeavor. However, following their own research experience, they recognize that PROs are as important as other clinical outcomes when they are well-matched and appropriately applied to the research question. As many PRO studies can be performed in pharmacy settings,[33,34,82] it is important that learners are familiar with PRO research. We also recognize that it is helpful to provide clear instruction with appropriate resources to help students learn the concepts and the process of conducting proper PRO research. Regular research meetings to discuss literature throughout the project timeline are also valuable to help learners develop an understanding in PRO research. We hope that this chapter will serve as an introduction to PRO research to learners.

Future of PRO Research

Patients are the center of healthcare as they are the recipients of the care. Therefore, PROs should be the focus for PCC.[7] PROs are essential indicators of the effectiveness of patient-centered care.[6] Though medical technology allows us to measure physical, physiological, and biochemical data of patients to diagnose, treat, and monitor disease conditions, there is some information that can only be obtained from the patient. Importantly, measuring PROs also offer the opportunity to engage patients in meaningful and focused conversations during clinical encounters, improve quality of care, and enhance patient safety.[83,84]

Is a PROM *really* better than just asking: How is your (pain, walking, etc.) doing since I last saw you? This skepticism is common among many busy clinicians. PROs have been included in clinical practice long before there were instruments to measure them, simply by asking patients to report their illness and its impact on their lives. PROMs are a standardized, valid set of questions for collecting health status, functional status, symptoms, and problems directly from patients. Unfortunately, the vast heterogeneity of PROMs and paper-based administration have limited their successful use and implementation in clinical settings, delaying the adoption of PROMs within the medical community. However, electronic PROMs have several benefits over paper-based PROMs, such as reducing the administrative burden for data management, scoring, and interpretation and reducing wastes in the paper, printing, and storage. More importantly, automated PROM data are incorporated directly into the EHR and can be used in real-time during clinic visits.

The future of value-based healthcare delivery depends on PROs.[39,85] PROs have been used as quality metrics (e.g., patient satisfaction, process of care) and one of the outcomes for evidence-based practice (e.g., HRQoL, functions). PROs are increasingly recognized by clinicians, regulators, and patients as valuable outcomes as they provide unique information on the impact of a medical condition and its treatment from the patient's perspective. To conduct high-quality PRO research, it must begin with improved, PRO-specific education for the research team about the core principles and methods for PRO research. We believe that routine collection of longitudinal PRO data across disease conditions will be crucial for value-based care and evidence-based practice in the near future.

Summary and Conclusions

PROs are established as a central and indispensable outcome for evaluating healthcare and treatments. PROs can be used by clinicians, patients, and policymakers to assess treatment choices, form guidelines, enable regulatory decisions for drug approval, and inform policy decisions for pricing and reimbursement. This chapter highlights the importance of PROs and provides an overview of PRO research. We also supply important considerations for conducting PRO research, as well as examples, with the hope that they will give researchers and learners the needed introduction and overview of how PROs have been used in clinical studies and practice. Lastly, the opportunity exists for learners to participate in PRO research if they desire.

Key Points and Advice

- PROs are one of the essential outcomes that can be used in clinical and observational research in pharmacy settings.
- PROs should be collected using valid instruments that are purposefully developed to capture intended concepts or perspectives of health.
- PROMs are standardized sets of questionnaires that are used to capture desired PRO concepts.
- Learners should be knowledgeable about how to select appropriate PROMs to best serve their study's objectives as well as PROM scoring and interpretation.
- PRO researchers can help support the clinical research team in selecting outcomes that are relevant to patients even when PROs are not the primary outcomes. Additionally, PRO researchers are a great resource to help select appropriate PROMs for desired outcomes as well as interpret PRO data.

Chapter Review Questions

1. What are PROs, and how are they measured?
2. How do PROs contribute to pharmacy research?
3. How are psychometric properties used in developing PROs?
4. What are commonly used PROMs for measuring HRQoL and QoL?
5. What are the basic steps needed to conduct PRO research?
6. What key factors should be considered when conducting pharmacy research that includes PROs?

Online Resources

- Critical Path Institute (C-Path): Patient-Reported Outcome (PRO) Consortium used for finding PROMs used in clinical studies. https://c-path.org/programs/proc/
- Mapi Research Trust: PROQOLID database for identifying existing PROMs. https://eprovide.mapi-trust.org/about/about-proqolid

- HealthMeasures: Searching the Patient-Reported Outcomes Measurement Information System (PROMIS) toolset. https://www.healthmeasures.net/index.php
- Consensus-based Standards for the selection of health Measurement Instruments (COSMIN): Database of systematic reviews of outcome measurement instruments. https://database.cosmin.nl/
- Consensus-based Standards for the selection of health Measurement Instruments (COSMIN): Checklists for assessing the methodological quality of a study. https://www.cosmin.nl/tools/checklists-assessing-methodological-study-qualities/
- International Society for Quality of Life Research (ISOQOL): Implementing PROMs in clinical practice. https://www.isoqol.org/wp-content/uploads/2019/09/ISOQOL-Companion-Guide-FINAL.pdf

REFERENCES

1. Food and Drug Administration. Guidance for Industry, Patient-Reported Outcome Measures: Use in Medical Product Development to Support Labeling Claims. Accessed October 11, 2012. https://www.fda.gov/media/77832/download
2. Strimbu K, Tavel JA. What are biomarkers? *Curr Opin HIV AIDS*. 2010;5(6): 463-466.
3. Institute of Medicine Committee on the National Quality Report on Health Care D. Envisioning the national health care quality report. In: Hurtado MP, Swift EK, Corrigan JM, eds. *Envisioning the National Health Care Quality Report*. National Academies Press (US) Copyright 2001 by the National Academy of Sciences; 2001.
4. Gnanasakthy A, Mordin M, Evans E, Doward L, DeMuro C. A review of patient-reported outcome labeling in the United States (2011–2015). *Value in Health*. 2017;20(3): 420-429.
5. Gensheimer SG, Wu AW, Snyder CF. Oh, the places we'll go: patient-reported outcomes and electronic health records. *Patient*. 2018;11(6):591-598.
6. Black N. Patient reported outcome measures could help transform healthcare. *BMJ: British Medical Journal*. 2013;346:f167.
7. Epstein RM, Street RLJr. The values and value of patient-centered care. *Ann Fam Med*. 2011;9(2):100-103.
8. Cleeland CS, Ryan KM. Pain assessment: global use of the Brief Pain Inventory. *Ann Acad Med Singap*. 1994;23(2):129-138.
9. Dworkin RH, Turk DC, Farrar JT, et al. Core outcome measures for chronic pain clinical trials: IMMPACT recommendations. *Pain*. 2005;113(1-2):9-19.
10. Katz S, Ford AB, Moskowitz RW, Jackson BA, Jaffe MW. Studies of illness in the aged: the Index of ADL: a standardized measure of biological and psychosocial function. *JAMA*. 1963;185(12):914-919.
11. Lawton MP, Brody EM. Assessment of older people: self-maintaining and instrumental activities of daily living. *Gerontologist*. 1969;9(3):179-186.

12. World Health Organization. *WHOQOL-BREF: Introduction, administration, scoring, and generic version of the assessment.* 1996.

13. Hays RD, Sherbourne CD, Mazel RM. The rand 36-item health survey 1.0. *Health Econ.* 1993;2(3):217-227.

14. Herdman M, Gudex C, Lloyd A, et al. Development and preliminary testing of the new five-level version of EQ-5D (EQ-5D-5L). *Qual Life Res.* 2011;20(10):1727-1736.

15. Diener E, Emmons RA, Larsen RJ, Griffin S. The satisfaction with life scale. *J Pers Assess.* 1985;49(1):71-75.

16. Kaplan RM, Anderson JP, Ganiats TG. The quality of well-being scale: rationale for a single quality of life index. In: Walker SR, Rosser RM, eds. *Quality of Life Assessment: Key Issues in the 1990s.* Springer; 1993.

17. Eton DT, Yost KJ, Lai JS, et al. Development and validation of the Patient Experience with Treatment and Self-management (PETS): a patient-reported measure of treatment burden. *Qual Life Res.* 2017;26(2):489-503.

18. Cleary PD, Crofton C, Hays RD, Horner R. Introduction: advances from the Consumer Assessment of Healthcare Providers and Systems (CAHPS®) Project. *Medical care.* 2012;50.

19. Marshall G, Hays R. *Patient Satisfaction Questionnaire Short Form (PSQ-18).* RAND Corporation; 1994: 7865.

20. Cleeland CS. Symptom burden: multiple symptoms and their impact as patient-reported outcomes. *J Natl Cancer Inst Monogr.* 2007;(37):16-21.

21. Cohen ME, Marino RJ. The tools of disability outcomes research functional status measures. *Arch Phys Med Rehabil.* 2000;81(12 Suppl 2):S21-S29.

22. Katz S. Assessing self-maintenance: activities of daily living, mobility, and instrumental activities of daily living. *J Am Geriatr Soc.* 1983;31(12):721-727.

23. World Health Organization. Development of the WHOQOL: Rationale and Current Status. *Int J Ment Health.* 1994;23(3):24-56.

24. Mayo N. Dictionary of Quality of Life and Health Outcomes Measurement. *International Society for Quality of Life Research*; 2015.

25. Seligman M. *Authentic Happiness: Using the New Positive Psychology to Realize Your Potential for Lasting Fulfillment.* Free Press; 2002.

26. Diener E, Lucas RE, Oishi S. Advances and open questions in the science of subjective well-being. *Collabra: Psychology.* 2018;4(1).

27. Bull C, Byrnes J, Hettiarachchi R, Downes M. A systematic review of the validity and reliability of patient-reported experience measures. *Health Serv Res.* 2019;54(5):1023-1035.

28. Cleary PD. Evolving concepts of patient-centered care and the assessment of patient care experiences: optimism and opposition. *J Health Polit Policy Law.* 2016;41(4):675-696.

29. Anhang Price R, Elliott MN, Zaslavsky AM, et al. Examining the role of patient experience surveys in measuring health care quality. *Med Care Res Rev.* 2014;71(5):522-554.

30. Kingsley C, Patel S. Patient-reported outcome measures and patient-reported experience measures. *BJA Education.* 2017;17(4):137-144.

31. Barnett MJ, Frank J, Wehring H, et al. Analysis of pharmacist-provided medication therapy management (MTM) services in community pharmacies over 7 years. *J Manag Care Pharm*. 2009;15(1):18-31.

32. Truong HA, Layson-Wolf C, de Bittner MR, Owen JA, Haupt S. Perceptions of patients on Medicare Part D medication therapy management services. *J Am Pharm Assoc*. 2009;49(3):392-398.

33. Snyder ME, Chewning B, Kreling D, et al. An evaluation of the spread and scale of PatientToc™ from primary care to community pharmacy practice for the collection of patient-reported outcomes: a study protocol. *Res Soc Admin Pharm*. 2021;17(2): 466-474.

34. Al-Jumah KA, Qureshi NA. Impact of pharmacist interventions on patients' adherence to antidepressants and patient-reported outcomes: a systematic review. *Patient Prefer Adherence*. 2012;6:87-100.

35. Lindenmeyer A, Hearnshaw H, Vermeire E, Van Royen P, Wens J, Biot Y. Interventions to improve adherence to medication in people with type 2 diabetes mellitus: a review of the literature on the role of pharmacists. *J Clin Pharm Ther*. 2006;31(5):409-419.

36. Davis EM, Packard KA, Jackevicius CA. The pharmacist role in predicting and improving medication adherence in heart failure patients. *J Manag Care Pharm*. 2014;20(7):741-755.

37. Rasmussen AA, Wiggers H, Jensen M, et al. Patient-reported outcomes and medication adherence in patients with heart failure. *Eur Heart J - Cardiovasc Pharmacother*. 2021;7(4):287-295.

38. Gagné M, Boulet LP, Pérez N, Moisan J. Patient-reported outcome instruments that evaluate adherence behaviours in adults with asthma: a systematic review of measurement properties. *Br J Clin Pharmacol*. 2018;84(9):1928-1940.

39. The AMCP Partnership Forum. Building the foundation for patient-reported outcomes-infrastructure and methodologies. *J Manag Care Spec Pharm*. 2019;25(4):501-506.

40. Caraballo C, Desai NR, Mulder H, et al. Clinical implications of the New York Heart Association Classification. *J Am Heart Assoc*. 2019;8(23):e014240.

41. Aparasu R, Chatterjee S. The scientific approach to research and practice. In: Aparasu R, Bentley J, eds. *Principles of Research Design and Drug Literature Evaluation*. 2nd ed. McGraw-Hill; 2020.

42. PCORI Methodology Committee. PCORI Methodology Standards. Accessed April 23, 2015. https://www.pcori.org/research-results/about-our-research/research-methodology/pcori-methodology-standards

43. Ishaque S, Karnon J, Chen G, Nair R, Salter AB. A systematic review of randomised controlled trials evaluating the use of patient-reported outcome measures (PROMs). *Qual Life Res*. 2019;28(3):567-592.

44. Oldsberg L, Garellick G, Osika Friberg I, Samulowitz A, Rolfson O, Nemes S. Geographical variations in patient-reported outcomes after total hip arthroplasty between 2008-2012. *BMC Health Serv Res*. 2019;19(1):343.

45. Brooks R. EuroQol: the current state of play. *Health Policy*. 1996;37(1):53-72.

46. Riazi A, Hobart JC, Lamping DL, et al. Using the SF-36 measure to compare the health impact of multiple sclerosis and Parkinson's disease with normal population health profiles. *J Neurol Neurosurg Psychiat.* 2003;74(6):710.

47. Cohen RM, Greenberg JM, Ishak WW. Incorporating multidimensional patient-reported outcomes of symptom severity, functioning, and quality of life in the Individual Burden of Illness Index for Depression to measure treatment impact and recovery in MDD. *JAMA Psychiat.* 2013;70(3):343-350.

48. Ishak WW, Greenberg JM, Saah T, et al. Development and validation of the Individual Burden of Illness Index for Major Depressive Disorder (IBI-D). *Adm Policy Ment Health.* 2013;40(2):76-86.

49. Lewis G, Duffy L, Ades A, et al. The clinical effectiveness of sertraline in primary care and the role of depression severity and duration (PANDA): a pragmatic, double-blind, placebo-controlled randomised trial. *Lancet Psychiat.* 2019;6(11):903-914.

50. Kroenke K, Spitzer RL, Williams JB. The PHQ-9: validity of a brief depression severity measure. *J Gen Int Med.* 2001;16(9):606-613.

51. Button KS, Kounali D, Thomas L, et al. Minimal clinically important difference on the Beck Depression Inventory-II according to the patient's perspective. *Psychol Med.* 2015;45(15):3269-3279.

52. Johnson SU, Ulvenes PG, Øktedalen T, Hoffart A. Psychometric properties of the General Anxiety Disorder 7-Item (GAD-7) scale in a heterogeneous psychiatric sample. *Front Psychol.* 2019;10:1713-1713.

53. Gandek B, Ware JE, Aaronson NK, et al. Cross-validation of item selection and scoring for the SF-12 health survey in nine countries: results from the IQOLA Project. International Quality of Life Assessment. *J Clin Epidemiol.* 1998;51(11):1171-1178.

54. Moczygemba LR, Barner JC, Brown CM, et al. Patient satisfaction with a pharmacist-provided telephone medication therapy management program. *Res Soc Admin Pharm.* 2010;6(2):143-154.

55. Germain A, Shear MK, Hall M, Buysse DJ. Effects of a brief behavioral treatment for PTSD-related sleep disturbances: a pilot study. *Behav Res Ther.* 2007;45(3):627-632.

56. Buysse DJ, Reynolds CF3rd, Monk TH, Berman SR, Kupfer DJ. The Pittsburgh Sleep Quality Index: a new instrument for psychiatric practice and research. *Psychiatry Res.* 1989;28(2):193-213.

57. Lavallee DC, Chenok KE, Love RM, et al. Incorporating patient-reported outcomes into health care to engage patients and enhance care. *Health Aff.* 2016;35(4):575-582.

58. Basch E, Deal AM, Kris MG, et al. Symptom monitoring with patient-reported outcomes during routine cancer treatment: a randomized controlled trial. *J Clin Oncol.* 2016;34(6):557-565.

59. Wohlfahrt P, Zickmund Susan L, Slager S, et al. Provider perspectives on the feasibility and utility of routine patient-reported outcomes assessment in heart failure: a qualitative analysis. *J Am Heart Asso.* 2020;9(2):e013047.

60. Calvert M, Kyte D, Mercieca-Bebber R, et al. Guidelines for inclusion of patient-reported outcomes in clinical trial protocols: the SPIRIT-PRO extension. *JAMA.* 2018;319(5):483-494.

61. Snyder CF, Aaronson NK, Choucair AK, et al. Implementing patient-reported outcomes assessment in clinical practice: a review of the options and considerations. *Qual Life Res.* 2012;21(8):1305-1314.

62. Varni JW, Seid M, Rode CA. The PedsQL: measurement model for the pediatric quality of life inventory. *Med Care.* 1999;37(2):126-139.

63. Cella DF, Tulsky DS, Gray G, et al. The functional assessment of cancer therapy scale: development and validation of the general measure. *J Clin Oncol.* 1993;11(3):570-579.

64. Juniper EF, Buist AS, Cox FM, Ferrie PJ, King DR. Validation of a standardized version of the asthma quality of life questionnaire. *Chest.* 1999;115(5):1265-1270.

65. Brady MJ, Cella DF, Mo F, et al. Reliability and validity of the functional assessment of cancer therapy-breast quality-of-life instrument. *J Clin Oncol.* 1997;15(3):974-986.

66. McQuellon RP, Russell GB, Cella DF, et al. Quality of life measurement in bone marrow transplantation: development of the Functional Assessment of Cancer Therapy-Bone Marrow Transplant (FACT-BMT) scale. *Bone Marrow Transplant.* 1997;19(4): 357-368.

67. Basch E, Abernethy AP, Mullins CD, et al. Recommendations for incorporating patient-reported outcomes into clinical comparative effectiveness research in adult oncology. *J Clin Oncol.* 2012;30(34):4249-4255.

68. Patel N, Ferris M, Rak E. Health and nutrition literacy and adherence to treatment in children, adolescents, and young adults with chronic kidney disease and hypertension, North Carolina, 2015. *Prev Chronic Dis.* 2016;13:E101 [Retraction].

69. Sarker SK, Bt Kamal AAI, Bin Rohazaki AA, et al. Prevalence of patients compliance among hypertensive patients and its associated factors in Klinik Kesihatan Botanic Klang, Malaysia. *Int J Intg Med Sci.* 2016;3(7):345-349 [Retraction].

70. Reeve BB, Hays RD, Bjorner JB, et al. Psychometric evaluation and calibration of health-related quality of life item banks: plans for the Patient-Reported Outcomes Measurement Information System (PROMIS). *Med Care.* 2007;45(5 Suppl 1):S22-S31.

71. Cella D, Riley W, Stone A, et al. The Patient-Reported Outcomes Measurement Information System (PROMIS) developed and tested its first wave of adult self-reported health outcome item banks: 2005-2008. *J Clin Epidemiol.* 2010;63(11):1179-1194.

72. Grossman LV, Mitchell EG. Visualizing the Patient-Reported Outcomes Measurement Information System (PROMIS) measures for clinicians and patients. *AMIA Annual Symp Proc.* 2018;2017:2289-2293.

73. Guinn D, Wilhelm EE, Lieberman G, Khozin S. Assessing function of electronic health records for real-world data generation. *BMJ Evid Based Med.* 2019;24(3):95.

74. International Council on Harmonization. Guidance for Industry: E9 Statistical Principles for clinical trials. Accessed August 4, 2016. https://www.fda.gov/media/71336/download

75. Coens C, Pe M, Dueck AC, et al. International standards for the analysis of quality-of-life and patient-reported outcome endpoints in cancer randomised controlled trials: recommendations of the SISAQOL Consortium. *Lancet Oncol.* 2020;21(2):e83-e96.

76. Collaborative Institutional Training Initiative. CITI Program. Accessed December 10, 2020. https://www.citiprogram.org/index.cfm?pageID=14

77. Calvert M, Blazeby J, Altman DG, Revicki DA, Moher D, Brundage MD. Reporting of patient-reported outcomes in randomized trials: the CONSORT PRO extension. *JAMA*. 2013;309(8):814-822.

78. Payakachat N, Hadden KB, Ragland D. Promoting Tdap immunization in pregnancy: Associations between maternal perceptions and vaccination rates. *Vaccine*. 2016;34(1):179-186.

79. Payakachat N, Hadden KB, Hanner J, Ragland D. Maternal knowledge of pertussis and Tdap vaccine and the use of a vaccine information statement. *Health Educ J*. 2018;77(3):322-331.

80. Gladden ME, Hung D, Bhandari NR, et al. Arkansas community's attitudes toward the regulation of medical cannabis and the pharmacist's involvement in Arkansas medical cannabis. *J Am Pharm Assoc*. 2020;60(1):235-243.

81. Lee CM, Neighbors C, Hendershot CS, Grossbard JR. Development and preliminary validation of a comprehensive marijuana motives questionnaire. *JSAD*. 2009;70(2):279-287.

82. Wuyts J, Maesschalck J, De Wulf I, De Lepeleire J, Foulon V. Studying the impact of a medication use evaluation by the community pharmacist (Simenon): Patient-reported outcome measures. *Res Soc Admin Pharm*. 2020;16(12):1760-1767.

83. Nelson EC, Eftimovska E, Lind C, Hager A, Wasson JH, Lindblad S. Patient reported outcome measures in practice. *BMJ*. 2015;350:g7818.

84. Greenhalgh J, Gooding K, Gibbons E, et al. How do patient reported outcome measures (PROMs) support clinician-patient communication and patient care? A realist synthesis. *J Patient-Rep Outcomes*. 2018;2(1):42.

85. Squitieri L, Bozic KJ, Pusic AL. The Role of Patient-Reported Outcome Measures in Value-Based Payment Reform. *Value Health*. 2017;20(6):834-836.

13

Chapter Thirteen

Quality Improvement Research in Pharmacy Settings

Ana L. Hincapie, PhD, MS and
Elizabeth Schlosser, PharmD, BCPS, BCACP

Chapter Objectives

- Define quality improvement research in pharmacy settings
- Discuss various sources for quality improvement research in pharmacy settings
- Identity common research questions in quality improvement research
- Understand the practical considerations for quality improvement research
- Understand the technical considerations for quality improvement research
- Discuss the strategies for harnessing the expertise for quality improvement research
- Describe an example of learner involved quality improvement research project
- Understand the dissemination framework for quality improvement research

Key Terminology

Quality, quality improvement (QI), QI research, model for improvement, plan-do-study-act cycle (PDSA)

Introduction

In healthcare, achieving quality is one of the most important goals for institutions caring for millions of patients each year. Although the definition of quality of care has evolved over the years, a widely accepted definition is the one suggested by the Institute of Medicine (IOM), declaring healthcare **quality** as "the degree to which healthcare services for individuals and populations increase the likelihood of desired health outcomes and are consistent with current professional knowledge."[1] Moreover, the IOM has identified six domains that characterize the quality of care, including effectiveness, efficiency, equity, patient-centeredness, safety, and timeliness.[1] Thus, quality of care is a multidimensional construct where all of its components guide efforts for its improvement to yield better patient outcomes.

Since the 2010 Patient Protection and Affordable Healthcare Act (ACA) enactment, healthcare has been transformed in the United States. This law not only allowed the expansion of healthcare coverage but also introduced significant changes on how healthcare services are reimbursed to hospitals, community pharmacies, and healthcare plans, among others.[2] For example, ACA expanded existing value-based performance programs for hospitals. In these programs, reimbursements are adjusted based on the levels of quality of the services as measured by specific quality metrics such as 30-day mortality rates, readmission rates, and surgery complications, among others.[3] Value-based performance models have been implemented beyond inpatient care settings. For instance, the Centers for Medicare & Medicaid Services (CMS) reimburses Medicare Drug Prescription Plans based on the level of quality achieved in the five-star rating program.[4] There are multiple quality metrics in this five-star rating program that can be impacted directly by the work of pharmacists, including medication adherence, medication safety, and medication therapy management (MTM). Pharmacy students and residents are often asked to support or lead projects that seek to improve healthcare quality across settings, contribute to positive patient outcomes, and help improve these value-based quality metrics. Therefore, there is a need for learners to understand and utilize healthcare principles and tools that seek to improve quality. This chapter will focus on defining **quality improvement** (**QI**) in the context of pharmacy practice research. It provides examples of QI pharmacy practice projects, compares the concept of QI projects versus QI research, and delineates practical steps to plan and initiate a QI project, including the assembly of the QI team, selection of a problem, selection of a research methodology, use of a QI framework, and setting specific aims. Finally, this chapter summarizes considerations for the dissemination of QI project findings.

Quality Improvement and Quality Improvement Research

Healthcare **QI** is the systematic and continuous approach to change and improve healthcare delivery and outcomes. The improvement can target patients' outcomes; patients' experiences with care; or change in system processes and efficiency to offer more effective and safer care.[5] To generate change, QI can utilize a wide range of evidence-based or theory-driven interventions and frameworks to guide QI, including the Model for Improvement (MFI), Lean, and Six Sigma, among others.[6] These frameworks originated from other industries such as the automotive field before their widespread application in healthcare.[6] All of these approaches, however, share similar principles. First, they all focus on continuous testing overtime to find the best solution that fixes a problem. In QI, interventions are adopted and tested in a repetitive series of steps prompting for a constant evaluation of results and modification of aims based on results. Second, improvement is data-driven. Data, both quantitative and qualitative, are collected to establish how systems and processes work and respond to changes. With data, a baseline can be established, and specific, quantifiable goals can be set. Data allows the QI team to identify variations in a process and take corrective actions accordingly. Third, QI frameworks focus on teamwork. This implies that QI activities, from planning to execution, involve a multidisciplinary healthcare team to promote the success and sustainability of the improvements. Finally, QI focuses on incorporating the patient voice, values, and preferences into its design.[7]

It is important to distinguish QI from QI research. QI research is a scientific investigation to generate generalized knowledge or evidence for QI. Although there is overlap in the principles and methods used by both, their goals and scope are different (see Table 13–1). The use of QI principles alone to produce a change in healthcare cannot be considered research. The main difference is that QI research implements and evaluates interventions to yield generalizable knowledge broadly applicable outside the primary institution. That is, the results are shared via peer-reviewed outlets, i.e., manuscripts, posters, etc., and can be applied to populations and settings beyond those studied. By contrast, QI aims to generate local change using interventions deemed already effective or accepted.[7] For example, a QI project might entail the implementation of a new evidence-based clinical guideline for prescribing statins in a specific ambulatory care clinic.[8] A QI research project in the same area might focus on testing the hypothesis that a pharmacist intervention increases adherence to statins.[9] Both projects improve the quality of care for patients receiving statins, but the latter aims to generate evidence applicable to and intended to be shared broadly outside the primary institution. Finally, QI research projects are subject to the oversight and Human Subject Research approval of local Institutional Review Boards (IRB).

If your QI project fits any of the following descriptions, it might be considered research. First, the project utilizes methodologies of typical experimental designs such as randomization to assign the intervention. Second, the main goal of the project is to generate new evidence rather than to evaluate the implementation of existing knowledge in a local setting. Third, the risk of the intervention to participants is greater than minimal. And finally, the potential

TABLE 13-1. **CHARACTERISTICS OF QUALITY IMPROVEMENT RESEARCH VERSUS QUALITY IMPROVEMENT PROJECTS**

Consideration	Quality Improvement Research	Quality Improvement Projects
Goal	To contribute to new knowledge, test a specific hypothesis.	To assess or improve a clinical care process or program. It addresses a specific problem
Benefits	Designed to contribute to generalizable knowledge and answer a research question	Designed to improve a process, program, or system. Results are only relevant to study site
Ethics	Requires Human Subject Research approval from local Institutional Review Board (IRB). Informed consent may be required.	QI projects do not require IRB approval.
Risks	May place subjects at risk and stated as such	By design, does not increase a subject's risk
Design	Use of experimental and nonexperimental research designs to test the intervention	Use of continuous assessment of process measures
Analysis	Statistically prove or disprove a hypothesis	Compare a program/process/ system to an established set of standards.
Results Dissemination	Primarily aim to externally disseminate results through publication of journal articles and poster/podium presentations	Findings are disseminated internally to the institutions' stakeholders.

funding for the project is external to the organization where the project will be conducted, or there is a commercial interest in the results. It might be difficult as a pharmacy student or resident to determine whether the project is QI research or an improvement project. Therefore, it is highly recommended that you consult with a representative of the IRB overseeing your organization regarding QI and QI research project policies before you start the project. Most IRB offices at Academic Institutions and Academic Health Centers have internal processes that guide investigators in such determination. Additionally, your local IRB may evaluate QI research differently than traditional clinical research.

Considerations Before Starting a QI Project

QI projects in pharmacy are exceptionally diverse, spanning operations, clinical improvements, and patient outcomes in a variety of settings, including community hospitals, academic medical centers, outpatient facilities, community pharmacies, and ambulatory care settings, to name a few. Examples of QI projects or research are readily available through pharmacy organizations and peer-reviewed literature and may help to develop your area for improvement or research questions. A few examples in diverse pharmacy settings include: integrating de-prescribing practices into community pharmacists' daily workflow through training and workflow strategies;[10] utilizing lean principles to decrease time to first dose of antibiotics for patients presenting with sepsis,[11] and promoting the appropriate use of intravenous acetaminophen using the **Plan-Do-Study-Act** (PDSA) framework.[12] A consideration to bear in mind while contemplating a QI initiative in pharmacy practice is that in healthcare, multifaceted problems might require complex solutions, including rigorous scientific hypothesis testing of new interventions.[13] The next sections describe the steps to guide you in the development of the QI project. Additionally, a case example is weaved throughout the remaining sections of the chapter.

Case example

■ INCREASING NEW PRESCRIPTION VOLUME AT AN OUTPATIENT PHARMACY

A PGY1 pharmacy resident in an outpatient pharmacy within a pediatric community-based hospital is planning for her residency research project. The pharmacy director is concerned with the limited use of the pharmacy by the pediatric hospital patients and shared the results of an internal patient survey from the previous year revealing that 43% of respondents who visited the pediatric hospital were unaware of the onsite outpatient pharmacy. Of those who were aware, 62% have used the pharmacy either to fill a prescription, purchase over-the-counter (OTC) medications or both. Statements received from the survey suggested a lack of patient-family awareness of pharmacy services available. The pharmacy personnel agreed that the outpatient pharmacy was not being given the priority needed to reach the full potential to serve the hospital's patients. Therefore, the PGY1 was tasked to propose and implement a QI project to address this problem.

*Used with Permission of author Dr. Nicholas Michel

CREATING THE QI TEAM

One of the first and most important steps in a QI project is to identify the QI team. The team is likely to be interdisciplinary (depending on your setting and the scope of the project) and include important stakeholders for the process being improved. A stakeholder is not only someone who is affected by a change but anyone who has an interest in the change. Involving stakeholders in project brainstorming and then approaching them about getting formally involved in the project is a great way to recruit for the QI team. It may be tempting to only include those stakeholders who are already familiar with the problem and may already be on board with your proposal. However, including people resistant to change will help move the project forward. Engaging resistors early allows you to identify and better prepare to address potential barriers based on their feedback, thus avoiding potential organizational delays. Another strategic team member you will want to engage if available is the organization's QI department.[14]

The core working team should consist of a team lead, technical experts, an improvement advisor, clinical/system leaders, and an executive sponsor. There is no set number of an appropriate QI team size; what is more relevant is the diversity of perspectives and experience in the healthcare process of the stakeholders.[15] The team lead is responsible for the everyday management of the project and must be a part of the system undergoing change. It is important to note here that as a student/resident, your role may be as the team-lead, or it may be as a team lead assistant depending on the project and your role within the system undergoing change. Technical experts are also very important to the team as they are persons that are highly knowledgeable and involved in the process being improved and can offer many different perspectives. For example, if the project requires the implementation or modification of existing software, involving a representative of the IT department should be considered. Another example might be that you want to shorten the time it takes to start antibiotics in patients presenting with sepsis. In this scenario, you would want to consider including physicians as they are likely the ones ordering the antibiotics and nurses as they will be administering them.

Quality Improvement advisors are well versed in QI projects and can act as a resource or a guide through the process. They may be employed within the organization or may have to be consulted but their expertise is invaluable. Finally, clinical and executive leaders should be a part of the research team. Clinical leaders are typically intermediate-level managers who bring a more global perspective of the organization as a whole and also have the authority to authorize changes within processes. A clinical pharmacy manager or director of pharmacy, nurse manager or medical directors are examples of clinical leaders. Executive sponsors are higher-level managers who may not be directly involved in the process regularly but who can secure resources and remove barriers when they arise. Executive sponsors include "C-suite" executives such as Chief Medical Officers, Chief Financial Officers, Chief Executive Officers, Assistant Vice-Presidents, etc. Additionally, a group that may often be overlooked but is highly important are patients or patient advocates. Patient advocacy groups may already be a part of the organization and can easily be engaged in the project.[14]

DEVELOPING A QI COMMUNICATION PLAN

Once the team is established, it is important to develop a communication strategy in order to disseminate your QI plan within the organization to keep stakeholders informed about project progress as an accountability tool and to ultimately broadly disseminate the results and success. This plan should be tailored to each team member's specific role. For example, those with the most interest in the project and the highest influence will want to be kept in close contact with regular meetings or e-mails. In addition to variations based on role in the project, frequency of communication will also vary based on project timeline and deliverables. During the early days of project implementation, you may want to have more frequent meetings/emails and decrease frequency over time. Those with lesser influence, lesser interest, or simply peripheral to the project can likely remain informed through established communication channels such as quarterly staff meetings or newsletters. Prioritizing team members and stakeholders according to their influence and interest will help establish the strategy that is most appropriate for each group.[16] In general, the communication plan should include the audience for the message (front-line staff pharmacists, managers, patients, etc.), the purpose of the communication (informative, feedback requested, share progress, sustain engagement, etc.), timing (before project initiation, at specific project milestones, etc.), methods (e-mails, in-person meetings, flyers, etc.), and the QI team member responsible.

Selecting a QI Design Methodology

After assembling your team and developing a communication strategy, you will need to define the QI methodology for your project. Although traditional clinical study research designs such as randomized control trials are applied in QI research, sometimes randomization of interventions for QI projects is prohibitively time and resource consuming.[17] Due to this limitation of randomization, QI projects often use alternative study designs to help address potential concerns with internal validity without randomization. These include but are not limited to Before-and-After Designs, Interrupted Time Series, Before-and-After with Nonequivalent and Mixed-Methods designs.[18]

BEFORE-AND-AFTER DESIGN

In this design, the QI team collects data for the outcome before the QI intervention implementation and after the implementation.[18] It is assumed that any outcome changes occurred due to the intervention. This is the simplest study design but also is the most prone to potential confounding because even with extensive planning, it is likely impossible to control for all external factors that could potentially influence the outcome, such as organizational trends, other interventions that run in tandem to your intervention within the organization, etc. For example, in a study that aims to implement a medication reconciliation program to reduce the heart failure 30-day readmission rate, patients may be affected by other institutional interventions such as discharge planning and discharge patient education, among others. Despite these limitations, the Before-and-After design is commonly used in circumstances where it is not possible to obtain data from a control group. There are multiple examples readers can review in the pharmacy literature of QI projects applying this design.[19–22]

INTERRUPTED TIME SERIES

One way to improve the Before-and-After design is to obtain multiple data points, typically at equal intervals before and after the intervention.[18,23] This approach is useful to establish the trend of the outcome measure, which is then interrupted by the intervention. The hypothesis is that the outcome trend will change after the intervention implementation. For instance, in a QI study that evaluated the impact of expanding pharmacist services in a pediatric intensive care unit, investigators collected the prevalence of medication errors per 100 prescriptions six times before the intervention and six times after the intervention at one-month intervals. Using interrupted time series statistical analyses, the authors' demonstrated a change in the slopes of the medication error rates using a regression model after the QI intervention.[24]

BEFORE-AND-AFTER DESIGN WITH NONEQUIVALENT CONTROL GROUP

This study design compares the effect of the QI intervention on the outcome before and after its implementation in a group that received the intervention and in a control group that did not.[18] The control group is called nonequivalent because these individuals are not randomly assigned to the groups. This design helps address the potential effect of organizational trends. For instance, a pharmacist-led QI project that aims to optimize the prescribing of opioids may be affected by institutional opioid-related policies implemented at the same time of the study. Using before and after with nonequivalent control group study design, in this case, may help better differentiate the effect of the institutional policies from the QI project on study outcomes.[25] To minimize potential biases introduced by having nonequivalent groups, control groups are often selected based on baseline characteristics of demographics and outcomes of interest. For example, if a QI intervention wants to increase medication adherence rates, the control group baseline level for adherence should ideally be similar to the intervention group. Statistical strategies like multivariable regression analyses can then be used to control for potential differences in baseline characteristics between groups. Detailed descriptions of these strategies can be found in the companion book *Principles of Research Design and Drug Literature Evaluation.*[26]

MIXED-METHODS DESIGN

A mixed methods design collects, analyzes, and integrates both quantitative and qualitative data during the research process. Qualitative data are nonnumerical, typically in the form of text, which can be obtained from interviews, group interviews (e.g., focus groups), observations, and questionnaires.[18] In QI, mixed methods may help investigators obtain a deeper understanding of why a QI intervention is successful or not or to gather the point of view of patients and other stakeholders.[27] For instance, a QI study in the United Kingdom sought to reduce prescribing errors by implementing a multimodal intervention based on modified feedback to junior prescribers. As part of the evaluation plan, investigators used mixed methods using qualitative data through focus groups to assess pharmacists' and prescribers' views on the interventions. Ultimately, the qualitative data in this study helped identify a variety of unintended consequences associated with implementing the interventions.[28]

Selecting a QI Framework

In addition to selecting the research design for a QI project, the QI team should select a QI framework. QI frameworks assist investigators in understanding the gaps in quality of care and plan for sustainable interventions that can seamlessly be integrated into practice over time. This chapter will focus on the three most common QI frameworks driving continuous QI in pharmacy practice: The MFI, Lean, and Six Sigma.

MODEL FOR IMPROVEMENT

The **MFI** is a systematic and data-driven framework widely used in healthcare to speed up quality improvement efforts. MFI is intended to supplement change models that organizations may already use and focuses on developing, testing, implementing, and spreading changes. The Institute for Healthcare Improvement (IHI) adapted this framework for use in healthcare in 1996.[29] In the MFI, the QI team starts the QI process by answering three global questions, followed by the process of testing changes (i.e., Interventions). The three questions are:

1. What are we trying to accomplish?
2. How will we know that a change is an improvement?
3. What changes can we make that will result in improvement?

The first question yields measurable, quantifiable, time bound, and place-specific goals. The second question helps identify which measures will be used to determine whether an intervention is successful or not. Finally, the last question guides the QI team in selecting the interventions to be implemented and tested. After answering these questions, the QI team will test the intervention using the PDSA Cycle.

The **PDSA** is a four-step cycle for the design, implementation, and evaluation of a quality improvement project. In the Plan stage of the cycle, the QI team specifies the goals for the project; determines who, what, when, and where for the intervention to be tested; and plans for data collection. In the Do stage the intervention is tested, and data are collected, and the plan is carried out. Subsequently, during the Study stage, the data are analyzed, and conclusions/lessons learned are identified and summarized. Finally, in the Act stage, the QI team decides whether to adopt, adapt, or abandon the intervention and plan for the next cycle. There is no set number of PDSA cycles anticipated for any QI project as it is highly variable and will depend on the nature of the intervention and results. For example, a resident or student researcher might participate in one PDSA cycle during their time in the learning program, but subsequent PDSA cycles may be needed to fully address the gaps in care based on the data collected. The next section expands on the MFI model as MFI is a relatively simple tool that is typically viewed as an accompaniment to a broader change strategy which will be discussed below. MFI has widespread application in healthcare, including pharmacy practice and a variety of free online resources available for its implementation.[30,31]

LEAN

The lean manufacturing model originated in the automotive industry, most notably Toyota but has since experienced extensive application to other areas of business and healthcare.[32] Lean focuses on identifying and reducing waste through continuous improvement. In Lean, each step of a process is evaluated to determine whether it adds value or does not add value (i.e., waste) to the overall process. In healthcare, waste can be observed in multiple ways, for example, inefficient discharge processes, unnecessary diagnostic tests, incorrect medication administration, inefficient processes that increase waiting times for care, etc. For instance, in a hospital pharmacy, Lean was used to reduce the rate of missing doses and production errors in the sterile product area.[33] The QI pharmacy team analyzed walk patterns, area floor plans and observed staff workflows. Using a simulation room, the team evaluated different models to optimize workflow. The overall results of the QI included enhanced workload sharing, pharmacy technicians' work redistribution, and reduction in production errors, among others.[33]

SIX SIGMA

Another QI methodology typically used in conjunction with Lean is Six Sigma.[34] Compared to Lean, which focuses on waste, Six Sigma focuses on eliminating quality problems and reducing variability in operational processes. It utilizes statistical tools to assess and monitor the variability of processes. Six Sigma follows a five-step process for QI implementation: (1) Define the problem, (2) measure outcomes and quantify the problem, (3) analyze the data to identify quality problems and their causes, (4) improve the process through tested interventions, and (5) control the new process with constant monitoring and correction of process deviations to maintain success. These steps are commonly abbreviated as DMAIC (Define, Measure, Analyze, Improve, and Control). One Example of the Six Sigma application in pharmacy involved a group of investigators who reduced the rate of medication errors in a home delivery pharmacy service.[35] In the Define step, the QI team operationalized the definition of medication errors. In the Measure step, the team created an electronic database to collect any medication errors reported in the different stages of the dispensing and delivery service and made modifications to the error reporting process to consistently collect data. During the Analyze step, the team reviewed medication error data from the medication error database for the initial five months after implementation and found that 96% of errors originated at the prescription processing stage versus 4% at the dispensing stage. For the Improve step, the QI team implemented a multimodal intervention that included the development of standard operating procedures, enhanced pharmacists' training, and improved storage of sound-alike-look-alike medications. Finally, for Control, the team utilized charts and established error rate targets and a monitoring plan to assure sustained success.[35]

The selection of a QI framework, whether it is the MFI, Lean, or Six Sigma, will depend on the familiarity of the QI team with the different frameworks and the resources available within the organization for its use. Multiple professional organizations maintain access to free online resources, including training videos, checklists, and worksheets to conduct a QI project using these models. Some useful websites to consult include the American Society of Health-System Pharmacists (ASHP) Quality Improvement Resource Center (https://www.ashp.org/Pharmacy-Practice/Resource-Centers/Quality-Improvement), the American Society for Quality (ASQ) (https://asq.org/quality-resources), and the IHI site (http://www.ihi.org/resources/Pages/Tools/Quality-Improvement-Essentials-Toolkit.aspx).

Case Example

■ QI TEAM, METHODOLOGY, AND IMPROVEMENT FRAMEWORK CHOICES

The resident assembled a QI project team of stakeholders who typically interact with new patients at the beginning of their visit, including certified pharmacy technicians, hospital registration leaders, marketing representatives, the outpatient pharmacy manager, and a patient-family representative. A communication plan was developed to ensure that all stakeholders would be informed of the project from its conception. The plan included an initial in-person meeting followed by biweekly emails during the first two months of the project. The QI team decided to apply the MFI framework because it was the approach most known by the QI team.

Starting Your QI Project

IDENTIFYING THE PROBLEM

In order to get started on your QI project, the specific problem being addressed must be clearly defined. Some considerations that will help identify a quality problem include evaluating current gaps in performance and strategic connections for the organization. Often gaps in performance are identified through evaluations from accreditation surveys such as the Joint Commission Pharmacy Accreditation survey,[36] internal self-assessments, audits of findings from other regulatory bodies such as state boards of pharmacy, or current performance on value-based measures in contracts with health plans. In many pharmacy practice settings, organizations enter into contracts with payers that provide incentives and payment for meeting certain quality metrics dubbed "value-based measures." An example of a common measure is patient adherence rates for antihypertensive medications. If reporting indicates that performance on this measure is low within the organization and not meeting predetermined goals, this likely would be a good area for a QI project. Electronic medical records and "dashboards" have made collecting and analyzing data to identify gaps and plan QI targets and projects much easier and accessible for organizations as a whole.

　　Strategic connections for the organization are highly important, as you will want to align your project with the organization's strategic goals. Fortunately, with the shift of focus both in healthcare and pharmacy practice to quality rather than quantity of care, there are many opportunities to align QI projects with payment models and gain additional buy-in using strategic goals for an organization. For example, hospital reimbursement for inpatient care is now linked to 30-day readmission rates from initial discharge for patients initially admitted with certain conditions (i.e., chronic obstructive pulmonary disease or COPD, acute myocardial infarction, heart failure) through the Medicare Hospital Readmissions Reduction Program. If you are interested in improving care for COPD patients and your organization is participating in this program, including readmission rates in your project outcomes will demonstrate additional project value to the organization by potentially improving hospital reimbursement, which can help generate greater stakeholder buy-in. Many organizations participate in payment models like this example, but variation certainly exists, and it is important for researchers to discuss and have a solid understanding of current reimbursement models used within the organization to best position your QI project for success. This can be done by examining the strategic goals of the organization or discussing reimbursement incentives with the management team members of your QI team.

　　Additionally, consider the six domains of quality of care mentioned in the introduction and assess whether there are problems or gaps in the pharmacy department around any of these domains. See Table 13–2 for examples.

　　After identifying a problem, it is necessary to understand factors that may be contributing to the problem. In QI, there are multiple tools that can be used to understand the root cause of a problem. A root cause analysis is a way of understanding what is currently happening and why it is happening.[43] A variety of tools such as the Fishbone diagram, The 5-Whys process, Process Mapping, and Pareto Charts are available to help perform

TABLE 13−2. QUALITY OF CARE DIMENSION AND EXAMPLES OF GAPS IN CARE IN PHARMACY PRACTICE

Dimension	Examples of Gaps in Care
Safety	Unintentional continuation of medications intended for acute illness after hospital discharge[37]
Effectiveness	Lack of optimized guideline directed medical therapy (GDMT) in heart failure patients[38]
Patient-centered	Poor patient satisfaction with comprehensive medication review[39]
Timeliness	Treatment delays associated with Prior Authorizations[40]
Efficiency	Expired medications in automated dispensing cabinets[41]
Equitable	Racial and socioeconomic disparities in pharmacy access and services[42]

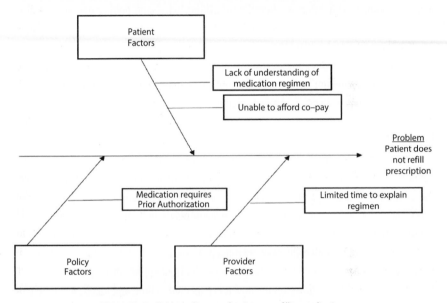

Figure 13−1. Fishbone diagram of patient not refilling medication.

a root cause analysis. These tools are complementary to each other and commonly used together in root cause analysis.

Fishbone Diagram

In the Fishbone diagram, also known as the Case and Effect or Ishikawa diagram, the QI team brainstorms and maps out possible causes of a quality problem.[43] To create a Fishbone diagram, the problem is written on the right side of a horizontal line (see Figure 13–1). The causes of the problems are then listed along this line. Subsequently, the QI team proceeds to brainstorm the causes or contributing factors of the problem and write them along the horizontal line. Typically, causes are grouped in general themes such as patients, providers, policies, processes and procedures, and equipment. Each theme or group represents a branch (or spine) in the diagram. After completing the diagram, the QI team should select one area as the focus of the improvement. Although all areas are worthy of inquiry, the QI team may narrow their focus in a variety of pragmatic ways, such as selecting a cause that appears repeatedly across multiple categories, one that is considered the most likely to occur, or the cause that seems the easiest to fix.

The 5-Whys

The 5-Whys tool consists of asking the simple question of "Why?" five times until the real cause of the problem is identified. If a root cause is not revealed after five whys, the QI team continues asking additional whys until a root cause becomes evident.[43] Although it may be easy to stop after one iteration of asking "why" and getting one answer, it is recommended to ask "why" at least five times to dig deeper into the cause of the problem as often the surface why is not the root cause but simply a byproduct of another problem upstream. In the antibiotics administration delay example shown in Figure 13–2, stopping at the first why would not have revealed a root cause that could be addressed by an intervention focused on a system or process change.

Process Mapping

Process mapping is a tool that uses flowcharts to depict each sequential step of a particular process.[44] Steps are represented using different shapes and symbols. For example, the beginning or start of a process uses an oval (see Figure 13–3), tasks or activities are represented by boxes, and steps where a decision needs to be made use diamonds. All these shapes are connected with arrows indicating the direction of the process. There are multiple benefits of formally drawing out a process. First, it ensures that the entire QI team has a baseline understanding of the process; it also identifies discrepancies between how the process actually flows versus how it is expected to flow, and finally, it can help to visually highlight steps that cause problems (i.e., delays, work duplication, illogical step sequence, unclear lines of responsibility, or failure of communications). Once the process map is completed in detail, the QI team can more easily identify opportunities for improvement. For example, the QI team may discuss if there are unnecessary tasks that can be eliminated or combined with other tasks; the QI team may also use process inconsistencies to help identify training and education that might resolve these inconsistencies; lastly, the QI team may identify resource needs such as additional personnel to complete certain steps in the process.

Pareto Charts

Pareto charts are another root cause tool that uses diagrams to analyze and summarize quantitative data on causes of problems.[44] These charts have two components: a bar chart with the classification of the causes of problems, ordered from the most frequent to the

Problem: Antibiotics were delayed for a septic shock patient, increasing her risk of death.

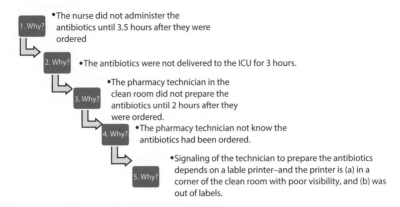

Figure 13–2. Example of the 5-Whys process. (Adapted from Howell MD, Stevens JP. *Understanding Healthcare Delivery Science.* New York: McGraw Hill; 2020.)

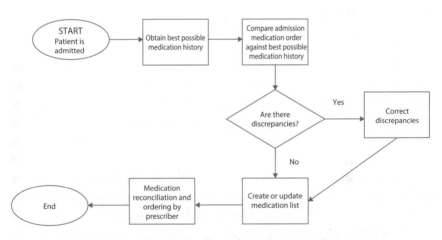

Figure 13–3. Example of a flowchart diagram for a medication reconciliation process.

least frequent, and an overlapped line graph of the cumulative percentage of all the problem causes. For example, Figure 13–4 is a Pareto chart of data about causes of medication errors in community pharmacies using a new electronic prescribing system. A Pareto chart is used to assess the 80/20 Pareto Rule, which indicates that 80% of the problems or outcomes can be attributed to 20% of the causes. In Figure 13–4, 80% of the cumulative frequency of medication errors (outcomes) are accounted for by three error types: incorrect date selection, incorrect patient directions, and wrong dose selection (causes). This information can be used by the QI team to develop an intervention targeting these three causes. A Pareto chart can help prioritize which problems should be addressed first.

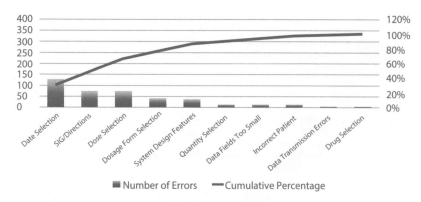

Figure 13–4. A Pareto chart of data on causes of medication errors in community pharmacy.

After identifying the problem and its causes using any of the tools described above, the next steps for the QI team are to establish the aims for improvement and select an intervention that closely aligns with the root causes of the problem.

Establishing the QI Aims

After completing a root cause analysis, researchers should establish the specific aims of the project. In the MFI, the QI team is prompted to address the question *what are we trying to accomplish?*[26] To answer this question, an aim statement or project goal should be defined. A good approach to develop an aim statement is to write it following the SMART guidance, that is, the statement should be Specific, Measurable, Achievable, Relevant, and Time-bound.

Specific: Aims should be well-defined, identify the problem, and specify the overall goal by using active verbs such as reduce or increase. Additionally, aims should identify the target population, and the setting where the project will be conducted.

Measurable: Aims should indicate a target number that will prompt the QI team to know when the goal has been accomplished or to monitor progress. Targets may be informed by internal or external benchmark goals that are not being met. For example, the national median for the percentage of long-stay residents who got an antipsychotic medication in nursing homes was 14.4% in 2019,[45] thus projects targeting this outcome should aim for a decrease below this threshold value.

Achievable: The QI team should consider the resources, leadership support, and time available before setting up the project aims.

Relevant: A relevant aim fits the mission and goals of the pharmacy department and the overall organization.

Time-Bound: The aim should specify a completion date or time frame. The following template can help drafting the aim: By [specific date], we will [increase or decrease]

TABLE 13–3. EXAMPLES OF QI AIMS RE-WRITTEN TO FIT THE SMART CRITERIA

Aim	SMART Aim
Improve immunization rates among healthcare workers in a nursing home.	By June of this year, we will increase influenza vaccination rates in the nursing home from 30% to 60%.
We will train pharmacy technicians on a new medication refill process at an ambulatory care clinic.	By the end of July 2020, the pharmacy resident team will have trained 90% of pharmacy technicians on a new medication refill process at an ambulatory care clinic.
Implement a double-check process to prevent dispensing errors at a community pharmacy.	By the end of 2021, we will decrease the percentage of dispensing errors at a community pharmacy by 20% with the implementation of a double-check process.

the [specific QI outcomes] by [add target number] %. Table 13–3 displays examples of QI aims statements re-written to follow the SMART criteria.

CHOOSING QI MEASURES

Selecting appropriate measures is an essential aspect in QI to evaluate whether an intervention is yielding expected results or not. In the MFI, this is addressed by answering the question, *how will we know a change is an improvement?*[29] For QI projects, it is useful to select a mix of measures to provide a comprehensive assessment of the impact of the interventions. Measures can be classified into four categories: structure, process, outcomes, and balancing measures.[46] Structure measures indicate the presence of structural elements such as equipment, software, personnel, and so on. An example of a structure measure is the ratio of pharmacists to patients or the presence of an electronic health record system. Process measures assess how the work is performed while providing patient care or conducting other pharmacy operations. For example, the proportion of patients with diabetes that receive a statin evaluates the process of following recommended clinical guidelines. Outcome measures focus on clinical and patient-centered indicators that reflect the impact of the intervention on patients' health status. Examples of outcome measures include mortality rates, number of hospital readmissions, percent of patients with uncontrolled hypertension, etc. Finally, balancing measures help monitor the potential unintended consequences of implementing a QI project. For example, by implementing an activity to increase the efficiency of the dispensing process, pharmacists might have less time for verification or checking of prescriptions resulting in the potential increase of percent of dispensing errors (balancing measure).

In pharmacy practice, good places to start looking for quality measures are the Pharmacy Quality Alliance (PQA) and the National Quality Forum (NQF) websites.[47,48] On the PQA's website, there is an array of pharmacy quality measures focused on six domains.[47] These domains include medication adherence (e.g., Proportion of Days Covered: Renin Angiotensin System Antagonists), appropriate medication use (e.g., Use of Medications to Prevent Major Cardiovascular Events in Persons with Diabetes), medication safety (e.g., Antipsychotic Use in Persons with Dementia), medication management services (e.g., Completion Rate for Comprehensive Medication Review [CMR]), opioid use (e.g., Concurrent Use of Opioids and Benzodiazepines), and specialty drug-related measures, (e.g., Treatment of Chronic Hepatitis C: Completion of Therapy). The NQF website offers a comprehensive list of quality measures focusing on a wide range of areas of healthcare, including inpatient/hospital, ambulatory care, behavioral health, post-acute care, and home care.[48] During the process of selecting the QI measures, the QI team should consider measures that align with the organizations' goals and other quality activities. This will help determine if there are measures already in place in the organization with automated mechanisms to obtain and report results.

Case Example

■ ESTABLISHING QI AIMS AND MEASURES.

The QI team established an aim to increase the new prescription capture rate (process measure) among new patients from 23% to 33% over a six-month period. Baseline data had shown that prescription volume variation was present, suggesting that prescription volume is dependent on hospital census. Therefore, the new prescription capture rate defined as a first fill prescription was used. A Fishbone diagram was developed to identify possible factors preventing the utilization of the pharmacy. After this process, it was concluded that pharmacy advertisement was needed to increase the new prescription capture rate.

Selecting a QI Intervention

Once the measures have been defined, the next step is to select an intervention. This pertains to the last question in the MFI: *what changes can we make that will result in improvement?* A good initial approach to answer this question is to hold a brainstorming session with the QI Team. To prepare for this session, the QI team should be first presented with an overview of the current problem, and the entire team should have a clear understanding of the existing processes or systems related to the quality problem. Tools such as process mapping or flow diagrams can assist in this task by communicating essential details, stakeholders involved, and steps of a process to the team. In addition to gathering potential solutions or interventions in the brainstorming session, other resources should be consulted, such as published evidence-based guidelines, practices, or innovations.

The QI team should discuss the timeliness of expected preliminary and final results and identify available resources while selecting an intervention. For example, consider identifying whether there are value-based purchasing and other financial contracts with healthcare plans due dates for achieving quality goals and work around those timelines. Other timelines to consider include due dates to submit final research reports to residency directors or preceptors, or submission deadlines for conference abstracts. Resources needed for QI projects might include money for printing materials or acquiring new equipment, personnel time for data collection and analysis, statistical analysis software, and technology.

Small improvements that can be seen quickly will help to generate buy-in among stakeholders and drive the project forward. In general, evidence has shown that education or training and the development of rules and policies have the least impact. Interventions of this type may be necessary as first steps for the organization are generally easy to implement, but they might not have a sustained impact and lead to organizational change. Thus, if feasible, they should be used in combination with other approaches such as the simplification, standardization, computerization, or automation of processes and systems.[49] For example, processes can be evaluated to reduce their number of steps, or existing organizations' rules or policies can be simplified. Standardization is the act of developing and implementing uniform technical specifications and methods for a process to increase consistency and repeatability and decrease variability. Examples of standardization interventions include the implementation of standardized medication ordering and administration protocols.[50] Computerization and automation refer to the use of computers and information technologies in tasks or processes. For example, health information technologies such as electronic health records, barcoding systems, smart infusion pumps, and electronic prescribing have been implemented to improve the quality of care.[51] Regardless of the intervention selected, it is always better to start with a smaller, more feasible QI project and intervention than to plan a large project and fail to complete it. Finally, the QI team should capitalize on the resources available within the organization, including information technology, QI departments, personnel, etc., to maximize project feasibility.

APPLYING THE PDSA CYCLE

After answering the three key questions of the MFI, the next step is to test the intervention using the PDSA cycle. As mentioned above, the total number of cycles and the length of each cycle needed to establish whether an intervention is successful may vary depending on the number and nature of interventions being tested, outcome measures, and project scope. However, small-scale testing (e.g., one intervention in one unit) in short time periods is preferred. This approach gives the flexibility to move on faster if there are no results or new issues are raised after the intervention implementation. For example, if a proposed intervention is causing tension among providers and it is not being adopted, it is better to modify or discard it sooner (after a month) and move to test another intervention.

PDSA CYCLE STAGE: PLAN

In the Plan stage of the cycle, the QI team determines who will be involved and defines details of the intervention implementation, such as when and where the intervention will be tested. Additionally, a plan for data collection is created. The data collection plan should include the source of data, frequency of data collection, individuals responsible for data collection, and data analysis for each measure. In QI, data should be collected and analyzed as close to real-time as possible to facilitate timely continuous feedback and action.

There are multiple sources and ways in which you can obtain QI data. First, identify if any of the measures are already monitored by the organization, and therefore the data are already collected on an ongoing basis. For example, in community and ambulatory care pharmacy, the Proportion of Days Covered (PDC) measure of medication adherence is routinely monitored. Electronic medical records and other information systems also have the capability of generating a variety of automated data reports. A good starting point is to identify and consult the department manager, such as the pharmacy manager, about existing automatically generated reports of quality measures because multiple stakeholders within organizations routinely collect data for QI at the patient or system level. You can also reach out to the information technology department to generate reports that are not already routinely monitored. In the event that manual data collection is required, for example, extracting limited, specific patient data from electronic medical charts or paper records, it is useful to create a data collection sheet that will have all data that you will want to be pulled from each patient. Additionally, you will want to develop and maintain a spreadsheet with detailed instructions of where and how data will be transcribed. This is particularly relevant if multiple members of the pharmacy team will assist in the data collection process. Standardization will reduce time on data cleaning later in the project. Features of certain computer programs may be able to assist with this standardization by only allowing data within the spreadsheet to be formatted in a specific way. Depending on the intervention and measures, data may need to be collected more or less frequently. One key point is to determine how soon change is expected to occur. For instance, in clinical outcome measures such as PDC, changes can be observed between one and three months. In-process measures such as Completion Rate for CMR, change can be observed within weeks. This will help you determine how often data collection will need to occur.

Finally, qualitative data may be useful in understanding certain aspects of care quality and should be considered in QI projects. Qualitative data can provide a deeper knowledge on how an intervention was adopted, provide insights about patients' experiences with care and identify future directions for the QI intervention being tested. Qualitative data can be collected via open-ended questions in surveys, interviews, and focus groups.

The goals of the QI project inform the sample size determinations. If the main goal of the project is to test the efficacy of an intervention to produce generalizable knowledge, sample size calculations will adhere to principles for hypothesis testing in research design. A good summary for sample size calculations can be found in the companion book *Principles of Research Design and Drug Literature Evaluation*.[26] When the main objective of the QI project is to evaluate improvement and variance over time, the sample size is determined by some practical considerations. Performance trends of a measure over time can be discerned with approximately 30 to 100 data points.[52] This range is suggested as general guidance. Similar to determinations of sample size in hypothesis testing, anticipated large intervention effects and low variation in processes might reduce the number of data points needed. Additionally, QI projects that require long periods to obtain data might be constrained in the number of data points available. The QI project team must ascertain and balance the burden of data collection and overall project costs against the study aims. For example, if it is determined that the data collection must be done manually for 700 patients by only one individual student or resident and must be completed within three months, it is not likely feasible to proceed with this data collection plan. In this example, you could consider reducing the sample size and/or engaging other members of the team to assist with data collection. In addition, if the impact of the project is expected to be small, time spent on data collection should not outweigh the potential benefits.

PDSA CYCLE STAGE: DO

In this stage, The QI team carries out all the activities planned for project implementation and data collection. It is also relevant to document any problems or issues revealed during this stage, such as whether the intervention was not implemented or executed as planned, the intervention did not yield the expected results or any issues or delays with data collection. These problems could be raised during staff meetings or unsolicited electronic or personal communication with members of the QI team. This feedback will become important in the Act stage of the PDSA cycle to decide if the intervention should be modified or discarded for the next cycle.

PDSA CYCLE STAGE: STUDY

In this stage, the QI team analyzes and interprets the data collected during the Do stage. Similar to the sample size determinations, data analysis techniques for QI projects focused on hypothesis testing about intervention efficacy and requiring the comparison of before-after or intervention versus control group data must apply statistical techniques (i.e., *t*-tests of two means). In QI specifically, there are additional graphical tools that provide a quick overview of data and changes. Several of these are discussed in the "Identifying the Problem" section previously, and other examples are provided in the toolkit at the end of this chapter. Instead of comparing aggregated data points such as the mean of an outcome before and after the intervention (two data points), QI Run Charts and Control Charts ascertain variation in data points over time.[53] For example, in a QI project aimed at increasing the number of patients scheduled for a CMR appointment, investigators can evaluate the number of weekly appointments for three months before and three after the intervention. This approach yields approximately 24 data points for 24 weeks. This contrasts to only two data points generated by comparing the mean number of appointments for the entire three-month period before and after intervention implementation.

Run charts are simple and practical graphics that allow the QI team to assess two types of variation of a measure over time.[53] The first one is the common cause variation, which is produced by random variation; that is variation normal to the process. The second variation type is called special cause (nonrandom) variation, which is produced by specific and identifiable causes such as a clinical intervention. To create a run chart, time intervals are depicted on the X-axis, a measure for each time point is plotted on the Y-axis, the points are connected through a line, and the median is calculated and displayed as a horizontal line (see Figure 13–5). The median can be calculated with the baseline data, so any changes due to the intervention will be more prominent on the chart. Additionally, it is common to annotate in the Run Chart the time interval for the start of a cycle or when the intervention was implemented.

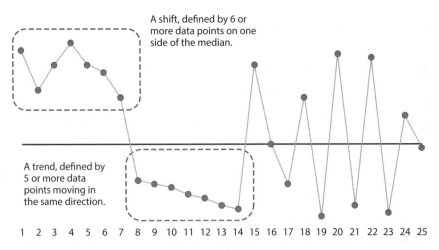

Figure 13–5. A sample run chart with a shift and a trend illustrated. (Reproduced, with permission, from Howell MD, Stevens JP. *Understanding Healthcare Delivery Science.* New York: McGraw Hill; 2020: Figure 14–6.)

Three probability-based rules are used to establish whether results displayed in a run chart indicate a change due to special cause (not-random) variation. First, "Shifts" of an outcome measure occur when there are six consecutive data points above or below the median, excluding any point located in the median. Second, "Trends" occur when all five consecutive points move upward or downward. If two consecutive points have the same value, only one is counted. Finally, "Runs" represents a series of sequential points on one side of the median (see Figure 13–5). To estimate the number of runs on a chart, the investigator can count the number of times the line connecting the points crosses the median and add one to this number. When only random variation is affecting the outcomes, there should be a regular pattern in the number of points above and below the median.[23]

Control charts are run charts to which upper and lower level limits are included.[54] They provide additional statistical information to detect the change and are better for monitoring variance. The lower and upper limits represent one, two, or three standard deviations (SD) (see Figure 13–6). Similar rules applied in run charts can be used to detect changes and suggest that special cause variation has occurred. First, when a data point falls beyond a control limit (typically three SDs); second, when two out of three consecutive points occur beyond two SDs; third, any four out of five consecutive points fall beyond one SD from the mean; and finally, when eight consecutive points fall above or below the average. If after the intervention implementation there is an expected change in measures, but there are no special causes variations observed in run charts or control charts, the QI team needs to investigate reasons (e.g., intervention not being implemented properly) and move on modifying the intervention or testing a different one.

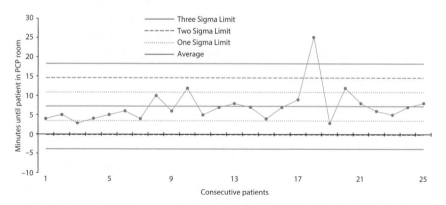

Figure 13–6. A control chart, plotting the number of minutes it takes to room each consecutive patient in an outpatient primary care office. (Reproduced, with permission, from Howell MD, Stevens JP. *Understanding Healthcare Delivery Science*. New York: McGraw Hill; 2020: Figure 14–7.)

PDSA CYCLE STAGE: ACT

In this stage, the QI team should review the data findings and the summary of unintended consequences or problems raised during the implementation. Using this data, the QI team must decide whether to Adopt, Adapt, or Abandon the intervention before moving into a new PDSA cycle.[29] The intervention can be *Adopted* if there is evidence of change after the first cycle and the findings are what the team expected. The team may choose to continue testing the same intervention to gather more data or to scale up the intervention to a bigger group, or implement it under different conditions, such as in a different unit or pharmacy. Alternatively, the intervention can be *Adapted* or modified before the next PDSA cycle. Ideas for adapting the intervention can be generated from a review and discussion of the issues and problems information collected in the Do stage. Finally, the intervention can be *Abandoned* if it is determined that it cannot be modified, and there is no foreseeable possibility that expected results can be obtained with further testing. In this case, the QI team may want to select another intervention and start a new PDSA cycle.

Case Example

■ IMPLEMENTING A PDSA CYCLE

Three advertisement interventions were tested in various areas of the hospital applying five PDSA cycles, each three weeks in length. Data included information generated Monday through Friday during pharmacy business hours. Baseline data of new prescriptions per new patient capture rate was determined to be 23%. A report documenting all prescriptions written at the hospital over the course of a month was obtained, and a chart was generated. The chart showed hospital department areas with the highest prescription generation, indicating opportunities for increasing pharmacy new prescription volume. The emergency department (ED) was determined as one of the main departments with 14% prescription generation.

New prescriptions per new patient data collection occurred on the Monday of each week. A report generated by the prescription processing system provided the number of new prescriptions. A new patient census was provided by the hospital. All data were collected in Excel, and a run chart was produced for each PDSA cycle to evaluate interventions impact on prescription volume over time. At the completion of interventions, a patient survey was administered to new patient-families who filled a prescription. The patient-family was able to select the word and image of the advertisement type that led pharmacy usage.

- *Cycle 1-Impact of Electronic Advertisement*: A one-slide advertisement displayed on patient facing televisions in the waiting rooms of the ED, Same Day Surgery (SDS), and specialty clinic areas. The advertisement contained a large photo of an outpatient pharmacist providing medication counseling along with a short detail of pharmacy services provided, hours and location. The pharmacy ad cycled with other hospital promotions and was visible six times per hour and stayed on the television screen for 30 seconds.

- *Cycle 2-Impact of Electronic Advertisement*: To further test the impact of pharmacy advertisement on patient facing televisions, the marketing team adapted the advertisement to include a free product enticement: "Receive a FREE product when filling a new prescription if you mention this ad (Limit 1 per patient)." The advertisement again included a picture of an outpatient pharmacist providing medication counseling along with pharmacy hours and location.

- *Cycle 3-Impact of Physical Advertisement*: The QI team designed and produced two types of physical advertisement: (1) A 2 foot by 3 foot–sign placed outside the pharmacy containing a picture of a child with large verbiage stating "Fill prescriptions here" along with pharmacy services and hours; and (2) smaller (8.5"×11") easel standing signs which were placed at all greeter/registration desks and near surgery provider-patient consultation rooms. The signs contained a picture of a child and pharmacists, along with pharmacy services, location, and hours. Additionally, a statement in Spanish was included.

- *Cycle 4-Impact of Electronic Advertisement (Inpatient Unit—GetWellNetwork)*: The GetWellNetwork is an interactive patient care system that delivers patient education and entertainment at the bedside right to their television. The GetWellNetwork is in the inpatient unit of the hospital. An application was created for the pharmacy, and once accessed, it provided a short description of pharmacy services (including Meds to Beds prescription delivery) and outlined hours and location.

- *Cycle 5-Verbal or Word-of-Mouth Advertisement (in the ED)*: ED registration representatives are one of the first individuals in contact with patient-families in the ED, making them an ideal vehicle for pharmacy verbal or word-of-mouth advertisement. Additionally, ED representatives document patient pharmacy preferences in the hospital electronic medical record. With ED registration leadership involvement, verbiage of ED registration representatives during pharmacy preference questioning of patient-families was changed from "What pharmacy do you use?" to "If you were to get a prescription today, would you like to get it filled with our pharmacy upstairs? Your medication(s) will be ready when you arrive or within a few minutes." Additionally, representatives were provided with details of pharmacy services and offerings in case additional questions were asked. The training was provided by email communication and side-by-side instruction.

Disseminating QI Findings

Once your project is completed or even while it is ongoing, it is important to be able to communicate your findings to a wider audience. This audience may be within or outside your organization, depending on the applicability of the project to other institutions. Within your organization, consider regular meetings for groups that may be interested in your project. This could include committees focused on quality of care; groups of physicians, nurses, or other healthcare professionals; meetings of organizational leadership; and so on. Thinking more broadly, consider presenting a poster or podium presentation at local or national conferences. Explore conferences hosted by local chapters of national pharmacy organizations like the ASHP, the PQA, or the American Pharmacists Association (APhA). Other professional organizations focused on quality include the International Society for Quality in Healthcare (ISQUA) and the ASQ. Many of these conferences, both locally and nationally, will have the opportunity to present posters and podium presentations. Remember, your QI team can assist you in preparing and delivering these presentations as well.

You should also consider publishing the findings of your QI project and QI research. Others would be interested in learning about your activities and lessons learned. There are journals specifically focused on QI to consider, such as *BMJ Quality Improvement Reports*, *BMJ Quality and Safety*, *American Journal of Medical Quality*, *Journal for Healthcare Quality*, and *Joint Commission Journal on Quality and Patient Safety*. You can also publish in journals specific to certain populations or practice settings. For example, if your project involved pediatric medication safety, consider journals focused on pediatrics. The SQUIRE (Standards for Quality Improvement Reporting Excellence) provides a framework for writing QI project reports and has been endorsed and co-published by many prominent journals.[55] Similar to other manuscript reporting guidelines, the SQUIRE guidelines give reporting recommendations for each general section of the manuscript, including the title and abstract, introduction, methods, and results. However, there are specific elements relevant to QI projects. In the introduction, investigators are prompted to clearly define the problem and to include a rationale section that justifies why the chosen intervention, model, or framework was expected to work, be sustainable, and replicable. In the methods section, investigators should provide a description of the contextual factors (e.g., local environment, organization's dynamics, and resources) that were essential for the success of the project and might have an impact on the generalizability of the intervention. The intervention should be described in sufficient detail to facilitate reproducibility. In the discussion section, investigators should address the intervention's sustainability and the potential for adoption in other contexts. Following the SQUIRE guidelines while writing the QI report may ensure all critical elements are specified and documented.

Case Example

■ COMMUNICATING FINDINGS

After the QI implementation, the new prescription capture rate per new patient increased by 10%. Prescription capture rate from the emergency department increased by 33%. Ninety-one percent of patient-families indicated verbal or word-of-mouth advertisement by hospital staff led to outpatient pharmacy use. The findings were first communicated to key internal stakeholders, including the ED director, to emphasize the importance of their staff letting patients know about the outpatient pharmacy. Additionally, the resident created a poster presentation for the annual meeting of the local pharmacists' association.

Summary and Conclusions

This chapter presented a stepwise approach to conduct a QI project to systematically and continuously change and improve healthcare delivery. QI projects and QI research have common elements, and both aim to improve patient care outcomes. Before starting an initiative, the QI team should define the scope of the project and establish whether it is considered QI research, and obtain appropriate regulatory approvals. There are multiple frameworks to use for QI projects, but they all share the same principles of systematic testing of ideas, reduction of variance, and use of data. Pharmacy students and professionals can contribute to the overall goals of their organization in achieving high quality of care by implementing a wide range of QI activities.

Key Points and Advice

- QI methodologies can be utilized in pharmacy research projects to provide high-quality pharmacy services.
- When undertaking QI projects:
  - Ensure a variety of perspectives in the QI team to increase support for the project.
  - Establish mechanisms for regular communication with stakeholders based on their interests and influence on the project.
  - Consult whether the QI project requires Human Subject Research approval with the local IRB office.

○ Develop project aims that are SMART (Specific, Measurable, Achievable, Relevant, and Time-bound) and make sure they align with the organization's mission and vision.

○ Select a QI methodology and framework that fits the QI team's training. Develop a plan for implementation, tasks, data collection, and analysis.

○ Aim to disseminate your findings internally and externally through presentations and publications.

Chapter Review Questions

1. Define quality in the context of the healthcare system.
2. What are the core principles of Quality Improvement?
3. What are three characteristics that differentiate a QI project from QI research?
4. What are the steps of the Model for Improvement to implement a QI project?

Online Resources

- American Society of Health-System Pharmacists (ASHP) Quality Improvement Resource Center. https://www.ashp.org/Pharmacy-Practice/Resource-Centers/Quality-Improvement
- American Society for Quality (ASQ). https://asq.org/quality-resources
- Instituted for Healthcare Improvement (IHI). http://www.ihi.org/resources/Pages/Tools/Quality-Improvement-Essentials-Toolkit.aspx
- Model for Improvement template. https://www.pocqi.org/wp-content/uploads/2017/08/Quality-improvement-project-template.pdf
- The NHS Quality, service improvement and redesign (QSIR) tools. https://www.england.nhs.uk/sustainableimprovement/qsir-programme/qsir-tools/

REFERENCES

1. IOM. *Crossing the Quality Chasm: A New Health System for the 21st century, Institute of Medicine*. National Academies Press; 2001.
2. Obama B. United States health care reform: progress to date and next steps. *JAMA*. 2016;316(5):525-532.
3. Tompkins CP, Higgins AR, Ritter GA. Measuring outcomes and efficiency in Medicare value-based purchasing: Medicare's value-based purchasing plan could be a transformational agent of change. *Health Aff.* 2009;28(Suppl 2):w251-w261.

4. Reid RO, Deb P, Howell BL, Shrank WH. Association between Medicare Advantage plan star ratings and enrollment. *JAMA*. 2013;309(3):267-274.

5. Batalden PB, Davidoff F. What is "quality improvement" and how can it transform healthcare? *Qual Saf Health Care*. 2007;16(1):2-3.

6. Picarillo AP. Introduction to quality improvement tools for the clinician. *J Perinatol*. 2018;38(7):929-935.

7. Roussel L. Differentiating quality improvement projects and quality improvement research. In: Harris JL, Roussel L, Thomas, PL, Catherine Dearman C, eds. *Project Planning and Management: A Guide for Nurses and Interprofessional Teams*. 2016:31-50.

8. Martin C, Phillips R, Johnson C. Improving provider awareness to statin prescribing guidelines: A quality improvement project. *J Vasc Nurs*. 2020;38(1):25-28.

9. Ma Y, Ockene IS, Rosal MC, Merriam PA, Ockene JK, Gandhi PJ. Randomized trial of a pharmacist-delivered intervention for improving lipid-lowering medication adherence among patients with coronary heart disease. *Cholesterol*. 2010;383281.

10. Farrell B, Clarkin C, Conklin J, et al. Community pharmacists as catalysts for deprescribing: an exploratory study using quality improvement processes. *Can Pharm J (Revue des Pharmaciens du Canada)*. 2020;153(1):37-45.

11. Horng M, Brunsman AC, Smoot T, Starosta K, Smith ZR. Using lean methodology to optimize time to antibiotic administration in patients with sepsis. *Bull Am Soc Hosp Pharm*. 2018;75(5_Supplement_1):S13-S23.

12. Nguyen LP, Nguyen L, Austin JP. A quality improvement initiative to decrease inappropriate intravenous acetaminophen use at an academic medical center. *Hosp Pharm*. 2020;55(4):253-260.

13. Gutiérrez Ubeda SR. An approach to identify "right" problems for initial quality improvement projects. *Global J Qual Saf Healthcare*. 2020;3(1):1-5.

14. Silver SA, Harel Z, McQuillan R, et al. How to begin a quality improvement project. *Clin J Am Soc Nephrol*. 2016;11(5):893-900.

15. Module 14. Creating Quality Improvement Teams and QI Plans. Accessed June 15, 2021. https://http://www.ahrq.gov/ncepcr/tools/pf-handbook/mod14.html

16. Randall S. *Using Communications Approaches to Spread Improvement: A Practical Guide to Help You Effectively Communicate and Spread Your Improvement Work*. Health Foundation; 2015.

17. Portela MC, Pronovost PJ, Woodcock T, Carter P, Dixon-Woods M. Republished: How to study improvement interventions: a brief overview of possible study types. *PMJ*. 2015;91(1076):343-354.

18. Mormer E, Stevans J. Clinical quality improvement and quality improvement research. *Perspect ASHA Spec Interest Groups*. 2019;4(1):27-37.

19. Deyo JC, Smith BH, Biola H, et al. Reducing high-risk medication use through pharmacist-led interventions in an outpatient setting. *JAPhA*. 2020;60(4):e86-e92.

20. Heavner MS, Rouse GE, Lemieux SM, et al. Experience with integrating pharmacist documenters on cardiac arrest teams to improve quality. *JAPhA*. 2018;58(3):311-317.

21. Chowdhury TP, Starr R, Brennan M, et al. A quality improvement initiative to improve medication management in an acute care for elders program through integration of a clinical pharmacist. *J Pharm Prac*. 2020;33(1):55-62.

22. Coleman M, Hodges A, Henn S, Lambert CC. Integrated pharmacy and PrEP navigation services to support PrEP uptake: a quality improvement project. *J Assoc Nurses AIDS Care*. 2020;31(6):685-692.

23. Penfold RB, Zhang F. Use of interrupted time series analysis in evaluating health care quality improvements. *Acad Pediatr*. 2013;13(6):S38-S44.

24. Maaskant JM, Tio MA, van Hest RM, Vermeulen H, Geukers VG. Medication audit and feedback by a clinical pharmacist decrease medication errors at the PICU: an interrupted time series analysis. *Health Sci Rep*. 2018;1(3):e23.

25. Rohan VS, Taber DJ, Patel N, et al. Impact of a multidisciplinary multimodal opioid minimization initiative in kidney transplant recipients. *Clin Transplant*. 2020;34(10):e14006.

26. Aparasu RR, Bentley JP. *Principles of Research Design and Drug Literature Evaluation*. Jones & Bartlett Publishers; 2014.

27. Austin Z, Sutton J. Qualitative research: Getting started. *Can J Hosp Pharm*. 2014;67(6):436.

28. Reynolds M, Jheeta S, Benn J, et al. Improving feedback on junior doctors' prescribing errors: mixed-methods evaluation of a quality improvement project. *BMJ Qual Saf*. 2017;26(3):240-247.

29. Langley GJ, Moen RD, Nolan KM, Nolan TW, Norman CL, Provost LP. *The Improvement Guide: A Practical Approach to Enhancing Organizational Performance*. John Wiley & Sons; 2009.

30. Taylor MJ, McNicholas C, Nicolay C, Darzi A, Bell D, Reed JE. Systematic review of the application of the plan–do–study–act method to improve quality in healthcare. *BMJ Qual Saf*. 2014;23(4):290-298.

31. Nicolay C, Purkayastha S, Greenhalgh A, et al. Systematic review of the application of quality improvement methodologies from the manufacturing industry to surgical healthcare. *Database of Abstracts of Reviews of Effects (DARE): Quality-assessed Reviews [Internet]*. 2012.

32. Liker JK. *Toyota Way: 14 Management Principles from the World's Greatest Manufacturer*. New York: McGraw Hill Education; 2004.

33. Hintzen BL, Knoer SJ, Van Dyke CJ, Milavitz BS. Effect of lean process improvement techniques on a university hospital inpatient pharmacy. *Am J Health Syst Pharm*. 2009;66(22):2042-2047.

34. DelliFraine JL, Langabeer JR, Nembhard IM. Assessing the evidence of Six Sigma and Lean in the health care industry. *Qual Manage Healthcare*. 2010;19(3):211-225.

35. Castle L, Franzblau-Isaac E, Paulsen J. Using Six Sigma to reduce medication errors in a home-delivery pharmacy service. *Joint Commission J Qual Patient Saf*. 2005;31(6):319-324.

36. The Joint Commission Accreditation and Certification-Pharmacy. Accessed June 15, 2021. https://www.jointcommission.org/accreditation-and-certification/health-care-settings/pharmacy

37. Gadkari AS, McHorney CA. Unintentional non-adherence to chronic prescription medications: how unintentional is it really? *BMC Health Services Res*. 2012;12(1):98.

38. Al-Bawardy R, Cheng-Lai A, Prlesi L, et al. Heart failure postdischarge clinic: a pharmacist-led approach to reduce readmissions. *Curr Probl Cardiol.* 2019 Oct;44(10):100407.

39. Cardosi L, Hohmeier KC, Fisher C, Wasson M. Patient satisfaction with a comprehensive medication review provided by a community pharmacist. *J Pharm Technol.* 2018;34(2):48-53.

40. Wallace ZS, Harkness T, Fu X, Stone JH, Choi HK, Walensky RP. Treatment delays associated with prior authorization for infusible medications: a cohort study. *Arthritis Care Res.* 2020;72(11):1543-1549.

41. Nanni AN, Rana TS, Schenkat DH. Screening for expired medications in automated dispensing cabinets. *Am J Health-System Pharm.* 2020;77(24):2107-2111.

42. Chisholm-Burns MA, Spivey CA, Gatwood J, Wiss A, Hohmeier K, Erickson SR. Evaluation of racial and socioeconomic disparities in medication pricing and pharmacy access and services. *Am J Health-System Pharm.* 2017;74(10):653-668.

43. Andersen B, Fagerhaug T. *Root Cause Analysis: Simplified Tools and Techniques.* Quality Press; 2006.

44. Harel Z, Silver SA, McQuillan RF, et al. How to diagnose solutions to a quality of care problem. *Clin J Am Soc Nephrol.* 2016;11(5):901-907.

45. Medicaid. Percentage of Long-Stay Nursing Home Residents who got an Antipsychotic Medication. 2019. Accessed June 15, 2021. https://www.medicaid.gov/state-overviews/scorecard/long-term-nursing-home-residents-antipsychotic-medication/index.html

46. Urick BY, Urmie JM. Framework for assessing pharmacy value. *Res Soc Admin Pharm.* 2019;15(11):1326-1337.

47. PQA. Pharmacy Quality Alliance. Accessed January 2012. http://www.pqaalliance.org/

48. NQF. National Quality Forum 2012. http://www.qualityforum.org/Home.aspx

49. Cafazzo JA, St-Cyr O. From discovery to design: the evolution of human factors in healthcare. *Healthcare Quart (Toronto, Ont.).* 2012;15(spec no):24-29.

50. Saad A, Der-Nigoghossian CA, Njeim R, Sakr R, Salameh P, Massoud M. Prescription errors with chemotherapy: quality improvement through standardized order templates. *APJCP.* 2016;17(4):2329-2336.

51. Cunningham TR, Geller ES, Clarke SW. Impact of electronic prescribing in a hospital setting: a process-focused evaluation. *Int J Med Inform.* 2008;77(8):546-554.

52. Perla RJ, Provost LP, Murray SK. Sampling considerations for health care improvement. *Qual Manage Healthcare.* 2014;23(4):268-279.

53. Perla RJ, Provost LP, Murray SK. The run chart: a simple analytical tool for learning from variation in healthcare processes. *BMJ Qual Saf.* 2011;20(1):46-51.

54. Koetsier A, van der Veer SN, Jager KJ, Peek N, de Keizer NF. Control charts in healthcare quality improvement. *Methods Inf Med.* 2012;51(03):189-198.

55. Ogrinc G, Mooney S, Estrada C, et al. The SQUIRE (Standards for QUality Improvement Reporting Excellence) guidelines for quality improvement reporting: explanation and elaboration. *BMJ Qual & Saf.* 2008;17(Suppl 1):i13-i32.

Chapter Fourteen

Secondary Data Research in Pharmacy Settings

Sujith Ramachandran, PhD and Kaustuv Bhattacharya, PhD

Chapter Objectives

- Define secondary data research in pharmacy
- Discuss various secondary data sources in pharmacy
- Identity common research questions in secondary data research
- Understand the practical and technical considerations for secondary data research
- Discuss the strategies for harnessing the expertise needed for conducting secondary data research
- Describe an example of learner-involved secondary data research
- Understand the dissemination framework for secondary data research

Key Terminology

Primary data research, secondary data research, electronic health records, provider surveys, administrative claims, automated systems, patient registries, cohort, case-control, cross-sectional design

Introduction

When presented with a research question, most investigators look to collect or gather their own data to best answer that question. However, sometimes the data required to answer a given research question may already exist—collected by another investigator or by an external entity. When such data are employed to answer a research question, it can be called secondary data research. Secondary data is merely pre-existing data that was collected by an entity for purposes other than to answer your research question. Primary and secondary data research are differentiated by the purpose of data collection and the research question. In primary data research, data are collected for the purpose of answering specific research questions. Therefore, the research purpose is perfectly aligned with the data collection. In secondary data research, data are not collected for the specific purpose of answering your research questions but can be used for the purpose of your research. Therefore, the data collection purpose is not perfectly aligned with the purpose of your research.

Examples of secondary data include national population surveys, provider surveys or encounter audits,[1] administrative claims,[2] electronic health records (EHRs),[3,4] pharmacy records, and patient registries.[5] Secondary data research has seen widespread use in pharmacy practice, with applications such as evaluation of characteristics of pharmacy use,[6–8] medication use,[9,10] and the economic and clinical outcomes associated with medication use.[11–13] In addition, secondary databases have also been used to study pharmacy-based vaccinations,[14,15] and the impact of policies on medication use and patient outcomes.[16,17] This chapter gives an overview of the various secondary data sources used in pharmacy practice, common research questions in secondary data research, and practical and technical considerations of secondary data sources. It also discusses expertise and resources for learner-involved secondary data research, examples of learner-involved secondary data research, and dissemination of secondary data research.

Secondary Data Sources in Pharmacy Practice

NATIONAL POPULATION SURVEYS

Population surveys are usually conducted by various government agencies to generate national-level estimates of population health. These surveys employ complex survey designs with population-based weighting so that the survey samples can be generalized to the entire population. The attractive feature of these databases is that most of them are available to researchers at low or no cost and include rich information not otherwise captured by other data sources. Examples of population surveys that are commonly used in secondary data research include the Medical Expenditure Panel Survey (MEPS), Behavioral Risk Factor Surveillance System (BRFSS), and National Health and Nutrition Examination Survey (NHANES).

The MEPS, conducted by the Agency for Healthcare Research and Quality (AHRQ), surveys the noninstitutionalized civilian population in the United States (U.S.).[18] It collects information on the respondents' health status, demographic and clinical characteristics, healthcare utilization and expenditures, and health insurance coverage.[19] Studies examining economic, behavioral, and humanistic aspects of healthcare are ideal for the use of MEPS data. The BRFSS is an annual, telephone-based survey conducted by the Centers for Disease Control and Prevention (CDC) and state health departments. It collects data from the noninstitutionalized U.S. population on risky behaviors, preventive health practices, and healthcare utilization and access related to chronic conditions, in addition to demographic, clinical, and economic characteristics.[20] Studies looking at health behaviors will benefit from using BRFSS data. The NHANES is a survey conducted in two-year cycles by the National Center for Health Statistics (NCHS), with the purpose of evaluating the health and nutritional status of the noninstitutionalized, civilian U.S. population. It collects physical examination, laboratory, and other clinical examination data, in addition to survey interview data, which enables researchers to combine self-reported health behavior and demographic data with clinical information to answer the research question of interest.[5]

PROVIDER SURVEYS

Provider surveys contain nationally representative data on provider visits across a wide spectrum of healthcare settings, including inpatient hospitalizations, physician office visits, and home healthcare agencies, among others. The main purpose of conducting these surveys is to generate national estimates of population health. Data usually collected in these surveys include information on general health, nutritional status, insurance status, sociodemographic information, healthcare utilization, and costs, among others. Common examples of such data sources used in research include the Healthcare Cost and Utilization Project (HCUP), National Ambulatory Medical Care Survey (NAMCS), and the National Hospital Ambulatory Medical Care Survey (NHAMCS).

The HCUP, sponsored by the AHRQ, and conducted with the help of Federal-State-Industry partnerships, contains inpatient, emergency department, and ambulatory surgery encounter data from U.S. hospitals and is useful for estimation population-level trends in hospitalization events.[21] The NAMCS and NHAMCS are annually conducted by the National Center for Health Statistics of the CDC and collect information on the healthcare providers, services used, and patient characteristics from physician office-based practices and hospital outpatient departments, respectively.[22] Compared to the population surveys that had the person or individual as the sampling unit, provider visit or inpatient hospitalization event are the sampling unit for provider surveys or encounter audit databases.

ADMINISTRATIVE CLAIMS

Administrative claims are one of the most common sources of secondary data. They are generated by every payer whenever an insurance billing claim is submitted. Most commonly collected information in administrative claims includes payment information, clinical diagnosis codes and procedure codes for the service rendered, and the date for the service rendered. Because claims data include all healthcare services paid for by an insurer, they allow for tracking the healthcare utilization and outcomes for a large number of individuals over a long time. They are often used for conducting outcomes research.

All health insurance payers, including Medicare and Medicaid, have their own administrative claims data, with some sources such as MarketScan aggregating claims across several private insurers.[23] Medicare is the largest payer in the United States, and Medicare claims data have widely been used for secondary data research. The Medicare claims data consists of claims information from various inpatient, outpatient, and other settings such as skilled nursing facilities, home healthcare, and hospice. Of particular interest to students is the availability of the Prescription Drug Event file, which contains information about drug utilization such as date of prescription fill, drug dispensed, quantity dispensed, days supplied, total cost, and out-of-pocket cost. Medicare and other administrative claims data are very useful for conducting studies focusing on economic and clinical aspects of healthcare, owing to the ability to be able to follow patients longitudinally over time—something that is not possible with most other secondary data sources.

ELECTRONIC HEALTH RECORDS

EHRs are clinical information repositories that collect patient healthcare information during healthcare delivery.[3,4] They contain patient demographic and clinical information, vital statistics, in addition to patient and caregiver reported information. They also contain information on medical diagnoses ascertained, procedures and services rendered, medications prescribed, along with provider information. Billing for healthcare service provided is the main purpose of EHRs, with research being a secondary use of the data.[24] An EHR system may comprise of data from a single healthcare center or linked networks such as integrated delivery networks or inter-hospital systems.[4]

EHR systems have seen widespread adoption in the past decade, largely due to the Health Information Technology for Economic and Clinical Health (HITECH) Act with providers incentivized to develop electronic data capturing and sharing capabilities under the Center for Medicare & Medicaid Services' meaningful use EHR initiative.[25] Epic, Cerner, and Meditech are some of the most commonly used EHR systems in the United States, with Epic being the commonly used EHR system in both inpatient[26] and outpatient[27] settings. Implementation of EHR systems such as Epic has led to better identification of poor compliance to clinical guidelines[28] and monitoring of outcomes associated with medical procedures.[29] Further, it has resulted in increased adherence to prescribing guidelines,[30] facilitation of genomic counseling,[31] and improvement in patient safety.[32]

EHR data have widespread use in studies focusing on medical service or drug utilization, incidence or prevalence of particular conditions, examination of the natural history of a disease, post-marketing safety surveillance,[4] and performance improvement.[33] Emerging use of EHRs in secondary data research includes active surveillance (Sentinel programs)[34] and comparative effectiveness research (e.g., Patient-Centered Outcomes Research Institute's PCORnet),[35] among others.

AUTOMATED SYSTEMS

Automated systems are software systems designed to ensure that medication management can be performed in a safe and effective manner and can be used at multiple stages of the medication use process.[36] The medication use process consists of six different stages—selection and procurement, storage, ordering and verification, preparation and dispensing, administration, and patient monitoring and assessment—involving a wide array of stakeholders, including manufacturers, patients, providers, pharmacists, and other healthcare professionals.[37] This interrelated network of medical use involves several handoffs among a variety of healthcare providers and can often lead to medication errors.[38] These errors can occur at various stages of the medication use process, ranging from more than 10% in the dispensing and verification to almost 40% in the administering and prescribing.[39]

Automated systems such as computerized prescriber order entry and clinical decision support systems are commonly used at the prescribing stage, whereas order management systems and pharmacy information management systems are used at the order verification stage. Further, automated systems such as workflow and inventory management systems, automated dispensing devices, among others, are commonly used at the preparation and dispensing stage, while electronic medication administration systems and bar code medication administration systems are used at the administration stage. Health information technology (IT) frameworks containing prescription fill and fill history information, in addition to patient clinical information such as diagnoses, laboratory tests, and allergies, allow for improved communication at various stages of the medication use workflow and help toward building a safe and effective medication management system. The most common automated medication management system in the United States is Pyxis (San Diego, CA) that offers support both in inpatient and outpatient settings across various stages of the medication use process. Some examples of research conducted using automated data are provided here.[40,41]

PATIENT REGISTRIES

Patient registries contain information for a specific disease, specifically collected to help improve the understanding of a given condition. The information available in patient registries include sociodemographic characteristics (race, gender, age or date of birth, education, and income), enrollee address information, preenrollment medical history (clinical conditions, onset/duration of the disease, treatment history, and genetic information).[42] Further, information is collected on genetic information, disease stage or severity, and other patient characteristics such as health insurance coverage. Certain patient registries also collect information on patient characteristics (health status, health literacy, health behaviors, well-being, marital status, and family history) and provider characteristics. Patient registries are commonly used in studies focusing on the natural history of the disease, clinical disease progression, effectiveness and safety of treatments, surveillance of rare events, heterogeneity of treatment effects, access to treatments, and real-world treatment patterns. Additionally, patient registries are often used in studies that employ historical controls in diseases where randomization may be unethical.[43] The most common examples of patient registries in the United States are the Surveillance, Epidemiology, and End Results (SEER) and the National Cancer Database (NCDB).

The SEER is a federally funded surveillance system developed by the collaboration of CDC, National Cancer Institute, and regional cancer registries.[44] It aggregates information from 18 states representing all regions of the United States. Local/regional cancer registries report information on all cancer cases within a specific region to SEER, making the SEER data population-based. The information available in the SEER registry includes patient sociodemographic characteristics, clinical information, including the history of cancer, cancer site, stage, pathological and treatment information, as well as information on death and cause of death.[45] The NCDB is a cancer-specific registry sponsored by the American Cancer Society and the American College of Surgeons; it collects data from hospital-based cancer cases from more than 1,500 hospitals accredited by the Commission on Cancer.[46] Similar to SEER, NCDB collects cancer-specific clinical information and overall survival data.[47-49] However, unlike SEER, NCDB is collected from hospitals only and cannot be considered population-based.[5,50] Depending on the information available in a specific patient registry, patient registry data can be used in studies focusing on trends in treatment or survival, disparities in health outcomes, and comparative effectiveness of various treatment modalities.[47,51,52] A summary of the various secondary data sources are provided in Table 14–1.

COMMON RESEARCH QUESTIONS IN SECONDARY DATA RESEARCH

Secondary data has been widely used to answer research questions related to the structure, process, and outcomes of pharmacy-based services as per the Donabedian model.[53]

TABLE 14–1. TYPES OF SECONDARY DATA SOURCES WITH EXAMPLES

Data Source	Examples	Sources
National Population Surveys	Medical Expenditure Panel Survey; Behavioral Risk Factor Surveillance System	https://www.meps.ahrq.gov, https://www.cdc.gov/brfss
Provider Surveys	Healthcare Cost and Utilization Project; National Ambulatory Medical Care Survey	https://www.hcup-us.ahrq.gov/, https://www.cdc.gov/nchs/ahcd
Administrative claims	Medicare; MarketScan	https://resdac.org/, https://www.ibm.com/products/marketscan-research-databases
Electronic health records	Epic; Allscripts	https://www.epic.com/, https://www.allscripts.com/
Automated systems	Pyxis; Cerner	https://www.bd.com/en-us/offerings/brands/pyxis, https://www.cerner.com/
Patient registries	Surveillance, Epidemiology, and End Results; National Cancer Database	https://seer.cancer.gov/, https://www.facs.org/quality-programs/cancer/ncdb

The research questions are based on the extent of data captured by the secondary data sources under three categories—structure, process, and outcomes to assess the quality of healthcare. While structural measures examine characteristics of health systems or provider organizations related to care delivery, process measures assess provider-patient interaction with regard to care performance. Outcome measures include assessment of the result of the care delivered and include all measures of patients' health status and well-being that are impacted by the care provided. Table 14–2 presents examples of common research questions for the Donabedian Model components.

Understanding the secondary data sources is critical in formulating research questions. Administrative claims data contain payment information, clinical diagnosis and procedure codes for care rendered, medication fill dates, and the date of inpatient or outpatient care provided. As they include information on all healthcare services paid for by the insurer, they are well suited for tracking healthcare utilization and outcomes for individuals over time. Given the type of data captured by administrative claims, they are ideally suited for understanding process measures such as medication dispensing, co-prescribing of medications, and others; and outcome measures such as healthcare utilization, medication adherence, safety and effectiveness, and others. The EHRs contain information on medical diagnosis, procedures performed, and medication prescribing, in addition to provider information, patient clinical and demographic characteristics, vital statistics, and other patient or caregiver reported information. Given the type of information available in EHR systems, they are very well suited for research aimed at the understanding process (medication prescribing) and outcomes (clinical outcomes) of care.

TABLE 14–2. EXAMPLES OF COMMON RESEARCH QUESTIONS UNDER THE COMPONENTS OF THE DONABEDIAN MODEL

Donabedian Model Component	Research Question	Data Source	Literature Examples
Structure	Impact of pharmacy and provider characteristics	EHR	Sessoms et al., 2015[54]
		Administrative claims	Gani et al., 2015;[55] Schwab et al., 2019[56]
	Impact of state and Federal policies	Administrative claims	Munshi et al., 2018;[57] Tak et al., 2019[17]
		EHR	Karter et al., 2018[16]
Process	Rates of medication use, co-prescribing, and concomitant use	Administrative claims	Jeffery et al., 2019;[58] Paulsen et al., 2020;[59] Han et al., 2020[60]
		EHR	Nimbal et al., 2016;[61] Saxon et al., 2019[62]
	Rate of treatment initiation	Administrative claims	Bonafede et al., 2018;[63] Lind et al., 2019[64]
Outcome	Factors associated with medication adherence and its impact on the clinical and economic burden	EHR	Hood et al., 2018[11]
		Administrative claims	Lynch et al., 2009;[65] Ivanova et al., 2012[66]
		EHR linked with administrative claims	Ma et al., 2020;[67] Romanelli et al., 2014[68]

Steps in Secondary Data Research

The scientific research process involves the following steps: (1) pose a research question and hypothesis, (2) develop and implement a research plan, (3) perform data collection and analysis, and (4) prepare a research report.[69] The first step in any research study is to pose a research question that is feasible and makes a significant contribution to existing literature.[70] The next step is to formulate a hypothesis based on the literature and the latest understanding of scientific evidence. For secondary data research, considerations of feasibility need to take into account the availability of appropriate data sources that allow for capturing all the variables and the nuances necessary for answering the research question in the population of interest. Similarly, the formulation of a research plan requires understanding the principles of secondary data research design. More information about commonly used designs in secondary data research is provided in the following section. Once a research plan is formulated, the secondary data of interest must be acquired, with careful consideration for ethical and legal principles of data use, and the actual project must be carried out, followed by preparing a research report. Finally, it is important to remember that the formulation of the research question must always precede the choice of the research plan, including whether or not the proposed project is best addressed using primary or secondary data research. After a robust research question is posed, the investigator must consider all available options, evaluate their feasibility, strengths, and weaknesses before choosing to pursue any one approach. The practical and technical considerations of secondary data research that allow investigators to make such decisions are provided below.

Practical and Technical Considerations of Secondary Data Sources

ADVANTAGES AND DISADVANTAGES OF SECONDARY DATA RESEARCH

One of the major advantages of using secondary data is the sample size. Secondary databases generally offer much larger sample sizes as compared to other methods of research,[71] and therefore have greater power and are able to detect smaller differences in effect. They are also an attractive option for research questions involving rare events.[72] Another advantage of secondary data research is methodologic ease. Studies with multiple control groups can be easily conducted without having to embark upon prospective data collection, and study design changes can be easily incorporated.[73] The cost of conducting secondary data research is often much lower than other types of research, especially when compared to randomized control trials. Additionally, secondary data research using real-world data is often much more generalizable than other types of research.[71,74]

However, there are certain limitations of secondary data research that need to be considered. Most secondary databases do not contain all clinical information required for research purposes since these data sources are often not developed for the purpose of research. For example, administrative claims data do not contain information on disease severity or laboratory test values.[75,76] Billing coding issues can also bias study findings.[77] Most secondary data sources contain information only for a particular group of individuals (e.g., older adults or those who are enrolled in Medicaid), and results from studies using these data sources cannot be generalized to other populations.[78] Additionally, population surveys and provider surveys are limited by the cross-sectional nature of the data and the inability to follow individuals over time.[19] Moreover, they can lead to additional technical challenges due to the complex sample design. For example, studies using the MEPS data may lead to higher variance in study estimates due to its multistage sampling design.[79] EHRs also suffer from various limitations due to inconsistencies in documentation, incomplete data capture, and lack of standardization between different EHR systems.[4]

STRUCTURE OF DATA AND DATA COLLECTION METHODS

The data structure and collection methodology of a database vary based on the type of secondary data. Administrative claims data are collected from insurance billing systems, which are developed for the purpose of documenting billing and payment for healthcare services provided. EHRs were designed to collect data at the time of healthcare delivery for efficient delivery of care. Population and provider surveys, and encounter audits, on the other hand, are designed for the purpose of evaluating several health factors at the population level, whereas patient registries collect data from several local/regional registries for effective surveillance of disease incidence prevalence and survival. The structure of a database is closely tied to its data collection methodology. Databases that are intended to be made publicly available for the purpose of research, such as population and provider surveys, are generally easier to analyze as they are set up in a manner that allows for easier data management and analysis. Other databases such as EHRs, administrative claims, and other datasets that include longitudinal follow-up may include multiple research files and need extensive data management prior to analysis. When multiple data files are present within a given secondary database, they are usually connected to each other through a common linking variable. Such datasets are termed as relational databases.

The concept of relational databases is particularly useful in secondary data research, with many of the healthcare information systems relying on this infrastructure to eliminate data redundancy. In a relational database framework, a linking variable can be used to aggregate data from multiple sources containing different information. For example, Figure 14–1 outlines the relational database structure for Medicare. As we can see in this example, the unique linking variable (BENE_ID) can be used to combine data from different Medicare files pertaining to demographic and Medicare enrollment information (Master Beneficiary Summary File), inpatient admissions (MedPAR), physician office-based visits (Carrier/NCH file), and prescription drug event (Part D file).

The scope of secondary data also varies depending on the data source used. The scope of EHR data or administrative claims data is limited to the network from which these data are gathered. For example, Medicare data is limited to most individuals who are 65 years of age or older, with a few exceptions for additional eligibility.[78] Population surveys are generalizable to non-institutionalized population, and provider surveys, such as NAMCS, are generalizable at the event level (all physician office-based visits, in this

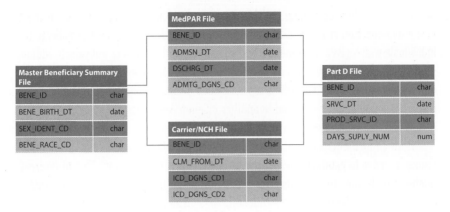

Figure 14–1. Example of a relational database framework for Medicare data.

case). To ensure that the surveys are generalizable on such large scales, these data are collected with careful survey methodology, and each response is assigned a sample weight. MEPS, for example, employs a probability-weighted complex survey design with multistage sampling using three weight variables—primary sampling unit, strata, and person weight.[80]

STUDY DESIGN

Before conducting any secondary data research, investigators should prepare a robust study design carefully designed to best answer their research question and/or test their a priori hypotheses. The study design for a given secondary data project depends on several considerations and must be rooted in principles of epidemiology.[81–83] Most learner-involved secondary data research utilizes cohort, case-control, and cross-sectional designs.

The first group of designs, called cohort studies, are the most commonly used method for the investigation of epidemiological questions.[81] A cohort is defined as "a group of people who have something in common when they are first assembled"[82] and are then followed along to identify or capture other characteristics. Given adequate follow-up and adequate information about potential confounders, cohort designs are really powerful tools for answering research questions. In fact, the often-cited upper tier of the evidence hierarchy,[84] the randomized clinical trial, is a cohort study that includes a random component to decide which cohort gets the treatment of interest.[81,82] Some examples of cohort studies can be found elsewhere.[15,85]

A useful contrast to the cohort design is the case-control study.[81] The classical case-control studies usually begin by first selecting individuals with and without the outcome of interest and then examining individual history to identify the presence or absence of the hypothesized risk factor. In this context, the word "case" is used to indicate the individuals with a given outcome of interest, and "controls" refers to individuals without the outcome.[82] Some examples of case-control studies can be found elsewhere,[86,87] and more information about the various types of study designs applicable to secondary data research can be found here[88] and in another chapter. A summary of some examples of cohort and case-control studies can be found in Table 14–3.

Both cohort and case-control studies involve collecting data across various time points in order to estimate the temporal relationships between variables of interest. Such study designs may be described as being longitudinal in nature. In contrast, a **cross-sectional design** involves collecting data on all variables of interest at a single point in time.[81] Cross-sectional studies are a snapshot of a population at any given time and are intended to describe the characteristics of a population or correlations between observed characteristics at the same time. Cross-sectional studies require fewer resources and time than longitudinal studies and are ideal for capturing characteristics such as disease prevalence. Cross-sectional studies that use secondary data either involve data collected at a single time point or those collected with no temporal information to construct a cohort or a case-control design. Popular examples of cross-sectional studies using secondary data may utilize several years of data from

TABLE 14–3. EXAMPLES OF SECONDARY DATA RESEARCH USING COHORT AND CASE-CONTROL STUDY DESIGN

Study	Design	Data Sources	Research Objective	Key Findings
Gatwood et al., 2020[15]	Cohort	Insurance claims linked with publicly available data	Examine the potential influence of social determinants of health on rates of pneumococcal vaccination in older American adults	Social determinants of health such as health literacy, poverty, internet access, and political affiliations were correlated with pneumococcal vaccine hesitancy.
Ganz et al., 2014[86]	Case control	Electronic health records from the Geisinger Health System	Identify the association of body mass index (BMI) and risk of type 2 diabetes	A positive association was found between BMI and risk of diabetes, with increasing BMI correlated with incrementally greater risk.
Ray et al., 2019[9]	Cross-sectional	2015 National Ambulatory Medical Care Survey	Estimate the prevalence of antibiotic use without documented indication in the outpatient setting	An estimated 18% of ambulatory care visits in 2015 (corresponding to 24 million visits) involved an antibiotic prescription without documented indication.

cross-sectional surveys such as the NAMCS or MEPS but are still considered cross-sectional because they do not include any follow-up information on the eligible population. Some examples of cross-sectional designs are available elsewhere,[89] and more information about such studies is provided elsewhere.[81]

OPERATIONALIZATION

Once the study has been designed, it is important to consider how the key study variables will be operationalized within the framework of the available data. While operationalizing variables can always be tricky, doing so when using data from secondary sources—which may not contain all the data points exactly as needed—is particularly challenging. Because of this reason, secondary data researchers should rely on literature to ensure that their operationalization of a given construct is valid and test their assumptions carefully with sensitivity analyses in order to minimize potential misclassification bias.[90] Previous research has shown that some methods of identifying chronic conditions such as diabetes in administrative claims data have better accuracy than other approaches.[90] For example, constructs such as exposure to drugs may be operationalized as the presence of medication fills in pharmacy records or as the presence of a medication administration record in the inpatient records. Other constructs such as the occurrence of a clinical event such as a diagnosis of a condition may be identified using diagnosis codes present on administrative claims or electronic medical records. Further variations in operationalizing drug exposure or disease exposure may involve identifying repeated records for medications or conditions in order to confirm the presence of these variables.

GENERALIZABILITY

Among other key considerations in conducting secondary data research is the eligible population for the study. It is important to understand what populations are captured by the selected data source and how any inclusion or exclusion criteria might affect the composition of the study population. Identifying these criteria will allow researchers to make inferences about the generalizability of study findings. For example, data about patients with diabetes from a nationally representative survey such as MEPS may provide results widely generalizable to all patients with diabetes, but the same data collected from a given hospital medical records may only be applicable to that hospital and not even to the community living in that neighborhood. Understanding and recognizing these differences helps not only with interpreting results but also with selecting a data source and a study design that can best answer the research question.

UNAVAILABLE INFORMATION

Secondary data researchers need to be keenly aware of not just what information is captured in their data source of choice but also what information is not available. This nuance of recognizing unavailable information can make a critical difference in carrying out a robust study. Lack of information can affect a study in several ways. First, a given data source may not capture variables that may be important covariates or confounders of the effect of interest. For example, data sources like EHRs do not capture potential follow-up visits occurring outside of the hospital system, and administrative claims data do not capture constructs such as disease severity, which may confound the effect of interest. Second, the presence of missing data in secondary data sources can cause significant bias, especially when the reason for the missingness is not completely random. Researchers must carefully account for missing data in their study analytic plan to make sure their findings are robust.[91,92]

DATA LICENSING AND INSTITUTIONAL APPROVALS

Perhaps the most nuanced resource consideration for secondary data research is with respect to data security, privacy, and approvals. Some secondary data sources such as population and provider surveys are publicly available and do not contain any sensitive or identifiable information. For such data, few approvals are necessary for research as the use of these datasets for research is usually considered exempt by an institutional review board. However, other data, such as administrative claims and medical records, include sensitive information such as identifiable patient data such as names, dates of birth, and other health information. Sharing and use of such information, called protected health information (PHI), is covered by the Health Insurance Portability and Accountability Act of 2009.[93,94] When PHI data are being used, it is important to ensure that all research procedures—including where the data are stored, how they are accessed, used, and disposed of after the research—are approved by an institutional review board. Some data sources, such as administrative claims or patient registry data, may also require the investigator to establish new data use agreements with the data providing entity in order to ensure that adequate security policies are in place. Such data use agreements, when applicable, must be closely followed in order to protect patient privacy.[95]

Expertise and Resources for Learner-Involved Secondary Data Research

There is wide variability in the degree of expertise and resources needed for learner-involved secondary data research. While not all of these skills and resources may be directly taught during the course of a typical PharmD curriculum, they can be gathered by seeking the right mentors and building a collaborative team that can make the research practically feasible. When relying on the expertise and resources of the team, it is important that the investigator engage the team early in the process to get the most out of their collaborators and to ensure the best probability of a successful project.

EXPERTISE NEEDED FOR LEARNER-INVOLVED SECONDARY DATA RESEARCH

Information Technology Expertise

Depending on the data source chosen, students may need some expertise in IT in order to extract, store, and convert the data into research-analyzable files. When publicly available data sources are used, the IT expertise required may be minimal as the data provider generally makes user guides available to assist with IT needs. But in the case of electronic medical records or medical charts, students may need to work with a faculty member, or the health system's IT department to query the EHR interface or search through available electronic datasets to narrow the records to be examined. If a unique secondary data source is used, such as data from scraping social media posts or aggregating other content, IT experts can assist in the automation of the data gathering process and save time.

Statistical Software Expertise

Depending on the data source chosen for the project, the use of specialized statistical software may be needed for the successful completion of a secondary research project. Commonly available resources such as Microsoft Excel may be adequate in some instances but is nevertheless not recommended because it is not tuned specifically for the purpose of research and may lead to errors in data management and analysis. More specialized software offerings such as SPSS, SAS, STATA, or R may be the more useful choice. However, all of this software needs additional training and expertise before a student pharmacist can successfully use them for the project. While expertise in this software may be available through their research team, there is also an abundance of online learning materials that can help with learning this expertise. For example, publicly available data sources such as MEPS provide guidance for how to import and analyze their data in a variety of statistical packages.[96] For software such as SAS and STATA, freely available online courses are put together by either the software developer themselves or by other users.[97-100] The open-source software, R, has several online user forums specifically for learning and applying the software for research projects.[101]

Research Team

There is no resource more important to completing a successful research project for a student pharmacist than putting together the right research team. Selecting the right mentor and ensuring that the team provides all the needed expertise can make a significant difference in the project's success. While there are no strict guidelines on the number of people needed for a successful project, there are few core areas of expertise that must be provided by the team. These areas are: (1) clinical expertise, (2) study design expertise, (3) statistical expertise. Every student pharmacist research project should include an appropriate clinician mentor to ensure that the research questions are meaningful, significant, and have the potential to make an impact in the scientific or clinical communities. Expertise in study design or training in epidemiology can help with the selection of an appropriate study design and avoiding bias. While most student pharmacists should at least develop a familiarity with the fundamentals of biostatistics, including null hypothesis statistical testing, for the purpose of interpreting and critically evaluating literature, it is strongly recommended that statistician consultation is sought for any secondary research projects. Depending on the nature of the research question driving the project, the statistical analysis may involve simple descriptive analysis, bivariate tests of significance, multivariable adjustment, or perhaps even more complex statistical procedures. Relying on a statistician's expertise to approve the analytic plan is critical prior to the start of the project. Further assistance to conduct the analyses or interpret the results may also be useful on an as-needed basis.

Resources Needed for Learner-Involved Secondary Research Projects

In addition to gathering expertise from collaborators, several specialized resources may be required for successfully executing secondary data research projects. The first resource is a computer or server that can house the data being used to conduct the research. There are several important considerations in the selection of a computer for secondary research. They are: (1) data storage space, (2) processing power capability, (3) compatibility of research software, and (4) data security and privacy concerns. Considerations of data storage space may be the simplest to assess and can be evaluated by comparing available data storage space with the estimated size of the research dataset. Assessing the required processing power for a given dataset may be more complicated and may require reaching out to IT experts. Most statistical software companies provide assistance with processing power on a computer. While this may seem like an intimidating challenge, the growing availability of faster and cheaper processors today allows for processing very large datasets on most personal computers today. The processing power is also related to what software is actually being used to conduct the statistical analysis. It is important to ensure that the latest versions of the statistical software are compatible with the computer being used. The choice of statistical software (such as Excel, SPSS, SAS, STATA, or R) and clinical tools (such as Micromedex, Lexicomp, AHFS Drug Information, and others) used for the project is a critical decision that must be made prior to starting research procedures. The decision for selecting a software should depend not only on compatibility with the computer platform but also cost, the capability of conducting the required analysis, and the ability of the investigator to correctly use the software.

Dissemination of Secondary Data Research

Several avenues exist for the dissemination of peer-reviewed, learner-involved, secondary data research. These avenues allow students to publish in journals that are either focused on a specialized audience of clinicians, policymakers or more generalized audiences that have wider readerships. When attempting to publish in peer-reviewed outlets, students should follow commonly used reporting frameworks as a guideline for their reports. The most popular reporting frameworks for reporting findings from observational studies include the REporting of studies Conducted using Observational Routinely-collected health Data (RECORD) Statement for Pharmacoepidemiology (RECORD-PE)[102] and the Strengthening the Reporting of OBservational studies in Epidemiology (STROBE)[103] statement. Both frameworks are available in the form of checklists[104,105] online and encourage reporting of findings in a way that is transparent, clear, and allows for replication of study findings. While a thorough description of these reporting guidelines is beyond the scope of this chapter, both frameworks encourage transparent reporting of study design, setting, participants, data sources, data access, cleaning, linkage, and statistical methods. These frameworks are unique to the reporting of observational research studies, and RECORD-PE is specifically aimed at capturing the complexity of pharmacoepidemiologic research. More information about dissemination for learner-involved research is covered in another chapter.

Exemplars of Learner-Involved Secondary Data Research

This section will review two examples from student-led published research that uses secondary research. The goal of this review will be to gain an appreciation for the secondary data research and to identify key lessons about how a student pharmacist can put together a successful secondary data research project.

The first example is a research project that aimed to identify the correlation between the use of high-risk medications and hospitalization outcomes among older adults.[106] This research question was driven by previous literature that demonstrated that the use of these high-risk medications might result in avoidable hospitalizations.[107,108] Based on this evidence, the researchers hypothesized that the use of high-risk medications was associated with a higher risk of hospitalizations. The research employed a cohort design with administrative claims data from a 5% sample of Medicare beneficiaries from 2014 to 2016.[106] These data include all paid claims for healthcare services and medication fills received by older adults enrolled in Medicare. The data were licensed for use by the Centers for Medicare & Medicaid Services (CMS), and the project was approved by the institutional review board. In order to facilitate data security and management of the large dataset, all data were housed on high-performance, secure servers, and the research team was allowed to remotely access the data for the project. The rate of high-risk medication use was defined as per an established quality measure from the Pharmacy Quality Alliance (PQA). Patient characteristics, including the presence of comorbidities and occurrence of hospitalization, were identified using the medical claims. Data management and analysis were conducted using SAS version 9.4 (Cary, NC). Broadly, the study found that the rate of use of high-risk medications was 6.7%, 5.6%, and 4.7% in 2014, 2015, and 2016, respectively. Rates of use were higher for Black individuals and those enrolled in the Medicare low-income subsidy program, and individuals using high-risk medications had a higher risk of hospitalizations compared to those who did not use high-risk medications. Results were presented at a national conference as a poster session.

The second example involves a study that aimed to compare the rates of cefepime monotherapy failure between patients with and without obesity.[109] This research was driven by the knowledge that dosing of antibiotics such as cefepime depends on the pharmacokinetic characteristics of the patient, which are closely related to obesity. Patients with obesity often require greater doses in order to achieve successful treatment with cefepime, so the researchers hypothesized that obese patients would have greater rates of cefepime monotherapy failure compared to patients who were not obese. The study was conducted using EHRs from a large hospital system. These data include all hospital records on diagnoses, procedures, and treatment provided to patients receiving care from the hospital system. Since the researchers were affiliated with the hospital system that collects and aggregates these data, no additional data licensing was necessary. However, all study procedures were approved by an institutional review board. A cohort design was utilized to identify hospitalized patients who were administered cefepime monotherapy, and individuals were followed to identify clinical treatment failure, hospital length of stay, and mortality, among other outcomes. Individual demographics were also obtained from medical charts to identify BMI and classify patients as being obese or not. All data analyses were conducted using IBM SPSS version 24.0 (Chicago, IL). The researchers found that patients with obesity were more likely to experience treatment failure, but not greater length of stay, readmissions, or mortality. The findings were published in the Journal of Pharmacy Technology.

Summary and Conclusions

Secondary data is defined as pre-existing data that was collected by an entity for purposes other than to answer your research question. Examples of secondary data include national population surveys, provider surveys or encounter audits, administrative claims, EHRs, and patient registries. Each secondary data source has a unique structure, different strengths, and weaknesses and must be selected with careful consideration of research objectives and other considerations, as described above. Secondary data research can be an efficient way to maximize sample size for research projects at a low cost while still obtaining generalizable estimates of evidence. Successful student-led secondary data research requires putting together the right research team and resources in IT and statistical software. There are several broad avenues for the pursuit of learner-involved research in pharmacy. Student pharmacists must work to identify a mentor for their research experiences and work to find a research question of significance early in their time in pharmacy school. Upon identification of a research question, investigators must evaluate if an existing secondary data source can be used to efficiently answer their question and put together the right combination of expertise and resources needed to complete the project and disseminate findings. Ultimately, successful completion of any research project will involve a demonstration of leadership, persistence, and a curiosity to learn outside the classroom.

Key Points and Advice

- Secondary data research involves the use of previously existing data collected for purposes other than the investigator's research.
- A variety of secondary data sources—each with its own strengths and weaknesses—are available to investigators. Examples include national population surveys, provider surveys or encounter audits, administrative claims, EHRs, and patient registries.
- Successful secondary data research requires a variety of expertise in clinical knowledge, study design and statistical analysis, and IT.
- Investigators should ensure that required data use authorizations are obtained and data privacy and safety is safeguarded prior to embarking on secondary data research projects.

Chapter Review Questions

1. Define secondary data and list some examples of commonly used secondary data sources.
2. Compare and contrast the strengths and weaknesses of any three different secondary data sources.
3. Identify a research question from your area of expertise and identify a secondary data source that would be best suited to answer that question.
4. Imagine you are conducting a research study evaluating the impact of treatment adherence to bisphosphonate medications on the risk of future fractures among older women with osteoporosis. What are the advantages and disadvantages of conducting this study using data from administrative claims versus patient registries?
5. Take the example of the research question provided in the previous question. What are the advantages and disadvantages of conducting this study by collecting your own data versus using preexisting data? What aspects of the research question are important in making a choice between primary data research and secondary data research?

Online Resources

- Agency for Healthcare Research and Quality. Medical Expenditure Panel Survey Data Overview. Accessed January 1, 2021. https://www.meps.ahrq.gov/mepsweb/data_stats/data_overview.jsp
- Agency for Healthcare Research and Quality. HCUP Overview. Healthcare Cost and Utilization Project (HCUP). Accessed January 10, 2021. https://www.hcup-us.ahrq.gov/overview.jsp
- National Center for Health Statistics. NAMCS/NHAMCS—Ambulatory Health Care Data. Published January 4, 2021. Accessed January 10, 2021. https://www.cdc.gov/nchs/ahcd/index.htm
- IBM MarketScan. MarketScan Research Databases—Overview. Published December 16, 2020. Accessed January 10, 2021. https://www.ibm.com/products/marketscan-research-databases
- National Cancer Institute. Surveillance, Epidemiology, and End Results Program. SEER. Accessed January 11, 2021. https://seer.cancer.gov/index.html

- *HHS-AHRQ/MEPS*. Agency for Healthcare Research and Quality (AHRQ); 2021. Accessed January 24, 2021. https://github.com/HHS-AHRQ/MEPS
- Stata. Learn. Accessed January 24, 2021. https://www.stata.com/learn/
- SAS Bootcamp Week 1—YouTube. Accessed January 24, 2021. https://www.youtube.com/playlist?list=PLyiJ8xo-a2jO27wBPaF2ELIm69JaPePux
- IDRE Stats—Statistical Consulting Web Resources. Accessed January 24, 2021. https://stats.idre.ucla.edu/
- Free SAS e-Learning for Academics. Accessed January 24, 2021. https://www.sas.com/en_us/learn/academic-programs/resources/free-sas-e-learning.html
- RStudio. Open source & professional software for data science teams. Accessed January 24, 2021. https://rstudio.com/

REFERENCES

1. CDC. National Center for Health Statistics. NCHS. Published December 23, 2020. Accessed December 28, 2020. https://www.cdc.gov/nchs/index.htm
2. CMS. Medicare. Accessed December 28, 2020. https://www.cms.gov/Medicare/Medicare
3. Häyrinen K, Saranto K, Nykänen P. Definition, structure, content, use and impacts of electronic health records: a review of the research literature. *Int J Med Inf*. 2008;77(5):291-304.
4. Cowie MR, Blomster JI, Curtis LH, et al. Electronic health records to facilitate clinical research. *Clin Res Cardiol*. 2017;106(1):1-9.
5. Cole AP, Friedlander DF, Trinh Q-D. Secondary data sources for health services research in urologic oncology. *Urol Oncol: Seminars and Original Investigations*. 2018;36(4):165-173.
6. Look KA. Patient characteristics associated with multiple pharmacy use in the U.S. population: findings from the Medical Expenditure Panel Survey. *Res Soc Admin Pharm*. 2015;11(4):507-516.
7. Wu J, Davis–Ajami ML, Noxon V. Patterns of use and expenses associated with mail-service pharmacy in adults with diabetes. *JAPhA*. 2015;55(1):41-51.
8. Wang J, Thomas J, Byrd D, Nola K, Liu J. Status of diabetes care among community pharmacy patients with diabetes: Analysis of the Medical Expenditure Panel Survey. *JAPhA*. 2010;50(4):478-484.
9. Devraj R, Deshpande M. Demographic and health-related predictors of proton pump inhibitor (PPI) use and association with chronic kidney disease (CKD) stage in NHANES population. *Res Soc Admin Pharm*. 2020;16(6):776-782.
10. Kantor ED, Rehm CD, Haas JS, Chan AT, Giovannucci EL. Trends in prescription drug use among adults in the United States from 1999-2012. *JAMA*. 2015;314(17):1818-1830.
11. Hood SR, Giazzon AJ, Seamon G, et al. Association between medication adherence and the outcomes of heart failure. *Pharmacotherapy: J Human Pharmacol Drug Ther*. 2018;38(5):539-545.

12. Watanabe JH, Ney JP. Association of increased emergency rooms costs for patients without access to necessary medications. *Res Soc Admin Pharm.* 2015;11(4):499-506.

13. Gellad WF, Donohue JM, Zhao X, Zhang Y, Banthin JS. The financial burden from prescription drugs has declined recently for the nonelderly, although it is still high for many. *Health Aff.* 2012;31(2):408-416.

14. Inguva S, Barnard M, Ward LM, et al. Factors influencing human papillomavirus (HPV) vaccination series completion in Mississippi Medicaid. *Vaccine.* 2020;38(8):2051-2057.

15. Gatwood J, Shuvo S, Hohmeier KC, et al. Pneumococcal vaccination in older adults: an initial analysis of social determinants of health and vaccine uptake. *Vaccine.* 2020;38(35):5607-5617.

16. Karter AJ, Parker MM, Solomon MD, et al. Effect of out-of-pocket cost on medication initiation, adherence, and persistence among patients with type 2 diabetes: The Diabetes Study of Northern California (DISTANCE). *Health Serv Res.* 2018;53(2):1227-1247.

17. Tak CR, Gunning K, Kim J, et al. The effect of a prescription order requirement for pharmacist-administered vaccination on herpes zoster vaccination rates. *Vaccine.* 2019;37(4):631-636.

18. Agency for Healthcare Research and Quality. Medical Expenditure Panel Survey Data Overview. Accessed January 1, 2021. https://www.meps.ahrq.gov/mepsweb/data_stats/data_overview.jsp

19. Armbrecht E, Shah A, Schepman P, et al. Economic and humanistic burden associated with noncommunicable diseases among adults with depression and anxiety in the United States. *J Med Econ.* 2020;23(9):1032-1042.

20. Bhattacharya K, Joshi N, Shah R, Nahar VK. Impact of depression on health-related quality of life among skin cancer survivors. *SKIN: J Cutaneous Med.* 2019;3(6):381-394.

21. Agency for Healthcare Research and Quality. HCUP Overview. Healthcare Cost and Utilization Project (HCUP). Accessed January 10, 2021. https://www.hcup-us.ahrq.gov/overview.jsp

22. National Center for Health Statistics. NAMCS/NHAMCS—Ambulatory Health Care Data. Published January 4, 2021. Accessed January 10, 2021. https://www.cdc.gov/nchs/ahcd/index.htm

23. IBM MarketScan. MarketScan Research Databases—Overview. Published December 16, 2020. Accessed January 10, 2021. https://www.ibm.com/products/marketscan-research-databases

24. Kim E, Rubinstein SM, Nead KT, Wojcieszynski AP, Gabriel PE, Warner JL. The evolving use of electronic health records (EHR) for research. *Semin Radiation Oncol.* 2019;29(4):354-361.

25. U.S. Department of Health and Human Services Centers for Medicare & Medicaid Services 42 CFR Parts 412, 413, 422 et al. Medicare and Medicaid Programs; Electronic Health Record Incentive Program; Final Rule. Published July 28, 2010. Accessed May 2, 2021. https://www.govinfo.gov/content/pkg/FR-2010-07-28/pdf/2010-17207.pdf

26. Health Leaders. In EMR Market Share Wars, Epic and Cerner Triumph Yet Again. Published April 30, 2019. Accessed May 2, 2021. https://www.healthleadersmedia.com/innovation/emr-market-share-wars-epic-and-cerner-triumph-yet-again

27. Definitive Healthcare. Top 10 Ambulatory EHR Vendors by 2019 Market Share. Published December 11, 2017. Accessed April 23, 2021. https://blog.definitivehc.com/top-ambulatory-ehr-systems

28. Grigoryan L, Zoorob R, Wang H, Trautner BW. Low concordance with guidelines for treatment of acute cystitis in primary care. *Open Forum Infect Dis.* 2015;2(4):159.

29. DeBoer EM, Prager JD, Kerby GS, Stillwell PC. Measuring pediatric bronchoscopy outcomes using an electronic medical record. *Ann Am Thorac Soc.* 2016; 13(5):678-683.

30. Adelson KB, Qiu YC, Evangelista M, et al. Implementation of electronic chemotherapy ordering: an opportunity to improve evidence-based oncology care. *J Oncol Prac.* 2016;10(2):e113-e119.

31. Sonstein L, Clark C, Seidensticker S, Zeng L, Sharma G. Improving adherence for management of acute exacerbation of chronic obstructive pulmonary disease. *Am J Med.* 2014;127(11):1097-1104.

32. Kullar R, Goff DA, Schulz LT, Fox BC, Rose WE. The "epic" challenge of optimizing antimicrobial stewardship: the role of electronic medical records and technology. *Clin Infect Dis.* 2013;57(7):1005-1013.

33. Peterson ED, Shah BR, Parsons L, et al. Trends in quality of care for patients with acute myocardial infarction in the National Registry of Myocardial Infarction from 1990 to 2006. *Am Heart J.* 2008;156(6):1045-1055.

34. Ball R, Robb M, Anderson SA, Pan GD. The FDA's sentinel initiative—A comprehensive approach to medical product surveillance. *Clin Pharmacol Ther.* 2016;99(3):265-268.

35. Fleurence RL, Curtis LH, Califf RM, Platt R, Selby JV, Brown JS. Launching PCORnet, a national patient-centered clinical research network. *J Am Med Inform Assoc.* 2014;21(4):578-582.

36. California HealthCare Foundation. Addressing Medication Errors in Hospitals: A Framework for Developing a Plan. Published July 2001. Accessed April 21, 2001. https://www.chcf.org/wp-content/uploads/2017/12/PDF-addressingmederrorsframework.pdf

37. Zgarrick DP, Alston GL, Moczygemba LR, Desselle SP. *Pharmacy Management: Essentials for All Practice Settings.* New York, NY: McGraw-Hill Education; 2016.

38. Institute of Medicine Committee on Quality of Health Care in America. *To Err Is Human: Building a Safer Health System.* Washington, DC: National Academies Press; 2000.

39. Bates DW, Cullen DJ, Laird N, et al. Incidence of adverse drug events and potential adverse drug events: implications for prevention. *JAMA.* 1995;274(1):29-34.

40. Pavlin JA, Murdock P, Elbert E, et al. Conducting population behavioral health surveillance by using automated diagnostic and pharmacy data systems. *MMWR.* 2004:166-172.

41. Fishman PA, Shay DK. Development and estimation of a pediatric chronic disease score using automated pharmacy data. *Med Care.* 1999:874-883.

42. Gliklich R, Dreyer N, Leavy M, eds. Registries for Evaluating Patient Outcomes: A User's Guide. Third edition. Two volumes. (Prepared by the Outcome DEcIDE Center [Outcome Sciences, Inc., a Quintiles company] under Contract No. 290 2005 00351 TO 7.) AHRQ Publication No. 13(14)-EHC111. Rockville, MD: Agency for Healthcare Research and Quality. Published April 2014. Accessed April 21, 2021. https://effectivehealthcare.ahrq. gov/sites/default/files/related_files/registries-guide-3rd-edition-vol-2-140430.pdf

43. Ghadessi M, Tang R, Zhou J, et al. A roadmap to using historical controls in clinical trials–by Drug Information Association Adaptive Design Scientific Working Group (DIA-ADSWG). *Orphanet J Rare Dis.* 2020;15(1):1-19.

44. National Cancer Institute. Surveillance, Epidemiology, and End Results Program. SEER. Accessed January 11, 2021. https://seer.cancer.gov/index.html

45. Doll KM, Rademaker A, Sosa JA. Practical guide to surgical data sets: Surveillance, Epidemiology, and End Results (SEER) database. *JAMA Surgery.* 2018;153(6):588-589.

46. American College of Surgeons. National Cancer Database. Accessed January 11, 2021. https://www.facs.org/quality-programs/cancer/ncdb

47. Seisen T, Sun M, Leow JJ, et al. Efficacy of high-intensity local treatment for metastatic urothelial carcinoma of the bladder: a propensity score–weighted analysis from the National Cancer Data Base. *J Clin Oncol.* 2016;34(29):3529-3536.

48. Seisen T, Sun M, Lipsitz SR, et al. Comparative effectiveness of trimodal therapy versus radical cystectomy for localized muscle-invasive urothelial carcinoma of the bladder. *European urology.* 2017;72(4):483-487.

49. Seisen T, Krasnow RE, Bellmunt J, et al. Effectiveness of adjuvant chemotherapy after radical nephroureterectomy for locally advanced and/or positive regional lymph node upper tract urothelial carcinoma. *J Clin Oncol.* 2017;35(8):852-860.

50. Janz TA, Graboyes EM, Nguyen SA, et al. A comparison of the NCDB and SEER database for research involving head and neck cancer. *Otolaryngol Head Neck Surg.* 2019;160(2):284-294.

51. Cole AP, Dalela D, Hanske J, et al. Temporal trends in receipt of adequate lymphadenectomy in bladder cancer 1988 to 2010. *Urol Oncol: Seminars and Original Investigations.* 2015;33(12):504.e9-504.e17.

52. Hanna N, Sun M, Meyer CP, et al. Survival analyses of patients with metastatic renal cancer treated with targeted therapy with or without cytoreductive nephrectomy: a National Cancer Data Base study. *J Clin Oncol.* 2016;34(27):3267.

53. Donabedian A. Evaluating the quality of medical care. *The Milbank Memorial Fund Quarterly.* 1966;44(3):166-206.

54. Sessoms J, Reid K, Williams I, Hinton I. Provider adherence to national guidelines for managing hypertension in African Americans. *Int J hypertens.* 2015.

55. Gani F, Lucas DJ, Kim Y, Schneider EB, Pawlik TM. Understanding variation in 30-day surgical readmission in the era of accountable care: effect of the patient, surgeon, and surgical subspecialties. *JAMA Surgery.* 2015;150(11):1042-1049.

56. Schwab P, Racsa P, Rascati K, Mourer M, Meah Y, Worley K. A retrospective database study comparing diabetes-related medication adherence and health outcomes for mail-order versus community pharmacy. *J Manag Care Spec Pharm.* 2019;25(3):332-340.

57. Munshi KD, Mager D, Ward KM, Mischel B, Henderson, RR. The effect of Florida Medicaid's state-mandated formulary provision on prescription drug use and health plan costs in a Medicaid managed care plan. *J Manag Care Spec Pharm.* 2018;24(2):124-131.

58. Jeffery MM, Hooten WM, Jena AB, Ross JS, Shah ND, Karaca-Mandic P. Rates of physician coprescribing of opioids and benzodiazepines after the release of the Centers for Disease Control and Prevention Guidelines in 2016. *JAMA Network Open.* 2019;2(8):e198 325-e198325.

59. Paulsen R, Modestino AS, Hasan MM, Noor-E-Alam M, Young LD, Young GJ. Patterns of buprenorphine/naloxone prescribing: an analysis of claims data from Massachusetts. *Am J Drug Alcohol Abuse.* 2020;46(2):216-223.

60. Han Y, Balkrishnan R, Hirth RA, Hutton DW, He K, Steffick DE, Saran R. Assessment of prescription analgesic use in older adults with and without chronic kidney disease and outcomes. *JAMA Network Open.* 2020;3(9):e2016839-e2016839.

61. Nimbal V, Segal JB, Romanelli RJ. Estimating generic drug use with electronic health records data from a health care delivery system: implications for quality improvement and research. *J Manag Care Spec Pharm.* 2016;22(10):1143-1147.

62. Saxon DR, Iwamoto SJ, Mettenbrink CJ, et al. Antiobesity medication use in 2.2 million adults across eight large health care organizations: 2009-2015. *Obesity.* 2019;27(12):1975-1981.

63. Bonafede M, Johnson BH, Shah N, Harrison DJ, Tang D, Stolshek BS. Disease-modifying antirheumatic drug initiation among patients newly diagnosed with rheumatoid arthritis. *Am J Manag Care.* 2018;24(8):SP279-SP285.

64. Lind BK, McCarty D, Gu Y, Baker R, McConnell KJ. Predictors of substance use treatment initiation and engagement among adult and adolescent Medicaid recipients. *Subst Abuse.* 2019;40(3):285-291.

65. Lynch WD, Markosyan K, Melkonian AK, Pesa J, Kleinman NL. Effect of antihypertensive medication adherence among employees with hypertension. *Am J Manag Care.* 2009;15(12):871-880.

66. Ivanova JI, Bergman RE, Birnbaum HG, Phillips AL, Stewart M, Meletiche, DM. Impact of medication adherence to disease-modifying drugs on severe relapse, and direct and indirect costs among employees with multiple sclerosis in the US. *J Med Econ.* 2012;15(3):601-609.

67. Ma X, Jung C, Chang HY, Richards TM, Kharrazi H. Assessing the population-level correlation of medication regimen complexity and adherence indices using electronic health records and insurance Claims. *J Manag Care & Spec Pharm.* 2020;26(7):860-871.

68. Romanelli RJ, Segal JB. Predictors of statin compliance after switching from branded to generic agents among managed-care beneficiaries. *J Gen Intern Med.* 2014;29(10):1372-1378.

69. Aparasu RR, Satabdi C. The scientific approach to research and practice. In: Aparasu RR, Bentley JP, eds. *Principles of Research Design and Drug Literature Evaluation*. 2nd ed. McGraw Hill; 2020. https://accesspharmacy.mhmedical.com/content.aspx?bookid=2733&sectionid=226710549

70. Hulley SB. Conceiving the research question. In: Hulley SB, Browner WS, Grady D, Hearst N, Newman TB, eds. *Designing Clinical Research*. 2nd ed. Baltimore: Williams & Wilkins; 2001:17–24.

71. Gandhi S, Salmon JW, Kong SX, Zhao SZ. Administrative databases and outcomes assessment: an overview of issues and potential utility. *J Manag Care Pharm*. 1999;5(3):215-222.

72. Motheral BR, Fairman KA. The use of claims databases for outcomes research: rationale, challenges, and strategies. *Clin Ther*. 1997;19(2):346-366.

73. Harpe SE. Using secondary data sources for pharmacoepidemiology and outcomes research. *Pharmacotherapy: J Human Pharmacol Drug Ther*. 2009;29(2):138-153.

74. Suissa S, Garbe E. Primer: administrative health databases in observational studies of drug effects—advantages and disadvantages. *Nat Clin Prac Rheumatol*. 2007;3(12):725-732.

75. Spitzer WO, Suissa S, Ernst P, et al. The use of β-agonists and the risk of death and near death from asthma. *N Engl J Med*. 1992;326(8):501-506.

76. Suissa S, Blais L, Ernst P. Patterns of increasing beta-agonist use and the risk of fatal or near-fatal asthma. *Eur Respir J*. 1994;7(9):1602-1609.

77. Peabody JW, Luck J, Jain S, Bertenthal D, Glassman P. Assessing the accuracy of administrative data in health information systems. *Med Care*. 2004:1066-1072. Published online.

78. Strom BL, Carson JL. Use of automated databases for pharmacoepidemiology research. *Epidemiol Rev*. 1990;12(1):87-107.

79. Chowdhury S, Machlin S, Gwet K. Sample designs of the medical expenditure panel survey household component, 1996-2006 and 2007-2016. Published online 2019. https://meps.ahrq.gov/data_files/publications/mr33/mr33.shtml#15meps

80. Machlin S, Yu W, Zodet M. *Computing Standard Errors for MEPS Estimates*. Rockville, MD: Agency for Healthcare Research and Quality. Retrieved January 2005;28:2006.

81. Rothman KJ. *Epidemiology: An Introduction*. 2nd ed. Oxford University Press; 2012.

82. Fletcher R, Fletcher SW, Fletcher GS. *Clinical Epidemiology: The Essentials*. 5th ed. Lippincott Williams & Wilkins; 2013.

83. Lash TL, VanderWeele TJ, Haneuse S, President KJRV. *Modern Epidemiology*. 4th ed. LWW; 2021.

84. NHMRC. Guidelines for the Development and Implementation of Clinical Guidelines. Published online 1995.

85. Koller D, Hua T, Bynum JP. Treatment patterns with antidementia drugs in the United States: medicare cohort study. *JAGS*. 2016;64(8):1540–1548.

86. Ganz ML, Wintfeld N, Li Q, Alas V, Langer J, Hammer M. The association of body mass index with the risk of type 2 diabetes: a case–control study nested in an electronic health records system in the United States. *Diabetol Metab Syndr*. 2014;6(1):1-8.

87. Mapel DW, Hurley JS, Frost FJ, Petersen HV, Picchi MA, Coultas DB. Health care utilization in chronic obstructive pulmonary disease: a case-control study in a health maintenance organization. *Arch Intern Med.* 2000;160(17):2653-2658.

88. Pearce N. Classification of epidemiological study designs. *Int J Epidemiol.* 2012;41(2):393–397.

89. Ray MJ, Tallman GB, Bearden DT, Elman MR, McGregor JC. Antibiotic prescribing without documented indication in ambulatory care clinics: national cross sectional study. *BMJ.* 2019;367:l6461.

90. Funk MJ, Landi SN. Misclassification in administrative claims data: quantifying the impact on treatment effect estimates. *Curr Epidemiol Rep.* 2014;1(4):175-185.

91. Graham JW, Cumsille PE, Shevock AE. Methods for handling missing data. In: Schinka JA, Velicer WF, Weiner IB, eds. *Handbook of Psychology.* 2nd ed. John Wiley & Sons; 2012;109-141.

92. Norris CM, Ghali WA, Knudtson ML, Naylor CD, Saunders LD. Dealing with missing data in observational health care outcome analyses. *J Clin Epidemiol.* 2000;53(4):377-383.

93. Perakslis ED. Cybersecurity in health care. *N Engl J Med.* 2014;371(5):395-397.

94. Kruse CS, Smith B, Vanderlinden H, Nealand A. Security techniques for the electronic health records. *J Med Sys.* 2017;41(8):127.

95. ResDAC. Federal Regulations Governing the Release of CMS Data. Accessed January 17, 2021. https://www.resdac.org/articles/federal-regulations-governing-release-cms-data

96. *HHS-AHRQ/MEPS.* Agency for Healthcare Research and Quality (AHRQ); 2021. Accessed January 24, 2021. https://github.com/HHS-AHRQ/MEPS

97. Stata. Learn. Accessed January 24, 2021. https://www.stata.com/learn/

98. SAS Bootcamp Week 1 - YouTube. Accessed January 24, 2021. https://www.youtube.com/playlist?list=PLyiJ8xo-a2jO27wBPaF2ELIm69JaPePux

99. IDRE Stats – Statistical Consulting Web Resources. Accessed January 24, 2021. https://stats.idre.ucla.edu/

100. Free SAS e-Learning for Academics. Accessed January 24, 2021. https://www.sas.com/en_us/learn/academic-programs/resources/free-sas-e-learning.html

101. RStudio. Open Source & Professional Software for Data Science Teams. Accessed January 24, 2021. https://rstudio.com/

102. Benchimol EI, Smeeth L, Guttmann A, et al. The REporting of studies Conducted using Observational Routinely-collected health Data (RECORD) Statement. *PLoS Med.* 2015;12(10):e1001885.

103. von Elm E, Altman DG, Egger M, et al. The Strengthening the Reporting of Observational Studies in Epidemiology (STROBE) statement: guidelines for reporting observational studies. *Epidemiology.* 2007;18(6):800-804. [published Online First: 2007/12/01].

104. Reporting of studies conducted using observational routinely-collected data. RECORD-PE Checklist. Published 2019. Accessed May 2, 2021. http://www.record-statement.org/checklist-pe.php

105. STROBE statement. STROBE checklists. Published November 2007. Accessed May 2, 2021. Available at https://www.strobe-statement.org/index.php?id=available-checklists.

106. Wittman M, Ramachandran S. PQA2020 abstracts of contributed papers. *JAPhA*. 2020;60:e241-e248.

107. Fick DM, Cooper JW, Wade WE, Waller JL, Maclean JR, Beers MH. Updating the Beers criteria for potentially inappropriate medication use in older adults: results of a US consensus panel of experts. *Arch Intern Med*. 2003;163(22):2716-2724.

108. Fick D. Potentially inappropriate medication use in a Medicare managed care population: association with higher costs and utilization. *J Manag Care Pharm*. 2001;7(5):07-413.

109. Morrison AR, Loper JT, Barber KE, Stover KR, Wagner JL. Effect of obesity on clinical outcomes of patients treated with cefepime. *J Pharm Technol*. 2020:8755122520967398. Published online.

Chapter Fifteen

Qualitative Research in Pharmacy Settings

Kimberly M. Kelly, PhD, MS and Trupti Dhumal, MS

Chapter Objectives

- Define qualitative research in pharmacy settings
- Discuss the goals and importance of qualitative research in pharmacy settings and healthcare
- Understand the methodology of qualitative research and its scope
- Identify common research questions addressed with qualitative research in pharmacy settings
- Understand the practical and technical considerations for conducting qualitative research in pharmacy settings
- Describe various sources of qualitative data that can be used for research in pharmacy settings
- Discuss the strategies for harnessing the expertise needed for conducting qualitative research in pharmacy settings
- Describe examples of learner-involved qualitative research project in a pharmacy setting
- Understand the dissemination framework for qualitative research in pharmacy settings

Key Terminology

Action research, constructivism, constant comparison, content analysis, epistemologies, ethnography, faithful reporting, framework analysis, grounded theory, immersion/crystallization, interpretivism, inter-rater reliability, key informants, member checks, methodological triangulation, mixed methods, narrative analysis, nominalism, ontology, objectivism, positivism, purposive sampling, qualitative theories, realism, reflexive notes, subjectivism, saturation (theoretical saturation, data saturation), thematic analysis, theoretical sampling, transferability, unit of analysis

Introduction

Depending on your experience, many things may come to mind when someone says, "qualitative analysis." To the inexperienced, it may bring to mind anything that is not done at the bench, something that happens when you talk to people or do surveys or something that is loose and unscientific. To the experienced, it brings to mind a rigorous, effortful process that is distinct yet interactive with quantitative analysis. There is no single definition for qualitative research, but it can be viewed as an iterative process focused on gathering rich but interpretive data.[1] It allows researchers to understand the inner experience of participants and enables us to describe complex phenomena and processes in greater depth, which may be challenging due to the small number of people affected.[2] It is important to note at this point that the use of the term "Qualitative Research" is controversial among some scholars in the field. The preferred term among these individuals is "Qualitative Inquiry." No distinction is made in the current chapter, and the terms are used interchangeably.

The goal of this chapter is to provide an overview of qualitative analysis in the context of pharmacy. The chapter on qualitative research in the companion book[3] was designed to provide support in the review of qualitative research publications, while the current chapter is a primer to assist pharmacists and new investigators in conducting qualitative analysis in the pharmacy context. In this chapter, we touch on critical elements to consider in designing and conducting qualitative inquiry and also provide examples of learner-involved qualitative analysis to serve as a building block for future efforts. As we are unable to go into depth on some approaches, we offer additional resources to explore more detailed information.

Qualitative and Quantitative Research: Similarities and Differences

An important distinction for qualitative analysis may be its difference from quantitative analysis. Table 15–1 helps to contrast qualitative from quantitative analysis. At its simplest, qualitative is descriptive. Rather than looking at the number of people that feel or think a certain way, we are trying to sample the range of ideas and experiences. For example, with qualitative analysis, we can understand an individual's story about why they are not adherent with their blood pressure medication. Whether or not a person spontaneously mentions a particular response to your question does not indicate whether s/he might hold that belief; thus, frequencies of mention of something is not the purview of

TABLE 15–1. COMPARISON BETWEEN QUANTITATIVE AND QUALITATIVE RESEARCH APPROACHES

	Quantitative	Qualitative
Purpose	Represented by numbers; examine relationships among variables	Represented by words; explore people's experiences, underlying perceptions, and opinions
Questions	Analytical; confirms/test assumptions or hypotheses	Exploratory; generates in-depth insights concepts, thoughts, or perspectives
Sampling	Usually random sampling or cluster sampling	Usually purposive or theoretical sampling
Data source	Instruments/measurements, secondary datasets, interviews, and surveys (closed-ended questions)	Interviews and surveys (open-ended questions), documents, and observations
Analysis	Statistical methods to analyze causation or correlation	Thematic analysis for patterns, relationships, and contextual meaning
Results	Trends and statistical significance with a goal of generalizability	Codes and themes that reflect the researcher's understanding of a group

qualitative research. However, to position qualitative as the opposite of quantitative analysis is not exactly true. The two are integral to one another and have a complex interplay in our search for knowledge. Qualitative can be formative, serving as a building block to quantitative analysis. For example, we conduct focus groups to identify barriers to smoking cessation, which we can later measure in a quantitative survey. It may also be concurrent or explicative to help interpret quantitative analyses. This complex way of learning, integrating both qualitative and quantitative analysis to explore a phenomenon, is termed mixed methods.

Qualitative methods aim to answer questions, which are beyond the realm of quantitative research. The main goal is to let the results emerge from the participants. This is accomplished by gathering more subjective and less quantifiable data by assessing opinions, perceptions, attitudes, and beliefs. The variety of methods and rich data offer a window into the mindset of participants. Most importantly, it aims to explain phenomena and the reason behind their occurrence.

Qualitative Research in Healthcare

Qualitative inquiry consists of an array of techniques adapted from philosophy, anthropology, sociology, and other social sciences.[4] The extension of qualitative methods to healthcare has been gradual, being widely applied in nursing, health services, pharmacy practice, medicine, and health policy (see Table 15–2 for examples). These methods go

TABLE 15–2. EXAMPLES OF PUBLISHED QUALITATIVE RESEARCH IN HEALTHCARE

Discipline	Author	Study Objective	Data Collection Method	Qualitative Approach Employed	Application
Nursing	Olsen et al.[5]	To generate a theory by assessing processes and strategies of oncology nurses aiming to support young patients with cancer and their partners through a nursing program	Telephone interviews	Thematic analysis	Patient care
	Jennings et al.[6]	To elucidate the impact of patient turnover as a source of workload through ethnography	Participant observation, in-person interviews, document analysis, and fieldnotes	Ethnography	Workflow and care management
Health services	Bradby et al.[7]	To explore attitudes and experiences of underrepresented South Asian service-users of the Child and Adolescent Mental Health Services (CAMHS)	Focus groups and in-person interview	Thematic analysis	Mental illness
	McAlearney et al.[8]	To explore issues associated with leadership development in healthcare	In-person interviews	Grounded theory	Quality of life
Pharmacy practice	Benson et al.[9]	To describe and explore patient perceptions regarding antihypertensive drugs	In-person interviews	Thematic and relational analysis	Medication taking behavior
	Shiyanbola et al.[10]	To explore African Americans' perceptions of type 2 diabetes	Focus groups	Phenomenology and content analysis	Illness perceptions
Medicine	Chou et al.[11]	To collect women's views on the impact of operative delivery in the second stage of labor	Clinical interactions	Discourse analysis	Patient knowledge
	Florian et al.[12]	To assess the perceived and actual presence of community assets to aid diabetes control	Photovoice session	Community-based participatory research and thematic analysis	Diabetes management
Health policy	Lasseter et al.[13]	To understand public preferences regarding childhood vaccination and help inform future policy related decisions	In-person interviews	Thematic analysis	Public preferences
	Ono et al.[14]	To generate evidence regarding functions of healthcare extension for providing quality improvement support to primary care practices	In-person interviews and document analysis	Immersion crystallization	Program evaluation

beyond numbers, seeking an in-depth evaluation of phenomena outside the scope of quantitative research. It aims to capture an individual's perception regarding health and enables healthcare professionals to understand their feelings and experiences. It allows an improved recognition of treatment effectiveness, quality of care, and patient satisfaction. Qualitative inquiry often focuses on understanding health beliefs and health behaviors. In pharmacy practice, qualitative methods may identify issues with current practices and assess patient's reflections on pharmacy visits and their encounter with pharmacists.[15,16] Qualitative methods are also widely applicable to understand pharmacist-patient communication. For example, a qualitative study was performed to understand care-taking behaviors that foster a good pharmacist–patient relationship.[17] "Knowing the patient" is key to fostering the pharmacist-patient relationship through identifying unmet needs, explaining medications, and assisting with patient navigation. With the recognition of patient-centered care, ensuring the incorporation of patient preferences and values in treatment is critical.

Qualitative Methodologies for Pharmacy Practice-Based Research

To help set the stage for qualitative methods, we must reflect on our own biases in approaching a topic. People have different beliefs about ontology, the nature of reality (e.g., the extent that the world around is real and knowable). In realism, reality exists independently of how any one person perceives it, but in nominalism, the reality is subjective and dependent on the individual.

People also may consider different epistemologies or "ways of knowing." From the standpoint of objectivism, we can observe the truth and meaning within an object. In constructivism, the truth is constructed by interactions with an object, whereas the truth is imposed on the object by a person in subjectivism. In other words, if we are talking about adverse drug reactions, objectivism says that we can directly assess symptoms, but other epistemologies would say that symptoms are highly dependent on the person experiencing them.

Finally, people may use different qualitative theories (methodologies), which at its most basic is the relationship among things or how things work. Science is dominated by positivism, that we can assess and measure reality through our interactions with the external world (e.g., weight on a scale). However, other theories are important in qualitative research, such as interpretivism, which says that reality is highly dependent on the person experiencing the world, and thus to understand these different realities, we must understand the different ways of experiencing the world. For example, a person participating in a Phase II study of chemotherapy for liver cancer may indicate that nausea is minor, but for a healthy volunteer in a Phase II study for a shingles vaccine, nausea may be very problematic. Ontologies, epistemologies, and theories serve as the framework for qualitative inquiry, the ways we collect information about reality. Many methods of qualitative inquiry are available,[18,19] but in this section, we focus on five commonly used in the health sciences. Often, successful qualitative researchers may use the techniques of more than one approach.

ETHNOGRAPHY

Ethnography is a qualitative approach commonly associated with anthropology. The most distinctive feature of ethnography is its immersive quality. In other words, an ethnographer typically goes to an area for an extended time period (perhaps years) and tries to live and interact with a group to understand them. Ethnography relies on multiple sources (e.g., documents, interviews, observations, objects). They also talk to key informants, individuals who have a holistic understanding of the group (e.g., social worker, pastor), and may refer back to these individuals from time to time for additional information or clarification. Ethnographers keep reflexive notes, similar to a chemist's log, but these also include the feelings of ethnographers and thoughts about how their own background may be influencing their experience. Ultimately, when the researcher has an understanding of the group, they write an ethnography, which includes a synthesis of the many resources they collected. An example of this approach can be found in an ethnography of women with human immunodeficiency virus (HIV) or AIDS.[20] Similar to ethnography, immersion/crystallization recognizes the challenges of traditional qualitative analysis in clinical care.[21] In immersion/crystallization, the researcher immerses himself/herself in the data but then takes time away to crystalize or reflect on the data gathered. A recent study utilized immersion/crystallization to explore lay understandings of pertussis and vaccination.[22]

GROUNDED THEORY

Grounded theory gets its name from its goal: to generate a theory that is grounded in data.[2] The methodology is rooted in sociology, and its goal is to identify all the elements that make up a theory to explain why something happens. Data are collected, analyzed, and then new data are collected based on the existing data and what the needs are (this is called theoretical sampling). As data are collected, codes are assigned to discrete units of data (e.g., sentences). Axial coding is conducted that involves identifying relationships or linkages between codes and themes developed through open coding.[23] Data analysis is complete when theoretical saturation is reached, i.e., no new information is collected to further refine the model. For example, a study assessing patient satisfaction in substance use disorder rehabilitation treatment utilized axial coding to understand the relationships between codes emerging from the interview text.[24] These inductive codes were assessed to understand their context and how they relate to patient satisfaction.

CONTENT ANALYSIS

Content analysis is a method utilized to examine data and patterns by exploring visual, written, or verbal information quantitatively or qualitatively. The qualitative content analysis goes beyond quantification, wherein researchers focus on the contextual meaning of a text or subjective interpretation by identifying codes and themes. The quantitative content analysis counts the presence or occurrence of a phenomenon. Overall, the aim is to condense the data into structured categories either by developing a framework using themes identified from your data (an inductive process) or by using an existing theory or coding scheme to interpret the data (a deductive process).[25] The information is bracketed as a code or theme and labeled within a category. Then occurrences of words or terms may be counted in a text. The coding is continued until data saturation is reached, i.e., no additional new codes can be identified. Thematic analysis is an approach to analyzing qualitative data, which involves the identification of themes and patterns in data.[26] The procedure of thematic analysis may be distinct from or overlapping with content analysis. Framework analysis may be considered a specialized form of qualitative content analysis.[27]

NARRATIVE ANALYSIS

Narrative analysis can be thought of as a form of discourse analysis (i.e., an analysis of conversations). Narrative analysis is a way of understanding people's stories (narratives). Stories are unique to the individual and the context in which they are elicited. For example, when talking about a difficult interaction with a pharmacy technician, we may have different versions of the event for our friends, for our preceptor, and with the pharmacy technician years later. Narrative analysis fits well within a qualitative theory of interpretivism because it says that individuals have their own perspectives of the world and reality. Stories can be oral or written and may be extracted from a larger discussion (a discourse). A narrative typically focuses on an experience of an individual. Numerous forms of narrative analysis exist, but a dramaturgical narrative analysis is helpful in the context of healthcare. Labov proposes that individuals are narrators of their own dramas, and each story (narrative) that a person tells has multiple components,[28] just like a theatrical play with a beginning, middle, and end, and this approach has been used to understand familial opioid misuse.[29]

ACTION RESEARCH

Action research is an approach that embeds research into solving social problems. Hallmarks are participation in the research process by members of the population that are being studied. These members of the population are people who do not traditionally have the opportunity to engage in research. This approach has its origins in Paulo Freire's work in education in poor communities in Brazil.[30] The goal was to help people in these communities solve their own problems. In the medical literature, more recent iterations of Action Research underpin community-based participatory research (CBPR).[31] At the initiation of CBPR, a group of interested members of the community join together in a group and meet together at typical intervals (e.g., monthly). The group works together to identify a common problem, collects data to understand the problem, processes the data, develops an action plan, and implements it. Major distinctions with typical research are the iterative process where multiple actions can be taken over time and the sustainability of action because the solution was generated by the community. Such approaches can enhance service-learning experiences.[32]

Steps in Qualitative Research

The basic steps of the scientific research process also apply to qualitative research. These steps include: (1) pose a research question and hypothesis, (2) develop and implement a research plan, (3) perform data collection and analysis, and (4) prepare a research report.[33] In qualitative analysis, which is sometimes used for hypothesis generation and is often descriptive and attempts to provide a rich description of a phenomenon under investigation, there are special considerations for these steps. For example, in the first step, most advocate that qualitative studies be conducted without a predetermined hypothesis and rather be driven by a research question that is somewhat flexible.[18] Also, in the third step, great care should be taken to get rich data. Perhaps most challenging for individuals new to qualitative inquiry is to strategically use silence in interviewing to encourage participants to talk more and to explore issues not considered by the researcher. Further, data analysis typically proceeds throughout the data collection process enabling the researcher to be responsive to what new information needs to be collected. A clear take-home message is that qualitative inquiry is sometimes not a linear process, but like other approaches, the ultimate goal is to gain a better understanding of the phenomenon under study.

TABLE 15–3. EXAMPLES OF RESEARCH QUESTIONS IN PHARMACY ADDRESSED WITH QUALITATIVE RESEARCH

Focus Area	Author	Research Objective	Participants
Patients	Patwardhan et al.[34]	To explore tobacco users' perceptions regarding a brief tobacco cessation counseling program: ask, advise, and refer in community pharmacies	Patients
	Howren et al.[35]	To explore the engagement in disease management among patients with gout	Patients
Providers and pharmacists	Donovan et al.[36]	To understand the perceptions of pharmacy leaders about pharmacies and pharmacy staff dispensing naloxone	Pharmacists
	Silva-Suárez et al.[37]	To explore the coping mechanisms of community pharmacists during the COVID-19 pandemic in Puerto Rico	Pharmacists
Policymakers and stakeholders	Natafgi et al.[38]	To ascertain stakeholders' receptivity for the Learning Healthcare System model to a novel evidence-based healthcare delivery framework	Community members, healthcare professionals, patients, stakeholders
	Zhao et al.[39]	To qualitatively explore influencing factors of the plan selection process by Medicare beneficiaries	Community members

The next two sections explore different types of qualitative research questions specific to pharmacy along with some practical and technical considerations that can be used to support decisions regarding the steps and procedures when conducting qualitative research.

Common Research Questions for Qualitative Research in Pharmacy

With advances in healthcare, the field of pharmacy is experiencing significant growth. Accordingly, more emphasis has been given to the inclusion of pharmacy-related qualitative research to provide new perspectives and knowledge. The pharmacist's role includes several aspects of healthcare, such as dispensing medications, facilitating patient services, providing counseling, and ensuring safety. The interactive nature of the qualitative approach provides opportunities to explore these areas and improve pharmacy services. In pharmacy settings, qualitative research can be valuable in addressing research questions focused on patients, providers, and pharmacists, policymakers, as well as other stakeholders. Moreover, achieving research objectives often relies on the integration of these focus areas. The following sections provide further details concerning each of these focus areas, and Table 15–3 provides some additional examples from the published literature.

PATIENTS

Qualitative research has wide applications, and perhaps the most important is providing a medium for patients to voice their opinions. The methods can be applied to address problems concerning patients and identify strategies that motivate them to change.[40] For example, medication nonadherence is an ongoing problem in the United States. A pharmacist can use individual or focus group interviews to understand a patient's medication-taking behavior. Emerging themes can be utilized to recognize barriers to adherence.[41] Qualitative techniques are also applied to understand drivers to improve immunization rates, facilitate health screenings, and promote healthy behavior among patients. Various intervention strategies can be applied to initiate problem solving in these areas.

PROVIDERS

As much as qualitative research can provide a voice to vulnerable patients, qualitative inquiries are effective in answering questions for providers and pharmacists. In pharmacy practice, the most useful application is to improve current practices. Experiences of pharmacists or pharmacy staff can be captured regarding any newly employed prescription guidelines, counseling techniques, pharmacists' attitudes, etc. This can be accomplished by asking questions like: *Which practices work? How do you feel about current practices? What are your perceptions regarding your role?* The goal is to develop new approaches and intervention strategies that will support the practice and bridge any gaps. For example, a study utilized a qualitative approach to assess community pharmacist's perspective on the sustainability of their practice/service framework.[42]

POLICYMAKERS

Qualitative methods and related evidence are increasingly used to guide health policy development and intervention implementation. These methods prove essential by informing policymakers about system decisions and public perception. Unlike quantitative research that focuses on the efficacy of an intervention or change after a policy, qualitative methods seek answers to questions like: *Why was the intervention beneficial? How is it helpful?* Document analysis and in-depth interviews are effective in assessing the impact of a policy or intervention outcomes. For example, a qualitative study of pharmacists and primary care physicians in four states to understand the impact of prescription drug monitoring programs for controlled substances identified potential barriers to the implementation of such programs.[43] Another study used a qualitative approach to understand pharmacists' responses to an instant messaging application to communicate with patients after hours.[44]

OTHERS

Qualitative studies are appropriate to answer questions for payers and various professional organizations, as well as family members and communities. Qualitative data can inform pricing and reimbursement decisions and provide strategies to move practice forward. For health organizations, a qualitative inquiry has the ability to identify barriers and facilitators in an organizational framework and provide solutions to improve workflow.

Practical and Technical Considerations in Qualitative Research

SETTING

Context is important in understanding and interpreting qualitative data. The goal of qualitative research is not to be able to generalize to other groups; it is bound to the setting in which it was conducted. Thus, it is important to include information about the setting for individuals to understand the strengths and limitations of your approach. The audience can then determine the relevance of the results of your study. Qualitative researchers should provide details about the population under study, the time in which the study was conducted, and features of the environment. Qualitative research that is conducted in a unique environment in a unique time stands to make a greater contribution to the literature. However, simply because analysis has not been conducted in a population previously does not move science forward; indeed, we would expect qualitative research to have transferability, the ability of the findings to generalize from one setting to another. It is the rationale for choosing a particular setting that is more helpful.

SAMPLING

Like quantitative research, qualitative research has sampling strategies. For a review of sampling strategies in quantitative analysis, please refer to Chapter 11. Some qualitative sampling strategies are discussed in the chapter on evaluating qualitative research studies in the companion book.[3,45] Although convenience, quota and snowball sampling are sometimes used, two sampling strategies are more helpful for qualitative research. **Purposive sampling** helps to define the groups that you want to sample *a priori*. For example, you may be interested in segmenting your population such that you speak to individuals of certain ages and racial backgrounds. A table may be helpful to guide the types of people who need to be included. **Theoretical sampling** is more sophisticated; each interview provides insight into the next participant that is needed. When exploring a new field, it can be challenging to anticipate the types of people that will be needed to answer your research question; thus, decisions may be made after interviewing each participant. With such malleability, it is difficult to determine the number of people that you will need to speak with to answer your question at the outset of the study. It is highly dependent on the quality of the data you get from each participant (more is better) and how focused your research question is.

DATA COLLECTION

The most commonly used data collection methods for qualitative analysis include surveys, person-to-person interviews, and focus groups. Unlike in quantitative analysis, which may use a single word such as "agree" or a number on a scale such as a five-point response format, qualitative questions require more than a single word response. In quantitative terminology, qualitative questions are "open-ended" questions, having no predefined responses. Surveys and person-to-person interviews may be structured (static, everyone gets the same question), unstructured (the researcher has a general plan that may change based on the responses of the participant), or semi-structured (the researcher has a guide of questions to use with each participant but may explore certain areas). Focus groups are formalized group meetings of approximately 5 to 10 people who are gathered together to discuss a research topic chosen by the researcher. There are predefined questions for the focus group, and they last approximately one hour. Because focus groups are synergistic, they are considered a single data point for analysis, much like a single interview. Multiple interviews or focus groups are needed to be able to iterate or collect more data to answer the research question. Qualitative research also presents the opportunity to use other data for qualitative analysis, such as documents, written stories, conversations, websites, photographs, observations, and so on. Indeed, we have utilized audio recordings of genetic counseling sessions to understand the risk communication process.[46] Photovoice has been a useful tool to document the experience of medically underserved populations through photographs.[47]

DATA MANAGEMENT AND ANALYSIS

Confidentiality

Qualitative data has special data management concerns. Confidentiality and privacy are particular challenges, and investigators must carefully consider potential harms that may emerge, proceeding in the context of informed consent to research participants. Because there are few people and greater detail about those people in qualitative research, information may emerge that may be identifiable and unflattering for/harmful to the participant. For example, consider a study on barriers to pre-exposure prophylaxis, which included a teacher in a small community with undisclosed HIV. If it were somehow revealed through the study report that he had HIV, it could negatively affect his standing in his job and in his community. Thus, it is important that careful protections are put in place, working through and with your local Institutional Review Board. Other best practices include conducting qualitative interviews in private locations to protect participants. Also, data should be stored in protected areas and should be de-identified, which includes identifying participants by code number and may involve removing or changing identifying details such as names and locations. Even after removing these details, sensitive information may remain identifiable from context, and some advocate discussion of potential disclosures with participants[48] even sharing study reports before publication.[20]

Software

The qualitative analysis produces extensive data requiring appropriate management strategies. Traditional methods of data analysis include a review of textual data or the use of a spreadsheet. Although some researchers may prefer traditional methods, they can be burdensome and time-consuming. Researchers may utilize computer software to assist with more complex data. Electronic data analysis can be undertaken using a Computer Assisted Qualitative Data Analysis Software (CAQDAS). CAQDAS software provides a wide range of tools to support data analysis. Examples of CAQDAS include ATLAS.ti, MAXqda, and NVivo. ATLAS.ti (Scientific Software Development GmbH) and NVivo (QSR International) can manage and analyze extensive qualitative data; can systematically auto-code data, performing numerous operations to extract themes; and have multimedia functionality. While annotations and collaborations can be performed using ATLAS.ti, NVivo can be utilized for sentiment analysis (interpretation of subjective information/emotions).[49] Researchers are advised to have formal training before utilizing these software packages.

Coding (Words, Line by Line, Paragraph)

The unit of analysis is an important consideration in qualitative research. The most common units of analysis are individual words, phrases, lines, sentences, and paragraphs. Each unit of analysis is assigned one or more codes. In Figure 15–1, we illustrate the line as a unit of analysis for a quotation from a participant. The decision on the best unit of analysis will depend on your research question and the approach you are using. The code you assign will depend on the meaning you derive from the unit. The goal is to develop a list of common codes that you can repeatedly use through your analysis. As you are

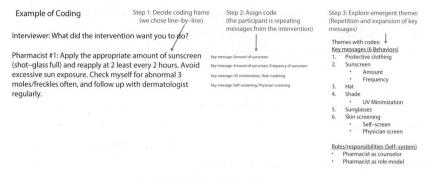

Figure 15–1. Coding example.

coding, you will start to see the codes start to form a hierarchy, with some codes being more general and some being more specific. Rather than waiting until you collect all of your data to analyze it as in quantitative analysis, in qualitative data analysis, you may start analyzing your data after the first interview. In fact, some approaches to qualitative analysis require you to do this. This method of **constant comparison**, comparing each new piece of data with previous data, is critical for qualitative analysis.

As you are building your hierarchy of codes, you will begin to see some "big picture" ideas that are notable from your analysis. Themes are "big picture" ideas that come out of or are **emergent** from your analysis. Indeed, qualitative analysis is notable for its emergent quality. These themes are the backbone of the results of qualitative analysis. The difficult part is to determine when you are finished collecting your data. Most approaches to qualitative data use **theoretical/idea/data saturation** as a stopping point. In this case, you have tried to find new ideas from your population; however, you are seeing more redundancy in codes and are getting no new information.

VALIDITY/TRUSTWORTHINESS

Validity and trustworthiness establish rigor in qualitative research. Over time, researchers have generated multiple strategies to assess the appropriateness of qualitative methodology, data, and other study processes. Various strategies are accepted to establish validity and trustworthiness.[50] **Reflexive notes** document how study results and other procedures are influenced by the researcher's own experiences and perceptions. The researcher can maintain a journal/diary to enter regular notes by reflecting upon the work process, thus preserving study credibility. **Faithful reporting** involves transparently conveying research findings. Researchers should use comprehensive descriptions to describe study results and also present any negative findings in the study. **Member checks** are generally a summary of findings or study reports shared with the research participants to check the legitimacy of the study data and overall work. **Methodological triangulation** entails using multiple methods to study a phenomenon (data collection/ data analysis). Converging multiple methods and sources serve better to support a conclusion and confirm findings compared to a single method or source. **Mixed methods** enable triangulation wherein both qualitative and quantitative approaches are utilized to augment the validity and trustworthiness of the study. For example, data is collected using both close-ended numerical questions (quantitative) and interviews or observations (qualitative). **Inter-rater reliability** is the extent to which multiple raters are consistent and agree with their ratings, assigning the same rating to the same variable. This level of agreement can be calculated using percentage agreement or kappa statistics.

Harnessing the Expertise

SKILLSET

Conducting qualitative research requires a specialized set of skills that are similar to skills utilized in routine pharmacy practice, and students can acquire such skills by taking qualitative methods courses. To provide an avenue for participants to speak, the researcher should be able to establish a rapport with the participants. Assuring a comforting but confidential environment for conversations is beneficial. It is important to proactively initiate conversations and use appropriate probes to collect rich data. While the researcher needs to guide discussions, the focus is overcoming the reticence of participants. Researchers can utilize reflective listening by repeating the ideas of the participant to confirm proper understanding. Generally, pharmacy researchers can utilize interpretative analysis (how a person makes sense of a phenomenon) both in qualitative research and in their practice. Lastly, the researcher can embrace the practice of reflexivity, constantly being reflective on their research and practice. These skills are developed with time; however, the researcher can exercise these techniques before undertaking any study.

EXPERTS NEEDED

Usually, a single qualitative methodologist has the expertise needed, who would guide data collection and analysis. Unlike in other fields, it is not obvious who has training in qualitative research methods. Further, some fields are more acquainted with certain types of qualitative analysis than others. Individuals in the social sciences are more likely to have qualitative training, especially in anthropology. Expertise in qualitative analysis can also be found in the health sciences, such as in nursing and public health. Importantly, individuals typically considered research methodologists in the health sciences (e.g., epidemiology and biostatistics) are not typically trained in qualitative analysis and, therefore generally would be unable to assist with qualitative research. If unable to identify qualitative researchers by word of mouth, reviewing relevant literature and course offerings can help identify experts.

WORKING WITH EXPERTS

If you are planning your own study, you will need to carefully review the literature to help formulate and solidify a research question. When meeting with a qualitative expert, you will discuss your research question, how you developed it, your relevant population, and how you will best interact with them. Through this process, they will assist in determining how best to answer your research question, given the constraints that you may have for your research. Whether you are initiating research or you are assisting with another investigator's research, you will likely play a role in data collection. One of the most challenging things for nascent qualitative researchers is to get complete, rich data; a qualitative expert may be able to provide helpful tips in this area. As you proceed through the data collection and analysis phases, having meetings with the qualitative expert can provide advice on how best to answer the research question and how your data to date is meeting your needs. Ultimately, qualitative experts can guide the development of reports from the data.

Exemplars of Learner-Involved Qualitative Research

SKIN CANCER AWARENESS NOW! (SCAN!)

The SCAN! project was a study of the feasibility and preliminary impact of a skin cancer prevention project in community pharmacy.[51] Preceptors and Advanced Pharmacy Practice Experience (APPE) pharmacy students were trained to deliver an intervention to individuals presenting for routine community pharmacy visits. APPE students recruited patients, confirmed eligibility, consented participants, administered surveys, and delivered the intervention. Immediately after the intervention, patients completed a survey to provide their feedback about the SCAN! At the end of the study, the preceptors and APPE students were interviewed by student pharmacists in an independent study research course and by PhD pharmacy students in Health Services and Outcomes Research to understand attention, liking, comprehension, self-efficacy, yielding, and action in response to the intervention. The PharmD and PhD students worked together to analyze the data using content analysis. Using a line-by-line approach, individual codes were developed from patient, student pharmacist, and pharmacist interviews to determine the strengths and weaknesses of our intervention, and emergent themes were identified.

As three different sources of data (patient, student pharmacist, pharmacist) and two different approaches to data collection (i.e., qualitative, quantitative) were used, we were able to triangulate emergent themes, enhancing the validity of our findings. Ultimately, the intervention evidenced improvements in skin cancer prevention behavior, and we learned ways to improve the intervention in the future.

PATIENT SATISFACTION IN SUBSTANCE USE DISORDER (SUD) REHABILITATIVE SERVICES

This project was developed by a graduate student in pharmacy administration and was focused on developing a patient satisfaction assessment for individuals in a SUD residential rehabilitation center.[24] Qualitative methods were utilized to understand the dimensions of satisfaction as ranked important by the individuals. The graduate student was trained in conducting semi-structured interviews with individuals seeking treatment and their counselors, learning to speak judiciously with the sensitive population, developing rapport, and reflexively evaluating her own biases. The student recruited individuals, recorded the interviews, transcribed them, and developed a codebook using preliminary data. The codebook was created inductively using Grounded theory, and the codes were applied to the remaining interview text.[23] The procedure identified five important aspects that influenced patient satisfaction. These dimensions were utilized to create a patient satisfaction assessment specific to SUD rehabilitation. The student later pilot tested the assessment on individuals seeking SUD treatment.

Dissemination Framework for Qualitative Research

Advancing science by sharing results should be the goal of qualitative inquiry. Ideally, multiple audiences should be considered (e.g., the general population, patients, pharmacists). Publishing qualitative research in professional journals can be challenging, as standards from quantitative research may be applied inappropriately to qualitative research. Increasingly, journals like the *Journal of American Pharmacists Association* have been a venue to showcase novel qualitative research to advance the science of pharmacy practice. Guidelines for publishing qualitative research are helpful, such as the Standards for Reporting Qualitative Research guideline (SRQR) and the Consolidated Criteria for Reporting Qualitative Research (COREQ) checklist.[52,53] COREQ is a 32-item checklist focused on improving the quality of reporting of qualitative approaches such as interviews and focus groups.[53] COREQ does not apply for other qualitative designs like case series, ethnography, or narrative research. It includes components categorized in three main domains: study design, analysis and findings, and details regarding study team and reflexivity.[54] Similarly, SRQR is a 21-item checklist of important considerations in the reporting of qualitative results.[52] The items in SRQR are organized consistently with the components of a research article. For example, the introduction should include the main research question; the methods should include the approach, researcher characteristics/ role, sampling strategy, context, data collection, and analysis; and the results section should include data synthesis and interpretation. Qualitative projects should be designed with reporting requirements in mind, as it is problematic to reach the end of the study and not be able to publish a manuscript due to missing information.

Future of Qualitative Research in Pharmacy

Some qualitative approaches have been less commonly used in the pharmacy context. We hope that pharmacy will increasingly move beyond the quantification of qualitative data to more exciting and novel qualitative approaches, such as immersion/crystallization, narrative analysis, and CBPR. Immersion/crystallization will become more important as pharmacists look inward on their practices and outward in terms of responses to the medical management that is being performed in community pharmacies. Further, we see a great opportunity to address medically underserved populations. Pharmacy can learn more about their practices from the stories of their patients; narrative analysis is a wonderful opportunity for pharmacy research. Finally, pharmacists have a significant contribution as trusted community healthcare providers and can work with community members to help them identify and act to improve health and well-being as in CBPR.

Summary and Conclusions

This chapter focused on the value of incorporating qualitative methods in pharmacy practice research. It included a systematic explanation of components of qualitative methods and various approaches undertaken in pharmacy practice, providing general but important insights with relevant examples. The methods also addressed common research questions and technical considerations in a pharmacy setting. The chapter explained the skills required to conduct research and highlighted the approaches adapted to gain expertise. Learner-based examples exposed readers to the potential for engaging in qualitative research as student pharmacists, residents, and fellows. Integration of these methods in a practice-based setting provides opportunities for pharmacists to explore patients' opinions or understanding and develop innovative intervention strategies.

Key Points and Advice

- Qualitative research is a rigorous way to answer questions related to pharmacy practice.
- Multiple approaches are available to conduct qualitative research. The choice of approach is based upon the best fit with your research question.
- Student pharmacists can play an important role in generating qualitative research questions, gathering and analyzing qualitative data, and generating conclusions.
- Begin with the end in mind: consider reporting guidelines at the outset of study design.

Chapter Review Questions

1. When should qualitative research be conducted?
2. What are the different methods for collecting qualitative data?
3. How can the validity of qualitative research be established?
4. How should qualitative data be reported?

Online Resources

Qualitative Research Methods: A Data Collector's Field Guide. https://www.fhi360.org/ sites/default/files/media/documents/Qualitative%20Research%20Methods%20-%20 A%20Data%20Collector%27s%20Field%20Guide.pdf

Qualitative Data Analysis Software. https://guides.library.illinois.edu/caqdas

Consolidated Criteria for Reporting Qualitative Research (COREQ). https://academic.oup. com/intqhc/article/19/6/349/1791966

Standards for Reporting Qualitative Research. https://journals.lww.com/academicmedi-cine/fulltext/2014/09000/Standards_for_Reporting_Qualitative_Research__A.21.aspx

REFERENCES

1. Merriam SB, Grenier RS. *Qualitative Research in Practice: Examples for Discussion and Analysis.* John Wiley & Sons; 2019.
2. Corbin J, Strauss A, eds. *Basics of Qualitative Research: Techniques and Procedures for Developing Grounded Theory.* 3rd ed. Thousand Oaks, CA: SAGE Publications, Inc.; 2008.
3. Rosenthal M. Evaluating qualitative research studies. In: Aparasu RR, Bentley JP, eds. *Principles of Research Design and Drug Literature Evaluation.* 2nd ed. New York: McGraw-Hill; 2020.

4. Denzin NK, Lincoln YS. Introduction: the discipline and practice of qualitative research. In: *The Sage Handbook of Qualitative Research*. 3rd ed. Thousand Oaks, CA: SAGE Publications Ltd; 2005:1-32.

5. Olsen PR, Harder I. Caring for teenagers and young adults with cancer: a grounded theory study of network-focused nursing. *Eur J Oncol Nurs*. 2011;15(2):152-159.

6. Jennings BM, Sandelowski M, Higgins MK. Turning over patient turnover: an ethnographic study of admissions, discharges, and transfers. *Res Nurs Health*. 2013;36(6):554-566.

7. Bradby H, Varyani M, Oglethorpe R, Raine W, White I, Helen M. British Asian families and the use of child and adolescent mental health services: a qualitative study of a hard to reach group. *Soc Sci Med*. 2007;65(12):2413-2424.

8. McAlearney AS. Leadership development in healthcare: a qualitative study. *J Organ Behav*. 2006;27(7):967-982.

9. Benson J, Britten N. Patients' decisions about whether or not to take antihypertensive drugs: qualitative study. *BMJ*. 2002;325(7369):873.

10. Shiyanbola OO, Ward EC, Brown CM. Utilizing the common sense model to explore African Americans' perception of type 2 diabetes: a qualitative study. *PLoS One*. 2018;13(11):e0207692.

11. Chou WS, Hamel LM, Thai CL, et al. Discussing prognosis and treatment goals with patients with advanced cancer: A qualitative analysis of oncologists' language. *Health Expect*. 2017;20(5):1073-1080.

12. Florian J, Roy NM, Quintiliani LM, et al. Using photovoice and asset mapping to inform a community-based diabetes intervention, Boston, Massachusetts, 2015. *Prev Chronic Dis*. 2016;13:E107.

13. Lasseter G, Al-Janabi H, Trotter CL, Carroll FE, Christensen H. The views of the general public on prioritising vaccination programmes against childhood diseases: a qualitative study. *PLoS One*. 2018;13(6):e0197374.

14. Ono SS, Crabtree BF, Hemler JR, et al. Taking innovation to scale in primary care practices: the functions of health care extension. *Health Aff (Millwood)*. 2018;37(2):222-230.

15. Amsler MR, Murray MD, Tierney WM, et al. Pharmaceutical care in chain pharmacies: beliefs and attitudes of pharmacists and patients. *J Am Pharm Assoc (Wash)*. 2001;41(6):850-855.

16. Sorensen TD, Pestka D, Sorge LA, Wallace ML, Schommer J. A qualitative evaluation of medication management services in six Minnesota health systems. *Am J Health Syst Pharm*. 2016;73(5):307-314.

17. McCullough MB, Petrakis BA, Gillespie C, et al. Knowing the patient: a qualitative study on care-taking and the clinical pharmacist-patient relationship. *Res Social Adm Pharm*. 2016;12(1):78-90.

18. Creswell JW, Poth CN. *Qualitative Inquiry and Research Design: Choosing among Five Approaches*. Thousand Oaks, CA: SAGE Publications; 2016.

19. Denzin NK, Lincoln YS. *The Sage Handbook of Qualitative Research*. 2017.

20. Lather PA, Smithies CS. *Troubling the Angels: Women Living with HIV/AIDS*. Boulder, CO: Westview Press; 1997.

21. Crabtree BF, Crabtree BF, Miller WL. *Doing Qualitative Research*. London: SAGE; 1999.

22. Garg R, Meraya A, Murray PJ, Kelly K. Illness representations of pertussis and predictors of child vaccination among mothers in a strict vaccination exemption state. *Matern Child Health J.* 2018;22(1):137-146.

23. Böhm A. Theoretical coding: text analysis in grounded theory. In: Flick Dans U, Kardorff E. von, Steinke I, eds. *A Companion to Qualitative Research.* London: SAGE; 2004: 270-275.

24. Dhumal T, Giannetti V, Kamal KM, et al. Patient satisfaction with substance use disorder rehabilitation services: a qualitative study. *J Behav Health Serv Res.* 2020.

25. Elo S, Kyngäs H. The qualitative content analysis process. *J Adv Nurs.* 2008;62(1):107-115.

26. Vaismoradi M, Turunen H, Bondas T. Content analysis and thematic analysis: implications for conducting a qualitative descriptive study. *Nurs Health Sci.* 2013;15(3):398-405.

27. Gale NK, Heath G, Cameron E, Rashid S, Redwood S. Using the framework method for the analysis of qualitative data in multi-disciplinary health research. *BMC Med Res Methodol.* 2013;13(1):117.

28. Labov W, Waletzky J. Narrative analysis: oral versions of personal experience. *J Narrat Life Hist.* 1997;7(1-4):3-38.

29. Alhussain K, Shah D, Thornton JD, Kelly KM. Familial opioid misuse and family cohesion: impact on family communication and well-being. *Addict Disorder Their Treat.* 2019;18(4):194-204.

30. Freire P. *Pedagogy of the Oppressed.* New York: Bloomsbury Publishing USA; 2018.

31. Bardwell G, Morton C, Chester A, et al. Feasibility of adolescents to conduct community-based participatory research on obesity and diabetes in rural Appalachia. *Clin Transl Sci.* 2009;2(5):340-349.

32. Davis LI, Wright DJ, Gutierrez MS, Nam JJ, Nguyen J, Waite AT. Interprofessional global service learning: a pharmacy and nursing practice experience in Botswana. *Curr Pharm Teach Learn.* 2015;7(2):169-178.

33. Aparasu R, Chatterjee S. The scientific approach to research and practice. In: Aparasu RR, Bentley JP, eds. *Principles of Research Design and Drug Literature Evaluation.* 2nd ed. New York: McGraw-Hill; 2020.

34. Patwardhan PD, Chewning BA. Tobacco users' perceptions of a brief tobacco cessation intervention in community pharmacies. *J Am Pharm Assoc (2003).* 2010;50(5):568-574.

35. Howren A, Cox SM, Shojania K, Rai SK, Choi HK, De Vera MA. How patients with gout become engaged in disease management: a constructivist grounded theory study. *Arthritis Res Ther.* 2018;20(1):110.

36. Donovan E, Bratberg J, Baird J, et al. Pharmacy leaders' beliefs about how pharmacies can support a sustainable approach to providing naloxone to the community. *Res Social Adm Pharm.* 2020;16(10):1493-1497.

37. Silva-Suárez G, Alvarado Reyes Y, Hernandez-Diaz A, Rodriguez Ramirez K, Colón-Pratts FM. The voices of community pharmacists during the COVID-19 pandemic in Puerto Rico. *J Am Pharm Assoc (2003).* 2022;62(1):202-208.

38. Natafgi N, Ladeji O, Hong YD, Caldwell J, Mullins CD. Are communities willing to transition into learning health care communities? a community-based participatory evaluation of stakeholders' receptivity. *Qual Health Res.* 2021;31(8):1412-1422.

39. Zhao Y, Diggs K, Chen ZX, Hohmann N, Kwon WS, Westrick SC. Qualitative exploration of factors influencing the plan selection process by Medicare beneficiaries. *J Manag Care Spec Pharm.* 2021;27(3):339-353.

40. Berkwits M, Inui TS. Making use of qualitative research techniques. *J Gen Intern Med.* 1998;13(3):195-199.

41. Kibicho J, Owczarzak J. Pharmacists' strategies for promoting medication adherence among patients with HIV. *J Am Pharm Assoc (2003).* 2011;51(6):746-755.

42. Crespo-Gonzalez C, Benrimoj SI, Scerri M, Garcia-Cardenas V. Community pharmacists' perspectives about the sustainability of professional pharmacy services: a qualitative study. *J Am Pharm Assoc (2003).* 2021;61(2):181-190.

43. Freeman PR, Curran GM, Drummond KL, et al. Utilization of prescription drug monitoring programs for prescribing and dispensing decisions: results from a multi-site qualitative study. *Res Social Adm Pharm.* 2019;15(6):754-760.

44. Rathbone AP, Norris R, Parker P, et al. Exploring the use of WhatsApp in out-of-hours pharmacy services: a multi-site qualitative study. *Res Social Adm Pharm.* 2020;16(4):503-510.

45. Aparasu RR, Bentley JP. *Principles of Research Design and Drug Literature Evaluation.* 2nd ed. New York: McGraw-Hill; 2020.

46. Chopra I, Kelly KM. Cancer risk information sharing: the experience of individuals receiving genetic counseling for BRCA1/2 mutations. *J Health Commun.* 2017;22(2):143-152.

47. PhotoVoice. Accessed December 11, 2020. https://photovoice.org/

48. Kaiser K. Protecting respondent confidentiality in qualitative research. *Qual Health Res.* 2009;19(11):1632-1641.

49. Zunic A, Corcoran P, Spasic I. Sentiment analysis in health and well-being: systematic review. *JMIR Med Inform.* 2020;8(1):e16023.

50. Amin MEK, Nørgaard LS, Cavaco AM, et al. Establishing trustworthiness and authenticity in qualitative pharmacy research. *Res Social Adm Pharm.* 2020;16(10):1472-1482.

51. Kelly KM, Dhumal T, Scott VG, et al. SCAN! A pharmacy-based, sun safety feasibility study. *J Am Pharm Assoc.* 2021;61(1):e69-e79.

52. O'Brien BC, Harris IB, Beckman TJ, Reed DA, Cook DA. Standards for reporting qualitative research: a synthesis of recommendations. *Acad Med.* 2014;89(9):1245-1251.

53. Tong A, Sainsbury P, Craig J. Consolidated criteria for reporting qualitative research (COREQ): a 32-item checklist for interviews and focus groups. *Int J Qual Health Care.* 2007;19(6):349-357.

54. Dossett LA, Kaji AH, Cochran A. SRQR and COREQ Reporting Guidelines for Qualitative Studies. *JAMA Surg.* 2021;156(9):875-876.

16

Chapter Sixteen

Drug Utilization Research in Healthcare

Varun Vaidya, PhD

Chapter Objectives

- Define drug utilization research in healthcare
- Discuss various data sources for drug utilization research
- Discuss general steps in drug utilization review
- Identity common research questions in drug utilization research
- Understand the practical considerations for drug utilization research
- Understand the technical considerations for drug utilization research
- Discuss the strategies for harnessing the expertise needed for conducting drug utilization research
- Describe an example of learner-involved drug utilization research
- Understand the dissemination framework for drug utilization research

Key Terminology

Drug utilization review, drug utilization research, defined daily dose, prescribed daily dose drug use evaluation, medication use evaluation, Anatomical Therapeutic Classification System, National Drug Code, Drug Identification Number, Generic Product Identifier, Systematized Nomenclature of Medicine, Unique Ingredient Identifier

Introduction

The rise of modern medicine has given us many new treatments and therapies. While we have an abundance of different treatments and medications, we must choose them correctly and economically. Along with all the benefits and desired effects, most drugs also produce unintended consequences, commonly known as side effects. Another challenge with the development and availability of new drugs is the consequent rising of costs. The process of new drug development is costly, affecting the price and affordability. With all the complexities in modern drug therapy, it becomes necessary to provide a mechanism to study prescribing and consumption of drugs to optimize this vital health resource. The multidisciplinary field of Drug Utilization Research (DUR) came into existence to study the appropriate and economical use of drugs.

The purpose of this chapter is to provide an introduction to the field of DUR, starting with its evolution. It will define DUR and discuss the multidisciplinary approach of DUR with some examples. It provides common questions and general steps in conducting learner-involved DUR. The practical and technical considerations for DUR are also provided in detail. The chapter also describes the methods and skills required to conduct and evaluate DUR. This chapter also provides the relevance of DUR to the pharmacy profession. Understanding DUR is helpful to a pharmacist providing clinical services.

Evolution of Drug Utilization Review

The DUR started in Europe in the early 1960s,[1] with many European countries recognizing the need to systematically evaluate the performance of drugs available to their patients. From a commercial point of view, the pharmaceutical industry was also interested in finding out their products' market performance by monitoring utilization to direct new drug development efforts. In DUR's early days, the focus was on standardizing the drug classification system and developing a unique measurement unit to study DUR.[1] Researchers came up with a new measurement unit called defined daily dose (DDD) that allowed to measure and compare drug utilization across different European countries. The early researchers focused on the following key questions to understand DUR:[2]

why drugs are prescribed;
who the prescribers are;
for whom the prescribers prescribe;
whether patients take their medicines correctly;
what the benefits and risks of the drugs are.

The DUR was formally defined by the World Health Organization (WHO) in 1977 as "The marketing, distribution, prescription, and use of drugs in a society, with special emphasis on the resulting medical, social and economic consequences."[3] Later as the field grew, this definition was not broad enough to capture all aspects of DUR. In 2008, the textbook *Pharmacoepidemiology and Therapeutic Risk Management* defined it to incorporate broader areas; "**Drug Utilization Research** *is an eclectic collection of descriptive and analytical methods for the quantification, the understanding and the evaluation of the processes of prescribing, dispensing and consumption of medicines, and for the testing of interventions to enhance the quality of these processes.*"[4] This definition reflects the current state of DUR more accurately.

Because of its need and perceived importance, DUR quickly spread to other countries and continents, including the United States and Latin America. In the United States, DUR was primarily driven by the federal government to curb Medicaid expenditure[5] without hurting the quality of care. Later it expanded to other programs and broader initiatives with the goal of increasing awareness of the risks and benefits of new and existing drugs. In the late nineties, the Centers for Education and Research on Therapeutics (CERTs) were funded by the Agency for Healthcare Research and Quality (AHRQ) to create awareness of benefits and risks of medications. The CERT is actively involved in conducting research addressing optimal and cost-effective use of drugs.

Drug Utilization Research and Drug Utilization Review

The adoption and growth of DUR also sparked the emergence of drug utilization review programs. Drug utilization review (not to be confused with drug utilization research) is a valuable process to identify issues with the proper use of drugs and prescribing patterns. Drug utilization review programs are commonly used by the Pharmacy Benefit Managers in the United States to optimize the appropriate use of drugs. They play an important role in improving prescribing and administration of drug use. Drug utilization reviews are also referred to as **drug use evaluation, medication use evaluation**, and medication use management.[6] Drug utilization review programs are a direct application of DUR. Research synthesized in the DUR field serves as a basis for drug utilization review. Pharmacist-conducted drug utilization reviews have shown significant improvements in the appropriate and economical use of medications. Due to their well-demonstrated utility, CMS requires every Medicare Part D plan sponsor to include drug utilization reviews available to all patients.[7]

Steps in DUR

Steps to conduct DUR follow a similar approach as typical scientific research. The scientific research process involves the following steps: (1) pose a research question and hypothesis, (2) develop and implement a research plan, (3) perform data collection and analysis, and (4) prepare a research report.[6]

POSE A RESEARCH QUESTION AND HYPOTHESIS

A research question is the first step in conducting any research project. It is crucial to formulate the research idea into an answerable research question. The research questions in DUR can inquire about if the drugs in a specific therapeutic class are appropriately being used. Are the intended drug therapies producing expected outcomes? Are certain drugs being overused or underused? Are we getting enough value from prescription drugs? Defining straightforward questions helps to come up with a hypothesis. Hypothesis gives more direction for the analytical approach that will be used in the research. However, the hypothesis is not needed if it is descriptive or exploratory research. Research question and hypothesis combined form the foundation needed for later stages of DUR.

DEVELOP AND IMPLEMENT A RESEARCH PLAN

After finalizing the research question and hypothesis, the next step is to formulate a research plan. A research plan is like a blueprint to conduct the project systematically, including specifics of study design. Often a cohort or cross-sectional designs are used in DUR. A carefully thought out research plan provides a critical framework needed for successfully implementation the study. Based on the study design, a typical research plan will provide step-by-step directions about data collection, statistical tests to be used, how every hypothesis will be tested, and results will be presented. It often includes dummy tables or empty shells, which help run statistical tests and data. The research plan also includes the timeline for the entire project with specific milestones and time points. Detailed timelines not only help in the overall organization of the project, but they also hold accountable all team members to complete their designated work.

PERFORM DATA COLLECTION AND ANALYSIS

The next step in the DUR is to perform data collection and analysis. The data collection will depend on whether the study uses primary data or secondary data, as defined above. Both primary and secondary data collection have their unique challenges, and the analysis plan will address if the data is being collected, primary or secondary. Data collection usu-ally takes more time when data is primary as it involves developing a data collection tool and processes like validating and testing it. The data analysis will involve descriptive and multivariable analyses. Descriptive analyses can help understand the study sample and drug utilization patterns, while multivariable analyses are useful to identify the factors associated with medication use or the effects of medication use on outcomes.

PREPARE A RESEARCH REPORT

This is the final step in the research project. The research report summarizes all work done and highlights major findings to communicate to the relevant audience. The research report should be written in an engaging format with very articulate narration and adequate details of methods employed and findings. There are two primary purposes of the research report: (1) Provide transparency so that others can replicate the study. (2) Convey the significant findings of the study. Careful attention should be given to both of these aspects while preparing a research report. Research reports need to be formatted into specifics of a journal or other venue where they are intended to be published.

Research Areas and Research Questions

With DUR's broad scope, DUR's application can be broadly categorized into three dis-tinct dimensions of drug utilization. It takes into consideration the medical, social, and economic aspects of drug utilization. In medical aspects, the focus is on clinical appro-priateness and clinical outcomes such as risk to benefit ratio of drugs. The social side of drug utilization typically studies the attitudes and beliefs of drug use, drug abuse and dependence, improper use of drugs, medication adherence disparities in use, etc. Finally, the third area is the economic aspects of drug utilization where we study costs effective-ness, value proposition of drugs, etc. This makes DUR a highly multidisciplinary field that borrows techniques from various fields. Scientific disciplines such as clinical pharmacy, health services research, pharmacoeconomics, outcomes research, and pharmacoepide-miology are often used for DUR.

The DUR has evolved into a much broader field from its early days, and it now touches on various aspects of general healthcare use. Research areas in DUR can address structure, process, and outcome aspects of the drug use process to address overall healthcare quality. Commonly known as the Donabedian model[8] (named after the physi-cian who coined the term), it was developed to evaluate healthcare quality.[9] DUR studies can address key questions in all three components of the Donabedian model.

STRUCTURE

This area of DUR deals with the evaluation of the structural components of healthcare delivery. Studies in this area evaluate systems and structures surrounding drug use, such as the process of ordering, delivering, or administering the drug in a hospital or healthcare facility. Such studies can be used to estimate the number of patients exposed to certain drugs within a specific time period. Additionally, the extent of use of a particular drug in a certain area (e.g., in a country, region, community, or hospital) can also be determined.

Imperfections in healthcare systems lead to major issues such as suboptimal and unequal access to healthcare resources. Patient access to medications has been a challenge in recent years. Lack of access to vital drugs is responsible for poor outcomes and reduced overall healthcare quality. According to a 2017 report by the WHO, nearly two billion people worldwide do not have access to essential medications.[10] When we look globally, access to essential drugs is largely suboptimal and changes considerably depending upon the country. Domestically, within the United States, where we have a fragmented healthcare delivery system with a patchwork of multiple payers at private and government levels, access to drugs is more complicated and vary greatly. DUR studies in this research area study drug utilization patterns with a focus on underutilization due to access issues and disparities in utilization. Typical research questions in this area deal with discrepancies in using essential drugs based on sociodemographic characteristics and geographic location.

PROCESS

The process is identified in the Donabedian model as the sum of actions that make up healthcare. These actions begin at the provider level (diagnosis, treatment, patient education) and extend to actions taken at the patient level. In order to understand optimum drug utilization, there are actions at both provider and patient levels. The actions such as appropriate prescribing and dispensing at the provider level and medication adherence and compliance at the patient level are studied in DUR. Researchers investigate prescribing patterns and study issues related to under/overprescribing, prescribing compliance with clinical guidelines, and regulatory recommendations. These studies are often interested in evaluating the determinants or factors associated with such use. DUR studies in this area determine the patterns of the drug followed over time along with separating the trends in drugs. Additionally, researchers can also estimate the extent of drug use, i.e., whether they are properly used, overused or underused. The comparison study of the observed patterns of the use of drugs for the treatment of certain diseases with current recommendations or guidelines is also a part of drug utilization studies. Studies can determine the pattern or profile of drug use and the extent to which alternative drugs are being used to treat particular conditions.

On the patient's side, medication adherence and compliance play a critical role in the appropriate utilization of drugs. Adherence is the last action in the process of healthcare delivery. No matter how accurate prescribing is done or how good the access is, if patients do not take their medications as directed or do not take it all, there will not benefit from the treatment. Medication adherence is a real-world phenomenon that does not get captured in protocol-driven clinical trials. A drug looking promising in clinical studies can fail to show its effectiveness if patients are not taking it in real-world settings. This is a common occurrence, and there are multiple reasons identified that affect patient's adherence. Routinely studying adherence is another crucial area to conduct DUR. Research questions in this area focus on measuring adherence to specific drugs or studying reasons behind low adherence to essential drugs. It is a growing body of literature that provides insights into improving drug utilization by addressing the underuse of drugs.

Drug utilization studies can help to evaluate the rational use of drugs. Irrational prescribing is a global problem, and bad prescribing habits lead to ineffective and unsafe treatment, exacerbation, or prolongation of illness, higher cost and distress, and harm to patients. Monitoring of drug utilization patterns helps to improve the therapeutic efficacy, provides feedback to the prescriber to assure rational use of medicines, and decrease the adverse drug reactions

OUTCOMES

Outcomes are the endpoints or the end results of treatments that ultimately demonstrate how effective any treatment is. Donabedian model defines outcomes as effects of healthcare on the health status of patients measured as health-related quality of life and patient satisfaction.[8] Along with the structural and process issues, outcomes evaluations complete the picture. Outcomes often depend on structure and process and are consequences of them. This is another area where DUR studies investigate the use of different medications and measure the impact on outcomes. If a drug is indicated for a specific condition or ailment, outcomes measure the success of controlling or curing that condition. Such studies also provide comparative data on multiple drugs that belong to the same class or are intended to treat a common condition. Although clinical trials are gold standards in establishing the efficacy of drugs, all clinical trials are performed in a controlled, experimental setting. The actual world is often different and messier compared to the clinical trial setting. DUR studies provide an important link between clinical trials and the real-world performance of the drugs. Outcomes could be safety, effectiveness, quality of life or other patient-reported outcomes, and economic outcomes. The research questions in this area compare the performance of drugs in terms of clinical endpoints, patient-reported outcomes, and also the affordability or cost-effectiveness of drugs. Outcomes data are fundamental to formulate guidelines, make recommendations, and ultimately optimize drug utilization. These studies also provide feedback to the pharmaceutical manufacturers to decide their focus on research and development.

Table 16–1 provides examples of studies focusing on structure, process, and outcome aspects of the drug use process.

TABLE 16–1. EXAMPLES OF DRUG UTILIZATION STUDIES FROM THE LITERATURE

Structure	• Briesacher B, Limcangco R, Gaskin D. Racial and ethnic disparities in prescription coverage and medication use. *Health Care Financ Rev*. 2003;25(2):63-76. https://www.ncbi.nlm.nih.gov/pubmed/15124378
	• Godman B, Shrank W, Andersen M, et al. Comparing policies to enhance prescribing efficiency in Europe through increasing generic utilization: changes seen and global implications. *Expert Rev Pharmacoecon Outcomes Res*. 2010;10(6):707-722. doi:10.1586/erp.10.72
	• Schumock GT, Stubbings J, Hoffman JM, et al. National trends in prescription drug expenditures and projections for 2019. *Am J Health Syst Pharm*. 2019;76(15):1105-1121. doi:10.1093/ajhp/zxz109
	• Wagner AK, Graves AJ, Reiss SK, Lecates R, Zhang F, Ross-Degnan D. Access to care and medicines, burden of healthcare expenditures, and risk protection: results from the World Health Survey. *Health Pol*. 2011;100(2-3):151-158. doi:10.1016/j.healthpol.2010.08.004
Process	• Braund R, Furlan HM, George K, Havell, MM, Murphy JL, West MK. Interventions performed by New Zealand community pharmacists while dispensing prescription medications. *Pharm World Sci*. 2010;32(1):22-25. doi:10.1007/s11096-009-9343-7
	• Cheung KC, van den Bemt PM, Bouvy ML, Wensing M, De Smet PA. Medication incidents related to automated dose dispensing in community pharmacies and hospitals--a reporting system study. *PLoS One*. 2014;9(7):e101686. doi:10.1371/journal.pone.0101686
	• Hersberger KE, Boeni F, Arnet I. Dose-dispensing service as an intervention to improve adherence to polymedication. *Expert Rev Clin Pharmacol*. 2013;6(4):413-421. doi:10.1586/17512433.2013.811829
	• Vaidya V, Gupte R, Balkrishnan R. Failure to refill essential prescription medications for asthma among pediatric Medicaid beneficiaries with persistent asthma. *Patient Prefer Adherence*. 2013;7:21-26. doi:10.2147/PPA.S37811
Outcomes	• Armour C, Bosnic-Anticevich S, Brillant M, et al. Pharmacy Asthma Care Program (PACP) improves outcomes for patients in the community. *Thorax*. 2007;62(6):496-502. doi:10.1136/thx.2006.064709
	• Ishida JH, McCulloch CE, Steinman MA, Grimes BA, Johansen KL. Opioid analgesics and adverse outcomes among hemodialysis patients. *Clin J Am Soc Nephrol*. 2018;13(5):746-753. doi:10.2215/CJN.09910917
	• Krska J, Morecroft CW, Poole H, Rowe PH. Issues potentially affecting quality of life arising from long-term medicines use: a qualitative study. *Int J Clin Pharm*. 2013;35(6):1161-1169. doi:10.1007/s11096-013-9841-5
	• Shah D, Vaidya V, Patel A, Borovicka M, Goodman MH. Assessment of health-related quality of life, mental health status and psychological distress based on the type of pharmacotherapy used among patients with depression. *Qual Life Res*. 2017;26(4):969-980. doi:10.1007/s11136-016-1417-0

Data Sources for DUR

Regardless of the research area within DUR, most research projects need a valid, reliable data source. Once the research area is chosen and a research question is narrowed down, the next step is to procure appropriate data to conduct DUR. About 50 years ago, the data were obtained directly from the patients or by abstracting medical records, and the quality of such data was questionable. Nowadays, the data used in health utilization research are large administrative databases generated from either electronic health record (EHR) systems or insurance claims processing. In DUR, the data sources used can be broadly categorized into primary and secondary data sources. Primary data is defined as the data that has been generated by the researcher through experiments, surveys, and interviews designed to understand and solve the research problems. For example, a study is trying to understand the utilization and effectiveness of certain prescription drugs; the researchers can create a structured questionnaire and survey patients taking those drugs. The data generated from this survey will be "primary data." It is collected solely for the research question on hand. Patient-reported data and healthcare providers reported data are two major sources for primary data collection in DUR.

Some of the main advantages of primary data are:

- Since the data is specifically collected for the purpose of research, it will have much detailed and organized information that is tailored for the specific research project.
- The researchers select the data collection tool themselves, giving them better control over the data collected for the research project. It saves time and effort to clean and format data, unlike secondary sources where data is not exclusively collected for the research project.
- Primary data collection provides an opportunity to not only design the data collection procedure; it also enables them to build quality control measures to improve the overall reliability and validity of the data.

With several advantages, there are also some disadvantages of primary data collection in DUR.

- Manually collecting data or conducting interviews is often an expensive and time-consuming endeavor.
- Getting an adequate sample size for quantitative analysis is more challenging with primary data collection. The response rate to surveys and questionnaires, especially when the study population is healthcare providers, is a common hurdle in conducting research based on primary data collection.

- Ethical issues such as protecting the privacy and anonymity of study participants need to address and require more rigorous review from Institutional Review Boards before collecting data compared to secondary data research where data is already deidentified and preprocessed for research.

In contrast to primary data, secondary data are defined as the existing data collected earlier by large government institutions, healthcare organizations, previous researchers, and other research organizations to meet their objectives. Secondary data are not collected for a specific research question. It is quite common to see a secondary data source in DUR. With improvements in technology and the increasing adoption of electronic medical records, it is becoming more convenient to design a DUR study by combining aggregate-level data to answer research questions. In DUR, secondary data can originate from pharmacy dispensing data records (community and hospital pharmacies), prescribing data (EHR systems, administrative claims data), and utilization data (patient registries, national surveys, and other publicly available datasets). Table 16–2 lists some of the commonly used datasets in the United States for DUR.

Since the researchers do not collect the data, secondary data are relatively quick, easy to use. If the data is available at no cost, it can also save on the research budget. However, some data are not publicly available, and researchers must pay certain amounts to access the data. Depending on the research's scope and subject matter, it may be significantly low

TABLE 16–2. EXAMPLES OF HEALTHCARE AND DRUG UTILIZATION DATA

Healthcare Utilization	Source
Electronic Medical Records	EPIC
	Allscripts
	Cerner
Administrative claims data	IBM Marketscan Commercial Claims and Encounters Database
	IQVIA Pharmetric
	OptumMedicare and Medicaid
Dispensing Data	IQVIA Xponent
	IQVIA National Prescription Audit
	Independent and Chain Pharmacies Data
National Surveys	National Ambulatory Medical Care Survey (NAMCS)
	National Hospital Ambulatory Medical Care Survey (NHAMCS)
	National Nursing Home Survey (NNHS)
	National Home and Hospice Care Survey (NNHS)
	Medical Expenditure Panel Survey (MEPS)
Registry	Surveillance, Epidemiology and End Results (SEER)-Medicare Linked Database

cost to purchase a data source rather than collect the primary data. It should be noted that the cost of obtaining specific proprietary commercial data could be prohibitive.

Along with all these advantages, there are some disadvantages of secondary data too. First, the data is not collected specifically for the research project, making it necessary to understand the structure and format of data. Often the data has quality issues and requires much effort in cleaning and reformatting data. It is also expected that the secondary datasets do not have all the variables needed for the analysis, and researchers must make adjustments to methodology to fit the data to the research question. A thorough understanding of data analytics research is important to have to use secondary datasets.

Both primary and secondary data have pros and cons. Depending on the budget, study design, and the required result from the health utilization research, one can determine the type of data used.

Practical Considerations of DUR

DUR requires detailed information about drugs and their use on multiple levels. Different drugs have different doses, indications, active ingredients, costs variations, and many other factors. Depending on the research question, all this information needs to be aggregated systematically. To standardize this process, DUR researchers need to be familiar with drug classification systems and common measurement systems. Both aspects are essential to aggregate the information gathered from varied sources across multiple systems to use in a DUR project.

DRUG CLASSIFICATION SYSTEMS

In order to conduct DUR, it is important to have a drug classification and pharmaceutical code system. Drug classification provides a common platform to describe various drugs in a country or a region. It must be collected and aggregated uniformly and is a prerequisite for comparing drug utilization data at the national and international levels. The drug classification's main objective is to ensure the drug's safe use to achieve the maximum benefit.

There are different ways drugs can be classified. Classification can be based on the chemical, pharmacological, biological, therapeutic, and biopharmaceutical properties of drugs. In chemical classification, drugs are categorized by their chemical structure—for example, beta-lactam antibiotics, opioids, and steroids. Similarly, in pharmacological classification, drugs are grouped according to action and mode of action. The mechanism of action is the type of activity of medicine at the biological target. The specific examples of drug classes based on the mechanism of action are 5-alpha-reductase inhibitor, angiotensin II receptor antagonist, ACE inhibitor, beta-blocker, etc.

Additionally, drugs can be classified according to the mode of action based on biological perspective and therapeutic class. In the mode of action, drugs are classified according to the anatomical and functional changes they induce. Drug classes defined by standard methods of action include diuretic, decongestant, bronchodilators, antimicrobials, antifungals, antithrombotic, etc. In therapeutic class, drugs are classified according to their therapeutic use. Some of the examples include antibiotic, antithrombotic, anticancer, sedative, and so on.

In the Biopharmaceutical Classification of Drugs, the drugs are classified into four classes based on their solubility and permeability.

- Class I: It has high solubility and high permeability; for example, metoprolol and paracetamol.
- Class II: Compounds under this group have high permeability and low solubility; for example, glibenclamide and ezetimibe.
- Class III: The drugs under this group has low permeability and high solubility; for example, cimetidine.
- Class IV: The drugs having low permeability and low solubility falls under this group; for example, bifonazole.

Within these classes of drugs, pharmaceutical codes are used to identify medication uniquely among other drugs. These coding systems assign a numeric value to each drug product to be identified and analyzed easily. Such systems uniquely identify active ingredients, drug systems in general, or a specific pharmaceutical manufacturer's specific product. An example include drug system identifiers (manufacturer-specific including inactive ingredients).

Anatomical Therapeutic Classification (ATC) System[11]

The **ATC** is a drug classification system that classifies the active ingredients of the drug according to the organ or system on which they act, along with therapeutic, pharmacological, and chemical properties. If they have the same active substance and indications but have different brands, they share the same code. It is a strict hierarchy, i.e., each code necessarily has one and only one parent code. As of May 7, 2020, there are 6,331 codes in ATC. World Health Organization Collaborating Centre controls it for Drug Statistics Methodology.

National Drug Code (NDC)[12]

The NDC is used in the United States to identify the unique product of drugs intended for human use. It consists of 10 or 11 digits, the three-segment numeric identifier assigned to each medication listed under section 510 of the U.S. Federal Food, Drug, and Cosmetic Act. The first segment of the code is the labeler code, which is around four, five, or six digits and is assigned by the Food and Drug Administration (FDA). The second segment is the product code with three or four numbers, and the third segment is the package code. The labeler sets these two segments.

Drug Identification Number (DIN)[13]

The DIN is an eight-digit unique number given to any product defined as a drug under the Canadian Food and Drugs Act. It provides the user information that the product has undergone and passed a review of its formulation, labeling, and instructions for use. It also helps in the follow-up of products on the market, recall of products, inspections, and quality monitoring.

Generic Product Identifier (GPI)[14]

The **GPI** is a 14-character hierarchical classification system that classifies drugs from their primary therapeutic use down to the unique interchangeable product regardless of the manufacturer or package size. The code consists of seven subsets, each increasingly providing more specific information about a drug available with a prescription in the United States.

Systematized Nomenclature of Medicine (*SNOMED*)[15]

The **SNOMED** is a computer-processable collection of medical terms in a systematic manner that provides codes, terms, synonyms, and definitions that cover anatomy, diseases, findings, procedures, microorganisms, substances, etc. It allows a reliable way to index, store, retrieve, and aggregate medical data across specialties and sites of care.

Unique Ingredient Identifier(UPI)[16]

The **UPI** is a nonproprietary, free, unique, unambiguous alphanumeric identifier linked to a substance's molecular structure or descriptive information generated by the Global Substance Registration System of the FDA. It is used to create permanent, unique identifiers for substances in regulated products. Proprietary database identifiers include those assigned by First Databank, Micromedex, MediSpan, Gold Standard Drug Database, AHFS, and Cerner Multum Cerner MediSource Lexicon; these are cross-indexed by RxNorm, which also sets a unique identifier (RxCUI) to every combination of the active ingredient and dose level.

In addition to drug classification, it is also helpful to have a basic understanding of disease classification systems. One commonly used disease classification is the International Classification of Diseases (ICD). This system developed by the WHO is widely used in research and by insurance companies. With the new diagnosis and advances in clinical sciences, ICD is revised regularly. The current version of this system is ICD-10.

MEASUREMENT OF DRUG UTILIZATION

While drug classification is essential to identify and describe drugs, researchers need to measure them systematically to analyze their utilization. A standardized metric is needed to aggregate the data coming from different sources into meaningful research. One of such standards is developed by the WHO and is called DDD.[2] The WHO developed it in collaboration with a center in Oslo, Norway, along with the International working group on drug statistics methodology. The DDD was developed along with the WHO's classification system (ATC), and every drug classified under the ATC system is assigned a DDD. A unique DDD is assigned to each ATC code and route of administration. This is a commonly used metric that provides a standard measurement across multiple drugs used in different countries.

The **DDD** is defined as the assumed average maintenance dose per day for a drug used for its main indication in adults. The DDD provides a common measurement regardless of the dosage form, package size, dispensing method, and strength. The DDD approximates the average dose based on the review of information around the world. It is useful in identifying population-level trends of drug utilization across different countries and population groups. However, it should be noted that this method is not to identify individual therapeutic doses. Patient-level dose differs based on the individual characteristics of a patient. DDD helps to see a broad picture of drug utilization, and it should not be considered as an exact reflection of actual use. Although a rough estimate, it provides a common measurement unit making it very useful in studying drug utilization changes over time, making comparisons between countries, and studying the comparative effectiveness of drugs.

To study the actual use of drugs, another method called prescribed daily dose (PDD) is used. **PDD** is the average daily amount of a drug that is actually prescribed to patients typically; it is calculated based on clinical data because it is an actual amount of dose prescribed. It has many variations based on different population groups, health systems, and cultures, and beliefs. It should be noted that due to the inherent differences in the way PDD and DDD are calculated, it can produce large discrepancies for the same drugs. Therefore, a good understanding of both methods is important before choosing an appropriate measure suitable for the research question. While PDD reflects more accurate prescribing at the patient level than the DDD, it is still prescribing data and not actual consumption. This distinction is important to acknowledge, especially when studying the medication adherence area of DUR. The research has shown that just because the record of the drug being prescribed does not guarantee that patients actually take it. When studying drug utilization patterns, it is important to understand these measures.

Analytical Considerations

The majority of the DUR is observational (nonexperimental) research. With any observational research, issues such as selection bias, information bias, and confounding are common to deal with in a DUR. Selection bias occurs when a study attempts to compare two groups without the random assignment commonly done in clinical trials. Observational retrospective studies do not have the ability to randomize groups, and therefore it is prone to selection bias. Statistical methods such as multivariable analyses and propensity score approaches can help to mitigate this issue. Confounding is another area where observational studies have a major challenge. Confounding occurs when studying an association between two variables, while the relationship can be explained by a third (confounding) variable. Such variables can be available in the data (measured confounding) and can be added to the analysis to adjust the results. However, the biggest challenge is when confounders are not available (unmeasured confounding) in the data. There is not much that can be done using a statistical adjustment to address it, and therefore, it is tough to establish any causal inference based on observational studies. Given the intricacies, one has to be cautious of the choice of statistical methods and analytical tools. A well-designed study should acknowledge and address these issues from conceptualization to analysis and drawing conclusions.

Expertise Needed to Conduct DUR

As DUR is a highly multidisciplinary and multi-professional field, researchers in this field need to be well versed in multiple areas. A solid foundation of pharmacotherapy, how drugs are classified, their chemical structures, risk, and benefits of various treatments is essential to research in this area. The clinical skills, particularly in clinical pharmacology (appropriate use of drugs, therapeutic guidelines, pharmacotherapy evaluation, etc.), are necessary to understand the process of prescribing, dispensing, and utilizing medications. Along with drug knowledge and clinical skills, it is also helpful to have a good grasp of analytical skills and database research. The DUR is often like a jigsaw puzzle where the puzzle pieces are coming from different data sources. The ability to see the big picture while focusing on details is crucial to leading a DUR project. The DUR often involves various descriptive and analytical methods for quantification. Different metrics and classification systems are often used in DUR, requiring a thorough understanding of biostatistical methods, pharmacoepidemiology methods, and terminology. In addition to quantitative methods and skills, it is also handy to understand qualitative methods. Qualitative techniques such as in-depth interviews, focus groups, purposive sampling, triangulation are used regularly when the DUR is based on primary data.

Due to this field's multidisciplinary nature, it is expected that a DUR project is done by assembling a team of experts in different areas. However, having foundational knowledge of pharmacoepidemiology, biostatistics, and pharmacoeconomics is important to be a part of such teams. This type of research is ideal for someone who is very knowledgeable and skilled in clinical expertise and has an analytical mind and problem-solving ability.

Reporting and Dissemination of DUR

Finally, after conducting analysis and finishing the results, it is important to find an appropriate venue to disseminate these results. Although DUR as a field does not have specific guidelines to report in publish, researchers usually follow the guidelines available for epidemiology and pharmacoepidemiology, which are closely aligned with DUR search guidelines. Examples of such guidelines include the Strengthening the Reporting of Observational Studies in Epidemiology (STROBE)[17] and the ISPE Guidelines for Good Pharmacoepidemiology Practice (GPP).[18] These guidelines provide essential checklists to follow to make sure all the critical components are appropriately addressed. The STROBE checklist provides 22 items detailing various components of the study. Several peer-reviewed journals recommend authors to follow STROBE guidelines while submitting their manuscript, and therefore a clear understanding of these guidelines is very helpful to publish findings successfully. Similarly, GPP also lays out clear directions (section V of the Guidelines) on how to communicate studies in pharmacoepidemiology applicable to DUR.

Exemplar of Learner-Involved DUR Research

As shown in Table 16–3, the study's main objectives were to examine the use of smoking cessation agents in COPD and lung cancer patients and predict the factors associated with the use of these agents among the patients. The hypothesis was whether the utilization of smoking cessation agents is influenced by various sociodemographic factors such as race and ethnicity. The study is a retrospective cohort study. The data used is sourced from the Medical Expenditure Panel Survey (MEPS). This is an example of a study based on a secondary data source. The MEPS data are collected yearly and can provide estimates on access, use, and healthcare expenditures on a national level. The information was extracted from 2006 to 2010 using the full-year consolidated medical conditions and the prescribed medicines files of MEPS. The years were selected because they were the most recent years. Since secondary data analysis, the data collection involved downloading existing data collected and published by AHRQ. A research plan was developed to include a detailed study design, variables needed for research, inclusion/exclusion criteria, and statistical tests to be implemented. The study subjects for this study were identified by using the ICD, Ninth Revision (ICD-9) codes of 490-492 and 162. COPD was defined as chronic bronchitis and emphysema. Asthma was excluded because treatment is different from COPD. Patients who responded to yes in the question, "do you currently smoke?" were considered active smokers and were included and observed. The smoking cessation agents were Chantix, Zyban, Wellbutrin, Budeprion, nicotine patches, and nicotine gums.

TABLE 16-3. EXAMPLE OF LEARNER-INVOLVED STUDY[19]

Research Question	What factors influence the use of smoking cessation agents among patients diagnosed with COPD or lung cancer?
Data source	Medical Expenditure Panel Survey (MEPS)
Key measures	Use of smoking cessation agents. Smoking status. Demographic characteristics associated with use of smoking cessation agents.
Operational definitions	*Smoking status*: Smoking status is based on the response on the MEPS questionnaire regarding current smoking yes/no.
	Use of smoking cessation agents: Smoking cessation agents use is defined based on responses to the prescribed medication file in MEPS. (The smoking cessation agents included all prescription as well as OTC drugs [Chantix, Zyban, Wellbutrin, Budeprion, nicotine transdermal patches, and nicotine gums] classified by Multum therapeutic sub-classification used by MEPS to categorize prescription and nonprescription.)
	COPD or lung cancer patients: COPD and/or lung cancer diagnosis is defined based on the ICD-9 codes for COPD and Lung cancer in MEPS data COPD (ICD-9: 490–492) or lung cancer (ICD-9).
Analysis	Retrospective cross-sectional analysis

Those who responded that they were taking smoking cessation agents were also included. Those who were not taking these agents were labeled as nonusers. A suitable venue to publish the findings was selected to prepare the manuscript and abstract accordingly. The study's primary variable was the utilization of smoking cessation agents by COPD and lung cancer patients who smoke. A theoretical framework called the Andersen Behavioral Model was used to identify prevalent factors that led to non-utilization. According to the model, there are predisposing factors, enabling factors, and need-based factors that determine patient utilization of health services. Predisposing factors are sociocultural characteristics of individuals such as age, gender, race, ethnicity, education, and patient knowledge. Enabling factors are resources were insurance and income. Need-based factors are the perception of a need for services due to problems.

Descriptive statistics were used to obtain the number of patients, their smoking status, and utilization of cessation agents. A logistic regression model was constructed to determine the odds of smoking cessation agents according to characteristics. The research results showed that around 73 million noninstitutionalized persons suffer from COPD, and three million patients with lung cancer during the five-year study period. This was passed on unweighted data on 6,713 individuals with COPD and 256 with lung cancer. The data showed that 15.5 million COPD patients and 400,000 patients were current smokers. Only 8.83% of COPD persons and 12.65% of lung cancer patients were actively taking any forms of smoking cessation agents. Lung cancer patients were found to be mostly male Caucasians from the United States south.

Regression analyses revealed some predictive characteristics among COPD patients. Hispanics showed lower use of cessation agents, which can be supported by healthcare services' underutilization due to language barriers. Rates of quitting among Hispanic youth are low as well. Low utilization was also found in the African American population. Patients with insurance were found to have higher odds of using cessation agents compared to those without insurance. The study underlined the significance of providers' role in opening the conversation about the importance of smoking cessation and its benefits. The study's limitations include the information being from a secondary database, the smoking cessation and agents are self-reported, which may have recall bias and social desirability bias.

Summary and Conclusions

The DUR provides an excellent opportunity to participate in a practice-based research project that has real-world application. It is a multidisciplinary field that focuses on all aspects of drug use by combining expertise from many scientific areas. The use of drugs has evolved into a much complex system, and it will get even more complicated with the advancement of new drug development and the rise of personalized medicine. Rapid growth in technology in the fields of electronic data and advances in computational power are benefiting healthcare. The healthcare landscape is changing fast, providing conducive environments with rich datasets to conduct DUR. DUR is already impacting decisions related to the quality and affordability of healthcare. It is a growing field with much to learn and research.

Key Points and Advice

- DUR focuses on all aspects of drug utilization to improve appropriate and affordable use of drugs.
- DUR studies provide the evidence base to perform drug utilization reviews.
- Getting familiar with database research and understanding healthcare data is beneficial to work on a DUR study.
- Understanding DUR techniques and methodologies can help to conduct better research.
- DUR is a growing field with many possibilities to research and develop new methodologies.

Chapter Review Questions

1. Where did DUR originate, and how it is used in the United States?
2. What is DDD and can it be used to decide prescribing dose for individual patients?

3. What is the difference between DUR and drug utilization review?
4. What are the advantages and disadvantages of using primary versus secondary data sources in DUR?

Online Resources

NIH US National Library of Medicine. Unified Medical Language System (UMLS), SNOMED Clinical Terms. http://www.nlm.nih.gov/research/umls/Snomed/snomed_main.html

International Health Terminology Standards Development Organisation, SNOMED CT https://www.snomed.org/

WHO Collaborating Centre for Drug Statistics Methodology. Use of ATC/DDD. http://www.whocc.no/use_of_atc_ddd/

Academy of Managed Care Pharmacy—Drug Utilization Review https://www.amcp.org/about/managed-care-pharmacy-101/concepts-managed-care-pharmacy/drug-utilization-review

World Health Organization—Drug utilization studies: Methods and uses. https://apps.who.int/iris/handle/10665/260517

REFERENCES

1. Bergman U. The history of the Drug Utilization Research Group in Europe. *Pharmacoepidemiol Drug Saf.* 2006;15(2):95-98.

2. World Health Organization. *Introduction to Drug Utilization Research.* Oslo, Norway: World Health Organization; 2003.

3. World Health Organization. *The Selection of Essential Drugs. Report of a WHO Expert Committee.* World Health Organization; 1977.

4. Wettermark B, Vlahovic-Palcevski V, Salvesen Blix H, Ronning M, Vander Stichele RH. Drug utilization research. In: Hartzema AG, Tilson HH, Chan KA, eds. *Pharmacoepidemiology and Therapeutic Risk Management.* Harvey Whitney Books; 2008.

5. Kubacka RT. A primer on drug utilization review. *J Am Pharm Assoc (Wash).* 1996; NS36(4):257-261, 279.

6. Phillips MS, Gayman JE, Todd MW. ASHP Guidelines on Medication-Use Evaluation. *American Society of Health-system Pharmacists.* 1996;53(16):1953-1955.

7. Centers for Medicare & Medicaid Services (CMS). *Medicare Prescription Drug Benefit Manual.* Baltimore, MA: Centers for Medicare & Medicaid Services; 2008.

8. Donabedian A. The quality of care. How can it be assessed? *JAMA.* 1988;260(12):1743-1748.

9. McDonald KM, Sundaram V, Bravata DM, et al. *Closing the Quality Gap: A Critical Analysis of Quality Improvement Strategies.* Rockville, MD: Agency for Healthcare Research and Quality (US); 2007.

10. Chan M. *Ten Years in Public Health, 2007–2017: Report by Dr Margaret Chan, Director-General.* World Health Organization; 2017.

11. World Health Organization. *Anatomical Therapeutic Chemical (ATC) Classification.* https://www.who.int/tools/atc-ddd-toolkit/atc-classification

12. U.S. Food and Drug Administration. *National Drug Code Directory.* https://www.fda.gov/drugs/drug-approvals-and-databases/national-drug-code-directory

13. Government of Cananda. *Drug Identification Number (DIN).* https://www.canada.ca/en/health-canada/services/drugs-health-products/drug-products/fact-sheets/drug-identification-number.html

14. Wolters Kluwer. *The Medi-Span Generic Product Identifier (GPI).* https://www.wolterskluwer.com/en/solutions/medi-span/about/gpi

15. SNOMED. *SNOMED CT.* https://www.snomed.org/

16. U.S. Food and Drug Administration. *FDA's Global Substance Registration System.* https://www.fda.gov/industry/fda-resources-data-standards/fdas-global-substance-registration-system

17. Vandenbroucke JP, et al. Strengthening the Reporting of Observational Studies in Epidemiology (STROBE): explanation and elaboration. *PLoS Med.* 2007;4(10): e297.

18. Public Policy Committee, I.S.o.P. Guidelines for good pharmacoepidemiology practice (GPP). *Pharmacoepidemiol Drug Saf.* 2016;25(1): 2-10.

19. Vaidya V, et al. Utilization of smoking-cessation pharmacotherapy among chronic obstructive pulmonary disease (COPD) and lung cancer patients. *Curr Med Res Opin.* 2014;30(6):1043-1050.

17

Chapter Seventeen

Pharmacoepidemiology Research

Bryan L. Love, PharmD, MPH, FCCP, BCPS (AQ ID)

Chapter Objectives

- Define pharmacoepidemiology research
- Discuss potential data sources for pharmacoepidemiology research
- Identify common research questions in pharmacoepidemiology research
- Discuss practical considerations for pharmacoepidemiology research
- Identify technical considerations for pharmacoepidemiology research
- Discuss the strategies for harnessing the expertise needed for conducting pharmacoepidemiology research
- Describe an example of learner-involved pharmacoepidemiology research
- Summarize the dissemination framework for pharmacoepidemiology research

Key Terminology

Epidemiology, pharmacoepidemiology, pharmacovigilance, exposure, outcome, confounding, bias

Introduction

In 2020, as the world faced the pandemic related to COVID-19, the disease caused by severe acute respiratory syndrome coronavirus-2 (SARS-CoV-2) infection, the utility of observational research using methods derived from epidemiology was suddenly thrust into the forefront of our global society. **Epidemiology** is the study of the distribution and determinants of health-related states or events in specified populations and the application of this study to control health problems.[1] Within this definition, distribution refers to the frequency and pattern of events that occur in a population, and determinants are factors that influence the occurrence of disease and other health-related events.

Pharmacoepidemiology is a related area of research that uses principles of epidemiology to evaluate pharmaceutical products and services.[2] Typically, these studies evaluate the potential impact of medications or pharmacy services in large populations of patients using methods normally used by epidemiologists. Thus, pharmacoepidemiology lies at the intersection of research focused on pharmaceutical products or services and epidemiology methods of research. A variety of study designs are used to evaluate safety and efficacy related to medications or pharmacy services in large patient populations, including both randomized controlled trials and epidemiology study designs (e.g., cohort, case–control, case–crossover). Pharmacoepidemiology is a growing area of research, and it is one that trainees should be familiar with. This chapter will outline common elements, including typical research questions, practical and technical considerations, and sources of data for pharmacoepidemiology research. In addition, how to identify and harness the expertise needed for conducting this type of research will be addressed. Finally, an example of learner-involved pharmacoepidemiology research will be provided.

Pharmacoepidemiology and Pharmacovigilance

Pharmacoepidemiology research uses various epidemiologic study designs to measure relationships between *exposure* and an *outcome*. Typically, we think of **exposure** as being a receipt of medication, but it can also include the receipt of other types of interventions, such as a service like medication therapy management.[3] An equally important factor is the selection and measurement of the outcome. The **outcome(s)** will vary depending on the research questions but could include the occurrence of a health-related event, laboratory value, or death. Generally, it is not sufficient to collect data on the exposure and outcome only, as the relationship may be influenced or distorted by the presence of other factors termed *confounders*. By definition, a **confounder** is associated with both the exposure and outcome, has unequal distribution between groups being compared, and is not an intermediate step in the causal pathway between the exposure and outcome.[4]

Pharmacovigilance, the science related to the collection, detection, assessment, monitoring, and prevention of adverse events among licensed pharmaceutical products, is a specific type of research that falls under the heading of pharmacoepidemiology. Although the term "*pharmacovigilance*" was not coined until the 1970s, the work of formally investigating and identifying potential drug safety signals began as early as the 1950s.[5] In 1952, the

Food and Drug Administration (FDA) conducted a survey of hospitals, clinics, and medical schools to collect reports of serious and fatal blood dyscrasias, including aplastic anemia associated with chloramphenicol, a newly approved antibiotic derived from *Streptomyces venezuelae*. The value of this systematic approach to drug safety assessment led to legislation known as the Kefauver-Harris Amendments, which established processes used by the FDA to protect the public from unsafe and ineffective medications. Similar pharmacovigilance programs are in place throughout most countries. While pharmacovigilance is a key function of regulatory agencies, it remains a productive area of research for investigators.

Steps in Pharmacoepidemiology Research

The scientific research process for pharmacoepidemiology research is similar to the research process for other types of medical research. The basic steps for pharmacoepidemiology research include the following: (1) pose a research question and hypothesis, (2) select study design and data source, (3) perform data collection and analysis, and (4) prepare a research report. Each step is important and should be guided by a thorough review of the available literature. Ultimately, the research question or hypothesis should guide the research plans, including the selection of a data source and analysis.

DEVELOP A RESEARCH QUESTION OR HYPOTHESIS

An important first step in designing any research study is developing the research question or hypothesis to be examined. Ideally, a question should define the area of interest, identify the uncertainty or knowledge gap, and should be specified prior to beginning any analysis. Research questions often result from ideas garnered from a review of the medical literature, observations from clinical pharmacy practice, policy changes, discussions with mentors, or attendance at meetings or conferences. A well-developed research question can then be transformed into a testable hypothesis or a declarative statement suitable for statistical testing.

The PICOT framework is a recommended way of summarizing research questions that evaluate pharmacotherapy. Population refers to the sample of patients that will be included in the study. Intervention references the specific medication or therapy that is being investigated. Comparison describes the reference group that is used to compare with the intervention. Outcome identifies the expected results and intended measurements to examine differences between the intervention and comparison groups. Time represents the expected duration for follow-up or data collection. Examples of research questions for practice-based pharmacoepidemiology research using a PICOT framework are provided in Table 17–1.

TABLE 17–1. EXAMPLES OF PHARMACOEPIDEMIOLOGY RESEARCH QUESTIONS

Research Question	Population	Intervention	Comparison	Outcome	Time
What is the association between antidepressant used in early pregnancy and risk of congenital heart defects in young children?[6]	Danish mothers with singleton live births between 1995 and 2008 from the Danish Medical Birth Registry	Maternal prescription fill for SSRI prescription within the first trimester of pregnancy	Children whose mothers did not have SSRI prescription fill during the first trimester	Diagnosis of congenital heart defects according to ICD-10 coding	Development of outcome within the first five years of life
What are patient-level predictors for overuse of medications with sedative–hypnotic properties among U.S. Medicare beneficiaries?[7]	Fee-for-service US Medicare beneficiaries aged >65 years	High monthly drug burden index, a measure of a medication regimen's anticholinergic and sedative properties	Comparison: Low anticholinergic and sedative properties as measured by the drug burden index	Association between patient characteristics and high monthly drug burden index	Temporal changes in the drug burden index from January 2013 to December 2016
What is the impact of a community pharmacy-based transitions of care program on hospital readmission rates?[8]	Adults (> 18 years) hospitalized with primary diagnosis of congestive heart failure, chronic obstructive pulmonary disease, or pneumonia were recruited.	Medication therapy management appointment with a trained pharmacist following hospital discharge	Usual care following hospital discharge	Pharmacist interventions, medication-related problems, 30-day hospital readmission, patient satisfaction	Patients were recruited between April 2012 and June 2013; the intervention took place within three to seven days following hospital discharge

International Classification of Diseases, Tenth Revision (ICD-10) and Selective Serotonin Reuptake Inhibitor (SSRI)

STUDY DESIGN

A variety of study designs are used in pharmacoepidemiology research to answer research questions of interest. The two most common observational study designs are cohort and case–control studies. The companion textbook reviews these in more detail, but the primary difference in these study designs is the timing of when exposure and outcome are determined. In a cohort study, the exposure is determined first, and individuals are followed over time to see if they experience the outcome of interest. Conversely, in case–control studies, individuals are assessed for the presence of the outcome of interest first. An important determination for case–control studies is whether to use incident or prevalent cases. Incident cases are newly diagnosed during the defined time period. In contrast, prevalent cases include both newly diagnosed and existing patients with the outcome. Typically, incident cases are preferred to limit issues with recall bias and to avoid issues assessing the temporal sequence of exposure and outcome. Controls that did not have the outcome are then selected from the same population, and both cases and controls are retrospectively assessed to determine if they have a drug exposure.

Case–control studies are efficient when studying rare outcomes, quicker and less expensive to conduct, and usually require fewer subjects which can be advantageous for pharmacy learner-based studies. A key limitation with case–control studies is that they are prone to biases, particularly selection biases, which are discussed in more detail later in this chapter. The selection of controls from the same source population is an important consideration that deserves special attention during the planning process. If the source population that gave rise to cases is not the same population used for the selection of controls, it is likely that the estimates of the association between exposure and outcome will be biased.

Cohort studies are described as prospective or retrospective based upon when the exposure and outcome are assessed. Prospective cohort studies are dependent on screening, enrollment, and follow-up at regular intervals from exposure to the development of the outcome of interest. Thus, prospective cohort studies are usually not feasible for pharmacy learner research projects due to time constraints. Retrospective cohort studies conducted with existing data or specimens offer advantages inherent in cohort designs while shortening the time to complete the study. Other advantages of cohort studies include the ability to directly estimate risk, the ability to study multiple outcomes from one exposure, and decreased potential for biases.

DATA COLLECTION AND ANALYSIS

Data Sources

A variety of data sources are available to examine research questions in the field of pharmacoepidemiology. Data sources differ greatly based upon their intended use, patient population, variables available, and the longitudinal nature of data. In many cases, data sources are repurposed for research purposes, which creates advantages and disadvantages that the research team needs to consider. Examples of repurposed data sources include administrative databases, such as pharmacy dispensing records, which are primarily used for billing of medical services, and electronic health records (EHRs), which are primarily used for clinical documentation and patient care.[9] The largest limitation of these data sources is that they were not purposefully designed to capture data that may be necessary to answer a research question. Ultimately, the choice of data source for research purposes will depend on the specific research question, availability of data, study design, and advantages/limitations of the data source.[10] Guidance for the selection of a data source is available and endorsed by the International Society for Pharmacoepidemiology (ISPE). These guidelines discuss issues related to database selection, linking multiple databases, extraction and analysis, privacy and security, quality and validation procedures, and documentation for reproducibility of results.[11]

Administrative Databases

Administrative or claims databases are data sources that capture the extent of an individual's use of the healthcare system. Although this is primarily used for medical reimbursement for a submitted claim, these data repositories have also been used for pharmacoepidemiology research. These data have been evaluated extensively for validity (did the individual receive the medication according to what is recorded in the claims file?) and, therefore, are considered an excellent source of drug exposure data for research. Likewise, administrative databases are available for medical claims, including outpatient visits, hospitalization, procedures, and other ancillary care (e.g., home health, nursing homes). Typically, these administrative claims have specific coding formats, such as International Classification of Diseases, Tenth Revision (ICD-10), or Diagnosis Related Group methodology, to standardize within and across similar databases. For prescription claims, the biggest limitations are: (1) claims indicate that the medication was obtained, but there are no assurances that the medication was taken as prescribed, and (2) over-the-counter (OTC) medications are frequently not included as claims. For medical claims, the biggest limitation is that claims can vary by provider resulting incomplete or inaccurate diagnoses provided. Nonetheless, administrative claims represent a common source of data for pharmacoepidemiology research.

Electronic Health Records

Electronic health records (EHRs) represent longitudinal patient health data obtained and populated during the normal provision of clinical patient care. EHRs contain a variety of data elements useful for practice-based research, including: demographics, vital statistics, administrative data, medication profile information, clinical notes, and laboratory data. EHRs are ideal data sources for pharmacoepidemiology studies, including observational, pharmacovigilance, and clinical research.[12] The extent of data contained within EHRs will vary significantly, so the researcher will need to do their homework to ensure the EHR being considered contains the relevant data to answer their specific research question(s). Gaining access to an EHR would require approvals, which could be facilitated with input from mentors or collaborators.

Drug/Disease Registries

Similar to EHRs, registries are a potential data source for practice-based research. A registry is a postmarketing database designed to evaluate and improve outcomes for patients with a specific disease or patients with similar exposure, such as medications. Researchers can use these data to answer questions that evaluate certain treatments for a disease or how patients with specific characteristics respond to the treatment. This is important since Phase II/III studies used for regulatory approval often exclude patients with severe chronic conditions. A partial listing of registries is available in the Online Resources section of this chapter.

Randomized Clinical Trial Data Repositories

Randomized clinical trials (RCTs) are widely regarded as the gold standard for effectiveness studies involving medications. In addition, they are informative regarding common adverse events, but may not be large enough or of sufficient duration to detect rare or long-term adverse events. The planning, recruitment, and analysis of RCTs can take years to accomplish, so in most cases, these are not ideal for learner-directed mentored research projects. However, data generated through RCTs can be made available to researchers through an approval process and signed data use agreements (DUAs) for post-hoc research. Depending on the research question, these data sources may be considered for practice-based research involving students or residents. An example of research conducted using completed RCT data evaluated the effectiveness of a five-day course of levofloxacin for complicated urinary tract infections among males.[13] Additionally, these investigators have described their experience, which may be helpful for researchers considering this approach.[14]

Surveys/Questionnaires

Surveys are another option for learner-directed practice-based pharmacoepidemiology research. Although some surveys are longitudinal, most are considered cross-sectional or a snapshot in time. As a result, surveys have the advantage of efficiently assessing the prevalence of drug use in a population, both from a time and financial perspective. The main limitation of surveys is that due to their cross-sectional design, it is not possible to determine causal relationships because it is impossible to know whether the exposure preceded the outcome.

National health surveys such as the National Health and Nutrition Examination Survey (NHANES) are available to researchers at no cost. NHANES contains data on demographics, medical conditions, medications, physical examination, diet, labs, and other questionnaires. Surveys such as NHANES use complex, multistage, probability sampling designs to select participants' representative of the civilian, noninstitutionalized U.S. population. These surveys also oversample certain population subgroups to increase the reliability and precision of estimates for these subgroups. This complex sampling design requires specifying the sampling design parameters to analyze and interpret results appropriately. Additional information about NHANES, including data and tutorials, are available in the Online Resources section of this chapter.

Ad hoc Data Collection

An additional source of data for practice-based research includes ad hoc data, which can be considered as any data collected and curated by the research team specifically for the purpose of addressing one or more research questions. This could include collecting the entire data set or a specific variable that is missing from available data sources. The advantage of ad hoc data collection is that the research team can customize and often obtain variables that are not readily available through other data sources (e.g., administrative), but often this comes at the expense of additional time and effort to manually collect the data.

TABLE 17–2. COMMON DATA SOURCES FOR PHARMACOEPIDEMIOLOGY RESEARCH

Data Source	Advantages	Limitations
Administrative data	Potential for complete longitudinal data	Available data dependent on frequency of healthcare use
	Comprehensive medication coverage	Missing hospital and OTC medications
	Potential for large populations	
Electronic health records	Potential for complete longitudinal data	Available data dependent on frequency of healthcare use
	Often contains laboratory data	Medication profile represents prescribed, not filled prescriptions and OTC medications
	Potential for large populations	

Practical Considerations

TIME AND FUNDING

Time is often a primary consideration for pharmacy learner-based research since the goal for most is to complete the project while the student or resident is involved in their training program. For most pharmacy learner projects, funding is usually not needed. Although funding may not be required, the process of applying for and obtaining funding is an opportunity for pharmacy learners to gain additional experience in this area of the research process.

Time: The expression "time waits for no one" is especially true in the context of learner-directed practice-based research. For this reason, it is important to consider the scope of the project and ensure that the project can be completed in the time that is available. Fortunately, high-quality practice-based pharmacoepidemiology research studies are often completed in a short period of time, provided data are readily available. In the early stages of the research planning process, it is important to develop a realistic timeline to guide research activities through discussions with your mentor or research team. It is important to consider various steps, including literature review, development of a research question or hypotheses, development of the study protocol, submission for ethics review, obtaining data, analysis, interpretation of results, and dissemination of the study findings. Each of these steps takes time to accomplish and can vary among projects. It is recommended to build in additional time, when possible, to account for unexpected delays that can occur throughout the research process.

Funding: A second practical consideration is whether funding is needed to execute the research project. Learners should discuss with their project mentor whether funds are needed to support the project, potential sources of funding, and contingency plans if funding is not awarded. Examples of typical allowable uses of funding include obtaining data, compensating study personnel, or offsetting expenses related to the dissemination of the research. The funding source typically provides guidance on allowable expenses. Potential sources of funding for practice-based research include professional organizations, foundations, and other institutional sources.

ACCESS TO DATA SOURCES

Gaining access to data sources is a critical step in the execution of any pharmacoepidemiology study. The data source and study design should be complementary, and together, they should offer the best chance to answer the research question being considered. In most cases, student learners will need to work with their primary mentor to identify data sources available for the project. The most common data sources available to students, along with advantages and limitations, are listed in Table 17–2. In some cases, primary mentors may already have access to and experience with these data sources, which can expedite the research process. In order to use these data sources, many data providers require users to sign a DUA, which may include a description of the project, listing of data elements requested, security measures to protect data, confidentiality statements, any fees, and any terms of use, such as disclosure upon publication.

Regardless of which data source is chosen, the team will need to gain approval from the Institutional Review Board (IRB), which has the responsibility for ensuring that the privacy of individual research participants is not violated. Of particular importance for the IRB is the disclosure and use of protected health information (PHI), established by the Health Insurance Portability and Accountability Act (HIPAA). HIPAA establishes certain protections of privacy and confidentiality of health records and establishes conditions, including research, where PHI may be used or disclosed. This rule requires that participants be informed and agree to the disclosure of individually identifiable PHI. However, in most pharmacoepidemiology projects where existing deidentified data are used, a HIPAA waiver of authorization can be granted.

GOOD PHARMACOEPIDEMIOLOGY PRACTICES

The goal of pharmacoepidemiology studies is to provide important evidence of the effects of healthcare products and services in large populations. The ISPE publishes guidelines for Good Pharmacoepidemiology Practice (GPP) intended to aid researchers with matters related to planning, conduct, and interpretation of pharmacoepidemiology research.[15] The GPP addresses the following areas: protocol development, responsibilities of study personnel, study conduct, communication, adverse event reporting, and archiving.[15] All students considering a pharmacoepidemiology project are encouraged to carefully review this guideline document during the project planning stage.

DEVELOPMENT OF STUDY PROTOCOL

It is important that every study have a protocol developed to outline important facets of the research process. The GPP addresses specific areas in the research process, including protocol development, responsibilities, personnel, study conduct (human subjects protection; data collection, management, and verification; data analysis), reporting results, and communication of study findings.[15] An outline of important protocol contents with applicable descriptions is available to ensure important elements of the proposal are not overlooked. Your local IRB may also have template documents that can assist in the development of the study protocol.

OPERATIONALIZING EXPOSURE AND OUTCOME

It is very important in pharmacoepidemiology research to clearly define variables, particularly exposure, outcome, and key confounding variables. For example, if we are concerned with opioid use and overdose among young adults, then we need to clearly define each term. Thus, you would need to define the age range for young adults, how overdose is defined, and how opioid use is determined. The exposure, opioid use, could be operationalized as current, past, or any opioid use based on pharmacy prescription claims during a period of time. Often the standardized sources such as American Hospital Formulary Service or Micromedex are used to define and list all opioids. The dosing considerations may also require standardization-based morphine milligram equivalents or defined daily dose. Each of these exposure definitions would lead to different interpretations of the study's findings. Likewise, the definition of the outcome variable can influence the study's results and interpretation. In pharmacoepidemiology research, a systematic and standardized way of reporting diseases and health conditions, the ICD-10, is frequently used to define health outcomes. In the opioid example, there are codes available for opioid use disorder and poisoning due to opioids. Depending on the research question, either or both codes could be used to operationalize the outcome. Student learners should work closely with their mentor and other team members to determine whether the proposed variables are accurate measures of the exposure, outcomes, and confounders to answer the proposed research question.

Technical Considerations

SAMPLE SIZE CONSIDERATIONS

Extensive and technical reviews of power and sample size are available elsewhere and can be applied to pharmacoepidemiology studies. Formulas and calculators are available in textbooks or online to assist in estimates of sample sizes needed for the most common study designs (case–control and cohort) used in pharmacoepidemiology studies.[16] Since some pharmacoepidemiology studies use very large sample sizes, some additional considerations are often made. In every study, the research team will need to make decisions about the study significance level and power. By convention, a significance level or α of 0.05 or less is used for most medical research. Often, a more stringent α-level of 0.01 or even 0.001 may be used as the threshold for statistical significance when exceptionally large sample sizes are used. The threshold for power is customarily set at least 0.8, but in certain circumstances, such as when large sample sizes are expected, a higher value of 0.9 may be preferred. The magnitude of the effect (e.g., odds ratio) and variance expected in the measured outcome variable are important determinants to calculate sample size and power. Although the magnitude of the outcome is unlikely to be affected directly by very large sample sizes, a more precise measure of the outcome, as indicated by less variance, can be expected when very large samples are used.

BIAS AND APPROACHES TO MINIMIZE BIAS

The goal of pharmacoepidemiology research is to estimate drug effects on a particular outcome, but this can be met with many challenges as multiple factors can impact drug exposure and the outcome of interest. If not recognized and addressed appropriately, these factors can introduce measurement error into the study results. For example, the presence of a certain indication or comorbidity may predict drug exposure. Likewise, the degree of medication adherence can potentially impact the extent of drug exposure, which could affect the outcome. When an estimate of drug exposure on the disease does not represent the true effect of the exposure on disease outcome, this is called bias. There are different types of bias broadly categorized into three nonmutually exclusive types: (1) *selection bias*, (2) *information bias*, and (3) *confounding*. Bias can be introduced during the design phase or occur during the analysis phase of a research study. Common types of biases that occur are briefly described below, but the reader is referred to the companion textbook, an epidemiology text, or other medical literature for a more in-depth discussion.[17]

Selection Bias

Selection bias occurs when there is a distortion of the true estimate of effect due to how study participants are selected, categorized, or retained throughout the study. Specific types of selection bias that are commonly encountered in pharmacoepidemiology research include prevalence bias, referral bias, protopathic bias, and censoring/missing data. Prevalence bias occurs when study participants are counted as having the outcome of interest when it was present prior to study initiation or exposure. Referral biases occur when the study participants are not representative of the population of interest. For example, studying the incidence of gastrointestinal bleeding associated with celecoxib among hospitalized patients may overestimate the incidence of bleeding compared to an ambulatory or outpatient population. Protopathic bias describes a situation where "an exposure was started, stopped, or changed because of the baseline manifestation caused by a disease or other outcome event." Type of bias is of particular importance in pharmacoepidemiology research since drug exposure can change over time and diseases attributed to the exposure may be identified much later. Finally, missing data are problematic in pharmacoepidemiology studies since multivariable analyses, including regression models, usually eliminate observations that are missing values for a variable included in the specified model. This has the potential to create biased estimates as the analytical sample may not represent the true population due to missing data.

Methods to adjust for selection bias in pharmacoepidemiology research include statistical methods such as covariate adjustment, inverse probability weighting (IPW), and sensitivity analyses. In cases where we can measure or determine factors that affect the exposure, or an individual's decision to participate, including these parameters in the statistical model, can reduce selection bias. Therefore, the measurement and adjusting of covariates are especially important in pharmacoepidemiology research. The IPW is a statistical technique that calculates the probability of being selected into the study for each individual and applies a weight equal to the inverse of the selection probability into the analysis. The IPW allows each participant to account for themselves but also for nonparticipants with similar characteristics. Sensitivity analyses are a common method to check for and control for bias if it cannot be mitigated by other methods. These can include the evaluation of the robustness of the study findings using multiple statistical approaches or study designs.

Information Bias

Information bias, sometimes referred to as measurement bias, results in a distortion in the measure of association caused by inaccurate measurements of study variables. This is a major concern when key variables, such as exposure, outcome, or confounding variables, are inaccurately measured, classified, or missing. For example, after a study is completed, you discover that the scale used to measure study participants' weight is inaccurate, resulting in weight measurements that are 5 to 10 pounds lower than the true value. In a study where weight or body mass index (derived from weight and height) are key variables, either exposure, outcome, or confounder, this could significantly bias the study results. Similarly, since medication records are often used to classify patients as exposed or unexposed in observational studies, incomplete or inaccurate records could result in misclassification of participants. When information bias occurs, it is important to consider whether the bias is equal among all participants, referred to as *nondifferential misclassification,* or if only one exposure group was affected, termed *differential misclassification.* The type of misclassification, whether differential or nondifferential, can assist the research team in determining how the bias may impact the overall results. Information bias can be difficult to detect in practice. Careful planning and execution during the research process may minimize bias. Measurement error may not be completely eliminated due to imperfect algorithms or lack of information to correctly classify individuals inherent in observational research. Specific techniques to minimize information bias may depend on the specific type of information bias anticipated. However, examples of strategies can include conducting validation studies, propensity score calibration studies, sensitivity analyses, or multiple imputations for missing data.[18,19]

Confounding Bias

Confounding is a special type of bias occurring between exposure and outcome due to a third variable referred to as a *confounder*. Confounding can occur with any study design, so identification of potential confounders is an important consideration for protocol development and database selection. As mentioned previously, potential confounding variables must meet specific criteria to be considered a confounder:

1. The potential confounder must be associated with the outcome of interest, either increasing or decreasing the risk of the outcome occurring. In other words, the confounding variable should influence the occurrence of the outcome in the absence of the exposure variable under study.
2. Second, the potential confounder should be associated with the exposure of interest but should not occur because of the exposure.
3. Finally, the potential confounder should not exist on the causal pathway (or be an intermediary step) between exposure and outcome.

Identification of potential confounders is important because, unlike other types of bias, confounders can be adjusted for during the analysis phase. Examples of analytic methods include multivariable regression and propensity score methods, including matching, weighting, stratification, or adjustment.[19] In the section that follows, we will review a relatively new method of graphically identifying potential confounders that require statistical adjustment.

INTRODUCTION TO DIRECTED ACYCLIC GRAPHS

Directed acyclic graphs (DAGs) are hypothesized causal diagrams increasingly used in epidemiology studies to describe relationships between important variables and to identify confounding. They are best utilized in the planning stage to make decisions about how to resolve confounding through statistical adjustment. We will use the example (Figure 17–1) to introduce some terminology and concepts related to DAGs for pharmacoepidemiology research. For a more detailed explanation of DAGs, the reader is referred elsewhere.[4]

The term *"directed"* indicates that all variables in the diagram are connected by arrows. Arrows in DAGs indicate direct causal effects between two factors, and this effect can be either protective or harmful. Arrows are mono-directional, indicating that one factor causes the other based upon prior knowledge. *Mediator* variables are variables that lie in the causal pathway as an intermediate variable between the exposure and outcome. A *collider* is a variable that is associated with two variables, and when graphed, the arrows appear to collide.

Paths in a DAG figure are sequences of arrows that connect the exposure and outcome being studied along with other variables associated with the exposure and outcome. *Direct paths* include those variables where all arrows point from the exposure to the outcome. DAGs are *acyclic* because paths cannot form a "loop." In other words, one cannot start with a variable, follow its direct path, and return to the original variable. *Backdoor paths* are those where the arrow from a factor points back to the exposure variable. Paths are considered "closed" if they contain a collider variable or if the statistical adjustment is applied appropriately to a confounder. If not appropriately addressed, open backdoor paths can introduce bias into the study results.

As mentioned previously, confounding, as indicated by open backdoor paths, can be addressed via statistical adjustment, also called conditioning. There are many methods of statistical adjustment to account for confounding, including stratification, restriction, matching, IPW, and multivariable adjustment. The decision about *how* to adjust for confounding depends on the research question and assessing the pros and cons of each approach. More importantly, the decision on *which* variables to condition on deserves great attention. Many researchers attempt to adjust for all potential variables; however, traditional statistical procedures that adjust for mediators (excluding mediation analysis) and colliders are an important source of bias. Alternatively, it is suggested to adjust for the minimally sufficient set of variables: all covariates that, when adjusted

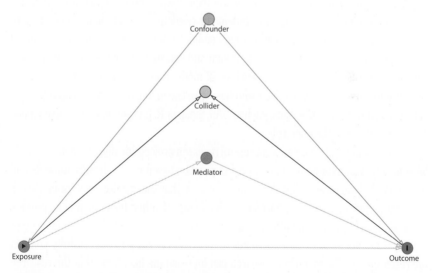

Figure 17–1. Example directed acyclic graph displaying the relationship between exposure, outcome, and other important variables. In this figure, there are four possible paths: (1) exposure, outcome; (2) exposure, mediator, outcome; (3) exposure, collider, outcome; and (4) exposure, confounder, outcome. This final path which includes the variable "confounder" is an open backdoor path, meets the criteria for a confounder, and should be adjusted using statistical methods appropriate to the study.

for, block all backdoor paths, but include no more or fewer covariates than needed. In the example provided, the minimally sufficient adjustment set includes only the "confounder" variable.

Needed Expertise

Team-based research has been responsible for some of the greatest scientific discoveries in the modern era. One need not look any further than the discovery, development, and distribution of mRNA vaccines to prevent COVID-19 infection within one year after the discovery of the virus. Many interdisciplinary teams have quickly been formed to address issues related to the testing, treatment, or consequences of SARS-CoV-2 infection. Although individual work can be more convenient, recent trends indicate an increase in team-based research due to significant advantages. For instance, team members from different scientific disciplines bring with them their unique perspective and complementary knowledge.

It is recommended that learners include personnel in their team to assist them in the planning, design, execution, analysis, and reporting of their research. It is suggested that team members with the following roles or expertise be considered for practice-based pharmacoepidemiology research by students or residents: project mentor, one or more clinicians familiar with the medications and condition under investigation, and personnel with experience in epidemiology study design and statistical methods. Since pharmacoepidemiology research involves the analysis of medications in large groups of people, it is critical to have someone involved who has expertise in extracting and analyzing large datasets with statistical programs, such as SAS, Stata, or R. It is possible that a team member can satisfy more than one role.

A project mentor is vital to a successful research project. Ideally, the mentor should be someone with experience in conducting practice-based research with students and residents. Although desirable, it is not necessary that the mentor have prior experience with epidemiology or pharmacoepidemiology if other team members possess these skills. The project mentor can assist students or residents in identifying other key team members with the experience and skills necessary to successfully conduct the research. Finally, mentored research can increase the likelihood that the research is impactful, resulting in the development of scholarly deliverables, including abstracts and published manuscripts.[20] Personnel with education, training, or experience in epidemiology methods are helpful for all aspects of study execution, including interpretation of the study findings. In addition, team members with statistical experience, particularly with the planned analysis, are recommended. Ideally, team members with epidemiology and statistical experience should be involved early in the planning process to avoid methodological issues and identify potential data sources necessary to answer the research question.

Dissemination of Pharmacoepidemiology Research

There are a variety of ways to disseminate relevant findings from pharmacoepidemiology research. These include presentations of research via abstracts and posters at local, regional, or national conferences. Additionally, publication in a peer-reviewed journal is another common dissemination format. For pharmacy residents, submission of a publication-quality final project report is a requirement of most accredited residency programs.

Historically, reporting of observational studies has been suboptimal, limiting the ability to understand key elements of the methodology used. This can lead to an inability to replicate studies and can explain disparate results between similar studies. Guidelines representing best practices for reporting observational studies using routinely collected health data have been developed to encourage complete and accurate reporting of research. These guidelines have evolved over time, and now there are several guidelines to assist researchers in sharing their study results. The STrengthening the Reporting of OBservational (STROBE) statement and Epidemiology checklists provide guidance based upon the type of study design used and is often required to be submitted along with a manuscript under consideration for many journals.[21] The REporting of studies Conducted using Observational Routinely collected Data (RECORD) was also developed to improve the dissemination of study results. Newer guidance, RECORD-PE (RECORD-PharmacoEpidemiology) was developed to improve the reporting of pharmacoepidemiology research, specifically.[22,23] RECORD-PE shares many similarities and many key improvements over prior guidance. One key aspect is the recommendation to include figures to illustrate important study design features such as exposure, washout periods, observation periods, and when covariates are determined. Additional guidance is provided on specifying how the drug exposure is operationalized and specifying the data sources used for drug exposure. RECORD-PE stresses the importance of defining the time window(s) when patients are considered exposed and how drug exposure is classified (e.g., current, prior, ever, or cumulative drug exposure). In addition, it is important to describe how individuals with more than one drug exposure are handled, as this can impact the interpretation of the study findings. A description of the health system where data are obtained should be included, especially as formulary restrictions may limit drug exposure between the target medication and comparators. It is highly recommended, and in many cases, it is required, that these checklists be used to ensure accurate and complete dissemination of research. Whenever possible, it is recommended to use the RECORD-PE guidance as it captures nuances in the reporting of pharmacoepidemiology-based research.

Exemplar of Learner-Involved Pharmacoepidemiology Research

Below is an example of a learner-involved pharmacoepidemiology research project. This project was conducted by a student who had prior knowledge and experience with epidemiology research. However, there are opportunities to participate in similar types of research without prior knowledge or experience.

Sepsis is a major public health problem affecting approximately 1.7 million adults in the United States each year. Sepsis is associated with prolonged length-of-stay (LOS), nearly 300,000 deaths, and accounts for more than $27 billion in total hospital costs annually. Hydroxymethylglutaryl-CoA (HMG CoA) reductase inhibitors, or statins, are primarily used for their potent cholesterol effects, but they also possess significant immunomodulatory and anti-inflammatory effects thought to be beneficial in patients with sepsis.[24] A brief description of the study in PICOT format is provided in Table 17-3. The major research question to be addressed was: In patients with sepsis requiring ICU care, does concomitant HMG-CoA reductase inhibitors, known as "statins," affect mortality and ICU LOS?

This study used data from adults within the Medical Information Mart for Intensive Care-III database, a large, freely available database comprising deidentified health-related data associated with over 40,000 patients who stayed in critical care units of the Beth Israel Deaconess Medical Center between 2001 and 2012. The receipt of statins (exposure) was determined from prescription records, and the outcome variables (mortality and LOS) were determined using medical records.

TABLE 17-3. EXAMPLE OF LEARNER-INVOLVED PHARMACOEPIDEMIOLOGY RESEARCH

Population	Adults admitted to intensive care unit (ICU) Beth Israel Deaconess Medical Center diagnosed with sepsis
Intervention	Receipt of statin prescription prior to ICU admission
Comparison	Patients without statin prescription prior to ICU admission
Outcomes	The two major outcomes of interest were ICU length-of-stay and 30-day ICU mortality
Time	The study considered patients admitted between 2001 and 2012

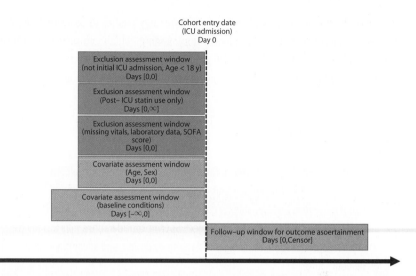

Figure 17–2. Graphical depiction of study design for pharmacoepidemiology research by a student learner.

We chose a retrospective cohort study, depicted in Figure 17–2, due to the importance of determining the temporal association between statin exposure and the development of the outcomes of interest. We did not pursue funding because the data were freely available, and it may have delayed the timeline for our project. The team included a graduate student, two research faculty, a statistician, and a clinical pharmacist with epidemiology training. In retrospect, it would have been ideal to include a critical care physician on the team. We took several steps to minimize bias and confounding in the study, including the selection of retrospective cohort study design. In addition, we used statistical methods, including multivariable regression and augmented IPW, to adjust for potential confounders.

Summary and Conclusions

Well-designed and executed pharmacoepidemiology research studies are increasingly being used to investigate pharmacy practice-based research questions. The PICOT framework is a recommended method to summarize research questions evaluating pharmacotherapy. Multiple data sources are available, and a variety of research methods can be used depending on the research question. A team-based approach with clinicians and researchers with epidemiology and/or biostatistics expertise is used for most successful pharmacoepidemiology research projects. Selection, information, and confounding biases are common threats to the validity of observational epidemiology research methods. DAGs are causal diagrams increasingly used in epidemiology studies to describe relationships between important variables and identify confounding, which can be resolved through statistical adjustment. The RECORD-PE guidance is a useful template for dissemination of results as it captures nuances in the reporting of pharmacoepidemiology-based research.

Key Points and Advice

- Pharmacoepidemiology is an area of research that uses principles of epidemiology to evaluate pharmaceutical products and services.
- Various data sources are available for pharmacoepidemiology research, but the choice of the data source will depend on the project. Specific considerations may include the specific research question, availability of data, study design, and advantages/limitations of the data source.
- Assembling a team with the needed expertise is a critical step when considering pharmacoepidemiology research. Student/resident learners should work with their mentor(s) to identify the expertise needed for their project.
- Selection, information, and confounding biases are major threats to the validity of non-randomized observational studies. DAGs offer a way to visualize relationships among variables and identify those that require statistical adjustment.

Chapter Review Questions

1. Identify three examples of pharmacoepidemiology studies from the recent literature.
2. Develop a pharmacoepidemiology research question using the PICOTS framework related to a topic of interest.
3. List potential data sources to address the research question. What are some advantages and disadvantages of each data source?
4. Select an appropriate epidemiology research study design and operationalize the exposure and outcomes for the research question.
5. Develop a DAG for exposure, outcome, and confounding variables planned for the research question.
6. Define the following terms:
   Selection bias
   Information bias
   Confounding bias

Online Resources

- National Institutes of Health listing of registries. https://www.nih.gov/health-information/nih-clinical-research-trials-you/list-registries
- National Health and Nutrition Examination Survey. https://www.cdc.gov/nchs/nhanes/index.htm
- International Society for Pharmacoepidemiology (ISPE). https://www.pharmacoepi.org
- Guidelines for Good Pharmacoepidemiology Practices. https://www.pharmacoepi.org/resources/policies/guidelines-08027/#1
- Developing a Protocol for Observational Comparative Effectiveness Research. https://effectivehealthcare.ahrq.gov/sites/default/files/related_files/user-guide-observational-cer-130113.pdf
- The REporting of studies Conducted using Observational Routinely-collected health Data (RECORD) Statement for Pharmacoepidemiology (RECORD-PE). https://www.pharmacoepi.org/pub/?id=1C8302DA-ACEA-29B1-7005-3CB91F9BCDDE
- Guidelines for Good Database Selection and use in Pharmacoepidemiology Research. https://www.pharmacoepi.org/pub/?id=1c2a306e-2354-d714-5127-9fd12e69fa66

REFERENCES

1. Last JM. (Ed.) *A Dictionary of Epidemiology*. 4th ed. New York: Oxford University Press; 2001.
2. Ferguson MC, Behnen EMT. Introduction to drug literature. In: Aparasu RR, Bentley JP, eds. *Principles of Research Design and Drug Literature Evaluation*. 2nd ed. New York: McGraw Hill Education; 2020.
3. Bluml BM. Definition of medication therapy management: development of professionwide consensus. *J Am Pharm Assoc*. 2005 Sep-Oct;45(5):566-572.
4. Roy J, Mitra N. Measured and accounted-for confounding in pharmacoepidemiologic studies: some thoughts for practitioners. *Pharmacoepidemiol Drug Saf*. 2021 Mar;30(3): 277-282.
5. Beninger P. Pharmacovigilance: an Overview. *Clin Ther*. 2018 Dec;40(12):1991-2004.
6. Sun Y, Pedersen LH, Wu CS, Petersen I, Sorensen HT, Olsen J. Antidepressant use during pregnancy and risk of congenital heart defects: a case-time-control study. *Pharmacoepidemiol Drug Saf*. 2019 Sep;28(9):1180-1193.
7. Shmuel S, Pate V, Pepin MJ, et al. Quantifying cumulative anticholinergic and sedative drug load among US Medicare beneficiaries. *Pharmacoepidemiol Drug Saf*. 2021 Feb;30(2):144-156.
8. Luder HR, Frede SM, Kirby JA, et al. TransitionRx: impact of community pharmacy post-discharge medication therapy management on hospital readmission rate. *J Am Pharm Assoc*. 2015 May-Jun;55(3):246-254.
9. Trevisan M, Fu EL, Xu Y, et al. Pharmacoepidemiology for nephrologists (part 1): concept, applications and considerations for study design. *Clin Kidney J*. 2021 May;14(5):1307-1316.

10. Hennessy S. Use of health care databases in pharmacoepidemiology. *Basic Clin Pharmacol Toxicol.* 2006 Mar;98(3):311-313.

11. Hall GC, Sauer B, Bourke A, Brown JS, Reynolds MW, LoCasale R. Guidelines for good database selection and use in pharmacoepidemiology research. *Pharmacoepidemiol Drug Saf.* 2012 Jan;21(1):1-10.

12. Cowie MR, Blomster JI, Curtis LH, et al. Electronic health records to facilitate clinical research. *Clin Res Cardiol.* 2017 Jan;106(1):1-9.

13. Mospan GA, Wargo KA. 5-Day versus 10-day course of fluoroquinolones in outpatient males with a urinary tract infection (UTI). *J Am Board Fam Med.* 2016 Nov 12;29(6):654-662.

14. Mospan GA, Wargo KA. Researchers' experience with clinical data sharing. *J Am Board Fam Med.* 2016 Nov 12;29(6):805-807.

15. Ispe. Guidelines for good pharmacoepidemiology practices (GPP). *Pharmacoepidemiol Drug Saf.* 2008 Feb;17(2):200-208.

16. Aparasu R, Bentley J. *Principles of Research Design and Drug Literature Evaluation.* 2nd ed. New York: McGraw Hill; 2020.

17. Prada-Ramallal G, Takkouche B, Figueiras A. Bias in pharmacoepidemiologic studies using secondary health care databases: a scoping review. *BMC Med Res Methodol.* 2019 Mar 11;19(1):53.

18. Althubaiti A. Information bias in health research: definition, pitfalls, and adjustment methods. *J Multidiscip Healthc.* 2016;9:211-217.

19. Fu EL, van Diepen M, Xu Y, et al. Pharmacoepidemiology for nephrologists (part 2): potential biases and how to overcome them. *Clin Kidney J.* 2021 May;14(5):1317-1326.

20. Osborne KW, Woods KM, Maxwell WD, McGee K, Bookstaver PB. Outcomes of student-driven, faculty-mentored research and impact on postgraduate training and career selection. *Am J Pharm Educ.* 2018 May;82(4):6246.

21. von Elm E, Altman DG, Egger M, et al. The strengthening the reporting of observational studies in epidemiology (STROBE) statement: guidelines for reporting observational studies. *Ann Intern Med.* 2007 Oct 16;147(8):573-577.

22. Harron K, Benchimol E, Langan S. Using the RECORD guidelines to improve transparent reporting of studies based on routinely collected data. *Int J Popul Data Sci.* 2018 Jan 10;3(1):2.

23. Langan SM, Schmidt SA, Wing K, et al. The reporting of studies conducted using observational routinely collected health data statement for pharmacoepidemiology (RECORD-PE). *BMJ.* 2018 Nov 14;363:k3532.

24. Chinaeke EE, Love BL, Magagnoli J, Yunusa I, Reeder G. The impact of statin use prior to intensive care unit (ICU) admission on critically ill patients with sepsis. *Pharmacotherapy.* 2021 Feb; 41(2):162-171.

18

Chapter Eighteen

Pharmacoeconomic Research

Khalid M. Kamal, MPharm, PhD

Chapter Objectives

- Define pharmacoeconomic research
- Discuss various types of pharmacoeconomic research
- Identify common research questions in pharmacoeconomic research
- Discuss steps in conducting pharmacoeconomic research
- Understand the practical considerations for pharmacoeconomic research
- Understand the technical considerations for pharmacoeconomic research
- Discuss the strategies for harnessing the expertise needed for conducting pharmacoeconomic research
- Describe an example of learner-involved pharmacoeconomic research
- Understand the dissemination framework for pharmacoeconomic research

Key Terminology

Pharmacoeconomic research, opportunity cost, cost minimization, cost-effectiveness, cost benefit, cost utility, perspective, costs, outcomes, direct costs, indirect costs, intangible, sensitivity analysis, discounting

Introduction

With the growing demand of healthcare coupled with rising healthcare costs, there is a need to prioritize efficient and equitable allocation of healthcare resources. Among

419

healthcare resources, allocation decisions are increasingly being made based on the value that includes quality and costs of new interventions. These interventions can include novel drug treatments, innovative clinical programs, new screening or diagnostic tests, and novel medical devices and procedures. **Pharmacoeconomic research** is a branch of health economics whose main goal is to quantify the value of a new intervention in terms of desirable outcomes such as better clinical evidence, economic savings, and improved patient outcomes compared to an alternative. These different outcomes generated by the intervention are then balanced against its costs, which represents the resources utilized in the delivery of the intervention.

Pharmacoeconomic research is a tool that determines the full impact of a new intervention by identifying, measuring, and comparing its costs and outcomes to an existing standard of treatment or usual care. This evaluation assists decision-makers in determining which intervention (versus an alternative) produces the best health outcomes for the resource invested (refer Figure 18–1). We need to keep in mind that pharmacoeconomic research is a prescriptive decision-making tool which assists in facilitating choices when allocating resources and should be used along with other tools such as safety, efficacy, quality, and equity assessments to inform medical decisions. This chapter outlines the importance of pharmacoeconomic research in pharmacy profession and the major components in pharmacoeconomic research. The chapter also offers a framework for

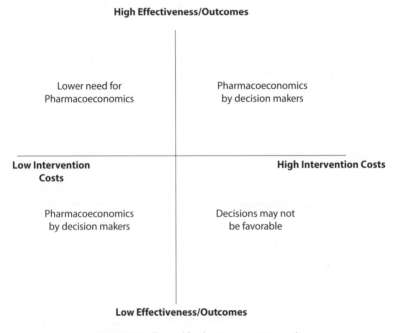

Figure 18–1. The need for pharmacoeconomic research.

conceptualizing and conducting pharmacoeconomic research by pharmacy students. The intention of the chapter is to help pharmacy students gain an understanding of the basics of conducting pharmacoeconomic research.

Importance of Pharmacoeconomic Research in Pharmacy Profession

The introduction of new interventions offers different opportunity costs to all healthcare stakeholders such as payers, providers, patients, and society as a whole. Opportunity cost is defined as the loss of potential benefit when an option is selected over its next best alternative. For example, in a pharmacy setting, when individualized patient counseling is offered by the pharmacist, the time allocated to the patient by the pharmacist cannot be used for another counseling and therefore, has a cost. If the appointment was canceled by the patient, the pharmacist could schedule a different patient and still generate revenue. Pharmacoeconomic research is utilized to assess the efficiency of these resource allocation decisions. Efficiency is defined as the allocation of resources in a way that maximizes or improves the outcomes. Efficiency can be of two types—allocative efficiency and technical efficiency.[1]

Allocative efficiency means that a particular mix or type of services that the healthcare system produces represents the maximum gain to the healthcare system. This type of efficiency is central to the decisions made by Pharmacy and Therapeutics (P&T) committees in managed care organizations and hospitals which use the drug outcomes as the benefits offered by the drug and the cost-effectiveness ratio as the criterion to decide the inclusion of the drug on the formulary when compared to a set of competing alternatives. Similarly, allocative efficiency is at play when deciding which pharmacy clinical service (e.g., diabetes clinic vs. smoking cessation) to invest in that will maximize health gains.

Technical efficiency, on the other hand, refers to the optimal delivery of an intervention when a decision has already been made on allocating resources to that intervention. An example of technical efficiency is a decision between the choice of biologic treatments versus traditional disease modifying antirheumatic drugs in the treatment of rheumatoid arthritis. Comparative performance is thus, central to assessing technical efficiency.

As discussed earlier, pharmacoeconomic research is utilized for efficient allocation of resources by all healthcare stakeholders. At a payer level (both public and private), this research is utilized to make informed decisions regarding formulary management, resource utilization, disease management, and health policy decisions such as product approvals and reimbursements. Pharmaceutical manufacturers use this research tool to determine launch prices for new products, identify investment in product development, and develop payer communication regarding the benefits of new interventions. Providers such as hospitals and clinicians use pharmacoeconomic research in selecting the best available treatments for their patients that improve both quantity and quality of life. Given the growing importance of pharmacoeconomics in healthcare decision making, knowledge of pharmacoeconomic research and its applications are essential to today's pharmacist. The role of pharmacists has evolved over the years, and today, they are not only involved in individualized patient care but also recognized as key members of interprofessional healthcare teams. Therefore In fact, pharmacoeconomic research presents a huge opportunity for pharmacists to showcase their role in not only reducing the overall cost of care but also in improving patient outcomes. For example, community pharmacists, through the delivery of cost-effective clinical pharmacy services, have played a major role in chronic disease management, medication adherence, drug utilization review, all of which have generated significant healthcare savings. Similarly, hospital pharmacists have enhanced patient care through programs such as antimicrobial stewardship, medication review, medication reconciliation, and transition of care programs, resulting in a direct impact on outcomes such as emergency visits, mortality, and length of stay. Pharmacoeconomic research has helped demonstrate the justification of resources needed for the clinical services and also allowed payers to decide reimbursements for such services based on the cost-effectiveness/benefit-to-cost ratios of these services.

Pharmacist's role will continue to evolve with the rapid advancement in technology such as gene therapies, artificial intelligence, and digital health. The introduction of expensive healthcare innovations will raise genuine concerns of affordability, access, and the demand to customize the services to patient's needs. In the not-so-distant past, pharmacists had adapted well to the introduction of expensive biologics by expanding their roles and responsibilities. Similarly, pharmacists will have to play a key role in identifying the opportunity costs of future innovations and in evaluating the capacity of their organization in optimally delivering these breakthrough treatments.

Steps in Conducting Pharmacoeconomic Research

A well-designed pharmacoeconomic research framework consists of 10 steps as outlined in Table 18–1. Figure 18–2 presents a more visual representation of the research framework. Once you put together the 10 steps of pharmacoeconomic research, these can be applied to diverse clinical areas and can also be customized to the specific needs of different healthcare stakeholders. Adhering to this framework increases the likelihood of obtaining valid and robust results. The next two sections will offer a more detailed description of each of these steps, including the practical and technical considerations in pharmacoeconomic research.

TABLE 18–1. PHARMACOECONOMIC RESEARCH FRAMEWORK

1.	Define the problem
2.	Identify alternatives
3.	Study perspective
4.	Patient population
5.	Time horizon
6.	Costs and outcomes
7.	Pharmacoeconomic methodology
8.	Study design
9.	Inflation and discounting
10.	Sensitivity analysis

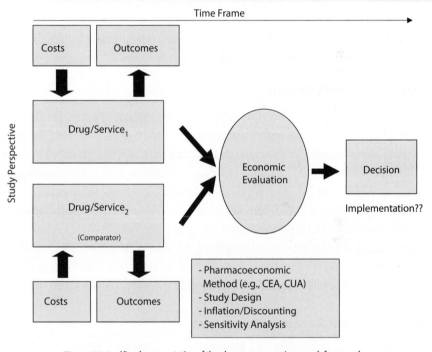

Figure 18–2. Visual representation of the pharmacoeconomic research framework.

Major Components in Pharmacoeconomic Research

DEFINING A PHARMACOECONOMIC QUESTION

Similar to any scientific research project, a pharmacoeconomic research must start with a well-defined research question. The goal is to identify a problem and focus on aspects of the problem that may need deliberate investigation. While deciding upon the research question, there are some essential elements that need to be considered. These include describing the interventions and the alternatives, study perspective, patient population, and selecting a time horizon, all of which will be discussed in detail in the next section.

RESOURCE AND OUTCOMES MEASUREMENT

The valid measurement of resource and outcomes are critical to the success of a pharmacoeconomic research. A basic structure of a pharmacoeconomic study includes comparing inputs and outputs of competing alternatives. The input reflects the resources consumed while delivering the intervention, while the output reflects the outcomes resulting from the use of the intervention. The input represents the difference in resources used to produce, distribute, and consume the intervention and the alternatives. These resources are reported in monetary units. The output, on the other hand, are of three types—clinical, economic, and humanistic. A pharmacoeconomic study should have a key outcome of interest but is not required to have all the three outcomes. If the goal is to study the problem from a broader perspective, all the outcomes can be included.

PHARMACOECONOMIC ANALYSIS

Once you identify the problem and set up the pharmacoeconomic structure, the next step is to select an analysis. The goal of a pharmacoeconomic analysis is to relate the costs (inputs) of implementing the interventions to the outcomes (outputs) generated by them. There are several analyses available, including cost analysis (CA), cost-minimization analysis (CMA), cost-benefit analysis (CBA), cost-effectiveness analysis (CEA), and cost-utility analysis (CUA). While each of these analyses measures costs in monetary terms, where they differ is the valuation of outcomes (refer Table 18–2). In CA, only costs are evaluated, and outcomes are not considered. A CMA is utilized to evaluate costs when the intervention and the alternatives have identical outcomes. The CBA involves evaluation of costs and benefits when all the outcomes are expressed in dollars. The outcomes

TABLE 18–2. **TYPES OF PHARMACOECONOMIC ANALYSES**

Analysis Type	Costs	Outcomes	Measure
Cost analysis	$$	None	None
Cost minimization analysis	$$	Equivalent	None
Cost benefit analysis	$$	Single or multiple outcomes	$$
Cost-effectiveness analysis	$$	Single outcome	Clinical units (life-years gained, blood pressure, fractures)
Cost utility analysis	$$	Single or multiple outcomes	Quality-adjusted life-years

expressed as natural units of clinical outcomes are evaluated in the CEA. Lastly, CUA is a type of CEA in which the outcomes incorporate a measure of the quality of life and are expressed as quality-adjusted life-years (QALYs). While the outcomes are measured differently, the costs could include direct, indirect, and intangible costs and their inclusion in the analyses depend on the study perspective.

RECOMMENDATIONS FOR HEALTHCARE STAKEHOLDERS

Pharmacoeconomic research is an important decision making tool that assists healthcare stakeholders on decisions related to the implementation of new interventions. These decisions can be in the context of formulary management, insurance coverage, reimbursements, practice guidelines, and clinical management guidelines. While pharmacoeconomic research presents the data in quantitative terms, the healthcare stakeholders' decisions are more subjective in nature. The subjective nature of the decision can be influenced by a number of factors such as unmet needs, resource constraints, affordability and budgetary controls, and scope of the analysis. Thus, it is extremely important for the stakeholders to interpret the study results within the context of their decision. Another point to keep in mind is that every decision does not need a new analysis. Evidence can be generated from existing literature; however, care must be taken to make sure that the evidence is of high quality and is generalizable to the decision at hand. In the next few sections, we will discuss how to set up a robust pharmacoeconomic study.

Developing a Pharmacoeconomic Question

IDENTIFYING A QUESTION

As with any research study, the process of identifying a pharmacoeconomic research question starts with articulating an idea that evolves into an important and relevant research question. This usually involves identifying an unmet need. The plan is to gather as much information on all relevant issues surrounding the question, including the motivation to perform the study. A possible source for an idea can be an evaluation of new technologies such as new treatments, novel clinical services, innovative medical devices, and even data management systems (e.g., electronic medical records). It is always good to narrow your problem into a specific question. For example, a problem with injectable oncolytic drugs is adherence. With the introduction of oral oncolytic agents, a CEA can be designed to estimate the cost per unit increase in adherence with the newer agents. Secondary questions can focus on improved quality of life and satisfaction in patients taking the new oral agents. Table 18–3 provides some sources of pharmacoeconomic research questions and published studies that may have utilized the suggested sources.

TABLE 18–3. PHARMACOECONOMIC RESEARCH SOURCES AND SAMPLE RESEARCH QUESTIONS

Sources of Pharmacoeconomic Research Questions	Published Study	Sample Research Questions
Introduction of novel treatments	Bensimon AG, Zhou ZY, Jenkins M, et al. An economic evaluation of pembrolizumab versus other adjuvant treatment strategies for resected high-risk stage III melanoma in the United States. *Clin Drug Investig.* 2020;40(7): 629-643.	To evaluate the cost-effectiveness of pembrolizumab versus other adjuvant treatment strategies for resected high-risk stage III melanoma from a U.S. health system perspective
Policy impact	Nianogo RA, Wang MC, Basurto-Davila R, et al. Economic evaluation of California prenatal participation in the Special Supplemental Nutrition Program for Women, Infants and Children (WIC) to prevent preterm birth. *Prev Med.* 2019;124:42-49.	To investigate the potential cost-savings that might result from prenatal infants and children participation
Current health issue	Neilan AM, Losina E, Bangs AC, et al. Clinical impact, costs, and cost-effectiveness of expanded SARS-CoV-2 testing in Massachusetts. *Clin Infect Dis.* 2020;18:ciaa1418.	To examine the clinical and economic impact of screening strategies in COVID-19 in Massachusetts
Clinical practice	Barlow S, Johnson J, Steck J. The economic effect of implementing an EMR in an outpatient clinical setting. *J Healthc Inf Manag.* 2004 Winter;18(1):46-51.	To estimate the financial impact of an EMR at a large, multispecialty and multisite ambulatory physician practice
Preventive care	Ruger JP, Abdallah AB, Ng NY, Luekens C, Cottler L. Cost-effectiveness of interventions to prevent HIV and STDs among women: a randomized controlled trial. *AIDS Behav.* 2014 Oct;18(10):1913-1923.	To assess the cost-effectiveness of behavioral interventions for reducing HIV and STDs infections among injection drug-using women
Pharmacist-led intervention	Tam-Tham H, Clement F, Hemmelgarn BR, et al. A cost analysis and cost-utility analysis of a community pharmacist-led intervention on reducing cardiovascular risk: The Alberta Vascular Risk Reduction Community Pharmacy Project (R$_x$EACH). *Value Health.* 2019;22(10):1128-1136.	To examine the short- and long-term cost of a pharmacist-led intervention to reduce cardiovascular risk compared to usual care
Study replication	Alshreef A, MacQuilkan K, Dawkins B, et al. Cost-effectiveness of docetaxel and paclitaxel for adjuvant treatment of early breast cancer: adaptation of a model-based economic evaluation from the United Kingdom to South Africa. *Value Health Reg Issues.* 2019;19:65-74.	To assess the cost-effectiveness of docetaxel and paclitaxel-containing chemotherapy regimens (taxanes) compared with standard (nontaxane) treatments

PERSPECTIVE

In pharmacoeconomic research, the **perspective** or the point of view has to be adopted as it dictates what types of costs and, in some instances, outcome measures are included in the study. As different stakeholders put emphasis on different costs depending on their needs and preferences, the results of these studies can look different when conducted from different perspectives. The typical perspectives include societal, payer, provider, patient, and employer. Given that the aim of a pharmacoeconomic analysis is to make the best use of all of society's resources, the societal perspective is considered the broadest perspective and usually includes all cost irrespective of who incurs them. Although this perspective is considered appropriate, there can be challenges in estimating all the different types of costs. In the literature, some studies may claim to use the societal perspective but exclude certain types of costs, and caution needs to be exercised in interpreting the results.

While societal perspective may lead to good outcomes and better decisions for the society, it may not be favored by stakeholders like providers and payers. Their perspectives are narrower in scope as compared to the societal perspective, and they put emphasis on mostly direct medical costs. A provider such as a pharmacist or a healthcare manager, with a limited budget, might include costs that are relevant to their practice setting, and a payer may include resources that they generally reimburse, which are mostly direct medical costs. From a patient's perspective, different costs include out-of-pocket costs, transportation or disease-related house remodeling costs, and wages lost due to time off work. This perspective is commonly employed if the patient is paying for the cost of the services. Given the different perspectives, it is possible to conduct a pharmacoeconomic study from multiple perspectives. The Second Panel on Cost-Effectiveness in Health and Medicine[2] recommends the use of two reference cases when conducting a pharmacoeconomic study—one from a healthcare sector perspective and another from a societal perspective. For example, an economic evaluation of a novel clinical pharmacy service is usually conducted from a provider perspective to justify investment in the service. The same study can also take a payer perspective to justify reimbursement for the services and a societal perspective to showcase the overall value of the novel clinical service. Table 18–4 provides a list of different costs included under different perspectives.

While the inclusion of certain types of cost is dependent on the perspective, the study time horizon is another element that is dependent on the choice of perspective. Studies with a payer perspective may be interested in short-term analysis (1-3 years) due to plan disenrollment rates or budgetary constraints. Societal perspective, on the other hand, usually considers a longer time horizon so as to account for different long-term costs and outcomes or costs and outcomes that occur in different time periods.[3]

TABLE 18-4. SELECTION OF TYPES OF COSTS BASED ON STUDY PERSPECTIVE

Perspective	Types of Costs
Societal	Broadest of all perspective, all costs (direct, indirect, and intangible), and consequences considered
Patient	Insurance copayments, out-of-pocket drug costs, indirect costs (work limitations), intangible costs (quality of life, anxiety, pain)
Provider	Direct costs (drugs, hospitalizations, laboratory tests), indirect costs are less important
Payer	Primary costs are direct costs; indirect costs *may* be included
Employer	Direct medical costs, indirect costs, intangible costs

ALTERNATIVES

As discussed earlier, the main goal of a pharmacoeconomic research is to determine the value of a new intervention by comparing its costs and outcomes to the most appropriate alternatives. Typically, alternatives are the most cost-effective option currently available (prior to the introduction of a new intervention) or those which will potentially be replaced by the new intervention. As the new intervention is generally more expensive but provides better outcomes, a key question that needs to be answered is how much we are willing to pay extra to get the extra benefits of the new intervention compared to its alternatives.

The selection of relevant alternatives is important in pharmacoeconomic research. The most commonly used alternative is the "standard of care" or "usual practice" which could be in the same or different therapeutic areas or even a nontherapeutic option (e.g., lifestyle modification). Interestingly, "do nothing" option can also be a valid alternative when introducing a novel drug or a unique clinical service. Ideally, all the alternatives that could potentially be replaced by the new intervention need to be considered and have to be described in detail. The inclusion of these alternatives, however, needs to be balanced against the data needs and the relative comparative effectiveness of these alternatives. If an alternative is not included, a rationale needs to be provided regarding its exclusion to increase the transparency of the analysis.

PATIENT POPULATION

The patient population in the study should be described in terms of their demographic (e.g., age, gender) and clinical characteristics (e.g., disease stage, severity, comorbidity). These characteristics have an influence on study variables such as baseline risk, treatment effect, treatment preferences, and resource utilization. For example, patients with varying severity of asthma (mild versus severe) will utilize different resources and also report different degrees of outcomes that can impact the study results. Another issue to consider is the generalizability of the patient population to the broader population. If patient data are taken from a randomized clinical trial, there is a need to assess the representativeness of the population to those seen in the real world. This can have a major impact on the results of the pharmacoeconomic study.

TIME HORIZON

The choice of time horizon has to be carefully considered and can range from a few weeks to several years. The selected time horizon should be able to capture the resource costs and both intended and unintended outcomes that will accrue over that time. A few factors need to be considered when choosing an appropriate time horizon. We have already discussed the importance of perspective and how it relates to the time horizon. Another important consideration is the number of years over which costs and outcomes accrue. If the study is conducted over several years, the future costs and outcomes have to be adjusted to reflect their present value. We will discuss discounting in the next section.

ASSUMPTIONS

In pharmacoeconomic research, most of the clinical data are obtained from randomized clinical trials which are then compared to the clinical data for the alternatives. As there are no head-to-head trials, assumptions have to be made in terms of baseline patient and clinical characteristics across the clinical trials. Another common assumption is that adherence to medications is 100%, which is not the case in the real world. Most clinical trials report intermediate outcomes, and in economic studies, we extrapolate these intermediate outcomes over time based on a number of assumptions, including long-term treatment efficacy rates, patient attrition, and long-term adverse events. Additionally, the economic data are collected from a variety of sources with an underlying assumption that the data quality is robust. Not surprisingly, the results of the pharmacoeconomic analysis will be dependent on the study assumptions and can vary considerably if not accounted for. Therefore, it is critical that we identify all the assumptions and test them using sensitivity analysis (discussed in the next section), which ultimately will increase the transparency of the study.

Practical Considerations: Resource and Outcomes Measurement

IDENTIFICATION, MEASUREMENT, AND VALUATION OF RESOURCE USE

So far, we have briefly discussed the types of costs and this section will help us understand how these costs are actually measured. The **cost** of an intervention includes the value of all the resources that are used to produce, distribute, and consume an intervention. For any new intervention, resource cost, whether directly or indirectly related to the intervention, are calculated in three stages—identification, measurement, and valuation. The first stage is to identify each component of the resources that are consumed during the provision of the intervention such as drug treatments, laboratory and diagnostic tests, physician visits, pharmacists' time, and hospitalization. The second stage deals with the measurement of resources in terms of frequency of use or units of resources used to produce the desired benefits such as doses of treatment administered, number of tests performed, and number of physician visits. The study perspective is critical when measuring resources. For example, a patient perspective may involve measuring the number of visits to physician's office and also the transportation costs for those visits. A payer perspective will only measure the number of physician visits. There are instances when some resources, especially in pharmacy clinical services, may be difficult to measure such as overheads (e.g., space). In such a case, you need to estimate the standard market rate of the space being used, which serves as a proxy for the resource. Another measurement issue arises when considering shared resources. Again, in a pharmacy clinical service example, shared resources can potentially include physician providing his/her expertise in a pharmacy clinic or an equipment being used for multiple disease areas. To measure shared resources, an allocation rate (e.g., cost of allocated physician time) is determined. This helps identify the amount of resource that is being used by the service under consideration. Failure to consider shared resources may result in inaccurate resource measurement.

The last stage of valuation involves applying unit cost to each resource that is consumed. For example, drug cost estimated from the Red Book and reimbursement rates for physician's office visits or diagnostic tests. At this stage, it is important to understand the difference between cost and charges. Cost refers to the actual cost associated with providing an intervention. Charges are not actual cost and in addition to the cost of the service, charges include profits and other resource costs that may be unrelated to the services billed. Thus, in a pharmacoeconomic analysis, we always use cost and not charges as charges overestimate the actual cost of an intervention. When planning a study, if you have access to charges, you will need to use standardized cost-to-charge ratios to convert charges into cost.

Resource Costs—Direct, Indirect, and Intangible

There is a need to understand the three main categories of costs employed in a pharmacoeconomic research. These include—direct costs, indirect costs, and intangible costs. Direct costs are incurred in the provision of medical care. These include drug costs, physician office visits, inpatient stay, diagnostic tests, and procedures. Some direct costs are nonmedical in nature and are generally incurred in the process of seeking medical care by the patients or their families. These include out-of-pocket costs, transportation costs, childcare expenses, and remodeling of house to disease condition. **Indirect costs** include productivity losses due to morbidity or mortality that may lead to loss or change of work hours. These include unpaid caregiving costs or loss of wages due to disease-related early retirement. Indirect costs should not be confused with overhead costs that are commonly reported in financial analysis. **Intangible costs** capture the social costs such as pain, grief, or anxiety that may be associated with the intervention. The challenge with intangible costs is that it is difficult to place monetary values, which makes it hard to include them in the analysis.

Overall, the costs generally fall in two categories—healthcare resources (direct medical costs) and patient and family resources (direct nonmedical, indirect, and intangible costs). When measuring the cost of the resources, a few factors such as study perspective and time horizon need to be considered.

OUTCOMES—ECONOMIC, CLINICAL, AND HUMANISTIC OUTCOMES

The **outcomes** include the benefits that an intervention offers and based on the ratio of benefits to costs, one can assess the cost effectiveness of the intervention. Most pharmacoeconomic research use the Economic, Clinical, and Humanistic Outcomes (ECHO)[3] model to quantify the value of an intervention in terms of the total resource utilization (direct and indirect costs), clinical-based outcomes (efficacy and safety data), and patient-reported outcomes (quality of life and satisfaction). When including outcomes in a study, intermediate- (e.g., clinical indicators such as glucose levels or blood pressure) or long-term outcomes (e.g., mortality, stroke) can be included depending on the study time horizon. Additionally, both positive and negative outcomes of the intervention should be included in the analyses otherwise the study could produce biased results. A key point to remember is that the selection of a pharmacoeconomic analysis is based on the type of outcomes incorporated in the study.

DATA SOURCES

Pharmacoeconomic research studies incorporate data from a variety of sources. Some of the data needed include incidence and prevalence data, treatment efficacy rates, resource utilization costs, and patient-reported outcomes. Broadly, the data sources can be categorized into external and internal data sources. The external data sources include published literature, healthcare databases, expert opinion, and unpublished sources. It is easy to find the data you need from published literature although you have to carefully consider the quality of the published studies. Data extracted from meta-analysis, systematic reviews and clinical trials are of high quality whereas data taken from case studies or expert opinions may not be of excellent quality. Healthcare databases (e.g., publicly available data, electronic medical records, administrative claims data) provide a wealth of data including information on disease incidence/prevalence, inpatient stays, mortality statistics, medication utilization, and patient characteristics. Similar to quality issues seen in published studies, healthcare databases can have some limitations. There could be errors in data due to misclassification bias (e.g., incorrect diagnosis), missing data, or lack of representative sample. Unpublished data (e.g., ongoing studies, data on file for pharmaceutical companies) can also be used, which can be obtained by contacting the author(s) of the study. Finally, data from expert opinion is used when no other data is available. However, data from experts are highly variable in nature and caution has to be exercised when using it. Internal data sources comprise of data that the organization conducting the research has access to. These include reimbursement data, resource utilization data, and clinical data. The advantage of using internal data is that it is readily available and provides good cost-effectiveness estimates compared to those based on external data.

Technical Considerations: Types of Economic Evaluation

Several analytical techniques are available when conducting economic evaluation, and it is important to understand the differences among them so as to select the most appropriate analysis (refer Figure 18–3). Before we learn the different types, we need to recognize the two categories of analysis—partial and full analysis. When deciding if an analysis is partial or full, two questions are important to ask—(1) were both costs and outcomes considered? (2) were two or more alternatives compared? If the answer to both the questions is a yes, it is a full analysis.

Cost analysis is a partial analysis as we include only costs and not outcomes. Similarly, an outcome analysis is a partial analysis as only outcome is compared between alternatives and not costs (e.g., randomized clinical trial). When conducting a CA, you simply have to identify, measure, and value the resources. When you compare the cost of two alternatives, you are trying to identify the least expensive option. If you are estimating the costs of one intervention with no alternatives, you are trying to calculate the cost of the intervention alone or how much is the investment in the intervention.

The four full analyses are CMA, CBA, CEA, and CUA. As mentioned earlier, these techniques measure costs in monetary terms, but they differ in the valuation of outcomes. A CMA is similar to CA except that outcomes are measured and proven equivalent across alternatives. Thus, the comparison is based on costs alone, and the goal is to identify the least expensive alternative. Some cases when CMA can

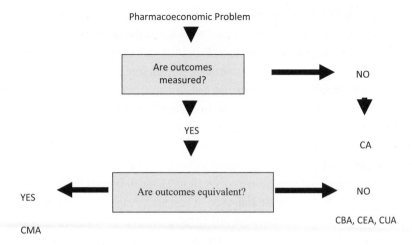

Figure 18–3. Selecting a pharmacoeconomic analysis.
CA, cost analysis; CBA, cost benefit analysis; CEA, cost-effectiveness analysis; CMA, cost minimization analysis; CUA, cost utility analysis

be used are when comparing brand drugs versus generic drugs (e.g., Lipitor versus Simvastatin), different practice settings (e.g., inpatient care versus home care), and different route of administration (e.g., intravenous versus intramuscular administration of levofloxacin).

A CBA measures both costs and outcomes in the same monetary units (e.g., dollars). When conducting a CBA for a single intervention, the question we are trying to answer is if the benefits produced outweigh the costs of the program. When conducting a CBA to compare two interventions, we are trying to identify which intervention produces the most benefits. Interestingly, a CBA can be used to evaluate single and multiple interventions. Also, as the benefits are measured in common units, we can compare intervention and alternatives with single or multiple outcomes. In CBA, the benefits are categorized as direct, indirect, and intangible benefits. Direct benefits are the cost avoided or potential savings because of the intervention. Indirect benefits are cost savings due to the increased earnings or productivity gains due to an intervention. Intangible benefits are the cost savings that result from a reduction in pain and suffering related to the intervention. Like intangible costs, intangible benefits are also difficult to measure. The major criticism for CBA is the challenge of placing a dollar value on benefits such as life-year gained. While clinical service evaluation often uses CBA, the analysis is limited when evaluating a treatment. The results of CBA are presented as net benefits, net costs, and benefit-to-cost ratio.

Both CEA and CUA estimate the monetary cost required to achieve a gain in health benefits. The difference between the two analyses is in how the health benefit is defined. In CEA, the outcomes are reported as clinical outcomes such as cases cured, blood pressure reduced, fracture avoided, or exacerbations averted. The use of clinical outcomes restricts the CEA from using a particular outcome that must be common across the comparators. When different outcomes are to be used, a more general outcome like life-years gained can overcome this requirement. A CUA is a type of CEA where the outcome is reported as QALYs. It is the only analysis where the outcome is adjusted for patient preferences or utility. Utility refers to the relative preference or value that a patient has for a particular health state and is measured on a scale of 0-1 with 0 = worst health state and 1 = best health state. Utilities are estimated in patients through the utility-based survey (e.g., quality of well-being, EuroQoL-5D) or rating scales (e.g., visual analog scale). Utilities can also be sourced from literature provided the patient population in the published study matches with that of your study. Once the utility is estimated, QALYs are calculated by multiplying the utility by the time spent in the given health state. For example, if a patient with moderate diabetes spends one year in the current health state and expresses a utility of 0.5 for his or her current health state compared to one year of life at ideal health state, then each year of current health is equivalent to 0.5 QALY (utility [0.5] × length of time in health state [one year]). The results of CEA and CUA are presented as incremental ratios, which are the change in costs associated with an intervention divided by the change in health benefits of the intervention. The incremental cost-effectiveness ratios (dollars per clinical effect) or incremental cost-utility ratios (dollars per QALY) express the relative efficiency of two interventions in producing health benefits.

Technical Considerations: Additional Techniques for Analysis

INFLATION

In general, prices of goods increase over time, and this includes medical costs as well. This rate of increase in prices is called inflation. The Bureau of Labor Statistics (BLS)[4] provides inflation value for different goods, including medical products and services, for each year. Using these values, you can adjust any old cost to present value using the formula:

$$\text{Present value} = \text{old price} \times \frac{\text{high year annual index value}}{\text{low year annual index value}}$$

The high and low year annual index value is taken from the BLS website. For example—most of the resource costs in a pharmacy can be calculated in present value (e.g., 2022 dollar value). If you are trying to calculate economic outcomes such as reduction in hospitalization costs or emergency visits, you would first need to find out the cost savings for hospitalization averted or emergency visits averted. If you have the present value (2022 dollar value) of the cost savings in your database or a recent study conducted in 2022 reported these numbers, you do not need to inflate these costs. If you do not have the present value and all you could find in the literature or claims database was an old estimate (for example, 2010 value), you will need to inflate the old cost to present value using the formula:

$$\text{Present value} = \text{old costs} \times \frac{2022 \text{ annual index value}}{2010 \text{ annual index value}}$$

A good practice is to always report the original year of the old costs that are being inflated to present value.

DISCOUNTING

An investment in novel interventions to improve patient health represents an investment of resources. These resources are utilized on a continuous basis (now and in the future) and result in health benefits (e.g., QALYs) that occur immediately and over a number of years. Therefore, to calculate the "net present value" of future resources and health gains, a mathematical procedure called **discounting** is utilized.

The two underlying premises of discounting are that individuals prefer to receive benefits today rather than in the future (think about lottery winners), and resources invested today in alternative interventions could earn a return over time. In other words, a dollar today is worth more than a dollar tomorrow. When a healthcare intervention extends over a period of several years, the present value of the intervention may be calculated by multiplying the future costs and future health benefits by a discount factor. The discount factor depends on the number of years into the future that the expense is incurred (n) and the discount rate (r).

Any future cost or health benefit can be converted to present value by using the formula:

$$\text{Discounted cost} = \frac{\text{cost of future event}}{(1 + r)^n}$$

For example, the costs associated with starting and maintaining an asthma clinic in the first year is $100,000 and $120,000 in the second year. Assuming a 5% discount rate, what is the net present value of the costs over the next two years? As discounting is not done on the costs in the first 12 months, the net present value will be calculated as:

$$100,000 + \frac{100,000}{(1+0.05)^1} = \$195,238$$

Discounting is usually conducted on costs or benefits that occur after one year using a discount rate of 3-5%.

SENSITIVITY ANALYSIS

As discussed earlier, a number of assumptions are made when estimating costs and outcomes in a pharmacoeconomic study. Also, these costs and outcomes are derived from multiple sources resulting in uncertainty which must be addressed. An example of uncertainty in a clinical pharmacy service that can affect your budget and planning includes estimating the number of patients who will potentially visit your pharmacy. If the number of patients change (increase or decrease), it has a direct impact on resource planning, such as the number of personnel or equipment needed. Sensitivity analysis is used to assess the impact of these uncertainties on the study results. By addressing these uncertainties, you are better prepared to understand how different study parameters affect the study results, and this will only increase the confidence in the overall study conclusions. When preparing the variable for sensitivity analysis, a range has to be defined, and then different cost-effective ratios are calculated for the range. If the final ratios do not change, the study results are pretty robust and are not affected by changes in the variable. For example, in a pharmacy clinic, if the cost purchase price of the Cholestech testing machine ranges between $2,000 and $3,000, you will conduct a sensitivity analysis to see the effect of the cost range on the overall study results. You will calculate your overall cost by using $2,000 purchase price of the Cholestech machine and then recalculate the overall cost using $3,000 purchase price of the Cholestech machine. This will help us understand if there are fluctuations in the overall budget and will help us understand the impact of Cholestech machine cost on the clinic's budget.

Recommendations for Decision Makers

INTERPRETATION OF RESULTS

A number of analyses can be used to assess the impact of a new intervention. When CA or CMA are utilized, the goal is to identify the least expensive alternative. In a CBA, once costs and benefits are calculated, a net benefit or net cost can be calculated using the formulas: Net benefit = total benefits – total costs and net costs = total costs – total benefits. If the net benefit ≥ 0 or the net cost < 0, the intervention is considered to be beneficial. A benefit-to-cost ratio can also be calculated by summing the total benefits of the intervention and dividing it by the total costs of the intervention. When the intervention is considered alone and if the benefit-to-cost ratio is ≥ 1, the intervention is considered beneficial, meaning it is generating more benefits for the cost invested. If the ratio is < 1, the recommendation is not to implement the intervention. When the intervention is being compared to an alternative, the one with the highest benefit-to-cost ratio is usually recommended for implementation.

When interpreting results from CEA or CUA, certain decision rules[5] are utilized against which the incremental ratios are assessed. The incremental ratios help us understand how much extra we are willing to pay for an intervention compared to alternatives to get an extra unit of health benefit. If the incremental ratios are $50,000/QALY or $110,000/QALY, what does that mean, and how are decisions made. In the United States, an incremental ratio in the range of $50,000-$100,000 is considered attractive, and a ratio above $100,000 is considered unattractive. As the incremental ratios involve trade-offs between costs and health benefits, the thresholds reflect the society's willingness to pay for the health benefit. Different countries like the United Kingdom (£20,000-£30,000) and Canada (CAD $20,000) have different thresholds than the United States, and the threshold merely reflects a public policy than a scientifically validated measure. Although we do not have a national threshold, most payers in the United States are not bound by these thresholds and base their decision on the affordability of the intervention.

AFFORDABILITY

Over the years, a substantial number of new interventions have been introduced that have transformed the way diseases are managed. Even though these new interventions are clinically superior to existing treatments, they are associated with high costs, and thus, affordability is a concern. For example, the introduction of sofosbuvir-based regimen[6,7] in the treatment of hepatitis C truly resulted in a paradigm shift in how the disease was treated. Prior to sofosbuvir, the cure rates with interferon were below 50%, and these injectables had poor patient outcomes. Sofosbuvir-based regimens were administered orally and have a cure rate of over 90%. These new treatments were cost-effective and also improved patient-reported outcomes such as satisfaction and quality of life. However, the major concern was affordability in terms of sustaining the high drug cost (sofosbuvir: $84,000 for 12-week treatment), thereby limiting its access to patients. Most payers in the United States implemented patient-related (e.g., prior authorizations, copays) and manufacturer-related policies (e.g., price discounts/rebates, outcomes-based risk-sharing agreements) to overcome affordability issues. One specific type of analysis that helps assess the affordability of new drugs is a budget impact analysis.[8] The analysis estimates the resource costs before and after the introduction of the intervention, and the change in costs is reported as per member per month (PMPM) cost. This helps the payer decide if the increase in PMPM can be absorbed in the budget or if there is a need to implement patient- and manufacturer-related policies to tackle the affordability issue. In healthcare decision-making, it is very likely for a treatment to be cost-effective but possibly being rejected based on the health plan's inability to afford it.

QUALITY ASSESSMENT

Over the last 20 years, the number of pharmacoeconomic studies reported in the literature has increased exponentially. A majority of these studies are conceptualized, implemented, and funded by the pharmaceutical industry, which can cause some concerns related to the validity of study results. To increase clarity and transparency, the studies need to comply with the recommendations of a number of published checklists.[9] We have discussed the 10 steps that define the pharmacoeconomic research framework. While some of the steps such as perspective, population, comparators, and time horizon may seem easy to evaluate, more attention is needed regarding the estimation and valuation of cost and outcomes input, data sources, and study assumptions. If the quality of the study is not scrutinized, there can be questions regarding the validity of the study results. Thus, to increase transparency and clarity of pharmacoeconomic research studies, a few instruments such as the Quality of Health Economic Studies (QHES)[10] and the Consolidated Health Economic Evaluation Reporting Standards (CHEERS)[11] have been utilized. The QHES is a quantitative instrument and provides a score from 0 to 100, with a higher score reflecting higher study quality. The CHEERS is a 24-item checklist that is used to provide guidance on how economic studies are reported. These instruments are quality assurance mechanisms that help in better conducting and reporting of studies resulting in reliable and valid healthcare decision making.

Expertise Needed for Conducting Pharmacoeconomic Research

RESEARCH MENTOR

A research mentor is key to successful mentee training, and you can work with a research mentor in a variety of settings—academia, industry, consulting organization, and government. One of the professional responsibilities of a research mentor is to train a student or a less-experienced researcher to become an independent researcher. The mentoring encompasses all the steps, including having an active research program, sharing knowledge and skills, developing expertise through research experiences, teaching dissemination strategies, and networking. Research mentors have doctoral degrees or have a pharmacy degree with advanced training in health economics and outcomes research.

PHARMACOECONOMIST

As a pharmacoeconomist, one has to have excellent expertise in the field. Most pharmacoeconomists have doctoral degrees in health economics and outcomes research and work for industry or clinical research organizations. Some also work in specialized centers in an academic setting. They help design clinical trials focusing on the measurement of economic and patient-reported outcomes, determine appropriate pricing of products, develop communication strategies to analyze, summarize and disseminate evidence and cater to both national and international healthcare stakeholders.

OTHER STAKEHOLDERS

Given the unique needs of different stakeholders, the level of expertise required by them is slightly different. Payers generally have individuals who have a good working knowledge of pharmacoeconomic research. They have to have the ability to critically evaluate the pharmacoeconomic studies submitted in support of access or reimbursement decisions. Those working for pharmaceutical industry or clinical research organizations are well trained in different pharmacoeconomic methods to generate evidence supporting the interventions. They also have the ability to understand the gaps and carefully plan their dissemination strategies to meet the unique needs of their stakeholders.

Exemplar of Learner-Involved Pharmacoeconomic Research

The goal of this case is to reinforce the 10 steps of the pharmacoeconomic research by providing an example of the use of oral disease-modifying therapies (DMTs) in multiple sclerosis (MS) and assessing the economic impact of these therapies. The case is based on a study conducted by pharmacy students who presented the results at the 2020 Academy of Managed Care Pharmacy (AMCP) Nexus meeting.[12] You have been working for a managed care organization for over two years, and you were recently appointed as the pharmacy representative on the P&T committee. The latest decision facing the P&T committee is approving the use of oral DMTs in patients with MS. DMT has become a mainstay of MS clinical care due to its benefits associated with disease progression and relapses. A number of DMTs are available in the United States, and oral DMTs are recommended as first-line for patients with relapse remitting MS (RRMS) who are reluctant to take self-injectable or intravenous infusion medications. However, the average annual wholesale acquisition cost of these oral therapies exceeds $80,000 in most cases. As someone who has studied pharmacoeconomic research, the committee expects you to calculate the cost per relapse avoided for approved oral therapies used in the treatment of RRMS so as to make a policy decision (refer Figure 18–4).

Dissemination of Pharmacoeconomic Research

Even before we think about dissemination strategies for pharmacoeconomic research, we need to make sure that the study adheres to the fundamental analytic principles (10 steps) as outlined in this chapter. The studies in the literature are either pharmaceutical industry-sponsored or are nonprofit sponsored like foundations and others. It is extremely important for students to understand the goals of these funders in terms of biases, generalizability, and inclusion of favorable/unfavorable conclusions. As discussed earlier, CHEERS[11] checklist consists of 24 recommendations that provide guidance on how economic studies are reported. The use of the checklist helps in improving the quality of the study and also the healthcare decisions. The 24 recommendations in the CHEERS checklist are subdivided into the following six main categories: Title and abstract (2), Introduction (1), Methods (14), Results (4), Discussion (1), and Other (2). The 14 recommendations in the "Methods" section consists of the major elements of pharmacoeconomic research such as study population, setting, time horizon, comparators, costs, outcomes, assumptions, analytical methods, choice of models, and price date. The "Result" section includes recommendations on study parameters, incremental costs, uncertainty, and heterogeneity while the "Other" section includes recommendations on funding source and conflict of interest. Based on the checklist, an average quality score can be calculated for a study and different pharmacoeconomic studies can be compared to see which performed better than others.

The AMCP Format for Formulary Submissions (Version 4.1) provides guidance to the manufacturers for formulary submission dossier development.[13] The payers require product clinical trials, disease burden, health economics, and other relevant patient outcomes data to make coverage and reimbursement decisions. The AMCP Format 4.1 provides guidance for submitting these evidences for unapproved products, approved products, and unapproved uses. The economic value of the product is presented based

STEP 1: Define the Problem
The Pharmacy & Therapeutics committee is evaluating patient safety and comfort against the cost of care when switching from intravenous to oral disease modifying therapies (DMTs) in relapse remitting multiple sclerosis (RRMS).

STEP 2: Identify Alternatives
Oral DMTs will include cladribine, dimethyl fumarate, diroximel fumarate, fingolimod, monomethyl fumarate, ozanimod, siponimod, and teriflunomide.

STEP 3: Study Perspective
The study will use a payer perspective and direct medical costs will be included in the analysis.

STEPS 4 & 5: Patient Population and Time Horizon
Patients with RRMS; One year time horizon

STEP 6: Cost and Outcomes
Costs to be considered include drug acquisition, monitoring, administration, and office visits. Outcomes will include relative relapse reduction and cost per relapse avoided.

STEP 7: Pharmacoeconomic Methodology
As the outcome is reported in natural units (relapse avoided), a cost effectiveness analysis will be conducted.

STEP 8: Study Design
A static decision model will be utilized to compare the approved oral disease modifying therapies for RRMS.

STEP 9: Cost Adjustment (Inflation and Discounting)
All costs will be adjusted to 2022 USD using the medical care component of the Consumer Price Index. As the study time horizon is only one year, discounting of future costs is not needed.

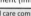

STEP 10: Uncertainty Analysis
A univariate sensitivity analysis will be conducted and a ±20% will be used for wholesale acquisition cost and relapse rate.

Other study considerations: Assumptions and reporting of results

The study will include some assumptions such as 100% adherence rate, patients taking the assigned DMTs over a one-year period, and no change in the disease condition in terms of severity. Once the study is set up, cost per relapse avoided for each oral DMT and incremental cost-effectiveness ratios will be calculated, which will assist in decision making and policy deliberations. Caution has to be exercised in making direct comparisons as the clinical efficacy data in this study will be taken from different clinical trials. Also, as the agents will have differing safety profiles, health plans need to weigh the clinical, economic, and humanistic data while making important coverage decisions.

Figure 18–4. Research case study.

on pharmacoeconomic research, which generally involves a decision-analytic-based cost-effectiveness model along with other economic models such as budget impact and financial models. As described in this chapter, transparency is extremely important when it comes to the synthesis of evidence on costs and outcomes, estimation of uncertainty, and providing explicit assumptions. The US Food and Drug Administration (FDA) via Section 114 of the FDA Modernization Act of 1997 (FDAMA)[14] regulates the dissemination of healthcare economic information by pharmaceutical manufacturers. Students should familiarize themselves with the USFDA and AMCP guidelines when it comes to disseminating these studies.

Another organization that is leading the mission to promote health economics and outcomes research at a global level is the International Society for Pharmacoeconomics and Outcomes Research (ISPOR).[15] The annual meetings provide plenty of opportunities to present the research studies and publish them in the society's journal, *Value in Health*.

Summary and Conclusions

Pharmacoeconomic research is a decision-making tool that assists in determining the value of interventions. A well-designed pharmacoeconomic research consists of 10 steps, and adherence to this framework increases the likelihood of obtaining valid and robust results. The three main categories of costs include—direct, indirect, and intangible costs and the three outcomes include economic, clinical, and humanistic outcomes. There are several analyses available, including cost analysis, cost minimization, cost-benefit, cost-effectiveness, and cost-utility analyses. While each of these analyses measures costs in monetary terms, where they differ is the valuation of outcomes. Budget impact analyses are also conducted to determine the affordability of interventions. Pharmacoeconomic research has numerous implications for diverse healthcare stakeholders and should be designed to meet their unique needs. Finally, these analyses should be carefully and critically evaluated to determine the relevance of the results to a specific decision.

The prospects of future growth of pharmacoeconomic research in pharmacy practice are quite good. The practice of pharmacy has started to shift from dispensing a product to providing personalized care. While the rates of chronic diseases and aging population are increasing, newer innovative interventions like gene therapies are rapidly diffusing in the market. Also, with the development of specialty pharmacy, there is an increased emphasis on coordination of care as a strategy to manage cost and improve patient outcomes. These innovations, however, come at a cost and have direct implications on pharmacy practice, especially in terms of resource allocations, reimbursement decisions, and drug evaluations.

Another area that is growing rapidly is the development and expansion of pharmacy clinical services, which have the potential to reduce risks and costs and improve patient outcomes. It is imperative that students not only become familiar with the scope and definition of pharmacoeconomic research but also develop critical skills in conducting these studies.

Key Points and Advice

- Pharmacoeconomics is the description and analysis of costs and outcomes of a drug or technology to the healthcare system.
- Several types of pharmacoeconomic analyses can be performed to assess the value of the drugs and technology.
- There is a need to balance the study rigor with the practical nature of the healthcare problem.
- Established approaches and frameworks should guide the development of pharmacoeconomic evaluations, including quality assessment using validated checklists.
- Pharmacoeconomic research has numerous implications for diverse healthcare stakeholders and should be designed to meet their unique needs.

Chapter Review Questions

1. Discuss the steps involved in conducting pharmacoeconomic research.
2. Identify the different types of costs and outcomes included in a pharmacoeconomic research.
3. Describe the different data sources used in an economic evaluation.
4. Compare and contrast the different types of pharmacoeconomic analysis.
5. Explain the concepts of inflation and discounting.
6. Discuss the application of pharmacoeconomic research from the perspective of different healthcare stakeholders.

Online Resources

- International Society for Pharmacoeconomics and Outcomes Research (ISPOR). www.ispor.org
- Academy of Managed Care Pharmacy (AMCP). https://www.amcp.org

REFERENCES

1. Lopert R, Lang DL, Hill SR. Use of pharmacoeconomics in prescribing research. Part 3: cost-effectiveness analysis—a technique for decision making at the margin. *J Clin Pharm Ther*. 2003;28(3):243-249.

2. Sanders GD, Neumann PJ, Basu A, et al. Recommendations for conduct, methodological practices, and reporting of cost-effectiveness analyses: second panel on cost-effectiveness in health and medicine. *JAMA*. 2016;316(10):1093-1103.

3. Kozma CM, Reeder CE, Schulz RM. Economic, clinical, and humanistic outcomes: a planning model for pharmacoeconomic research. *Clin Ther*. 1993;15(6):1121-1132.

4. Bureau of Labor Statistics. Published Dec 20, 2020. Accessed December 20, 2020. https://www.bls.gov/cpi/

5. Nanavaty M, Kaura S, Mwamburi M, et al. The use of incremental cost-effectiveness ratio thresholds in health technology assessment decisions. *J Clin Pathw*. 2015;2(1):29-36.

6. Linas BP, Barter DM, Morgan JR, et al. The cost-effectiveness of sofosbuvir-based regimens for treatment of hepatitis C virus genotype 2 or 3 infection. *Ann Intern Med*. 2015;162(9):619-629.

7. Chhatwal J, Kanwal F, Roberts MS, Dunn MA. Cost-effectiveness and budget impact of hepatitis C virus treatment with sofosbuvir and ledipasvir in the United States. *Ann Intern Med*. 2015;162(6):397-406.

8. Sullivan SD, Mauskopf JA, Augustovski F, et al. Budget impact analysis—principles of good practice: report of the ISPOR 2012 Budget Impact Analysis Good Practice II Task Force. *Value Health*. 2014;17(1):5-14.

9. Watts RD, Li IW. Use of checklists in reviews of health economic evaluations, 2010 to 2018. *Value Health*. 2019;22(3):377-382.

10. Ofman JJ, Sullivan SD, Neumann PJ, et al. Examining the value and quality of health economic analyses: implications of utilizing the QHES. *J Manag Care Pharm*. 2003;9(1):53-61.

11. Husereau D, Drummond M, Petrou S, et al. Consolidated health economic evaluation reporting standards (CHEERS)— explanation and elaboration: a report of the ISPOR health economic evaluations publication guidelines good reporting practices task force. *Value Health*. 2013;16:231-250.

12. Nedzesky J, Han M, Kamal KM. Cost per relapse avoided of oral therapies in relapsing-remitting multiple sclerosis. *J Manag Care Spec Pharm*. 2020;26(10-a):S87CP

13. Academy of Managed Care Pharmacy. Published May 11, 2021. Accessed May 11, 2021. https://www.amcp.org/sites/default/files/2019-12/AMCP_Format%204.1_1219_final.pdf

14. Neumann PJ, Lin PJ, Hughes TE. US FDA Modernization Act, section 114: uses, opportunities and implications for comparative effectiveness research. *Pharmacoeconomics*. 2011;29(8):687-692.

15. International Society for Pharmacoeconomics and Outcomes Research (ISPOR). Published December 11, 2021. Accessed Dec 11, 2021. www.ispor.org

19

Chapter Nineteen

Narrative and Scoping Reviews in Pharmacy Settings

Marie Barnard, PhD

Chapter Objectives

- Define narrative and scoping reviews in pharmacy settings
- Differentiate narrative and scoping reviews from other methods of evidence synthesis
- Identify resources for conducting narrative and scoping reviews
- Understand the practical steps for conducting narrative and scoping reviews
- Understand how to engage learners in narrative and scoping reviews
- Describe examples of learner involved narrative and scoping reviews
- Understand the dissemination framework for narrative and scoping reviews

Key Terminology

Evidence synthesis, narrative review, scoping review

Introduction

Evidence-based practice requires the development, synthesis, review, and utilization of evidence. Literature reviews are a method of evidence synthesis—identifying, organizing, synthesizing, and critiquing the published information on a particular topic or research question. Literature reviews can provide a summary of a topic, point to gaps in what we know, and identify questions that remain unresolved. Reviews can be helpful to both students and practitioners in that a current review is more up-to-date than a text-book. Reviews are helpful to researchers as they can identify gaps in knowledge, assist in developing a study hypothesis, and suggest areas in which study designs can be improved to increase the validity and reliability of the research in the field. Because pharmacists rely on research conducted in multiple disciplines, from lab sciences to health education to systems management, reviews can be helpful ways to gain quick insight into a topic.

Typologies of reviews have identified more than 20 different kinds of reviews and knowledge synthesis methods.[1-3] These range from overview reviews that simply summarize published literature to systematic reviews with meta-analyses (a statistical summary of quantitative studies). There are even reviews of reviews, so-called umbrella reviews.[2] Two commonly conducted and utilized reviews in pharmacy are narrative and scoping reviews. A **narrative review** is a broad term that refers to a review that summarizes evidence on a topic but does not utilize a standardized nor comprehensive search methodology. **Scoping reviews**, by contrast, use a systematic approach to search the literature with the goal of assessing and describing the potential size and scope of the research available on a topic, clarifying concepts and highlighting knowledge gaps.

This chapter introduces key issues related to conducting narrative and scoping reviews. It provides a brief description of each type of review. Guidance for how to develop a search strategy, conduct a search, review and select the articles for inclusion, and how to analyze and report the results are provided. Project management steps, including the use of reference management programs and data extraction tools, are also described. This chapter concludes by describing how to engage a team of researchers in narrative and scoping reviews and how to disseminate these reviews.

Narrative Reviews

Narrative reviews provide a qualitative synthesis of information on a topic. They are a bridge between the vast body of research on a topic and a reader who does not have the time, resources, or research knowledge to read a significant amount of original literature. Overviews, commentaries, critical reviews, consensus reviews, and meta-narrative reviews are all types of narratives reviews. When the term "narrative review" is used, it is most often referring to an overview, sometimes called a "narrative overview," an "unsystematic narrative review, or simply a "literature review."[1,4] These reviews synthesize previously published information and report the reviewers' findings in a condensed format. They can be useful as educational resources because they bring a lot of information together in a readable format.

Compared to other types of reviews, narrative reviews generally address broader topics and do not provide evidence for a specific research question. They are a useful methodology when there is a diverse collection of studies to be synthesized or when there are different types of methodologies or different theoretical approaches utilized, or different relationships between constructs examined. Narrative reviews do not provide any kind of statistical summary of the literature reviewed.

COMPONENTS OF A NARRATIVE REVIEW

A narrative review includes four main components: (1) introduction, (2) methods, (3) results, and (4) discussion. The introduction to a narrative review provides an overview of the topic and describes the aim or purpose of the review. The introduction provides a justification for why a review on this issue is warranted and may indicate the targeted audience for the review. The methods section describes the process the reviewers undertake to gather the literature included in the review. A narrative review is neither an exhaustive nor a systematic review of the literature. The goal of a narrative review is not to identify and incorporate every possible published study on a given topic. Instead, a narrative review incorporates literature that the authors feel is most relevant. In the methods section, the process and decision making for what information was reviewed are explained. The results section presents the summary of the literature. This can be presented as an article-by-article summary, organized by subtopics, or some other grouping that makes sense based on the purpose of the review. The discussion section provides a meaningful integration of all of the information in the review. The purpose of the review should guide the discussion section, connect the current review with the body of literature, identify any clinical or policy significance, and may offer the authors' interpretations or insights based on the information reviewed. The discussion should also include the limitations of the review.

REPORTING STANDARDS FOR NARRATIVE REVIEWS

There are publication reporting guidelines and standards for narrative reviews that can guide authors as they conduct and write up narrative reviews. The SANRA (Scale for the Assessment of Narrative Review Articles) provides six items to consider to evaluate the quality of a narrative review.[5] These include a justification of the importance of the review, a statement of concrete aims or formulation of questions, a description of the literature search, support for key statements by references, scientific reasoning, and presentation of data.

EXAMPLES OF NARRATIVE REVIEWS IN PHARMACY SETTINGS

Narrative reviews have been used in a variety of areas of interest to the pharmacy community. For example, Aggarwal and colleagues' narrative review on the challenges and opportunities related to multi-morbidity and polypharmacy was conducted to provide definitions and methods to recognize multi-morbidity and polypharmacy.[6] This review also describes for practitioners care models that have been shown to be effective and can be readily implemented in clinical practice. A narrative review by Bishop and colleagues described community pharmacy interventions to address inappropriate use of antibiotics.[7] They describe several community pharmacist-led interventions and highlight topics that may warrant additional attention for potential inclusion in pharmacy school curricula. Both of these reviews are examples of narrative reviews that can save a practitioner time by identifying interventions that can be implemented to address specific challenges.

Scoping Reviews

A scoping review is a method to synthesize evidence on a topic that follows a systematic approach to search, synthesize, and assess the scope of literature on a topic. The original scoping review framework was proposed by Arksey and O'Malley in 2005.[8] The goal of a scoping review is to map the key concepts of an area of research, including describing the extent, range, and types of evidence in the literature on a topic. Scoping reviews provide an overview of the evidence and do not usually assess the risk of bias in the evidence reviewed.[9] Scoping reviews can be useful for a variety of reasons.[9] Table 19–1 includes some of the reasons a scoping review may be conducted.

COMPONENTS OF A SCOPING REVIEW

The original framework proposed by Arksey and O'Malley has been expanded and refined, adding more detail to improve the clarity and rigor of the scoping review process.[8,10–13] See Table 19–2 for the components of the framework.[9] The framework provides guidance for each step in a scoping review. An introduction provides the background, justification,

TABLE 19–1. REASONS TO CONDUCT A SCOPING REVIEW

Reasons to conduct a scoping review include:
To examine emerging evidence, potentially identifying more specific questions that can be addressed in future research
To clarify definitions of concepts and/or establish conceptual boundaries for a topic
To examine a broad topic, identify gaps in the research in that selected area
To determine if a subsequent systematic review is needed
To delineate the types of evidence that has been published on a topic
To examine the research methods that have been used to study a topic, to guide future research

TABLE 19-2. SCOPING REVIEW FRAMEWORK

Components of the scoping review framework
Identifying the research question and objectives, linking the purpose and the research question/objectives
Identifying relevant studies, with inclusion criteria appropriate to the review objectives
Describing the plan to conduct the search, to select the studies, to extract the data and to present the evidence
Searching the evidence
Selecting the evidence
Extracting the evidence
Analyzing the evidence
Presenting the results
Summarizing the results, using the review purpose as a guide, drawing conclusions, and identifying implications

and purpose of the review. The methods section for a scoping review is more detailed than that of a narrative review, as it needs to report a more systematic and detailed search process. Details about how the articles to be included were selected, abstracted, and analyzed are reported. The results include a table of the data extracted and present a synthesis of the evidence to address the review's objectives. The discussion of a scoping review contextualizes the results in relation to the purpose of the review, current literature, and practice and policy.

REPORTING STANDARDS FOR SCOPING REVIEWS

The Preferred Reporting Items for Systematic Reviews and Meta-Analyses extension for scoping reviews (PRISMA-ScR) provides specific reporting guidance for scoping reviews.[12] The guidance includes a checklist of 20 items to report (e.g., including scoping review in the title, present the full electronic search strategy for at least one database, discuss the limitations of the review) and two optional items (rationale for and results of critical appraisal of individual sources of evidence).[12] The Joanna Briggs Institute (JBI) is another comprehensive resource that provides more focused methodological guidance for scoping reviews that also includes reporting standards.[14]

EXAMPLES OF SCOPING REVIEWS IN PHARMACY SETTINGS

Scoping reviews are regularly reported in the pharmacy literature. One such example is a review of the use and impact of telehealth medication reviews which was conducted to explore a gap in the literature.[15] The review found that while telehealth medication review may be feasible and has the potential to save money and improve care, the level of evidence was not yet sufficient to reliably inform practice and policy. Another scoping review conducted by Knott and colleagues investigated the literature related to pharmacy preceptor training programs.[16] They conducted this scoping review because the literature on this topic is broad and diverse. Their goal was to provide a comprehensive overview so that gaps and areas of interest could be identified. The review indicated that there is a need for an evidence-based approach to preceptor training and that programs should be evaluated on outcomes for students/trainees as well as for preceptors. Both of these scoping reviews followed the PRISMA-ScR reporting guidelines and reported information that can guide future investigations to answer important policy and practice questions.

Conducting Narrative and Scoping Reviews

IDENTIFY THE TOPIC, PURPOSE, AND TYPE OF REVIEW

Narrative and scoping reviews are approachable and valuable research projects that are ideal for student or resident researchers. To begin a narrative or scoping review, the first steps are to select a topic, determine if a review on that topic is needed, and, if so, what type of review is most appropriate. Ideas for review topics can come from many places, including personal interest, clinical need, and ideas arising from the discussion section of articles, among others. Identifying the target audience of the review is also helpful when developing the purpose and determining the type of review to be conducted.

Once you have a topic, search the literature to be sure a similar review has not been done recently to ensure that your review will provide new insight. To determine what type of review to do, consider both the purpose of the review and the skill and resources of the individuals who will conduct the review. If the purpose of the review is to simply summarize the literature on a topic, then a narrative review is appropriate. If the goal is to map the literature on a topic, to determine if a systematic review is needed, or to identify gaps and opportunities for further research, then a scoping review is appropriate. If the reviewer is going to work alone, has some limits on access to health sciences databases to systematically review the literature, or has limited time, then a narrative review is a more achievable goal. To conduct a scoping review, resources such as collaborators, access to health sciences databases, and time to conduct a thorough review are needed.

PREPARE TO CONDUCT THE REVIEW

For any type of review, a plan is needed for the review to be successfully executed. While narrative reviews do not require a protocol, they are recommended for scoping reviews and many of the components of a protocol are useful for any type of review. A scoping review protocol describes the objectives, methods, and reporting plans for the review.

By developing the protocol before conducting the review, there is greater transparency in the process. A scoping review protocol should be detailed, and any deviations from the protocol should be disclosed in the review. Both PRISMA ScR and JBI provide detailed guidance about what should be included in a scoping review protocol.[12,13]

While systematic reviews should be registered with PROSPERO or the JBI Systematic Review Register to reduce duplication of reviews and to limit reporting bias, scoping reviews are currently ineligible for registration. Protocols for scoping reviews can be placed in a publicly accessible repository such as Open Science Framework or Figshare.[17,18] If you do not register the protocol for a scoping review, you should provide details in the review about how to request it from the author.[12]

In addition to developing the protocol for a review, it is helpful to plan and prepare the organizational tools needed to conduct the review. First, identify the team members. Decide who will lead the project. Using your preliminary literature search mentioned above to estimate how much literature will need to be reviewed will help guide how many research team members will be needed to complete the project. Most scoping reviews have at least three authors so that when there is a disagreement between two reviewers about whether to include an article, a third team member can break the tie. Narrative reviews can be written by a single author, but a team approach helps ensure that key ideas are not left out of the review. Next, select a reference management system such as Zotero or Mendeley to help manage the literature that will be identified and considered for inclusion in the review. When searching databases, references can be automatically imported into these systems. They also support collaborative work as groups of references can be organized by folders that can be shared to team members. Both offer methods to add notes and tags to help organize and track the review teams' work. Finally, select a shared writing space such as Google Drive, Dropbox, etc., in which the team can share the articles selected for full text review and for the manuscript that will be developed.

DEVELOP AND IMPLEMENT THE REVIEW PROTOCOL

Once the purpose, the review type, the team members, and the organizational tools have been established, the review protocol can be developed and implemented.

Inclusion Criteria

Begin by clearly stating the primary question addressed by the review. Next, develop a list of criteria for what a study must include to be considered for inclusion in the review. This list should be based on the population, concept, and context of interest for the review.[9] The population are the types of participants for which literature would be included or excluded (e.g., children, patients with rheumatoid arthritis). The concept could be the intervention of interest (e.g., a therapeutic agent), a phenomenon, (e.g., quality of life), or

STUDENT HANDBOOK FOR PHARMACY PRACTICE RESEARCH

an outcome (e.g., smoking cessation). The context could include setting (e.g., community pharmacy), cultural factors, geographic location, or others based on the review objectives. Finally, specify the types of evidence that will be considered for inclusion and for exclusion. Types of evidence may include original research, systematic reviews, letters, guidelines, and so on. It is acceptable to use limits (e.g., no materials more than 10 years old), but if any limits are placed, especially for scoping reviews, they should be described.

Search Strategy

The inclusion criteria guide the search strategy. The search strategy describes how you will search for literature for potential inclusion in the review. For scoping reviews, the search strategy must be reported comprehensively. The specific databases searched, the specific search terms utilized, the time frame, any language restrictions, any search of unpublished research ("gray literature"—often conference proceedings or reports), and the number of articles identified must be reported. Narrative reviews should describe the search strategy but typically do not report the same level of detail as a systematic comprehensive search. Databases to consider searching include Pubmed, Embase, PsycInfo, Scopus, CINAHL (Cumulative Index to Nursing and Allied Health Literature), the Cochrane Database of Systematic Reviews, among others depending upon the topic of the review. Search terms should be carefully considered. Consultation with a librarian can be helpful. Utilize keywords, MeSH (medical subject headings) terms, Boolean operators (e.g., and, or, not), and the search options available in each database to best capture the relevant literature. The search terms will have to be customized for each database searched as the search structures can differ. Librarian assistance or the use of a search translator such as the Polyglot Search Translator can be helpful with this process.[19] The search strings can then be entered into each database, and the references identified and imported into the reference management system.

For scoping reviews, the PRISMA-ScR protocol calls for the inclusion of a figure in which the selection of articles is described in a flow chart.[12] The flow chart starts with the total number of articles identified and then describes how many articles are removed at each review step until the final number of articles selected for inclusion in the review is identified. A fillable version of this figure is available (http://www.prisma-statement.org/Extensions/ScopingReviews) and should be completed for every scoping review.

Title and Abstract Review

The next step is to review the titles and abstracts to determine if the articles should be included in the review. For narrative reviews, the authors will scan and identify the best articles to support the issues they wish to discuss in the review. For a scoping review, the title and abstract of every article identified in the search must be reviewed by at least two individuals. The team should review the inclusion and exclusion criteria for articles.

If there are two reviewers, each should independently read the title and abstract of every article. If there are more than two team members, the title and abstract review process can be divided among the team members so that every title and abstract is reviewed by at least two independent reviewers. Utilize the tagging function in the reference management system to mark articles that should be included. After each reviewer has completed reviewing all of the articles, search for the articles that have been tagged for inclusion by one or both of the reviewers. If only one reviewer tagged an article for inclusion, a third team member could break the tie, or the two reviewers can discuss and come to a consensus on whether the article should be included. Once this process is complete, the articles tagged for inclusion advance to the full-text review step. Moving all of these references into a new folder in the reference management system, sorting them alphabetically, and adding a tag with a unique number for each article can help keep the team organized. The full-text version of each reference needs to be procured at this step. Storing them either in the reference management system or in the shared digital folder by the unique number facilitates use by all team members.

Data Extraction

Once the titles and abstracts have been reviewed, and those marked for inclusion in the review are identified, it is time to conduct a review of the full text of each of these articles for a scoping review. The full-text review step is called data extraction or data charting. A table or form is used to systematically extract the same information from each article. Consider using a spreadsheet for reviewers to enter the data. Fields to include are the last name of the first author and publication year, the study objective, the number of participants in the study, a description of the participants in the study, variables related to the concept (as described above, this could be an intervention, phenomenon, outcome, etc.), and variables related to the context. Beyond these, add any other variables that would be useful based on the purpose of the review. These could range from study design (e.g., cross-sectional, case-control) to measurement tools (e.g., method of measuring medication adherence). Every review requires the creation of a new data extraction form as the variables will be different for each topic and purpose. Ideally, each article will be read and the data extracted by two team members. The data can then be compared, and any discrepancies can be resolved by a third reviewer or by a discussion to achieve consensus. The data extracted becomes the table of results for the review. Once this is ready, the information is ready for analysis. It is important to note that sometimes articles are excluded at the full-text review stage. While the title and abstract may have seemed appropriate, once the complete article is read, it may become clear it should not be included. The number of articles excluded at the full-text review stage and the reasons for exclusion should be noted on the PRISMA flowchart.

While narrative reviews can follow the structured scoping review process for both the title and abstract review and the data extraction, they usually follow a less formal process. Instead, reviewers may scan the articles identified in the search, select those that will be most helpful, and then take notes based on each article. Two common pitfalls in this step for narrative reviews are to include only the first few items identified or to include everything identified.

Analysis

Unlike a meta-analysis, a qualitative approach is utilized to analyze the data extracted for both narrative and scoping reviews. For both types of reviews, the extracted data should be reviewed, and a descriptive summary of the results should be developed. This summary should be organized by conceptual categories based on the purpose of the review. These could be methodologies utilized, key findings, gaps in the research, among others. Scoping reviews must include the table of extracted data.

PREPARING A REVIEW MANUSCRIPT

When preparing a manuscript for publication, the first step is to seek out the target journal's instructions or guidelines for authors. These will provide instructions for formatting, length, reference style, and other helpful information. Utilize these guidelines to set up a document with the required manuscript components. Typically, a manuscript includes the following components: title, keywords, abstract, introduction, methods, results, discussion, tables, figures, acknowledgments, and references. It is helpful to read similar reviews that have been published in the targeted journal to see how the manuscripts are structured, the length and depth of the various sections, and the writing style that has been successful for a particular journal.

The title should include the type of review, e.g., "narrative review" or "scoping review." The title page will include the list of authors who contributed to the manuscript. Most journals provide guidance as to who should be considered an author. This is especially important in a review. For some research projects searching for and summarizing articles may not qualify one for authorship; however, in a review project, that work is the "research" and may mean the individual should be included as a co-author. Make decisions regarding authorship at the beginning of the project. This ensures that no one is surprised that they are not included as an author or that they are an author and are expected to contribute at a level that they were not prepared for when the project started. Individuals who are not appropriate for inclusion as co-authors based on their contributions can be thanked in the acknowledgments. An abstract summarizing the review is usually included. Some journals want this to be broken into sections (e.g., background, methods, results, discussion), while others use a more narrative approach. Scoping reviews should provide the details of the databases and terms searched. Narrative reviews should also describe how the literature reviewed was identified but may be less detailed.

The body of the manuscript begins with an introduction that includes a comprehensive description of the topic of the review, provides a justification for the review, and makes explicit the purpose of the review. The methods section should provide the details of the search protocol and the analysis method. A statement indicating that the protocol was developed using PRISMA-ScR (or another source) and noting how to access the protocol should be included in the methods section for scoping reviews.

The results of a scoping review should include the search results, with a PRISMA flow chart included as a figure. For both types of reviews, a descriptive summary of the results by categories driven by the review purpose is then presented. The discussion section should not simply repeat the results. The discussion should contextualize the results. The section should start by providing a very brief summary as it relates to the review purpose. Next, discuss interesting findings in relation to the existing literature, as well implications for current practice, policy, and research. The limitations of the review should be noted. For narrative reviews it is important to note the limitations on the breadth of evidence reviewed. It is helpful to identify opportunities for future research based on the gaps in the current evidence base identified in the review. Some journals will also include a conclusions section. This should include an overall conclusion based on the findings of the review and should respond to the review's purpose. Briefly describe the key policy, practice, and/or research implications.

The references section is critical in a review. This provides full bibliographic information, which allows readers to find the original articles incorporated in the review. The use of a reference manager such as Zotero or Mendeley will make creating this section much easier. Be sure to select the reference style format required by the journal when generating the list of references and review them for accuracy.

Engaging Learners in Narrative and Scoping Reviews

Both narrative and scoping reviews are projects that novice researchers can contribute to and even lead. Reviews benefit from a team approach, and learners benefit by participating on a research team, gaining experience with how research projects are conceptualized, planned, executed, and communicated. One challenge novice researchers often encounter when developing a review is identifying a topic that is too broad. A review on "diabetes" will generate thousands of articles to review. Refining the topic and identifying a specified purpose is important to the success of the project. Learners often have great insight into topics that would be appropriate for a narrative review as they often easily identify the topics for which they were overwhelmed with the volume and variety of information available. Novice researchers often need to conduct the core activities of a scoping review as they develop an original research project making it simple to consider formalizing this process and publishing a scoping review, as it can help other researchers working in the area.

While reviews are projects well-suited for engaging learners with little to no research experience, mentorship and training can support their success. Novice researchers may need to learn how to search and read the literature, utilize reference management systems, utilize the expertise of a librarian, and work collaboratively. Co-reviewing a set of titles and abstracts and then full texts of articles as a team can help learners understand the thought process of how to apply inclusion/exclusion criteria and how to identify the data to extract.

Review projects are particularly well suited for engaging learners as the work of a review can mostly be done asynchronously, with team members working at their own pace and on their own schedule. Team meetings should focus on addressing key questions and developing specific action steps for each team member to complete before the next meeting. For example, when considering review topics, learners can search the literature to determine if a similar review has been conducted. When reviewing literature for potential inclusion, each team member can review a portion of the articles identified. A similar process can be utilized for data extraction. Team discussions of the extracted data are helpful for organizing and synthesizing the results for the discussion.

EXAMPLES OF LEARNER-ENGAGED NARRATIVE AND SCOPING REVIEWS

A study published in the *Journal of the American College of Clinical Pharmacy* in 2019 is an example of a narrative review in which students in both a doctor of pharmacy program and a doctor of medicine program were among the co-authors.[20] This narrative review examined pharmacists' practice roles related to the opioid crisis. The research team conducted a literature review to highlight pharmacist-driven practices, including prevention, harm reduction, treatment, and recovery-related care for patients affected by the opioid crisis. The authors describe their literature search methods and included seven articles. Of note, they did not systematically review nor report all of the possible literature on this topic. They selected articles that highlighted innovative programs and practices.

A 2016 review that sought to identify the literature that described the characteristics contributing to pharmacists' individual success in providing advanced patient care is an example of a scoping review that includes faculty and graduate students in the pharmaceutical sciences.[21] The review described the search strategy and identified ten articles that met the inclusion criteria for full-text review. A map of the literature is described, and content analysis identified and described two themes, "what successful pharmacists do" and "what successful pharmacists should be." This scoping review provided a description of what was known on these factors and identified the need for a more specific and practically oriented approach that accounts for individual and environmental factors to achieve individual-level success.

Dissemination of Narrative and Scoping Reviews

Dissemination of the results of scoping and narrative reviews is critical if they are to be useful to others. When preparing a review for dissemination, reporting guidelines (e.g., SANRA, PRISMA-ScR) should be utilized. The most common method of dissemination for a narrative or scoping review is via publication in a journal. It is helpful to identify a target journal to which the review will be submitted for publication consideration before a review project is executed. The review topic and the target audience (e.g., clinicians, researchers, decision-makers) are the most important factors to consider when selecting a potential journal.

Summary and Conclusions

Reviews are important methods to summarize and critically analyze the vast amount of literature on a topic or issue. Narrative and scoping reviews are two types of reviews that are valuable for practitioners, researchers, and decision makers. Narrative reviews provide summaries of selected literature on a topic and can be valuable educational resources. Readers must be aware of the potential for bias inherent to a narrative review. Scoping reviews utilize a systematic search and review process. They are useful for mapping the literature on a topic, determining if a systematic review is warranted, and identifying gaps and opportunities for further research. Both of these types of reviews are well suited to engage learners at all levels and can provide excellent experience in learning to critically evaluate and synthesize the literature.

Key Points and Advice

- Narrative and scoping reviews provide a synthesis of the literature on a topic.
- Narrative and scoping reviews are excellent team projects.
- Topic selection and purpose are critical decisions for narrative and scoping reviews.
- Narrative reviews are not comprehensive reviews of the literature.
- Scoping reviews systematically review and map the literature.

Chapter Review Questions

1. What are the benefits and limitations of a narrative review?
2. Describe when we should consider conducting a scoping review.
3. How do narrative and scoping reviews differ from systematic reviews?
4. Describe the resources needed to conduct a narrative or scoping review.
5. How can narrative and scoping reviews be disseminated?

Online Resources

Cochrane Training on Scoping Reviews. https://training.cochrane.org/resource/scoping-reviews-what-they-are-and-how-you-can-do-them
Figshare. https://figshare.com
JBI Manual for Evidence Synthesis. https://wiki.jbi.global/display/MANUAL
JBI Scoping Review Resources. https://joannabriggs.org/scoping-review-network/resources
Mendeley Reference Management. https://www.mendeley.com/guides/desktop
Open Science Framework. https://osf.io/
Polyglot search review translator. https://sr-accelerator.com/#/polyglot
PRISMA for Scoping Reviews. http://www.prisma-statement.org/Extensions/ScopingReviews
Zotero Reference Management. https://www.zotero.org/

REFERENCES

1. Grant MJ, Booth A. A typology of reviews: an analysis of 14 review types and associated methodologies. *Health Inf Libr J*. 2009;26(2):91-108.
2. Munn Z, Stern C, Aromataris E, Lockwood C, Jordan Z. What kind of systematic review should I conduct? A proposed typology and guidance for systematic reviewers in the medical and health sciences. *BMC Med Res Methodol*. 2018;18.
3. Tricco AC, Soobiah C, Antony J, et al. A scoping review identifies multiple emerging knowledge synthesis methods, but few studies operationalize the method. *J Clin Epidemiol*. 2016;73:19-28.
4. Green BN, Johnson CD, Adams A. Writing narrative literature reviews for peer-reviewed journals: secrets of the trade. *J Chiropr Med*. 2006;5(3):101-117.
5. Baethge C, Goldbeck-Wood S, Mertens S. SANRA—a scale for the quality assessment of narrative review articles. *Res Integr Peer Rev*. 2019;4(1):5.
6. Aggarwal P, Woolford SJ, Patel HP. Multi-morbidity and polypharmacy in older people: challenges and opportunities for clinical practice. *Geriatrics*. 2020;5(4).
7. Bishop C, Yacoob Z, Knobloch MJ, Safdar N. Community pharmacy interventions to improve antibiotic stewardship and implications for pharmacy education: a narrative overview. *Res Soc Adm Pharm*. 2019;15(6):627-631.

8. Arksey H, O'Malley L. Scoping studies: towards a methodological framework. *Int J Soc Res Methodol.* 2005;8(1):19-32.

9. Peters M, Godfrey C, McInerney P, Munn Z, Tricco A, Khalil H. Scoping Reviews (2020) version. In: *JBI Manual for Evidence Synthesis.* JBI; 2020: Chapter 11. Accessed January 1, 2021. https://synthesismanual.jbi.global/

10. Levac D, Colquhoun H, O'Brien KK. Scoping studies: advancing the methodology. *Implement Sci.* 2010;5:69.

11. Khalil H, Peters MDJ, Tricco AC, et al. Conducting high quality scoping reviews-challenges and solutions. *J Clin Epidemiol.* 2021;130:156-160.

12. Tricco AC, Lillie E, Zarin W, et al. PRISMA Extension for Scoping Reviews (PRISMA-ScR): checklist and explanation. *Ann Intern Med.* 2018;169(7):467.

13. Peters MDJ, Marnie C, Tricco AC, et al. Updated methodological guidance for the conduct of scoping reviews. *JBI Evid Synth.* 2020;18(10):2119-2126.

14. JBI Scoping Reviews Site | Joanna Briggs Institute. Accessed January 14, 2021. https://joannabriggs.org/scoping-review-network

15. Shafiee Hanjani L, Caffery LJ, Freeman CR, Peeters G, Peel NM. A scoping review of the use and impact of telehealth medication reviews. *Res Soc Adm Pharm.* 2020;16(8):1140-1153.

16. Knott GJ, Mylrea MF, Glass BD. A scoping review of pharmacy preceptor training programs. *Am J Pharm Educ.* 2020;84(10):ajpe8039.

17. Open Science Framework. Accessed January 17, 2021. https://osf.io/

18. Figshare. Accessed January 17, 2021. https://figshare.com/

19. Clark JM, Sanders S, Carter M, et al. Improving the translation of search strategies using the Polyglot Search Translator: a randomized controlled trial. *J Med Libr Assoc.* 2020;108(2):195-207.

20. Bratberg JP, Smothers ZPW, Collins K, Erstad B, Veve JR, Muzyk AJ. Pharmacists and the opioid crisis: a narrative review of pharmacists' practice roles. *J Am Coll Clin Pharm.* 2020;3(2):478-484.

21. Dikun JA, Crumby AS, Shahpurwala Z, Hall J, Charrois TL, Rosenthal MM. Understanding pharmacist success in practice: a scoping review. *J Am Pharm Assoc.* 2016;56(6):649-655.

20

Chapter Twenty

Systematic Reviews and Meta-Analysis in Pharmacy

Wei-Hsuan Lo-Ciganic, MSPharm, MS, PhD and
Juan M. Hincapie-Castillo, PharmD, MS, PhD

Chapter Objectives

- Define systematic review and meta-analysis in pharmacy
- Identify various sources for systematic reviews in pharmacy
- Describe proper research questions to address with systematic reviews and meta-analysis
- Identify the expertise needed for conducting systematic reviews and meta-analyses
- Describe the practical and technical considerations for conducting a systematic review
- Discuss the analytical considerations for carrying out a meta-analysis
- Describe the best practices for reporting findings of systematic reviews and meta-analysis
- Describe examples of learner-involved systematic reviews and meta-analysis
- Understand the dissemination framework for systematic reviews and meta-analysis

Key Terminology

Cochrane library, funnel plot, GRADE, grey literature, heterogeneity, meta-analysis, publication bias, and systematic reviews

Introduction

Over 2 million scientific pieces of literature are published in over 30,000 journals each year worldwide.[1] It is challenging to keep up with the overload of information. Well-conducted systematic reviews and meta-analyses are valuable to summarize evidence from the existing literature, may provide the strongest form of scientific evidence, and thus save one's time digesting information from numerous studies. Systematic reviews and meta-analyses provide a great opportunity and research experience for pharmacy students, residents, and fellows to learn how to search the literature, extract relevant information, evaluate the biases and quality of studies, synthesize findings, and work in a multidisciplinary research team. A systematic review can involve quantitative and/or qualitative synthesis when there is a sufficient number of good quality studies included. In pharmacy practice, systematic reviews may summarize the effects of interventions, policies, pharmacist management programs, or processes, such as evaluating the effects of different types of pharmacist-led interventions for improving medication adherence. **Meta-analysis** allows for the quantitative synthesis of results to produce a single pooled estimate of the intervention effects from studies included in a systematic review.

The goal of this chapter is to provide practical considerations and approaches to conducting a systematic review and meta-analysis using resources commonly available in pharmacy settings within a defined timeline of one year. This chapter will describe the proper research questions to address with systematic reviews and meta-analysis, the practical and technical considerations for conducting a systematic review, and the best practices for reporting them. It identifies the various sources for systematic reviews in pharmacy and the expertise needed for conducting such studies. Also, the analytical considerations for carrying out a meta-analysis are discussed.

Case Scenario

Mrs. M, a 65-year-old healthy woman with bilateral knee osteoarthritis (OA) came to your community pharmacy for consultation. She has been searching for information on glucosamine and chondroitin use in knee OA. Below are several examples of the information she identified:

- A local magazine: *"Overall, glucosamine and chondroitin sulfate were not significantly better than a placebo in reducing knee pain..."*
- Arthritis Foundation online: *"...Some people with mild to moderate OA taking either glucosamine or chondroitin sulfate reported pain relief..."*
- *The New York Times: "...Glucosamine has shown a benefit for those suffering from osteoarthritis. To discourage its use as a treatment option is ill-considered..."*

You conducted a quick literature search on PubMed on this topic, with over 500 studies identified. You may find an answer from each article, but the results appear to be conflicting. What should you do?

Details and key concepts of conducting systematic reviews and meta-analysis can be found in the companion book, *Principles of Research Design and Drug Literature Evaluation*. Briefly, a systematic review uses systematic and explicit methods that are reproducible and transparent to identify, select, extract, analyze, and critically appraise relevant information from the primary research included in the review to answer a well-formulated question.[2] As shown in the case scenario described above, systematic reviews are valuable for summarizing current evidence with conflicting findings from a large volume of literature to better guide patients, healthcare professionals, and policymakers on best practices.

Steps in Conducting a Systematic Review

Figure 20-1 summarizes the key steps of performing a systematic review including: (1) formulate a specific question using the "Population, Intervention or Exposure, Comparator, Outcome, Timing and Setting (PI[E]COTS)" elements; (2) develop a protocol including database sources, search strategies for each database, eligibility criteria (i.e., inclusion and exclusion criteria), relevant information and details to be collected and extracted, and methods to assess biases; (3) register the developed protocol at the International Prospective Register of Systematic Reviews (PROSPERO; https://www.crd.york.ac.uk/prospero/);[3] (4) conduct a literature search using all available database sources including grey literature, which includes reports, white papers, and other

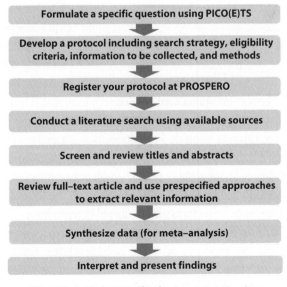

Figure 20–1. The key steps of performing a systematic review.

documents that are not peer-reviewed; (5) screen and review titles and abstracts from the initial search results; (6) review full-text articles and use prespecified approaches to extract relevant information (e.g., country, clinical outcomes); (7) synthesize quantitative and/or qualitative data (for meta-analysis) and conduct additional sensitivity and stratification analyses if needed; and (8) interpret and present findings.

Before Starting the Systematic Review

Before conducting a systematic review or meta-analysis, there are some guidelines that must be considered in the planning process. Planning ahead is the most important aspect of any research process as it allows the research team to move ahead efficiently and react timely to any unforeseen challenges presented throughout the process. Systematic reviews, and by extension, meta-analyses take a considerable amount of time given the breadth of information to synthesize and the coordination required by the research team members to undertake all tasks.

DEFINING THE RESEARCH QUESTION

Developing a good research question is the first step in conducting a systematic review. An explicit, relevant, and significant research question allows the team to have a clear direction in the research process and is a fundamental first step before engaging in any type of data collection. Sources or processes for generating a research question might include consultation with an expert (e.g., faculty, practicing pharmacists) knowledgeable in the field to identify existing gaps to address or ongoing public health issues (e.g., COVID-19 pandemic, opioid crisis). The specific purpose of a systematic review is to summarize the available evidence on a particular topic qualitatively, while conversely, the purpose of a meta-analysis is to summarize the evidence quantitatively, if feasible, by pooling effect estimates. While seeming straightforward, the research team should be explicit on what they want to "summarize" as simply saying so is not sufficient, nor appropriate, to produce reproducible and transparent research. Reproducibility is a mainstay of well-conducted research and should be prioritized in all decisions made from the point of study conception to dissemination and publication of results[4]—systematic reviews are no exception. The research question should follow the PI(E)COTS format, and the team should agree on each element to ensure the protocol will be adhered to accordingly.

While the PI(E)COTS format allows for an explicit research question, the research team must consider the question's relevance and importance. Given the extent of resources in time and manpower it takes to carry out a systematic review, the research team ought to consider whether the allocation of those resources is a worthwhile endeavor. Using knowledge of the specific needs and gaps in a given field, the senior members of the research team should make their first responsibility be to reflect on and justify the needs and significance of the research question. Once again, plainly summarizing the evidence is not a compelling enough reason to conduct a systematic review. It is also important to look up the particular research question in the PROSPERO[3] and Cochrane Library Reviews[5] websites to assess whether there is any registered systematic review and meta-analysis currently in process to avoid duplication of work done by other teams. The Cochrane Library is a collection of databases that contains different types of high quality, independent evidence to inform healthcare decision making. The prompts that the research team should consider in defining the research question are:

1. Has this research question been addressed previously with older evidence, and if so, is it important to update findings?
2. Will the clinicians, patients, regulators, and other stakeholders benefit from having a summary of results from this systematic review and meta-analysis, and will it have any meaningful contributions to patient care or policy?
3. Are the needed resources sufficient to complete the scope of this systematic review and meta-analysis? Is the return on time and effort investment worth it for the research team members?

Once the team has engaged in honest and thorough discussion, then it is time to define the research timeline.

RESEARCH TIMELINE

Although the specific time dedicated to conducting a proper systematic review and meta-analysis will vary as a function of the scope of research and the amount of evidence to synthesize, some general principles can be applied in defining milestones and time allocation in the planning process. The scope of the research question will primarily dictate the amount of evidence that will be retrieved in the initial search. While it is important to be broad in the initial search results in order to comprehensively capture all the relevant evidence, the research team should consider the resources available to them and the desirable timeline (e.g., one year) in which the team would like to complete the project. For example, a research question that aims to summarize the available evidence on the immune-related adverse events of immune checkpoint inhibitors in cancer patients will likely have a more time-consuming screening process than the same research question restricted to patients with a specific cancer (e.g., advanced melanoma).[6] Pharmacy-related systematic reviews and meta-analyses typically take at least 6 to 12 months to finish. The generalized activity normalization timetable (GANTT) presented in Table 20–1 outlines a few key milestones that a research team will want to meet over the time spent conducting

TABLE 20—1. GANTT CHART OUTLINING TASKS AND TIMELINE FOR A SYSTEMATIC REVIEW AND META-ANALYSIS

Tasks	6 to 12 months											
	M1	M2	M3	M4	M5	M6	M7	M8	M9	M10	M11	M12
Complete start up activities (e.g., IRB, obtain data)	x											
Discuss with research team to identify clinical and research gaps	x											
Determine the research question and list the scope of systematic review and meta-analysis	x											
Develop a systematic review and meta-analysis protocol such as defining databases and search strategies		x										
Register the protocol at PROSPERO			x									
Conduct literature search (initial and refined)			x									
Complete initial screening of title and abstracts				x								
Conduct full text reviews					x	x						
Extract information from eligible studies						x	x	x				
Summarize the findings from included studies									x			
Conduct meta-analysis when feasible										x	x	
Dissemination plans: presentations, abstracts/manuscripts, stakeholder dissemination of the study findings												x

GANTT: generalized activity normalization time table

the study, but the research team also needs to allow some flexibility for unforeseen circumstances (e.g., resolving conflicts on the articles screened by independent reviewers).

DEVELOPMENT AND REGISTRATION OF A PROTOCOL FOR SYSTEMATIC REVIEWS

To minimize biases and duplication of work, it is highly recommended to register the developed systematic review and meta-analysis protocols as early as possible with PROSPERO at https://www.crd.york.ac.uk/prospero/. PROSPERO is an international database of prospectively registered systematic reviews involving a health-related outcome in the fields of health and social care, welfare, public health, education, crime, justice, and international development.[3] PROSPERO does not accept registrations of scoping, narrative, or mapping reviews, reviews already registered in the Cochrane database, or mini or partial reviews done for a training course or for classwork that uses the PROSPERO system to teach students how to register. The Open Science Framework (OSF) tool does accept registrations of most of these review types. PROSPERO provides the guidance and helps for accessing and completing the registration form, which can be downloaded at https://www.crd.york.ac.uk/prospero/documents/PROSPERO%20registration%20form.pdf. It is worth noting that PROSPERO will not accept the initial registration of the protocol if the reviews have progressed beyond the point of completing data extraction. The registration template comprises mandatory fields including review questions (framed using PI(E)COTS where relevant), searches (including sources, dates, and any restrictions), condition or domain being studied (e.g., advanced melanoma), participants/population (e.g., adults), intervention(s) or exposure(s), comparator(s)/control(s), type of study to be included (e.g., phase III randomized controlled trials [RCTs]), main outcomes, risk of bias (quality) assessment, and strategy for data synthesis. The full list of required fields is given in the template. It may take at least 10 business days to get PROSPERO approval on the submitted protocol. After receiving the initial approval from PROSPERO, researchers can make changes, amendments, and updates of their protocol, and these modifications will appear as public records (all PROSPERO protocols remain permanently on PROSPERO). Once the systematic review is completed, the research team should provide the anticipated publication date with the bibliographic reference and electronic links to publications to PROSPERO. The research team is responsible for documenting the details of the availability of the systematic review's unpublished results or reasons for the termination of the review even when the team does not pursue publication.

Research Expertise and the Team

In a parallel process of developing a systematic review and meta-analysis protocol, the leading reviewer (e.g., pharmacy student) and his/her research mentor are highly encouraged to recruit a librarian, additional evaluators, and a biostatistician/statistician (especially when a meta-analysis is involved) to ensure the validity and accuracy of the study findings. It is also encouraged to include an expert in the conditions or clinical area of interest (e.g., oncologist or policy expert) to maximize the clinical utility or policy impact of study findings.

RESEARCH MENTOR

This person is usually the senior author in the research team who works closely with the leading reviewer and is in charge of the supervision of the study tasks. If the study is funded, the research mentor usually is in charge of managing the budget and administrative activities such as submitting progress and final reports to the sponsoring agency. During the data collection, the research mentor often serves as an arbitrator for discrepancies or when consensus has not been reached. The research mentor serves as the corresponding author for the dissemination of products (e.g., manuscript in a scientific journal).

LIBRARIAN

A well-conducted study can always benefit from the involvement of a librarian or an expert in library sciences to help with the literature review, in a systematic review and/or meta-analysis. This individual is well-versed in appropriate search strategies and the various databases available at your institution. The librarian in the team can facilitate efficient reference management and aid with technical tasks such as the deduplication of results from several databases. Typically, the librarian at your institution will collect some intake information from the team and will offer consultation during the search strategy building process. One often-overlooked task in budgeting time in the initial search strategy is the deduplication of findings from multiple databases. The librarian can help with the deduplication process and the building of a reference library in the citation manager software of preference (e.g., EndNote).

Given that a librarian might serve multiple departments or colleges at your institution, the leading investigator should maintain clear communications to make sure the librarian has the appropriate availability to be an active participant in the project within the expected timeline. It is also highly recommended to discuss the potential for authorship in the final manuscript with the librarian based on overall contribution and if the work product merits authorship or not. See Chapter 24, "Research Manuscripts," for a more detailed discussion of authorship.

EVALUATORS

Screening and data extraction or collection are the core tasks of the systematic review process. Depending on the scope of the research question, several evaluators may be needed to carry out these tasks effectively and to provide independent evaluation. It is up to the discretion of the leading investigator and research mentor to decide how many individuals to include. While a more "hands-on deck" could help to get the job done faster, it is important to recognize that having a larger team opens the door for potentially more discrepancies in the screening and data extraction process. It is also important for the lead investigator to provide comprehensive training for the evaluators not only before but also during the screening and data collection steps to ensure the quality of the evaluation process.

BIOSTATISTICIANS/STATISTICIANS

Specific to the conduct of meta-analysis, it is highly recommended to consult with a biostatistician/statistician to ensure the research team uses the correct statistical methods to obtain valid estimates from the included studies. This biostatistician/statistician can also provide important assistance in the summary of the results and guide the team on the best strategies to present the results. For example, the individual may suggest whether it is more appropriate to use random or fixed-effects models. Authorship should be negotiated and offered in accordance with his/her efforts at the beginning of the project for the biostatistician/statistician assisting with the statistical analysis.

Defining an Effective Search Strategy

KEY TERMS

Based on the prior literature and clinical expertise, the team should come up with a preliminary list of the key terms prior to meeting with the librarian. The research team can use each element in the PICO(E)TS to organize the key terms needed to build a comprehensive search strategy for a systematic review. With a librarian's help, the combination of these key terms along with the use of controlled vocabulary available in the selected databases (e.g., MeSH terms in PubMed database) and use of appropriate commonplace Boolean operators will allow the research team to obtain a broad and comprehensive range of results to begin their review. For example, when conducting a systematic review on renal adverse drug reactions related to the use of any nonsteroidal anti-inflammatory drugs (NSAIDs), the best strategy to include all medications in this pharmacological class in PubMed would be "Anti-Inflammatory Agents, Non-Steroidal" [pa], where "[pa]" specifies the search to include NSAIDs based on their pharmacological action.

DATABASES

Members of the research team should be familiar with the scope of resources available at their institution. Larger academic centers might have subscriptions to a larger number of databases, and the use of specific resources should be considered a priori in discussing the research protocol. Traditionally in the United States, the Medline (PubMed) database is the most likely source of information that a research team will consider first. While a single database might be deemed comprehensive enough in its indexing, all secondary data sources have inherent limitations on the scope of what can be retrieved. If available, the team should consider expanding their search to other relevant databases. Reviewers of the final report might question the appropriateness of conducting a systematic review using a single database. Depending on the institutional resources, common databases or sources that are often used for conducting a systematic review and meta-analysis in pharmacy research include: PubMed/MEDLINE, International Pharmaceutical Abstracts (IPA), Cumulative Index to Nursing and Allied Health Literature (CINAHL), Excerpta Medica dataBASE (Embase), ProQuest Thesis Dissertations, PsycINFO, Scopus, and Web of Science.

DOCUMENTATION

The best place to start and keep proper documentation when conducting a systematic review is the use of a PROSPERO protocol. For transparency and minimizing any biases, it is important that while conducting the search and data collection steps, each decision for modifying or refining search strategies and study eligibility criteria is documented accordingly. This information will later be used by the team in drafting the manuscript or study report. The most important elements to document are the decisions regarding conflicts on the evaluation of study eligibility and quality between the evaluators and other consensus-building discussions. Strong documentation is critical as the time between study conception, and final manuscript draft can be long, and the team might not recall all the decisions made during the research process.

Screening and Data Collection in Systematic Reviews

INCLUSION AND EXCLUSION CRITERIA

While the comprehensive initial search strategy can help in filtering out sources that are not appropriate (e.g., based on the study year or language of the manuscript), the research team needs to determine the specific criteria that will be used to include or exclude studies in the systematic review. For this purpose, it is important to go back to the PI(E)COTS research question in determining what studies to keep during the screening process. For example, a study could evaluate the specific type of cancer you are interested in, but it might be conducted in the pediatric population when you are interested in studies in adults. Likewise, the study title could be in English, but the body of the manuscript might be in another language that none of the research team members speaks proficiently. The inclusion and exclusion criteria should be determined prior to the start of the screening process, but revisions might be needed during the process based on feedback from the evaluators. The research team should document these revisions in the PROSPERO registration.

TITLE AND ABSTRACT SCREENING

The screening process begins with a simple review of the titles of the papers or sources obtained from the search. Remember that titles are not very explicit at times; therefore, the evaluators should be fairly liberal at this stage in deciding which papers to move forward and which ones to remove. For each source removed, the evaluators should document a reason as this information will be later reported in the creation of the Preferred Reporting Items for Systematic Reviews and Meta-Analyses (PRISMA) flowchart.[7] Managing the screening and selection processes can be challenging, especially for large-scale systematic reviews involving multiple reviewers. There are various free and subscription-based tools available to assist the screening and selection process, including Microsoft Excel, Covidence, RevMan, and SR ToolBox.[8] Each of these tools has unique features and advantages, and disadvantages. For example, Covidence is a user-friendly web-based tool for managing systematic reviews.[9] However, Covidence's title screening process currently provides a one-click mechanism to include or exclude references based on the inclusion and exclusion criteria without tracking the exact reason for exclusion. After the selection of titles, the evaluators should proceed with reading the abstracts of the selected papers. It is important to also be fairly liberal at this stage as many abstracts might not report all the specific components of interest in the PI(E)COTS research question. If there are more than two evaluators, the research mentor should ensure there are standardized screening criteria and procedures in place to ensure consistency. The procedures might include requiring the evaluators to consult with each other if needed to decide whether to keep or remove a certain reference prior to full-text screening.

FULL-TEXT SCREENING

Unarguably the most time-consuming step in a systematic review is the full-text screening step. This step inherently requires the most care by all research team members. As the name implies, this screening requires a thorough reading of the articles that were selected in the previous screening steps. The evaluators should be properly trained at recognizing the specific information that is needed for the purposes of the systematic review. The full-text screening allows the evaluators to find pertinent information that will be extracted in the next step. Due to the rather monotonous work involved for full-text screening, it is recommended that the evaluators take regular breaks while completing this task so that boredom and fatigue do not preclude them from capturing important information.

After the full-text screening, snowball methods may be undertaken to ensure a thorough literature review was conducted and no relevant citations were inadvertently missed. Forward snowballing involves citation searching, in which you start with an article you have included in your review and find the articles that have cited it. Citation searching in pharmacy may be conducted using Science Citation Index, Scopus, Web of Science Cited Reference Search, OvidSP MEDLINE, PubMed Central Citation Search, or Google Scholar, although these tools may produce different results. Reverse snowballing involves searching the references included in the bibliographies of your included studies. Snowballing methods can be time-consuming, and thus the research team needs to carefully consider if such searches will find additional unique citations and thus are warranted.[10,11]

DATA COLLECTION TOOLS

Once full-text screening is complete, the research team needs to perform the extraction of the information. The tools for data collection and extraction of the required information in the systematic review are varied, but they all share common features. The tools must list the "demographic" characteristics of the study, such as the year of publication and the first author's name. Depending on the specific research question, several items from the methods and the result sections of the study are extracted. All the information collected can be organized electronically in a simple Excel spreadsheet file, another database program, or Covidence. Data collection items should be determined a priori (i.e., prior to the data collection), but the team might modify or include additional fields depending on how the work progresses. Any deviation from the original protocol must be documented, and the evaluators should constantly check with each other to ensure consistency.

ORGANIZATION OF THEMES

After all the data is extracted, the information should be organized and synthesized in a way that is informative, and that answers the original research question. In turn, this is the qualitative step of the process where the evaluators identify common themes that arise from the data collection fields. The themes could be defined *a priori* or *post hoc* (i.e., after the data collection is complete). For example, when identifying different deprescribing methods for opioids, the themes can be categorized into pharmacist-based vs.

non-pharmacist-based interventions. A proper systematic review should probably have a balance of both, given that some themes that arise after the data collection might not have been thought of in the initial protocol development.

CROSS-VALIDATION AND RESOLVING CONFLICTS

Throughout the screening, data collection, and organization of themes, the research team members should consult with each other whenever there is ambiguity in any step. The research mentor and/or expert in the topic being studied can provide helpful guidance on resolving any conflicts that arise. When reporting results, the research team should be explicit on the processes and steps followed to reach a consensus.

SUMMARY TABLES

One way of presenting the information gathered in a systematic review is to include tables synthesizing the main findings. It is important to consider what tables will be included in the main body of the report or manuscript and which ones should be relegated to the appendix. While more information is preferred to offer a complete picture of the data extraction, the research team should avoid simply copying and pasting all the information from the original articles into summary tables. The tables should be easy to navigate but comprehensive enough to allow readers to gain insight into relevant information. The research team should keep in mind that readers can always refer to the listed references to obtain more information if desired. Therefore, the summary tables are mostly for presenting thematic analysis and information directly related to the research question.

VISUALIZATION OF RESULTS

Depending on the quantity and type of data summarized, it might be worth exploring ways to visualize the information graphically. "A picture is worth a thousand words" is really important when literally there are potentially thousands of words in the summary tables and the corresponding appendices. Any data visualization should be complementary to the report or manuscript and should stand-alone (i.e., interpretable without looking into texts). For example, a PRISMA diagram is recommended to visualize the flow of information through the different phases of the review.

ASSESSMENT OF RISK OF BIAS OR STRENGTHS OF EVIDENCE

A well-conducted systematic review not only summarizes the evidence and findings of the included studies but also quantifies the risk of biases from these studies. Risk of bias refers to the potential issues in the study that limit the validity and applicability of the results summarized. For example, potential biases to assess include the randomization process used, study deviations from the intended interventions, missing outcome data, measurement of the outcome, and selection of the reported outcome.[12] A common expression heard when conducting systematic reviews is "trash in, trash out," which refers to the inclusion of flawed studies that may bias the pooled results. To assess potential biases from the included studies, there are several tools available depending on the design of the included studies. Commonly used risk of bias assessment tools for included RCTs are the Jadad criteria[13] and RoB2 (a revised Cochrane risk-of-bias tool).[12] A popular risk of bias assessment tool for non-interventional studies is the ROBINS-I tool[14] that can be found at https://sites.google.com/site/riskofbiastool/welcome/home?authuser=0

Covidence's online tool also includes a risk of bias assessment component.[9] The Grading of Recommendations Assessment, Development and Evaluation (GRADE) assessment tool can be used to grade the quality (or certainty) of evidence and strength recommendation for each outcome and each comparison made.[15] The GRADE assessment tool evaluates the risk of biases, consistency (i.e., overall results similar to other studies), directness (i.e., with a single and direct link between the intervention and outcome), and precision of the findings.[15] Assessing the risk of bias and strengths of evidence requires careful consideration by the evaluators as there is room for ambiguity in these assessments. Similar to extraction and data collection, any conflicts regarding the score assigned to each of the bias and strength of evidence criteria must be discussed with the research team, and an arbitrator might be needed to reach a consensus.

Analytical Methods for Meta-Analysis

When a systematic review includes a sufficient number of studies (usually ≥ 3) with quantitative results, conducting a meta-analysis allows for calculating a single pooled estimate of treatment effects. Studies included should have good quality (i.e., no or low biases) and similar intervention and outcomes measures in representative populations. For continuous outcome measures (e.g., total cholesterol or depression scores), mean changes with standard deviation are extracted from each study, and the meta-analysis typically generates a pooled inverse variance of weighted mean changes. When the included studies use different scales (e.g., one depression scale ranges from 0 to 5 while another ranges from 0 to 100), these continuous data can be presented as standardized mean changes using a measure such as Hedge's g.[16] For dichotomous or binary outcomes (e.g., dead vs. alive, having a heart attack vs. not), the number of individuals having versus not having an outcome of interests and the effect estimates (e.g., relative risk) are extracted from each study. It is important to note that typical meta-analytic methods can only synthesize the same effect measures. For example, studies reporting odds ratios cannot be combined with studies reporting hazard ratios. It is also not recommended to combine the results from RCTs with the results from observational studies that may be inherently more biased. The biggest limitation of conducting a meta-analysis is indeed the fact that included studies very often have different designs and different measures of association. Hence, if the goal is to conduct a meta-analysis, the research team may limit the inclusion and exclusion criteria for the systematic review to specific study designs (e.g., RCTs) or conduct meta-analyses stratified by study design and type of effect estimates.

HETEROGENEITY EVALUATION

Commonly used software or tools typically report the V (statistics) reflecting the variation across study outcomes due to differences of studies included in the meta-analysis. The I-squared statistic (ranged 0–100%) is preferably reported in the meta-analysis, where the higher the I-squared value is, then the greater the heterogeneity is (e.g., 75% indicates a substantial heterogeneity).[17] The p-value of the heterogeneity chi-squared or Cochran's Q is also commonly reported,[18] whereas a p-value < 0.05 or p-value < 0.10 is generally considered as substantial heterogeneity across the included studies.

When there is a sufficient number of studies meeting the requirements for statistical pooling, then the research team must determine whether they will run a fixed or a random effects model. When there is significant heterogeneity across the included studies, it is more appropriate to use random effects models that account for both within and between variances of each study. A complete discussion on the methodology and math behind pooling estimates is outside the scope of this guide; therefore, we refer the research team to consult with a statistician who can provide technical assistance in calculations.

FIXED EFFECTS MODELS VERSUS RANDOM EFFECTS MODELS

Briefly, fixed effects models assume that any variation seen in different effect estimates (i.e., heterogeneity) is due to random error (i.e., chance) and only accounts for the within-study variance of each study. Conversely, random effects models recognize that different underlying characteristics and treatment effects across studies lead to heterogeneity. Random effects models include both between-study and within-study variation in the estimation of summary effect size and statistical significance (e.g., DerSimonian and Laird test). Because of this stricter assumption, random effects models are more conservative than fixed effects (i.e., providing wider confidence intervals).

FOREST PLOTS

The easiest way to summarize and visualize pooled estimates in a meta-analysis is the use of a forest plot such as shown in Figure 20–2,[19] which is a graph that represents the results of studies included in a meta-analysis.

PUBLICATION BIAS EVALUATION

Publication bias occurs when combining only the published studies without critical appraisal and may lead to an incorrect effect estimate and an overly optimistic conclusion. While including unpublished data and trial registries might overcome this issue, the research team should construct a funnel plot or other tests (e.g., Egger's test) to assess publication bias.[20] The funnel plot such as shown in Figure 20–3[19] is a scatter plot that graphs treatment effect estimates from each study with precision (e.g., standard error or variance of the estimate).[21] If there is a significant number of studies outside of the pyramid and the distribution is not symmetrical in a funnel plot, there is evidence for potential publication bias, and it must be discussed in the narrative of the report and manuscript.

SOFTWARE

There are software programs customized for conducting meta-analysis that can be purchased or that are freely available online. Some of these programs include Meta-win, Metaxis, RevMan, EasyMA, EpiMeta, and Meta-Analyst. Depending on the resources available to the team, specialized software might not be warranted, and statistical analysis can be conducted with the use of code in commonly used programs like Stata, SAS, Dstat, S+/R/R Studio, StatsDirect, and WinBUGS. Unless the research team members intend

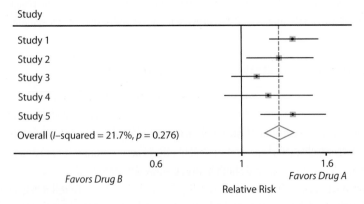

Figure 20–2. Forest plot of relative risk meta-analysis. (Reproduced, with permission, from Aparasu RR, Bentley JP, eds. *Principles of Research Design and Drug Literature Evaluation*. 2nd ed. McGraw Hill; 2020.)

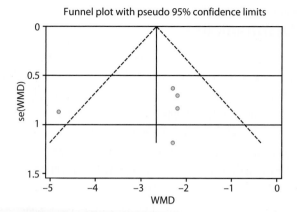

Figure 20–3. Funnel plot for test of publication bias in the weighted mean difference example. (Reproduced, with permission, from Aparasu RR, Bentley JP, eds. *Principles of Research Design and Drug Literature Evaluation*. 2nd ed. McGraw Hill; 2020.)

to acquire advanced statistical analysis skills with a particular piece of software, we recommend the use of statistical consulting services available at the home institution or the statistician in the team.

Dissemination of Systematic Reviews and Meta-Analyses

TARGET JOURNALS

The decision on where to publish the manuscript should be agreed upon by all members of the research team. In considering the available options, the team should decide the most appropriate fit that aligns well with the research question and the overarching goal and takeaways from the study. The web-based Journal/Author Name Estimator tool can quickly generate a list of journals whose audience and subject area fit well with your manuscript.[22] While it might be attractive to submit the final manuscript to a high-impact journal, the research team should approach the submission process strategically, considering that each journal has distinct requirements on formatting, different review times, and audiences. It is important to note that several journals will not publish a systematic review that has not been registered with PROSPERO and many publications require a risk of bias assessment in order to consider the manuscript.

MANUSCRIPT PREPARATION AND COMMON REPORTING GUIDELINES FOR SYSTEMATIC REVIEWS

It is prudent to read a published systematic review published recently in the target journal of interest. The research team should be mindful of word limitations and any restrictions on the number of tables or other exhibits allowed in the main body of the manuscript. Putting additional information in the appendix might be an option for a given journal, but the team must ensure that the main manuscript has enough information on its own to inform the readers. It is highly recommended the research team adhere to the PRISMA guidelines in preparing the final report and manuscript.[7] The current PRISMA statement and checklist are available at http://www.prisma-statement.org/. Key content areas of the PRISMA guideline include the study's rationale, objectives, eligibility criteria, search strategy, assessment of the risk of bias, data syntheses results, general results' interpretation, and limitations. There are several extensions to the PRISMA statement depending on the type of systematic review, such as network meta-analysis.

Exemplars of Learner-Involved Systematic Reviews and Meta-Analyses

EXAMPLE OF A SYSTEMATIC REVIEW

The study entitled "Effects of hydrocodone rescheduling on opioid use outcomes: A systematic review" aimed to summarize the changes reported in opioid prescribing, dispensing, and use associated with the rescheduling of hydrocodone-containing products.[23] The lead evaluator of this systematic review was a postdoctorate fellow at the institution who worked with five PharmD students to conduct screening, extraction, and data collection. The study was published in the *Journal of the American Pharmacists Association*. The investigators used five bibliographic databases and searched the gray literature following the guidelines of the Cochrane Handbook for Systematic Reviews of Interventions, conducted forwards and backwards snowball searches, and reported the results according to the PRISMA guidelines. After deduplicating the search results, two authors screened the titles. Then, two authors screened the full-text abstracts and articles. Two authors independently extracted data from the 44 identified studies after an additional team training exercise and using a data extraction sheet created for the study. All conflicts regarding study inclusion or data extraction were resolved by a third author. In addition to content experts in the field of pharmaceutical outcomes and prescription pain medications, this study included a pharmacy-liaison master's degree level research librarian in the team. This team successfully trained and systematized their screening processes and data extraction using gold standard techniques. The entire project took over a year, from study conception to the first submission. Research teams must account for the possibility of multiple submissions and revisions when trying to publish the manuscripts.

EXAMPLE OF A META-ANALYSIS

The study entitled "Effectiveness and safety of non-vitamin K antagonist oral antico-agulants for atrial fibrillation and venous thromboembolism: a systematic review and meta-analyses" aimed to examine the efficacy and effectiveness and safety of direct oral anticoagulants (DOACs) versus vitamin K antagonists by disease (atrial fibrillation vs. venous thromboembolism), study design (RCTs vs. observational studies), and individual DOAC (dabigatran, rivaroxaban, apixaban, and edoxaban).[24] The leading researchers of this study, a pharmacist fellow and a graduate student at the college of pharmacy at the institution, conducted screening, data collection and extraction, and statistical analyses. The researchers included 11 databases, conducted hand searches of gray literature using backward snowballing methods, and developed the methods, and reported the study using the PRISMA guidelines. The study team included content, clinical, and statistical experts and a research librarian. Two investigators conducted the literature search and title and abstract screening. Two reviewers screened the full text articles and abstracted the study data independently using a standardized data extraction form in Microsoft Excel. Conflicts between the reviewers were resolved by consensus and/or consultation with a third reviewer. The team obtained pooled estimates with 95% confidence inter-vals of the studies' outcomes using a random effects meta-analysis with inverse variance weighting and used two methods to assess publication bias (i.e., asymmetric distributions from the funnel plot, Duval and Tweedie nonparametric "trim and fill" model). The study was published in *Clinical Therapeutics*. The entire project took over a year and a half from study conception to the first submission.

Summary and Conclusions

Systematic reviews and meta-analyses combine the results of multiple studies in a mean-ingful and structured way to produce high-quality evidence regarding a phenomenon. Conducting a systematic review is a great way to involve pharmacy students, fellows, and residents in research, but members of the research team must be cognizant of the time commitment and resources required. Pharmacy students, fellows, and residents wish-ing to conduct a systematic review or meta-analysis should work with content experts and a research librarian. While it might be tempting to conduct their own statistical analysis, it is recommended that the pooling of estimates in a meta-analysis is done with guidance and consultation from a statistician. Individuals interested in conducting a systematic review and/or meta-analysis must follow strict procedures to ensure that the final product is transparent and reproducible. Rigorous methods for these types of studies include preregistration of the study, following the guidelines of the Cochrane Handbook for Systematic Reviews of Interventions, assessing for bias, and adhering to the PRISMA guidelines when developing the study methods and reporting the study results.

Key Points and Advice

- Before starting a systematic review or meta-analysis, assess the team for their availability to commit to the project, which may take at least six months.
- Work with content experts to develop an explicit, relevant, and significant research question.
- Preregister the study.
- Work with a research librarian to develop the search strategy and, if possible, to conduct your search.
- Have two investigators independently screen articles for inclusion and extract data. Involve a third investigator to resolve conflicts.
- Use a standardized form for data extraction.
- Train the investigators who will screen articles and conduct data extraction.
- Include a statistician in your team when conducting a meta-analysis.
- Assess biases of the studies included in your systematic review or meta-analysis.
- Adhere to the PRISMA guidelines when reporting the results of your study.

Chapter Review Questions

1. What is the name of the registration site for systematic review protocols?
2. What are the roles of each member in the research team when conducting a systematic review?
3. Why is a librarian an important member of a research team when planning systematic review?
4. What are commonly used tools used to assess risk of bias in a systematic review?
5. How should the final report and manuscript for a systematic review present the information from the included studies?
6. What conditions must be met before attempting to conduct a meta-analysis after obtaining all the necessary information from the systematic review?
7. In what circumstances should a fixed effects model be used for a meta-analysis?

Online Resources

Covidence. https://www.covidence.org

Journal/Author Name Estimator (JANE). https://jane.biosemantics.org

Preferred Reporting Items for Systematic Reviews and Meta-Analyses (PRISMA). http://www.prisma-statement.org/

PRISMA for Individual Patient Data systematic reviews (PRISMA-IPD). http://www.prisma-statement.org/Extensions/IndividualPatientData.aspx

PRISMA for Network Meta-Analyses (PRISMA-NMA). http://www.prisma-statement.org/Extensions/NetworkMetaAnalysis.aspx

PROSPERO: International prospective register of systematic reviews. https://www.crd.york.ac.uk/prospero/

REFERENCES

1. Landhuis E. Scientific literature: Information overload. *Nature.* 2016;535(7612):457-458.
2. *Undertaking Systematic Reviews of Research on Effectiveness. CRD's Guidance for those Carrying Out or Commissioning Reviews.* United Kingdom: University of York Centre for Reviews and Dissemination (CRD); March 2001.
3. National Institute for Health Research (NIHR): PROSPERO: International Prospective Register for Systematic Reviews. University of York, Centre for Reviews and Disseminations. Accessed January 26, 2021. https://www.crd.york.ac.uk/prospero/
4. Committee on Science E, Medicine, and Public Policy; Policy and, Global Affairs; National Academies of Sciences E, and Medicine, National Academies of Sciences E, and Medicine 2019. *Reproducibility and Replicability in Science.* Washington, DC: The National Academies Press; 2019.
5. Cochrane Library: Cochrane Reviews. John Wiley & Sons, Inc. Accessed January 26, 2021. https://www.cochranelibrary.com/cdsr/reviews
6. Chang CY, Park H, Malone DC, et al. Immune checkpoint inhibitors and immune-related adverse events in patients with advanced melanoma: a systematic review and network meta-analysis. *JAMA Netw Open.* 2020;3(3):e201611.
7. Moher D, Liberati A, Tetzlaff J, Altman DG, Group P. Preferred reporting items for systematic reviews and meta-analyses: the PRISMA statement. *PLoS Med.* 2009;6(7): e1000097.
8. The University of Tasmania. Systematic Reviews for Health: Systematic Review Tools. Accessed February 5, 2021. https://utas.libguides.com/SystematicReviews/Tools
9. Covidence. Updated February 4, 2021. Accessed February 5, 2021. www.covidence.org
10. Wright K, Golder S, Rodriguez-Lopez R. Citation searching: a systematic review case study of multiple risk behaviour interventions. *BMC Med Res Methodol.* 2014;14:73.
11. Horsley T, Dingwall O, Sampson M. Checking reference lists to find additional studies for systematic reviews. *Cochrane Database Syst Rev.* 2011;2011(8):Mr000026.

12. Risk of Bias 2 (RoB 2) A Revised Tool for Risk of Bias in Randomized Trials. Published 2020. Accessed February 8, 2021. https://www.riskofbias.info/

13. Jadad AR, Moore RA, Carroll D, et al. Assessing the quality of reports of randomized clinical trials: is blinding necessary? *Control Clin Trials*. 1996;17(1):1-12.

14. Sterne JA, Hernan MA, Reeves BC, et al. ROBINS-I: a tool for assessing risk of bias in non-randomised studies of interventions. *BMJ*. 2016;355:i4919.

15. Guyatt GH, Oxman AD, Vist GE, et al. GRADE: an emerging consensus on rating quality of evidence and strength of recommendations. *BMJ*. 2008;336(7650):924-926.

16. Hedges LV. Distribution theory for Glass's estimator of effect size and related estimators. *J Educ Stat*. 1981;6(2):107-128.

17. Higgins JP, Thompson SG, Deeks JJ, Altman DG. Measuring inconsistency in meta-analyses. *BMJ*. 2003;327(7414):557-560.

18. Fahmy T, Bellétoile A. Algorithm 983: fast computation of the non-asymptotic Cochran's Q statistic for heterogeneity detection. *ACM Trans Math Softw*. 2017;44(2): Article 20.

19. Lindsey WT, Olin BR, Hansen RA. Systematic review and meta-analysis. In: Aparasu RR, Bentley JP, eds. *Principles of Research Design and Drug Literature Evaluation*. 2nd ed. New York, NY: McGraw Hill; 2020.

20. Lin L, Chu H. Quantifying publication bias in meta-analysis. *Biometrics*. 2018;74(3):785-794.

21. Sterne JA, Egger M. Funnel plots for detecting bias in meta-analysis: guidelines on choice of axis. *J Clin Epidemiol*. 2001;54(10):1046-1055.

22. The Biosemantics Group. Journal/Author Name Estimator (JANE). https://jane.biosemantics.org

23. Usmani SA, Hollmann J, Goodin A, et al. Effects of hydrocodone rescheduling on opioid use outcomes: a systematic review. *J Am Pharm Assoc*. 2021;61(3): e20-e44.

24. Almutairi AR, Zhou L, Gellad WF, et al. Effectiveness and safety of non-vitamin K antagonist oral anticoagulants for atrial fibrillation and venous thromboembolism: a systematic review and meta-analyses. *Clin Ther*. 2017;39(7):1456-1478.e1436.

21

Chapter Twenty-One

Educational Research in Pharmacy

Adam N. Pate, PharmD, BCPS

Chapter Objectives

- Define educational research and the Scholarship of Teaching and Learning
- Discuss the goals and characteristics of educational research inquiry
- Understand the scope and limitations of educational research
- Understand the expertise and infrastructure needed for educational research
- Identify pillars and principles for developing sound methodology in educational research
- Discuss the importance of dissemination of educational research

Key Terminology

Scholarship of Teaching and Learning, educational research

Introduction

The Scholarship of Teaching and Learning (SOTL) is defined as research that has two primary goals: (1) deepening our understanding of how students learn and (2) exploring the effectiveness and desirability of one's teaching.[1] Although very similar, SOTL is not to be confused with educational research, which is a much more broad research area that looks beyond strictly teaching and learning, incorporating other important educational research topics like assessment, admissions practices, organizational inquiry, etc.[2] Unfortunately, both SOTL and educational research are often overlooked research areas that are frequently very fruitful and approachable for young researchers. Additionally, these research areas are especially appealing when research time constraints of completing a research project in one year during residency are considered.

When utilized appropriately, the SOTL provides a mental framework to scholarly evaluate any type of educational environment. This includes patient education, clinical education of colleagues or healthcare professional students, interdisciplinary team-based training, classroom education, and residency training in and of itself, to name a few. Literally, there are hundreds of areas that residents and students frequently are involved in that could benefit from greater SOTL efforts that would improve teaching and learning. Provided that all pharmacy students/residents in their career will be "teachers" in some fashion, the principles and theories that underpin SOTL will only enhance one's ability to effectively convey information in any situation.

This chapter will orient readers to the process and product of educational research beginning with a formal orientation to SOTL, including definitions and goals of SOTL. It will also cover a pragmatic approach to developing and publishing a SOTL project. Topics covered will include how to develop a research question, frameworks to enhance quality in SOTL research, common pitfalls and mistakes to avoid, and dissemination of the SOTL research findings.

Evolution of SOTL

SOTL is a relatively new area of scholarship that is most often attributed to the seminal work of Boyer in his book *Scholarship Reconsidered*.[3] Boyer argued for scholars to take a broader view of scholarship and suggested the traditional three areas of scholarship (discovery, integration, and application) be expanded to four and include teaching.[3] Since this humble beginning, SOTL has been a rapidly growing and evolving field of research that now has a large variety of professional organizations, journals, etc. Although encouraging, this rapid growth within the field presented challenges specifically related to scientific rigor, which resulted in some believing that SOTL is largely an atheoretical field of research that is a "methodological and theoretical mutt."[1,4]

Due to these methodological struggles in a rapidly evolving field, there have been small reckonings that are important for readers to fully contextualize their understanding of SOTL. One central concept that emerged from these reckonings is the differentiation of excellent teaching, scholarly teaching, and SOTL. Excellent teaching is what most would consider when thinking of a favorite professor/teacher and is identifiable via effective transferring of material, engaged learners, etc. However, excellent teaching is not SOTL, as it may not be informed by educational theory/research and is not shared broadly. Scholarly teaching, in contrast, is teaching rooted in sound educational theory or research-based teaching, but it is not systematic, nor is it disseminated via peer-reviewed publication. There are two major distinctions that define SOTL: (1) it is a systematic process focused on teaching and student learning and (2) aims to improve student learning not only in the researcher's classroom but also broadly with peers through the dissemination of findings in peer-reviewed journals. For excellent or scholarly teaching to become SOTL, it must be intentional, systematic, methodologically sound, and ultimately must be evaluated via peer review and disseminated.

Given the struggles of SOTL as it emerged as a research area, the paradigm of SOTL has recently shifted, emphasizing rigor and quality in SOTL research. This makes it critical for interested and incoming SOTL researchers to adhere to expected research standards and rigor of SOTL to continue to promote and advance its value and improve the chances of a project resulting in successful publication. Several authors have published a variety of helpful books and articles that focus on improving the methodological rigor of SOTL and educational research, which readers are encouraged to review as they start SOTL research projects.[2]

Developing the Research Question

SOTL ultimately involves taking a scholarly approach to teaching as a way to improve information delivery and student learning with the requirement of disseminating findings. Most often, this research begins from a very pragmatic problem-centric focus which often enhances the inherent appeal and approachableness for young researchers. This also makes students, residents, and recent graduates particularly adept at developing research questions to identify and develop areas of research inquiry as they have recent learning experiences from which to draw on.

The pragmatic nature of SOTL is one of its great qualities for many researchers. Oftentimes noticing a problem in one's personal teaching or learning and being curious if others have similar issues or hypothesizing about a potential remedy is the beginning of many SOTL research questions. Additionally, as many residents now complete teaching certificate programs as part of their residencies, there are ample opportunities to systematically institute and evaluate a SOTL project as part of the teaching requirements to complete a teaching certificate.

One commonly used framework to help in refining and choosing a research question is Hutchings' taxonomy, which is simply four broad categories that most SOTL research questions can be placed into. These categories are: (1) what works, (2) what is, (3) visions of the possible, and (4) new conceptual frameworks. Table 21–1 further elaborates on these and demonstrates what example research questions may be housed in each

TABLE 21–1. HUTCHINGS TAXONOMY EXPANDED WITH EXAMPLES AND REFERENCES

Hutchings' Taxonomy Category	Research Question Example and Reference
What works This question type generally seeks simply to identify if a new strategy or way of teaching "works" and is the most common category of SOTL inquiry	• Does a five-week reinforcement experience help students in their first year of pharmacy school?[5] • Do print or digital posters work better?[6]
What is This category seeks to describe in detail the situation, environment, etc., as it exists including its component elements, situational factors, etc.	• What is pharmacy students' perception of male faculty teaching female physiology, pathophysiology, and gender health?[7] • What is the coverage of the Science of Safety in experiential education?[8]
Visions of the possible Rather than seeing if something works or describing it in detail, this category views problems in teaching and learning through a new paradigm and seeks to reframe how we see or respond to common issues in teaching and learning.	• How will big data impact pharmacy practice, education, and research?[9] • Are there new opportunities for collaboration between academic and federal pharmacy?[10]
New conceptual framework This category involves the development and testing of new theories and mechanisms to explain teaching and learning. It is the least represented of all categories.	• Do situational judgment tests better assess new soft skill accreditation standard?[11] • Are there threshold concepts associated with learning the Pharmacists' Patient Care Process (PPCP) in a student's transition to practitioner?[12]

category. When viewing one's teaching requirements and activities as opportunities using Hutchings' taxonomy, it's easy to see how a variety of research projects become viable. These sources can include personal experience (what is), personal beliefs about teaching and learning (what could be), existing problems you're encountering (what works), ongoing initiatives (visions of the possible), new school or college initiatives (new conceptual frameworks/visions of the possible), and student/learner involved questions which could fit into multiple categories.

In addition to the wide variety of opportunities, the positive implications for personal improvement in teaching effectiveness should not be discounted. SOTL provides an optimistic lens to explore common issues in teaching and learning with a focus on improving the educational process. This makes teaching failures where learners do not learn as anticipated or learner feedback is largely negative, a rich source from which to develop SOTL research questions. Developing a research question in this area is particularly helpful for young educators as it provides a different perspective to view teaching failures through. SOTL provides an outlet to view these "failures" as opportunities to learn and further investigate. Researching best practices and learning new teaching methods allows an individual to view themselves as a great teacher in the making and dismantles the myth that only a select group of effective educators are simply born with an aptitude to teach.

After identifying a potential research area and drafting an initial research question, the refinement of this research question using the PICOTS (population, intervention, comparison group, outcomes, timeline, and setting) framework as discussed in Chapter 4, "Formulating Practice-Based Research Questions and Hypotheses," is one of the most critical components to establishing appropriate rigor in your research project. The research question refinement process in SOTL is very similar to clinical research in pharmacy practice. Thorough literature evaluation and research is the single best tool to help refine and adjust your research question as you learn more about the area you intend to research. Common search engines like PubMed, Google Scholar, etc., are helpful in this process, but particularly in SOTL readers may find at the Institute of Education Sciences (https://eric.ed.gov/), an educational research-specific search engine, very helpful.

Once a research question has been identified and refined, researchers must devote sufficient time and effort to understanding any educational, psychological, or other theories that may underpin or be related to the research question. This effort to describe and ground a project, in theory, is much more likely to create the caliber of research and methodological soundness that editors and reviewers will view favorably during peer review.[13] Granted, all SOTL questions may not have an educational theory to support them, but too often, a theory or other grounded basis is absent simply because researchers do not look broadly enough during their initial literature review. Researchers often ignore or are unaware of tangentially related research areas and theories such as psychology, sociology, communications, etc., that can inform educational research.

Understanding Underlying Theory

Once you've refined your research question and established a theoretical grounding, you are ready to move ahead to the methodological soundness of your SOTL project. A few helpful mental frameworks will aid you as you decide on your research methodology. One of the more expansive methodological and theoretical frameworks comes from Miller-Young and colleagues.[1] Miller-Young et al. combine methodology and theory into a single cohesive conceptual framework with the goal of helping stimulate theory-based SOTL and provide an example of how interconnected theory and methodology are. They utilize four broad learning theory categories of behaviorist, cognitivist, constructivist, and humanistic categories to help researchers frame their basic assumptions of how learning

METHODOLOGY							
	Quantitative	Qualitative	Naturalistic	Interpretive	Critical	Post Modern	Mixed Methods
THEORY Behaviorism							
Cognitivism							
Constructivism							
Social constructivism							
Humanism							

Figure 21–1. Research framework for SOTL. (Adapted from Miller-Young.[1] (SOTL, Scholarship of Teaching and Learning))

works. Behaviourism theory suggests that all behavior is based on an external stimulus. Many behaviourism theory-based studies have a strong psychological underpinning and seek to identify things like how to stimulate students to study more, change behavior, etc. Cognitivism views learning as the process of individuals creating mental schemas, structures, and models. Bloom's taxonomy of learning is a great example of a cognitivism theory-based perspective in education.

Constructivism theory focuses on the process of learning and emphasizes the construction of new knowledge in the context of prior knowledge and cultural factors that influence learning. Lastly, the humanistic theory focuses on the person in the learning situation and the freedom, dignity, and potential of human beings. Maslow's hierarchy is the predominant model within this theory. These four theories in Miller-Young's framework are then aligned with common methodological practices employed in SOTL, i.e., quantitative, qualitative, naturalistic, and so on, to help support increased rigor and methodological soundness within SOTL research (Figure 21–1).

Conceptual frameworks like Miller-Young and Hutchings are helpful when creating SOTL projects, but there are also other considerations that enhance SOTL quality that beginning researchers must be aware of. Felten outlines five principles of good practice in SOTL.[4] The first principle is that it is inquiry focused on student learning and is therefore inherently scholarly. It is not simply quality teaching or scholarly teaching, as mentioned previously. Second, it is grounded in both scholarly and local context, appropriately adding to and expanding the scholarly context while acknowledging the variation in the local context of classrooms, environments, faculty workloads, etc. Third, it must have substantial methodological rigor and validity with "intentional and rigorous application of research tools." Fourth, it should be conducted in partnership with students. This partnership may look different for each study, but it is very much akin to patient-involved research in the clinical realm and the renewed importance of viewing patients as partners in research rather than subjects.[14] Lastly, quality SOTL must be "appropriately public." Researchers should aim to share SOTL broadly through peer-reviewed publication as a means to continue to enhance the SOTL community and extend the research within the field.[4]

Types of Educational Research

The National Science Foundation and the U.S. Department of Education have identified six types of educational research to help researchers develop stronger educational research and "speed the pace of research and development in education."[15] These types include: (1) Foundational research, (2) Exploratory research, (3) Design and Development research, (4) Efficacy research, (5) Effectiveness research, and (6) Scale-up research. An understanding of these six types of research does not cover the complete spectrum of educational research, but is very useful to young researchers in generating and refining research ideas for education research.

Foundational Research: This research type contributes foundational knowledge that can be used to help build an intervention, measure, or evaluate relevant education outcomes. These studies are often beneficial for future educational research surrounding theory development and the evaluation of teaching and learning. Additionally, foundational research can be used in developing intervention and educational outcomes but is not required to have an explicit link to educational outcomes.

Exploratory Research: This type of research further explores the relationship of educational constructs in theory for further refinement and development of the theory or constructs. These correlational studies often help with the development of educational interventions aimed at specific outcomes of interest and may be some of the earliest work to link these outcomes to the particular teaching/learning activities.

Design and Development Research: This type of research design focuses on providing solutions to problems encountered in education and learning and develops educational interventions based on the theory. This is a highly iterative process as often this research type involves experimentation and analyzing of individual components with findings from this pilot work being used to further refine and develop the intervention. These findings from pilot tests can also be used for the evaluation and refinement of the theory itself.

Efficacy Research: This type of research evaluates the fully developed intervention to see if the intervention really "works" for improving educational outcomes in a controlled setting. It usually involves a specific population or setting based on convenience but requires strong study designs and methodologies to reduce biases in educational research.

Effectiveness Research: This type of research evaluates the intervention in normal settings to improve the generalizability of the intervention findings. It involves study populations and settings that are considered "typical." This research usually requires the evaluation of the interventions with minimum control on the settings.

Scale-up Research: This type of research requires evaluation of the intervention in multiple populations and settings to scale up or evaluate widespread application of the intervention. This research also requires minimum control on the settings to increase the scalability and generalizability of the intervention.

Common Research Designs and Methods

The scientific research process for SOTL is largely the same as many of those seen in other chapters in this text. Creating strong, specific, measurable research objectives that will answer or support a hypothesis or research question is an essential first step of any research project. This being said, there are specific research designs that likely will be encountered more frequently in SOTL than in other research areas. These common research designs often seen in pharmacy education research include quantitative, qualitative, mixed methods, and action research.[2]

Quantitative research involving experimental and nonexperimental designs is what most beginning researchers think of when first considering research. It simply involves research methodologies such as surveys that use numeric data such as counts and measures, i.e., student perception of learning using a seven-point scale. Qualitative research is also commonly used in SOTL and differs from quantitative in that it is a research methodology focusing on nonnumeric data such as focus group comments, recorded interviews, open text responses on surveys, and so on. Researchers may find that neither of these methodologies specifically answers their research question. In these situations, SOTL researchers often use mixed-methods research where both quantitative and qualitative methodologies are used in combination. Action research is a methodology that resembles continuous quality improvement in healthcare but focuses on groups of individuals making actionable teaching changes to improve a specific noted teaching problem. Other research design methodologies that are not as common in pharmacy education research but maybe encountered more broadly include naturalistic, interpretive, critical theory, and postmodern research study designs.

SOTL study design and methodology also inherently faces specific challenges unique to SOTL Provided that many SOTL studies utilize a prospective survey-based research method or involve a survey in some capacity, one of the most common challenges includes using appropriate survey-based methodology. Readers should refer to Chapter 11 for more information regarding how to conduct quality survey-based research that ensures the reliability and validity of the survey instruments. Experimental studies require randomization involving control and intervention groups; these often require more time and planning. Therefore, nonexperimental research is often used in education research. These often include pre and post, cross-sectional, and quasi-experimental studies. However, another challenge in SOTL is difficulty in having a clearly defined control and intervention group in nonexperimental studies, as often there is no sufficient comparator group. Researchers may be able to resolve this control/intervention group issue by comparing entire pharmacy class performance year over year (historical control) and performing statistical analysis to ensure that the two classes are similar enough to draw conclusions from the results. Lastly, when designing the methodology for a SOTL project, researchers need to ensure they are not inadvertently trying to solve multiple problems with one project. Being more narrow and focused typically results in better quality and more publishable studies. Please refer to Persky and Romanelli's article for help with navigating some of these challenges.[13]

Common Pitfalls in SOTL Research

It is important to understand how educational research, particularly in pharmacy education, has evolved. As compared to 20 years ago, pharmacy education now has a respectable amount of evidence-based research. This is significant as previously many early researchers would simply find a SOTL project from academic medicine, nursing, or some other related area and simply replicate its findings in pharmacy education. This has rightfully come under scrutiny. SOTL shouldn't simply replicate findings but rather contextualize and expand previous research. To help avoid this mistake before beginning the project, researchers should seek to clearly define how your subjects, research question, etc., are fundamentally different from the research found during the original literature review.[13]

Another common flaw in early SOTL research planning is wasting effort and studying common "SOTL myths." This failure is most often due to not challenging your research question and assumptions, evaluating if, indeed, your research question is a SOTL myth. One classic SOTL myth example is the impact of learning styles on how teachers should teach. Although appealing and implicitly something a young researcher may agree with, the evidence simply no longer supports that changing teaching strategies to appeal to a variety of learning styles has an impact on student learning.[16]

Other common pitfalls to avoid include having too broad of a scope for your project. This can be remedied by being very specific on what you're trying to accomplish and who you think your intervention will work for. The PICOT is a helpful framework used in the research process that can also be helpful here.[17] Single institution studies present another issue that is often problematic for publication if for no other reason due to limitations of generalizability and sample size. Readers are encouraged to collaborate with others in pharmacy, medicine, nursing, etc., for collaborative research opportunities that have a larger impact.

Practical and Technical Considerations in SOTL Research

Once the research question and the appropriate research design and methodology are finalized, the research protocol should be drafted for planning and approval of research. The key elements of the protocol for quantitative research include the research question and hypothesis, the theoretical basis for the study, study design details for experimental or nonexperimental study, data collection methods such as survey methodology details, sampling procedures, and data analysis, including statistical tests. The elements of the protocol for qualitative research include study aims and objectives, study design (action research, grounded theory, interpretative analysis), collection (surveys, interviews, and observation), and data analysis such as content, interpretive, or framework analysis. The mixed-method approach will involve all the elements discussed above.

Educational research often involves data collection from the students for both qualitative and quantitative approaches. Although informed consent from the students is needed, it is not cumbersome as a majority of SOTL research projects are deemed "exempt" by the Institutional Review Board (IRB). The IRB considers the following education research as exempt from full review as there is minimal risk to the respondents: (1) research involving normal educational practices in educational settings, and (2) research involving educational tests, surveys, interviews, or observations, including visual or auditory recording.[18] Although SOTL research projects are considered "exempt," IRB approval is still required to disseminate SOTL research. The research protocol, surveys, and any recruitment emails or materials are sent to the IRB in order to ensure adequate review and to receive IRB exemption.

After IRB approval, the educational research can be effectively implemented with appropriate planning. This requires planning for implementing any educational intervention and data collection for administering surveys or conducting interviews. Learner-involved research often involves cross-sectional or pre- and post-designs due to time and other considerations. If experimental designs are planned, more planning and resources are needed to implement the intervention in the courses. Approvals from the faculty and sometimes from the administrators are often needed for educational research. If electronic surveys are being planned, appropriate data collection tools such as Google Forms, Qualtrics, and Survey Monkey should be developed based on reliable and validated survey instruments. The mechanisms to reach the students should also be clearly delineated, such as the use of emails or listserv including the use of email reminders.

Common research designs that may be problematic include pre- or post-activity surveys which are commonplace in SOTL. The problem with this design is that depending on what you're trying to measure, this is likely an insufficient measure. For example, suppose you're measuring "learning" and plan to demonstrate that with a simple pre-post knowledge survey using multiple-choice questions; the evidence available now shows that demonstrating an improvement is highly likely. Seeing this improvement immediately after instruction does not ensure that learners have long-term retention of knowledge as learners may not fare any better when given these same questions in three months. Try to avoid these challenges by thinking of surrogate markers you may have access to, i.e., exam performance from year to year using similar or the same questions which aren't given pre/post, objective evaluations, i.e., objective structured clinical examination/advanced pharmacy practice experiences performance, etc.

After data collection, other considerations should include manipulation of data and practicing good data management. Young researchers should rely on their research mentors and others familiar with SOTL research methodology to help utilize data collection instruments that provide data output that is considered usable with minimal edits or data transformation. Familiarity with online survey tools, along with the functionality and formatting of data upon export, is important early in the research process. The usable data from the study are finally analyzed statistically for quantitative research and other interpretive tools for qualitative research to achieve the study objectives.

Expertise and Infrastructure Needed for SOTL Research

When beginning a SOTL project, you must consider what expertise and infrastructure you may need. The expertise needed may vary, but it is helpful to consider the stage learner or area in the curriculum your research will focus on. For example, if you're looking to evaluate fourth-year pharmacy students, having someone who is a preceptor, an experiential director, or has other intimate knowledge of the Advanced Pharmacy Practice Experience (APPE) process can make a significant contribution to brainstorming and refining a research question along with helping with access to research data. Other expertise needed depends on your research methodology. If you intend to retrospectively review large sets of data points from educational software, i.e., Examsoft, Blackboard, E*Value, etc., consider involving someone with expertise using the software as well as a statistician with experience manipulating big data sets. Often these researchers may be new to SOTL research but can play a critical role in fully evaluating and properly designing a SOTL study. Given that many SOTL projects involve survey research methodology, it is also prudent to either consult with someone well versed in survey research or invite them to be on the research team to leverage this expertise.

In addition to human capital and resources, it is important to have access to proper technical infrastructure to complete the project. Examples of this may include Qualtrics, Redcap, etc., for survey development and delivery. Microsoft Excel for data analysis is usually sufficient for most SOTL projects involving learners, but access to other statistics packages like SPSS (IBM Corp, Armonk, NY), STATA (StataCorp LP, College Station, TX), and R (R Foundation) can be helpful as well. Lastly, using a citation tracker for manuscript preparation, such as Zotero, Endnote, and so on, is incredibly helpful in the manuscript writing, submission, and revision phases of a project.

Dissemination Framework for Educational Research

The final step of any SOTL project is the dissemination of research. This is a critical element for your research to be truly considered SOTL and not simply scholarly teaching. The first dissemination of research findings is often via a poster presentation at an appropriate organization meeting, i.e., American Academy of Colleges of Pharmacy (AACP) annual meeting, American Society of Health-System Pharmacists (ASHP) midyear, American Pharmacists Association (APHA), etc.; refer to Chapter 22 "Research Abstracts and Posters" for more information on how to create quality poster abstracts and posters. After presenting your research as a poster, the second dissemination is most often in the form of a peer-reviewed manuscript. Manuscript preparation begins with researchers selecting a target journal of publication. Several popular journals within pharmacy education are the *American Journal of Pharmaceutical Education, Currents in Pharmacy Teaching and Learning* (CPTL), and *Pharmacy Education*. Each journal has different author guidelines that should be adhered to.

The authors should also consult guidelines for manuscript preparation such as (Standards for QUality Improvement Reporting Excellence in Education (SQUIRE-EDU), which is an extension to the SQUIRE guidelines used for healthcare improvement that, if followed, will help with completeness, transparency, and replicability of the research.[19] The Guideline for Reporting Evidence-based practice Educational interventions and Teaching (GREET) checklist is another tool that ensures authors avoid being too vague and are providing sufficient methodologic detail and transparency in describing local context to allow for study replication, therefore ensuring that the research is impactful and useful to the scientific community.[20] In addition to these guidelines and tools, readers can search the Enhancing the QUAlity and Transparency Of health Research (EQUATOR) network, a web-based resource created for the international audience of scholars solely aimed at improving the quality and value of research, to find relevant reporting guidelines.

Alternatively, to the traditional peer-reviewed manuscript and depending on the scope, sample size, and other potential limitations of a SOTL project, some journals are beginning to use alternate formats for peer-reviewed dissemination of findings. CPTL Pulses, which is a peer-reviewed blog post, is a great example of this as researchers can disseminate findings that may not be sufficient for a peer-reviewed manuscript but could still provide value to the community of educational scholars. Researchers can also now disseminate and publicize research work in addition to finding collaborators, etc., by posting ideas or research projects on social media sites such as Twitter and using common hashtags, i.e., #twitterrx, etc. After successfully publishing a research manuscript, researchers are encouraged to pursue dissemination via presenting findings as a podium at a national conference. This step allows you to more broadly share your findings but equally important is a great opportunity to identify collaborators and fellow researchers with similar interests.

Exemplars of Learner-Led Educational Research

There are several examples of learner-involved projects that showcase how to apply the concepts discussed in this chapter. We will take just one and demonstrate practices crucial for success using an example from an article published by Pearson, who was a third-year pharmacy student at the time of research and publication. Researchers initially were presented with a common problem in pharmacy education—students in a large, fixed seat classroom were participating in case-based learning during class, but only a handful of students were really answering faculty questions and participating in the case discussion. Identifying this problem allowed Pearson and colleagues to frame an initial research question of how to effectively conduct case-based learning in a large group fixed seating setting—Hutchings' visions of the possible. Now researchers began a literature review and analysis of educational research surrounding small group learning, case-based learning, etc., and began to refine their research question based on literature they found. One example was the identification of research on "fish bowls," which was a tool used in K-12 education which had recently been implemented and researched in some undergraduate courses.[21] After identifying a potential tool to help break the larger class into smaller functional groups, the authors began to look for theory to underpin their intervention and the outcome they wanted to evaluate. Researchers found a developmental psychology term/ theory of postformal thinking during their thorough review. In addition to identifying a theory, the authors found a validated, reliable survey that had been previously used to evaluate postformal thinking.

After this cursory literature search, researchers refined their research question adhering to PICOT as: are fishbowl activities effective for teaching pharmacotherapy and developing postformal thought in pharmacy students? Next authors discussed methodological options and how to initiate this research project. Ultimately, the authors used a cross-sectional pre- or post-survey design and administered the survey before and after class as they weren't directly evaluating knowledge. The research team used the validated, reliable survey (complex postformal thought [PFT]) questionnaire) and additionally added questions to assess student impressions of the activity. This was internally validated using review and edits based on feedback from other faculty who reviewed the survey. After revising and completing the review, authors submitted and received IRB exemption. Expertise was leveraged in this project by involving a faculty member who had a course with case-based teaching in it who also had previous experience with survey research. Additionally, the lead author leveraged content expertise as she reached out to one of the first authors on the literature found regarding post-formal thinking and had a quick call to discuss methodology and usage of the PFT questionnaire. Readers are encouraged to always consider reaching out to primary authors and others to ask permission for the use of scales not publicly available, etc. Data were collected via Google Forms and were analyzed in Microsoft excel. Lastly, to qualify as SOTL, dissemination must occur, and this research was presented as a poster presentation at ASHP midyear and subsequently published as a peer-reviewed manuscript in CPTL. This project demonstrates how to involve learners in SOTL research and how the pragmatic nature of SOTL creates conditions for creativity and finding solutions to common problems.

Summary and Conclusions

The SOTL and educational research are practical, approachable, and timeline-conducive research that may be appealing to both student and resident researchers. SOTL has evolved as a relatively new research category with a recent renewed focus on adhering to expected research design and methodological rigor to ensure research quality standards. Learning situations in which pharmacy students and resident researchers have the opportunity to conduct SOTL research are abundant, and most can easily be accomplished within one year. A proper understanding of education theory and common research methodology using frameworks and taxonomies is helpful to ensure rigor and quality when developing a SOTL research project.

Key Points and Advice

- SOTL is a relatively new research field that is often very approachable for new researchers, and many projects can be accomplished in one year.
- SOTL is distinct from scholarly teaching and effective teaching and should be systematic and disseminated broadly.

- SOTL has begun emphasizing methodological rigor and incorporation of theory where applicable as a standard for research in the field.
- Educational research is broader than SOTL and can encompass a variety of additional areas, including curricular assessment, organizational effectiveness, admissions, etc.
- SOTL is inherently a pragmatic and collaborative type of research that encourages the involvement of students in the research process.

Chapter Review Questions

1. What is the difference in SOTL, scholarly teaching, educational research, and effective teaching?
2. What are the five good principles for good SOTL?
3. Why is grounding SOTL research in appropriate theory important when defining a research question and what are some common theories?
4. What are some common methodological pitfalls and suggestions to avoid these when conducting a SOTL project?

Online Resources

- University of Minnesota Center for Educational Innovation. https://cei.umn.edu/sotl
- Center for Engaged Learning. https://www.centerforengagedlearning.org/studying-engaged-learning/what-is-sotl/
- American Journal of Pharmacy Education. https://www.ajpe.org/

REFERENCES

1. Miller-Young J, Yeo M. Conceptualizing and communicating SoTL: a framework for the field. *Learn Inq*. 2015;3:17.
2. McLaughlin JE, Dean MJ, Mumper RJ, Blouin RA, Roth MT. A roadmap for educational research in pharmacy. *Am J Pharm Educ*. 2013; 77(10):218.
3. Boyer EL. *Scholarship Reconsidered: Priorities of the Professoriate*. 1st ed. Princeton, NJ: Carnegie Foundation for the Advancement of Teaching; 1997.
4. Felten P. Principles of good practice in SoTL. *Learn Inq*. 2013;1:5.
5. Awuonda MK, Akala E, Wingate LT, et al. A pre-matriculation success program to improve pharmacy students' academic performance at a historically black university. *Am J Pharm Educ*. 2021;85(6):8214.

6. Newsom LC, Miller SW, Chesson M. Use of digital vs printed posters for teaching and learning in pharmacy education. *Am J Pharm Educ.* 2021;85(6):8307.

7. Johannesmeyer HJ, Dau NQ. Student pharmacists' perceptions of male faculty teaching female-specific sex and gender health topics. *Am J Pharm Educ.* 2021;85(6):8383.

8. Tang DH, Warholak TL, Slack MK, Malone DC, Gau C-S. Science of safety topic coverage in experiential education in US and Taiwan colleges and schools of pharmacy. *Am J Pharm Educ.* 2011;75(10):202.

9. Baldwin JN, Bootman JL, Carter RA, et al. Pharmacy practice, education, and research in the era of big data: 2014-15 Argus Commission Report. *Am J Pharm Educ.* 2015;79(10):S26.

10. Piascik P, Boyle CJ, Chase P, DiPiro JT, Scott ST, Maine LL. Reexamining the academic partnerships with federal pharmacy: 2018-19 Argus Commission Report. *Am J Pharm Educ.* 2019;83(10):7655.

11. DeLellis T, Noureldin M, Park SK, Shields K, Bryant A, Chen AMH. Development of a situational judgment test to assess ACPE Standards 3 and 4. *Am J Pharm Educ.* 2021 July 22:8511.

12. Kolar C, Janke KK. Aiding transformation from student to practitioner by defining threshold concepts for the pharmacists' patient care process. *Am J Pharm Educ.* 2019;83(8):7335.

13. Persky AM, Romanelli F. Insights, pearls, and guidance on successfully producing and publishing educational research. *Am J Pharm Educ.* 2016;80(5):75.

14. Husmann PR, O'Loughlin VD. Another nail in the coffin for learning styles? Disparities among undergraduate anatomy students' study strategies, class performance, and reported VARK learning styles: study strategies, learning styles, anatomy performance. *Anat Sci Educ.* 2019;12(1):6-19.

15. Common Guidelines for Education Research and Development: A Report from the Institute of Education Sciences, U.S. Department of Education and the National Science Foundation. Published September 13, 2021. Accessed September 13, 2021. https://nsf.gov

16. Solodky C, Chen H, Jones PK, Katcher W, Neuhauser D. Patients as partners in clinical research: a roposal for applying quality improvement methods to patient care. *Med Care.* 1998;36(8 Suppl):AS13-AS20.

17. Riva JJ, Malik KMP, Burnie SJ, Endicott AR, Busse JW. What is your research question? An introduction to the PICOT format for clinicians. *J Can Chiropr Assoc.* 2012;56(3):167-171.

18. Code of Federal Regulations. Title 45 Public Welfare Department of Health and Human Services; Part 46 Protection of Human Subjects. Published September 12, 2021. Accessed September 12, 2021. http://www.hhs.gov/ohrp/humansubjects/guidance/45cfr46.html

19. Ogrinc G, Armstrong GE, Dolansky MA, Singh MK, Davies L. SQUIRE-EDU (Standards for QUality Improvement Reporting Excellence in Education): publication guidelines for educational improvement. *Acad Med.* 2019;94(10):1461-1470.

20. Phillips AC, Lewis LK, McEvoy MP, et al. Development and validation of the guideline for reporting evidence-based practice educational interventions and teaching (GREET). *BMC Med Educ.* 2016;16(1):237.

21. Sutherland R, Reid K, Kok D, Collins M. Teaching a fishbowl tutorial: sink or swim? *Clin Teach.* 2012;9(2):80-84.

III

SECTION THREE

PRESENTING PRACTICE-BASED RESEARCH

22

Chapter Twenty-Two

Research Abstracts and Posters

Matthew A. Wanat, PharmD, BCPS, BCCCP, FCCM

Chapter Objectives

- Understand the goal of a research abstract and poster
- Explain the key elements of a research abstract
- Explain the key elements of a research poster
- Discuss common software packages for designing research posters
- Describe best practices in the visual design of research posters
- Develop key talking points for research poster presentations
- Create a poster template for future use
- Describe an example of a learner-involved research abstract and poster submission
- Understand the dissemination framework for research abstracts and posters

Key Terminology

Research abstract, research poster

Introduction

A central part of the research process is the dissemination of results. Sharing the results from a research project to a wide audience is important to build on what is currently known about a scientific area and to shape future research in that area. Most commonly, the initial dissemination of results is done in a poster presentation at a peer-reviewed scientific meeting. The purpose of presenting a research poster is multifactorial; first, posters provide a visual communication of your research findings in a succinct manner, to an audience interested in a specific scientific area.[1-3] Second, posters are an efficient method for facilitating the large-scale sharing of research findings and facilitation of networking among conference attendees, which allows for feedback, collaboration, and sharing of ideas.[4] Lastly, posters inherently increase the scholarly output of a researcher, which may help in several areas including obtaining a job that contains a research component (such as a Faculty appointment or Clinical Pharmacy Specialist position), securing future grant funding, promotion and tenure, or other recognition needed for career advancement.

Presenting a research poster usually occurs after the data collection and analysis phase, prior to the publication of complete results. The poster presentation process starts with the submission of an abstract, which is a short written summary of the project. The abstract is typically broken into four sections (IMRD—Introduction, Methods, Results, and Conclusions) with a separate paragraph for each section. The abstract submission deadline is typically several months before the meeting, which allows peer-review and acceptance for presentation at the meeting. Notification of abstract acceptance typically occurs one to two months prior to the meeting, allowing time for poster creation. An exception to this process may occur for pharmacy residents or fellows in postgraduate training programs, as the timing of professional meetings may occur at a point in the training year where they may not have final results. For this reason, several organizations that accept trainee posters, like the American Society of Health-System Pharmacists, American Pharmacists Association, and American Association of Colleges of Pharmacy, allow trainees to submit "in-process" abstracts and create posters that describe the project and methods but do not have complete results. In addition to poster presentations, researchers may be invited to present their work as a research snapshot presentation, virtual poster, or as a mini-podium or other type of oral presentation. Formal podium presentations are frequently reserved for top-rated abstracts and are further discussed in Chapter 23.

The purpose of this chapter is to discuss the process and best practices for creating research abstracts and posters for presentation at scientific meetings. This chapter will discuss the common terminology used in creating abstracts and posters, the process for writing a research abstract, designing and presenting a research poster, and the next steps in the research process after presenting a poster. Recommendations for best practices and data from peer-reviewed studies analyzing effective poster presentation strategies will be included. The chapter concludes by providing an example of a pharmacy learner-led research project and the subsequent abstract and poster generated from that project.

Research Abstracts

A research abstract is a concise summary of a project that is intended to allow the reader to quickly determine the purpose, scope, and main findings of the research.[5,6] Abstracts should be brief, focused, and contain powerful statements that draw the reader in to find out more about the project. Abstracts should state information related to the project but should not serve as a review or provide critical analysis of the project. An abstract can be written for several different reasons. The two most common uses for abstracts include review and selection for presentation or publication and indexing. Some examples of selection include when a manuscript is submitted to a peer-reviewed journal, when applying for a research grant, or when submitting research for presentation at a scientific conference.[6] Abstracts are an important part of the research process because they are frequently the first thing a reviewer or attendee will see. For scientific meetings, abstracts are the only information that reviewers will use to judge the appropriateness of the research to be presented at a specific conference. In addition to selection, abstracts are also used for indexing in research databases (i.e., PubMed, MedLine, Embase, and Scopus). By including an abstract in an indexed database, readers are afforded a chance to review the short synopsis to determine if obtaining and reading the full article would be helpful to them.

The two main types of abstracts are descriptive and informative abstracts. The type of abstract required will depend on the discipline and source the abstract is submitted to. Descriptive abstracts are usually shorter than informative abstracts and range from 50 to 100 words. A descriptive abstract paraphrases the sections of a project and does not provide details about methodology, results, statistical analysis, or conclusions. Descriptive abstracts require the reader to access and read the entire manuscript to better understand the project. In the discipline of pharmacy, journals and scientific meetings will typically request an informative abstract. An informative abstract is more detailed than a descriptive abstract with word count requirements ranging anywhere from 200 to 500 words. Informative abstracts provide specific details about a project, such as study design and inclusion/exclusion criteria, results and statistical outcomes, and conclusions of the research. Abstracts can also be structured or unstructured. Structured abstracts have a heading and paragraph for each section, while unstructured abstracts do not divide sections and present information in a single paragraph. Informative abstracts are usually written in a structured format, while descriptive abstracts are unstructured.

SECTIONS OF AN ABSTRACT

The required sections in an abstract may have small variations between disciplines, but most pharmacy-based research requires a structured informative abstract. The abstract should be broken into the following sections: title, introduction, methods, results, and conclusion. Some scientific meetings may have additional structured heading requirements where similar content is requested but broken into different sections. An example of this is the introduction section, where introduction and background may be used interchangeably, and study objectives may be included in this section or as a separate heading after the introduction. Content recommendations, including naming differences for what is included in each section, are summarized in Table 22–1. References should not be cited in an abstract due to a lack of space. The subsequent poster presentation or manuscript will have a section to provide references for the readers. Although uncommon, some organizations may request additional information in the abstract, including keywords, funding source, and trial registration number. There are several guidelines that peer-reviewed journals use as abstract submission requirements for randomized trials and systematic reviews that may be useful to review.[7,8] The Consolidated Standards of Reporting Trials (CONSORT) protocol is a 25-item checklist that helps authors report trial design, analysis, and interpretation of randomized-control trials. The Preferred Reporting Items for Systematic Reviews and Meta-Analysis (PRISMA) guidance is a 27-item checklist used to improve the reporting and transparency of systematic reviews and meta-analyses.

TABLE 22–1. SECTIONS AND CONTENT OF A RESEARCH ABSTRACT

Abstract Section	Select Examples of Content to Include
Title	Short, accurate title describing what was studied
	Identify trial design (randomized control trial, systematic review, cohort study)
Introduction (Background)	Statement about problem and existing research available
	The specific research question to be studied
Methods (Statistics)	Type of study design
	Data source used (health record, database)
	Timeline of study
	Intervention, randomization
	Study subjects—inclusion/exclusion criteria
	Study outcomes—primary/secondary
	Statistical tests to be used
Results	Discussion of results
	• Number of study subjects assessed and included
	• Results of primary outcome, including statistical test result
	• Results of secondary outcomes (harm, side effects), including statistical tests
	• Additional results as pertinent to the research (subgroup analysis, cost analysis, sensitivity analysis)
Conclusion (Discussion)	Overall interpretation of results
	Strength and limitation of evidence
	Recommended areas for future research

ABSTRACT SUBMISSION AND REVIEW PROCESS

A crucial step prior to writing an abstract is identifying the most appropriate scientific meeting to submit your research to. Things to consider when selecting a meeting are the timeline for submission and presentation, the overall goal of the meeting, the audience of clinicians or scientists who will be at the meeting, and whether it is more appropriate to submit to a pharmacy-centric meeting (like the American Society of Health-System Pharmacists or American Pharmacists Association) or a multidisciplinary specialty meeting (like the Society of Critical Care Medicine or American College of Cardiology).[4]

After a scientific meeting is chosen, the next step is to review submission requirements for the meeting. Most scientific meetings have rigid requirements that must be followed for presentation at their meeting. Authors should check to see if there are restrictions on research that has already been presented, including, for instance, previously at a smaller local or regional meeting. Many meetings will allow authors to present research that has already been presented at a local or regional meeting if it has not already been published. Authors should also look for the type of research the meeting is willing to accept. In addition to traditional research studies, some meetings accept case reports, descriptive studies, and other projects. Many organizations now require authors to upload an Investigational Review Board approval cover letter when submitting an abstract to ensure the study has institutional research approval. As discussed earlier, most meetings require complete results, but several pharmacy-centric conferences have a submission category for pharmacy trainees to submit projects without results. Authors should also look to see if the scientific meeting provides a copy of the rubric used to score abstracts to give them the best chance for a successful submission. Examples of criteria frequently evaluated by rubrics include originality of research, the importance of the research question, description of study methods, appropriateness of data analysis, and discussion of major results of the project.

The submission of an abstract to a scientific conference is almost always made online via a conference portal. Abstract submissions are made in online forms that usually have text fields for each section and incorporate word count restrictions. Most portals allow the author to cut and paste content from a word processing document into the portal. This can be a more efficient way to enter your abstract, but pay close attention to the formatting and symbol requirements to make sure it copies over successfully. When submitting, take note of all specific requirements. Many organizations will conduct an administrative review of abstract submissions before scientific review and reject abstracts not meeting word count, formatting, or other style requirements. Unless otherwise noted, English is the preferred scientific language used at national and international meetings.

After an abstract is submitted and passes administrative review, it is sent for peer-review. Peer-reviewers are usually volunteer members of the organization who have expertise in the category the research was submitted to. Abstracts may be reviewed by one to three peer-reviewers. Peer-review is different for each organization but typically involves the review and scoring of an abstract in multiple categories with a final numerical score or recommendation of acceptance or rejection. Common categories evaluated on abstracts include scientific approach or study design, originality, significance or impact, analysis, and study conclusions. Scores from peer-reviewers are then used by conference leadership to determine acceptance of the abstract, top research that deserves a podium presentation, and research awards. After peer-review is complete, you will be notified if your abstract is either accepted or rejected for presentation. Some organizations also provide peer-review scores and written feedback from the reviewers. Written feedback provides an excellent opportunity to incorporate these recommended changes into the poster presentation. Table 22–2 contains an example of a pharmacy learner-led research abstract that was submitted and accepted at the American Society of Health-System Pharmacists Midyear meeting in 2019. This abstract met all the submission criteria provided by the meeting and was peer-reviewed. The introduction set the stage for the purpose and need for the study, which was a lack of data with direct oral anticoagulants in the treatment of left ventricular thrombus. The methods section provided a specific search strategy and data sources that could be easily reproduced. The conclusion section was supported by the efficacy and safety results that were provided.

ADVICE FOR CREATING AN ABSTRACT

A well-written abstract accurately tells the story of a research project in a succinct, direct, straightforward manner. Authors should obtain feedback from study team members and mentors and expect to undergo several revisions before an abstract is ready for submission. The abstract should cover the main components of the project (IMRD).[9] Methods should be clearly written so they can be understood and reproduced by the reader. Results should provide specific outcome numbers for the primary and secondary endpoints, with statistical tests provided as appropriate. An abstract does not allow for the presentation of all study results, so prioritize the primary outcome and secondary outcomes that may be of interest to conference attendees.[4] The discussion should provide a brief conclusion of your main study results and should only make statements that are supported by the results. The discussion is a good place to highlight the need for future studies in the subject area if warranted.

There are common errors when writing an abstract that may lead to rejection of the submission. The most common error is not following submission requirements such

TABLE 22–2. EXAMPLE OF PHARMACY LEARNER-LED ABSTRACT

Title: Evaluating the efficacy and safety of the direct oral anticoagulants in left ventricular thrombus: a systematic review

INTRODUCTION: Left ventricular thrombus is often associated with left ventricular dysfunction and can lead to significant morbidity and mortality. Currently, vitamin K antagonists are recommended in patients with left ventricular thrombus due to limited evidence assessing the role of the direct oral anticoagulants in this patient population. With numerous drug-drug interactions, drug-food interactions, and heavy monitoring burden, warfarin use often poses a challenge to both patients and clinicians. Alternatively, direct oral anticoagulants do not require monitoring and have fewer interactions. With the recent release of a case series exploring direct oral anticoagulant use in patients with left ventricular thrombus, we conducted a systematic review to assess efficacy of these agents for left ventricular thrombus resolution.

PURPOSE: The purpose of this systematic review is to assess the efficacy and safety of direct oral anticoagulants for the treatment of left ventricular thrombus.

METHODS: A systematic search was conducted according to the Preferred Reporting Items for Systematic Review and Meta-Analyses guidelines for randomized controlled trials, cohort studies, case series, and case studies to evaluate the use of the direct oral anticoagulants in patients with a confirmed diagnosis of left ventricular thrombus. The primary efficacy outcome was resolution of left ventricular thrombus. The primary safety outcome was bleeding. Studies were excluded if left ventricular thrombus was not verified by imaging or were treated with anticoagulant other than a direct oral anticoagulant. Data sources utilized included PubMed and Embase. Search dates ran from January 1, 1999 to August 27, 2019.

RESULTS: A total of 6,791 articles were retrieved after removing duplicates. After title and abstract screening, 6,768 articles were excluded. Twenty-three full-text articles were assessed for eligibility. Seven of the twenty-three full-text articles were excluded as they did not meet predefined criteria. Two articles did not study patients diagnosed with left ventricular thrombus, and four articles did not use a direct oral anticoagulant for the treatment of left ventricular thrombus. Sixteen articles met the inclusion criteria. Of the 85 patients included, 49.4% were on rivaroxaban, 45.9% were on apixaban, 3.5% were on dabigatran, and 1.2% were on edoxaban. The mean follow-up time for LV resolution was 97 days. Resolution of LV thrombus occurred in 67.1% of patients. Bleeding occurred in 5.9% of patients. Of the 42 patients treated with rivaroxaban, 66.7% had resolution of thrombus and 9.5% had bleeding. Of the 39 patients treated with apixaban, 45.9% had resolution of thrombus and 2.56% had bleeding. Of the three patients treated with dabigatran, 66.7% had resolution of thrombus and no reported bleeding. Finally, the one patient on edoxaban had thrombus resolution with no bleeding.

CONCLUSION: Based on available literature, direct oral anticoagulants were shown to be effective in left ventricular thrombus resolution and had low rates of bleeding. These agents may pose an advantage to warfarin due to their minimal drug–drug interactions, diet modifications, and frequency of therapeutic monitoring. In patients who do not have a special indication for warfarin (e.g., prosthetic valve), direct oral anticoagulants may be considered for the resolution of LV thrombus. Large, prospective studies are needed to better assess the true efficacy and safety of the direct oral anticoagulants for this specific indication.

(LV, left ventricular)

as section headings, word count, or formatting for the title and body of the abstract. Since an abstract is concise, it should focus on the most important parts of the research project, with writing that is straightforward and to the point, avoiding excessive details. Abstracts should also avoid referencing studies and should not include graphs or figures. Remember that most conferences will publish abstracts in an issue of their companion journal, so the abstract will be available to read online.

Creating a Research Poster

POSTER OVERVIEW AND CREATION

Congratulations! Your abstract has been accepted. While a select few abstracts may be chosen for podium presentations, the majority of abstracts will be invited for presentation in a research poster format. A research poster is a visual summary of a project to communicate the research purpose, methods, and main findings to attendees at a scientific meeting. Research posters have evolved over the years, but they are typically large format print posters displaying your project. The primary goal of a research poster is to communicate your research efficiently and effectively to a wide audience at a scientific meeting. Additional goals may include obtaining feedback on your research methods, study design, or identifying potential future collaborators. Unlike in an oral presentation or seminar, audiences at poster sessions are not static; they move from poster to poster, trying to obtain as much knowledge as possible. The 10-10 rule is a good reference to use when creating your poster; the average attendee will spend 10 seconds scanning a poster from 10 feet away as they determine if they want to stop by for more information. With posters, the visual display is just as important as the content. There are many references available that contain suggestions for creating effective posters (Table 22–3).[1,4,5,9–15] Trainees may also be encouraged to utilize formats preferred by their research mentors. Effective creation of posters following these suggested recommendations and feedback from experienced mentors

TABLE 22–3. KEY ADVICE FOR CREATING A POSTER

A big mistake is trying to squeeze in too much information. A poster is not a manuscript—use it to summarize and discuss your key findings.

The title is important to draw the attendee in. The title should be in large and bold text, and concise.

Remember 10-10 rule—attendees will have 10 seconds to scan your poster from 10 feet away to decide if they want to stop by. Make key information easy to find and read.

Minimize lengthy text. Use bullet points and concise statements instead of full sentences/paragraphs.

Visual appeal is just as important as content. Strategically incorporate visuals such as charts, tables, graphs, and photos to draw the reader in.

Utilize a one- or two-color scheme for your poster. White backgrounds allow text to stand out best.

Make sure your conclusions/implications are backed up by the data you present.

Consider using poster templates from your institution. Ask for examples of mentor's posters to get an idea of expectations.

Edit your poster a lot. Start early, get frequent feedback, and make multiple rounds of changes.

Don't include the abstract on the poster—it is redundant. References are not usually needed, but if you do include them only choose a few major references to include.

will allow poster presenters to have the widest reach with their projects at scientific meetings.

The poster should contain most of the same sections used in the abstract. A large font, bolded, succinct title should appear at the top of the poster, with accompanying author names, credentials, affiliations, and logo. Be sure to use the correct name, spelling, and credentials of your study team members on the poster. The main body of the poster should have an introduction, objectives, methods, results, discussion, and conclusion. Most scientific meetings do not provide specific section criteria for posters as they do for abstracts. However, it is assumed that the poster will be an expansion of the abstract so often the key sections are duplicated and expanded upon with additional methods, results, and conclusions as appropriate. The results section should include data and statistical analysis and only provide results which are related to the stated study objective(s). Pharmacy trainee posters that do not contain results should provide a more detailed methods section and include a future implications section that predicts potential impacts based on the pending results. Posters may also include a reference section and may include a conflict of interest statement if required by the scientific meeting.

The most frequently used software to create a research poster is Microsoft PowerPoint, although Microsoft Publisher, Keynote, or Adobe software can also be used. PowerPoint allows you to create your poster in one slide and then expand that file into a larger size that can be printed as a poster. The PowerPoint file can be saved as a PDF so that the file does not become distorted when printed in a large poster format. It is important to check the poster size requirements for a specific meeting prior to starting the design of your poster. Presenters may also use poster templates provided by the scientific meeting or their home institution. Many students are familiar with editing functions in PowerPoint, leading to its frequent use. University librarians can also serve as a good source for help with providing feedback for creating and editing posters.[10]

POSTER FORMAT AND DESIGN

Effective formatting and visual design of a poster is crucial for a successful presentation. The visual imagery of a poster has been shown to be more influential than the actual content and the main driver in engaging viewers.[16] Unlike the rigorous criteria applied to abstracts or manuscripts, posters allow for the creative freedom to design them as the author sees best fit. There are many references that provide suggestions for creating successful posters, but almost all references agree on the following concepts. Posters should minimize the use of text and full sentences, providing just enough supporting text to provide context to the reader and summarize interpretations and conclusions.[17] When text is needed, avoid complex sentences and jargon, and instead utilize simplified writing. The body of the poster should have a logical flow of ideas, with clear and bold headings that are easily followed by the reader. Some authors have recently broken from the traditional flow of a poster to incorporate large, bolded summaries of their project in the center middle of the poster. When possible, visual graphics such as tables, graphs, and pictures should replace text.[2] Tempt the eye and let the pictures do the talking. Utilizing a flow-chart to describe the study timeline in the methods section, or a table of outcomes in the results section are great opportunities to incorporate visuals into the design. The use of infographics has also become a popular visual strategy to discuss results. Posters should be uncluttered and have some white space instead of being packed to the edges with content. These strategies will help draw the viewer to the poster for a more detailed conversation about the project. Remember that not every piece of information from the study needs to, or should be, displayed on the poster.

Font and text size are very important aspects of poster creation. Many conference attendees want the big take-home points from a poster, and font and text size can be helpful in providing this. While research has been conflicting, sans serif fonts such as Arial and Verdana may be easier to read than serif fonts such as Times New Roman.[1,18–21] It has also been proposed that sans-serif fonts may work better for headings and serif fonts for smaller text.[13] Font size was an important variable in the studies that analyzed the readability of font type. As most attendees will be about 5 to 10 feet away from your poster as they initially read it, use the largest size font that fits. The title should be easily viewed from 10 feet, so a font size of 50 to 80 is most appropriate. A font size of 40 to 50 is appropriate for section headings to allow attendees to quickly find sections they are interested in. The text in the body of the poster should have a font size no less than 24, but ideally between 30 and 40. The references section is an appropriate area to make the font smaller than 24 if more space is needed. The use of uppercase letters, bolded, and underlined font should be utilized in areas of the poster that you want to draw attention to. Examples of these areas may include the title, section headings, key results and interpretations, and conclusions.

ADVICE FOR CREATING A POSTER

Start creating the poster well before the deadline and plan for several revisions of the poster incorporating feedback from research mentors. Utilize peers who are not familiar with the project to get an understanding of what they take away from the poster after initial review. Check for grammatical and formatting errors that may distract the viewer from the purpose of the poster. The formatting should be verified by using gridlines and PowerPoint editing features to make sure all the sections are aligned and centered appropriately. Be creative and use pictures and color, but don't go overboard. Factors such as small fonts, wordy and cluttered posters, the inability to find key items, unclear study objectives, and conclusions that do not answer the objective have all been cited as examples present in poorly constructed posters.[13,15,17] Figure 22–1 is an example of a pharmacy learner-led research poster presented at the American Society of Health-System Pharmacists (ASHP) Midyear Clinical Meeting. This poster does a good job of utilizing a flow chart and table to provide a description of methods and results. Text is used throughout, but it is in a larger font and in bullet point format instead of complete sentences making it easier for the reader to digest. The author also used a large, bolded font in the middle of the poster to describe the study conclusion. This allows readers to quickly view a concise summary of the study to determine if they want to stop and discuss more in-depth.

Presenting a Research Poster

GENERAL PRESENTATION CONSIDERATIONS

Research posters are presented during poster sessions at a scientific conference. Poster sessions at large conferences may be scheduled during lunch or other times of the day when another educational programming is not scheduled to avoid conflicts. This allows many attendees to be present and presenters to have an adequate audience to present to. Smaller meetings or local conferences may have posters presented individually to the entire audience at once. Select organizations, like the Society of Critical Care Medicine, have replaced posters in lieu of three- to four-minute short PowerPoint presentations known as research snapshot presentations. Find the poster session hall prior to your session and familiarize yourself with the room. Show up in professional appearance and attire, which is most likely going to be a suit. If you are unsure, it is better to be overdressed for the session. The audience at a poster session spans a wide range of clinicians and scientists who are interested in new research findings to take back to their home institution, or attendees looking to find ideas to build upon for future research. The majority of visitors to a poster will come from interested attendees walking the hall and reviewing topics. Abstracts of all posters being presented will be published either online or in the meeting program. This allows attendees to review abstracts to determine which they want to stop by to obtain more information. Many meetings have structured "poster walk rounds," where a group of attendees is led by a moderator through a category of posters. Some scientific meetings may also assign attendees to visit select posters to ensure adequate discussion with presenters. Lastly, mentors, colleagues, and friends will likely stop by to see your poster. These supporters

Evaluating the efficacy and safety of the direct oral anticoagulants in left ventricular thrombus: a systematic review

Racha Kabbani, PharmD Candidate[1]; Matthew A. Wanat, PharmD, BCPS, BCCCP, FCCM[1]; Tracy E. Macaulay, PharmD, AACC, BCPS (AQ Cardiology), BCCP[2]; Rachel R. Helbing, MLIS, MS, AHIP[3]; Elisabeth M. Sulaica, PharmD, BCCP[1]

[1]University of Houston College of Pharmacy, Houston, TX [2]University of Kentucky College of Pharmacy, Lexington, KY [3]University of Houston University Libraries, Houston, TX

INTRODUCTION

- Vitamin K antagonists (VKA) are currently preferred in patients with left ventricular (LV) thrombus due to limited data assessing direct oral anticoagulants (DOACs) in this population[1,2]
- With numerous drug-drug interactions, drug-food interactions, and a heavy monitoring burden, warfarin use poses a challenge to patients and providers

OBJECTIVES

- To assess the efficacy and safety of DOACs in patients with LV thrombus
  - Efficacy - Resolution of left ventricular thrombus
  - Safety - Incidence of major bleeding events

METHODS

- A systematic search was conducted according to the Preferred Reporting Items for Systematic Reviews and Meta-Analyses guidelines
- Data sources utilized included PubMed & EMBASE
- Search dates ran from 1/1/1999 until 8/27/2019

Inclusion criteria
- Case studies, case series, case-control studies, cohort studies, and randomized control trials
- LV thrombus verified by imaging
- Oral DOAC use

Exclusion criteria:
- Left ventricular thrombus not verified by imaging
- Treatment with an anticoagulant other than a DOAC

> DOACs may be efficacious alternatives to VKAs with regard to LV thrombus resolution and overall low bleeding rates.
> Randomized control trials are needed to further evaluate the efficacy and safety of DOACs in these patients.

Study Selection Flow Diagram

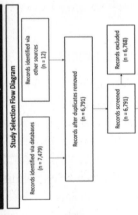

RESULTS

- A total of 85 patients were included in the systematic review
- Mean follow-up time for LV thrombus resolution was 97 days
- LV thrombus resolution was 67.1% (57/85)
- Bleeding incidence was 5.9% (5/85)

DOAC used (N=85)	LV Thrombus Resolution % (n/total)	Bleeding Incidence % (n/total)
Rivaroxaban (N=42)	66.7 (28/42)	9.5 (4/42)
Apixaban (N=39)	66.7 (26/39)	2.6 (1/39)
Dabigatran (N=3)	66.7 (2/3)	0 (0/3)
Edoxaban (N=1)	100% (1/1)	0 (0/1)

CONCLUSIONS

- This review indicates that DOACs may be efficacious alternatives to VKAs with regard to LV thrombus resolution
- Overall bleeding rates were low, but limited extrapolation due to the small sample size
- Large, prospective studies are needed to better assess the true efficacy and safety of DOACs compared to VKAs for this population

REFERENCES

(1) McCarthy CP, Vaidyanathan M, McCarthy KJ, et al. *JAMA Cardiol* 2018;3(7):642-9.
(2) Fleddermann A, Hayes CH, Magalski A, and Main ML. *Am J Cardiol* 2019;124(3):367-72.

Figure 22–1. Example of a pharmacy learner-led poster. The abstract was submitted to the 2019 ASHP Midyear Clinical Meeting and presented as a poster presentation in December 2019.

can serve as a positive start to the poster session and provide great support for your work. Ask mentors to invite colleagues in the field to attend your poster and provide feedback. Make sure to balance time spent with friends and visitors, and do not ignore attendees interested in talking more about your research.

POSTER PRINTING AND TRANSPORTATION

The logistics of getting the poster to the meeting is important to understand to minimize stress. Most presenters will have their poster printed prior to the meeting either via a third-party company or with a large printer if available at the local college or institution. This allows for the presenter to review the printed poster and potentially reprint it if needed. This option likely means that you will be traveling with your poster on an airplane. Do not check the poster in but rather carry it on the plane with your belongings. Poster tubes are odd-shaped and have been known to get lost. They are often retrieved at oversize luggage and can be another source of confusion. Hint: If you ask the flight attendant, they will often let you store it in the coat closet at the front of the plane. Another option is to use a printing service at or near the convention center or to have your poster shipped to your hotel. This option bypasses the stress of flying with another item but doesn't allow for the review of the poster prior to the meeting. Bring extra Velcro or push pins as the meeting may not provide them, or they may have been removed by the presenter from a previous session. Lastly, many attendees will bring a one-page printout of their poster to provide to attendees. Many meetings now recommend incorporating a QR code that attendees can scan which will allow them to download the poster in lieu of printouts. Bringing business cards is also a good idea to provide contact information for interested attendees who may want to contact you about your research.

PRESENTING YOUR POSTER

The most important aspect of presenting a poster is to be present. Poster sessions will usually last for 30 to 90 minutes, and this time is not only afforded to present your project but also when poster judging and walk rounds may occur. Presenting a poster is a chance to grow your reputation, increase networking, and obtain feedback on your project. It is imperative that you are present with your poster for the entire session to maximize these opportunities. You do not want to be absent from your poster when a prominent researcher in the field stops by to discuss. Stand to the side of the poster and maintain eye contact with attendees as they pass by. In addition to being present, be prepared to discuss your project. When an attendee approaches, start by introducing yourself and the title of your project. It's a good idea to have a two-minute summary of your work that you can present if the attendee wants more details. A great structure for the two-minute summary may include describing why the study was warranted, a brief overview of your methods, key results (primary endpoint and 1-2 secondary endpoints), and a concise conclusion that also provides thoughts on the next steps for research. The two-minute summary will suffice for most attendees, but it is likely you may have a few people who are really interested and may want to have a more detailed conversation. Poster sessions are often described as less stressful than an oral or podium presentation, but don't miss this crucial opportunity to present and network with peers.

Virtual poster sessions are becoming more common, opening up additional avenues for research presentation and real-time interaction with audiences. These sessions have been positively received by both presenters and attendees, often using breakout rooms where each presenter can share their poster and interact with attendees through a combination of text, audio, and video.[22-25] Poster session engagement and comfort level of presenting in a virtual setting have been described as positives with the virtual poster experience. Virtual sessions also have the benefit of no physical space limitations allowing more posters to be presented. Challenges to virtual poster sessions may include interacting with multiple people online at once, lack of nonverbal cues during communication, and technical difficulties related to technology and conference platforms, including audio and video issues.[25] The success of virtual poster sessions may allow for virtual presentations at future live conferences where attendees may not be able to attend in person.

AFTER THE POSTER SESSION

After presenting a research poster, there are several important final steps to optimize your scholarly work. Immediately following the meeting, sit down with your research team and discuss the feedback given during the poster session. This feedback can be very useful to improve the manuscript that will hopefully accompany the poster. Determine if any additional analyses could be run based on new ideas provided from the meeting. New analyses that provide additional data could also be used for a future poster presentation on the same topic. Additionally, it is very important to follow up with attendees who requested more information. Survey data from previous ASHP Midyear meetings have shown pharmacy poster presenters followed up with less than 30% of requests, and took an extended period of time to do so.[26] These follow-up opportunities may help improve the project or may result in networking that establishes long-term collaboration. A great tip is to utilize travel time (time at the airport, on the airplane) to draft emails and begin to follow up with conference attendees, especially while these interactions are fresh in your mind.

Scientific meeting abstracts and posters may be available to view online after a meeting, but these sources do not provide complete details about a research project. In order for your work to reach the widest audience, presenters should seek to transform their posters into peer-reviewed manuscripts. Transitioning posters into a peer-reviewed manuscript publication is arguably the most important step in the research process, but it does not happen as frequently as needed. Multiple studies analyzing pharmacy residents at regional and national meetings have found publication rates of 1.8 to 16% after poster presentation.[27–29] Publication rates for presenters at American Association of Colleges of Pharmacy (AACP) meetings, largely pharmacy faculty, was only 20%, with a median time to the publication of 15 to 24 months.[28,30] Barriers to publication may include lack of time or study team continuity on a project, responsibility for submitting publication, low priority or motivation, and lack of training program requirements to submit a manuscript for graduation.[29,31] Accepted publications were more frequently observational studies, had abstracts with results and statistics, involved multidisciplinary teams that included a physician, and were presented at a medical meeting instead of a pharmacy meeting.[27,30]

Summary and Conclusions

Poster presentations serve as an efficient and effective method for disseminating research results. They help to build on what is currently known about a scientific area, and to shape future research in that area. Presenting a poster is a great opportunity for a learner to share their research and broaden their professional network. Scientific conferences utilize abstracts, which are concise written summaries of a research project to evaluate the research's merit and appropriateness for poster presentation at a meeting. When writing an abstract, authors should focus on the most important parts of the research project. Follow the scientific meetings abstract requirements and utilize the scoring rubric, if available, to improve chances for acceptance. After an abstract is accepted, creating a visually engaging poster is important for an engagement at professional meetings. Utilize graphs, tables, and pictures in place of excessive wording to drive home key results and conclusions. After presenting a poster, the next important step in the research process is to incorporate feedback and prepare a manuscript for submission to a peer-reviewed journal. A manuscript allows for complete dissemination of the project that can easily be searched in indexed medical databases. An understanding of the abstract submission and poster presentation process, and tips for success, can improve research productivity and external visibility of research.

Key Points and Advice

- A research abstract is a concise summary of a project that allows the reader to determine the purpose and scope of the project. Common uses include conference presentations or publication summaries, and database indexing.
- When writing an abstract, authors should structure the writing into four main sections: introduction, methods, results, and discussion. Follow abstract requirements and utilize a scoring rubric to improve chances for acceptance.
- When creating a poster, utilize visuals such as pictures, charts, and graphs in place of excessive wording to highlight key aspects of research and increase engagement from attendees.
- Be present and prepared to discuss your research during the poster session. Prepare a two-minute synopsis of your research to discuss with interested attendees.
- After the poster presentation, meet with your research team and utilize feedback from the conference to improve your project. Submitting a manuscript after the presentation is important to make research available to a wide audience.

Chapter Review Questions

1. What are the key elements that should be included in an abstract?
2. What are some strategies you can use to increase the likelihood that your abstract gets accepted to a scientific conference?
3. What are some strategies you can use to create a poster that generates engagement from conference attendees?
4. What content should not be included in an abstract? What content should not be included in a poster?
5. What research activities should occur after presenting your poster? What should be the end goal of the research project?

Online Resources

- Research in Pharmacy: Professional Poster Presentations Advice for Students and New Practitioners. American Society of Health-System Pharmacists. https://www.ashp.org/Professional-Development/ASHP-Podcasts/Practice-Journeys/

Professional-Poster-Presentations-Advice-for-Students-and-New-Practitioners?login returnUrl=SSOCheckOnly

- Preparing a Poster Presentation. American College of Physicians. https://www.acponline. org/membership/residents/competitions-awards/acp-national-abstract-competitions/ guide-to-preparing-for-the-abstract-competition/preparing-a-poster-presentation
- How to Create a Research Poster. New York University Libraries. https://guides.nyu. edu/posters
- American College of Clinical Pharmacy Abstract Evaluation Criteria. https://www.accp. com/docs/meetings/abstracts/Abstract_Scoring_Original_Research.pdf
- American Society of Health-System Pharmacists Poster Presenter Handbook. https:// www.ashp.org/-/media/summer-meetings/docs/2019/Poster-Presenter-Handbook.ashx
- American Society of Health-System Pharmacists Professional Poster Submission Instructions. https://www.ashp.org/-/media/midyear-conference/docs/2020/MCM20-Poster-Submission-Instructions.ashx?la=en&hash=62EEA59152F7AF78EDC7E589DF1 E6102EA077E2A

REFERENCES

1. Persky AM. Scientific posters: a plea from a conference attendee. *Am J Pharm Educ.* 2016;80(10):162.
2. Hamilton CW. At a glance: a stepwise approach to successful poster presentations. *Chest.* 2008;134(2):457-459.
3. Young J, Bridgeman MB, Hermes-DeSantis ER. Presentation of scientific poster information: lessons learned from evaluating the impact of content arrangement and use of infographics. *Curr Pharm Teach Learn.* 2019;11(2):204-210.
4. Wood GJ, Morrison RS. Writing abstracts and developing posters for national meetings. *J Palliat Med.* 2011;14(3):353-359.
5. Nagda S. How to write a scientific abstract. *J Indian Prosthodont Soc.* 2013;13(3):382-383.
6. Abstracts. The Writing Center. University of North Carolina at Chapel Hill. Accessed December 7, 2020. https://writingcenter.unc.edu/tips-and-tools/abstracts/
7. Beller EM, Glasziou PP, Altman DG, et al. PRISMA for abstracts: reporting systematic reviews in journal and conference abstracts. *PLOS Med.* 2013;10(4):e1001419.
8. Hopewell S, Clarke M, Moher D, et al. CONSORT for reporting randomised trials in journal and conference abstracts. *Lancet.* 2008;371(9609):281-283.
9. Singh MK. Preparing and presenting effective abstracts and posters in psychiatry. *Acad Psychiatry.* 2014;38(6):709-715.
10. Gundogan B, Koshy K, Kurar L, Whitehurst K. How to make an academic poster. *Ann Med Surg.* 2016;11:69-71.
11. Boullata JI, Mancuso CE. A "how-to" guide in preparing abstracts and poster presentations. *Nutr Clin Pract.* 2007;22(6):641-646.
12. Rose TM. An illustrated guide to poster design. *AJPE.* 2017;81(7).

13. Pedwell RK, Hardy JA, Rowland SL. Effective visual design and communication practices for research posters: exemplars based on the theory and practice of multimedia learning and rhetoric. *Biochem Mol Biol Educ.* 2017;45(3):249-261.

14. Miller JE. Preparing and presenting effective research posters. *Health Serv Res.* 2007;42(1 Pt 1):311-328.

15. Willett LL, Paranjape A, Estrada C. Identifying key components for an effective case report poster: an observational study. *J Gen Intern Med.* 2009;24(3):393-397.

16. Rowe N, Ilic D. What impact do posters have on academic knowledge transfer? A pilot survey on author attitudes and experiences. *BMC Med Educ.* 2009;9:71.

17. Hess GR, Tosney KW, Liegel LH. Creating effective poster presentations: AMEE Guide no. 40. *Med Teach.* 2009;31(4):319-321.

18. Sheedy JE, Subbaram MV, Zimmerman AB, Hayes JR. Text legibility and the letter superiority effect. *Hum Factors.* 2005;47(4):797-815.

19. Kaspar K, Wehlitz T, von Knobelsdorff S, Wulf T, von Saldern MAO. A matter of font type: the effect of serifs on the evaluation of scientific abstracts. *Int J Psychol.* 2015;50(5):372-378.

20. Arditi A, Cho J. Serifs and font legibility. *Vision Res.* 2005;45(23):2926-2933.

21. Akhmadeeva L, Tukhvatullin I, Veytsman B. Do serifs help in comprehension of printed text? An experiment with Cyrillic readers. *Vision Res.* 2012;65:21-24.

22. Kazmierczak T, Bistany B. Setting up a research poster during COVID-19 lockdown: a reflection. *J Christ Nurs.* 2020;37(4):E45-E46.

23. Diegel-Vacek L, Carlucci M. An innovative virtual poster session for doctor of nursing practice student project presentations. *J Nurs Educ.* 2020;59(12):697-700.

24. Lamming DW, Carter CS. Maintaining a scientific community while social distancing. *Transl Med Aging.* 2020;4:55-59.

25. Holt EA, Heim AB, Tessens E, Walker R. Thanks for inviting me to the party: virtual poster sessions as a way to connect in a time of disconnection. *Ecol Evol.* 2020;10(22):12423-12430.

26. Bublin JG, Gales MA, Gales BJ. Response rates from poster presenters at ASHP meetings. American Society of Health-System Pharmacists. *Am J Health Syst Pharm.* 1999;56(3):277-278.

27. McKelvey RP, Hatton RC, Kimberlin CA. Pharmacy resident project publication rates and study designs from 1981, 1991, and 2001. *Am J Health Syst Pharm.* 2010;67(10):830-836.

28. Olson KL, Holmes M, Dang C, Patel RJ, Witt DM. Publication rates of abstracts presented by pharmacy residents at the Western States Conference. *Am J Health Syst Pharm.* 2012;69(1):59-62.

29. Weathers T, Ercek K, Unni EJ. PGY1 resident research projects: publication rates, project completion policies, perceived values, and barriers. *Curr Pharm Teach Learn.* 2019;11(6):547-556.

30. Spencer S, Majkowski C, Suda KJ. Predictors of publication rates for abstracts presented at the American Association of Colleges of Pharmacy Annual Meetings. *AJPE.* 2018;82(8).

31. Barriers to full-text publication following presentation of abstracts at annual orthopaedic meetings. Abstract. Europe PMC. Published Dec 9, 2020. Accessed December 9, 2020. https://europepmc.org/article/med/12533587

23

Chapter Twenty-Three

Podium and Other Oral Presentations

Kimberly Illingworth, PhD, BSPharm, FAPhA

Chapter Objectives

- Describe the structure of a typical oral scientific presentation
- Incorporate principles of storytelling into an oral scientific presentation
- Recognize how characteristics of an audience affect the structure and delivery of an oral presentation
- Discuss different viewpoints and techniques for presenting an in-person podium presentation, a seminar, a workshop, a TED-like talk, and an elevator speech
- Discuss various technologies to aid in the delivery of oral presentations
- Describe best practices in the delivery of a podium session or an oral presentation
- Describe an example of a learner involved podium presentation

Key Terminology

Podium presentation, research seminar, workshop, in-service, TED-like talk, elevator pitch

Introduction

Imagine looking at the computer and seeing the email message, "Congratulations! Your abstract has been accepted for a podium presentation." The first feeling may be elation in knowing that the hard work put into a research project will be shared with others. The second feeling, however, may be fear or anxiety from having to speak to strangers, including those who are more senior and experienced, in an unfamiliar environment. Fear and anxiety are reasonable and common responses to uncertainty and there may be quite a bit of uncertainty associated with presenting in such a scenario. However, presenting is simply telling a story—the beginning, middle, and end of a project of which the presenter is intimately familiar. Everyone has told a story at some point in their lives. To help alleviate some of the anxiety that may occur in the midst of preparing and presenting research, consider presenting as just telling a story.

One of the primary purposes of research is to advance knowledge in order to better understand the world and apply findings to benefit society. The key to advancing knowledge is the sharing of the processes used to conduct research projects and their results. Dissemination, or the sharing of the research findings, occurs through a variety of ways, but typically through publication in peer-reviewed journals and poster or oral presentation at scientific conferences. The goal of this sharing is to allow others to learn from the research so that they can add to knowledge through their own work or apply the research findings to practice. Further, it is also important to present one's research as a form of professional development. After the presentation, the investigator will frequently receive feedback from those in the audience. Feedback often focuses on future work, as well as how to address methodological challenges or alternative interpretation of results. The investigators have the opportunity to not only learn from this feedback but also use this information to improve future work. In addition, presenting at scientific conferences allows one to identify and network with potential collaborators. Presenting one's work also provides an opportunity for students, residents and fellows to demonstrate their skills, as well as network for employment opportunities.

The content and tools necessary to develop and deliver an effective oral presentation are reviewed in this chapter. In addition to best practices for preparing visual materials and presentation delivery, presentation types and formats will be highlighted. Ultimately, the goals of this chapter are to help the reader feel prepared and confident when delivering their presentation.

Oral Presentations: Breaking Down the Steps

Preparing and delivering a presentation to an unknown audience can seem overwhelming. However, there are steps that any speaker can follow to make it seem more manageable. Figure 23–1 outlines each of these steps and includes aspects about each of the following: (1) preparing an abstract or proposal for presentation, (2) preparing the

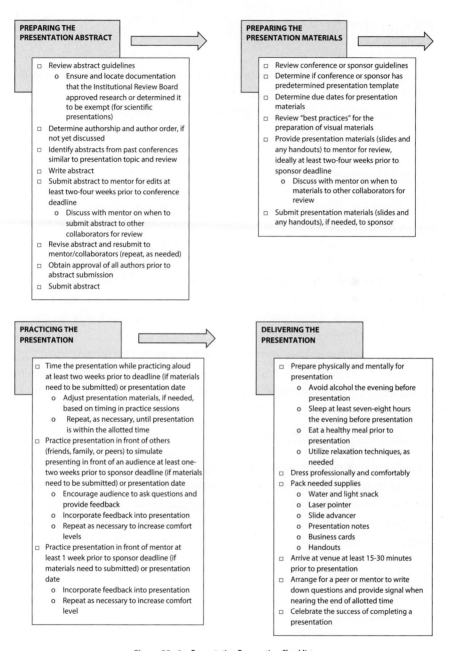

PREPARING THE PRESENTATION ABSTRACT

- ☐ Review abstract guidelines
  - o Ensure and locate documentation that the Institutional Review Board approved research or determined it to be exempt (for scientific presentations)
- ☐ Determine authorship and author order, if not yet discussed
- ☐ Identify abstracts from past conferences similar to presentation topic and review
- ☐ Write abstract
- ☐ Submit abstract to mentor for edits at least two-four weeks prior to conference deadline
  - o Discuss with mentor on when to submit abstract to other collaborators for review
- ☐ Revise abstract and resubmit to mentor/collaborators (repeat, as needed)
- ☐ Obtain approval of all authors prior to abstract submission
- ☐ Submit abstract

PREPARING THE PRESENTATION MATERIALS

- ☐ Review conference or sponsor guidelines
- ☐ Determine if conference or sponsor has predetermined presentation template
- ☐ Determine due dates for presentation materials
- ☐ Review "best practices" for the preparation of visual materials
- ☐ Provide presentation materials (slides and any handouts) to mentor for review, ideally at least two-four weeks prior to sponsor deadline
  - o Discuss with mentor on when to materials to other collaborators for review
- ☐ Submit presentation materials (slides and any handouts), if needed, to sponsor

PRACTICING THE PRESENTATION

- ☐ Time the presentation while practicing aloud at least two weeks prior to deadline (if materials need to be submitted) or presentation date
  - o Adjust presentation materials, if needed, based on timing in practice sessions
  - o Repeat, as necessary, until presentation is within the allotted time
- ☐ Practice presentation in front of others (friends, family, or peers) to simulate presenting in front of an audience at least one-two weeks prior to sponsor deadline (if materials need to be submitted) or presentation date
  - o Encourage audience to ask questions and provide feedback
  - o Incorporate feedback into presentation
  - o Repeat as necessary to increase comfort levels
- ☐ Practice presentation in front of mentor at least 1 week prior to sponsor deadline (if materials need to submitted) or presentation date
  - o Incorporate feedback into presentation
  - o Repeat as necessary to increase comfort level

DELIVERING THE PRESENTATION

- ☐ Prepare physically and mentally for presentation
  - o Avoid alcohol the evening before presentation
  - o Sleep at least seven-eight hours the evening before presentation
  - o Eat a healthy meal prior to presentation
  - o Utilize relaxation techniques, as needed
- ☐ Dress professionally and comfortably
- ☐ Pack needed supplies
  - o Water and light snack
  - o Laser pointer
  - o Slide advancer
  - o Presentation notes
  - o Business cards
  - o Handouts
- ☐ Arrive at venue at least 15-30 minutes prior to presentation
- ☐ Arrange for a peer or mentor to write down questions and provide signal when nearing the end of allotted time
- ☐ Celebrate the success of completing a presentation

Figure 23–1. Presentation Preparation Checklist

presentation materials, (3) practicing the presentation, and (4) delivering the presentation. The following sections provide additional details concerning various elements of these steps.

Planning for the Presentation

Even before preparing an abstract or a proposal for a presentation, speakers must engage in a number of planning considerations, such as determining the purpose and type of the presentation, evaluating the intended audience for the presentation, and deciding who else will be considered authors of the presentation.

IDENTIFY THE PURPOSE

Presentations have different purposes. The first step of planning is to determine the purpose, or goal, of the presentation. The purpose of the presentation often dictates the format. Depending on the presentation, the primary purpose may be to: introduce oneself, inform, instruct, stimulate, persuade, or entertain.[1,2] For example, the primary purpose of a 15-minute podium presentation at a scientific conference will be quite different from a 60-minute workshop focused on the application of scientific results to clinical practice scenarios. In addition, the presentation may have multiple goals, such as in the case of the continuing education presentations. In this case, the speaker's goals are to inform the audience of recent research and instruct them on how to apply it to their practice setting. Even if the primary purpose is not to entertain, the most effective presentations typically are both engaging and entertaining.[1]

DETERMINE THE PRESENTATION TYPE

The format of the presentation often is dictated by the type of presentation and its purpose. The most common types of professional presentations are described below. Although the preparation and submission of a formal abstract may not be required for all of these presentation types, some type of presentation proposal is helpful at this stage if a formal abstract is not utilized (see Chapter 22 for additional discussion of abstract preparation).

Scientific Podium Presentation

The purpose of podium presentations, sometimes referred to as platform presentations, is to inform, where the presenter communicates research findings, usually at a conference. Podium presentations are selected through a peer-review process, which begins months before the presentation occurs. The process involves investigators submitting an abstract, or summary, of their research approximately four to six months prior to the scheduled conference (see Figure 23–1). All investigators should review and approve the abstract prior to its submission. Two to three independent reviewers evaluate the abstract and make the determination of whether it should be accepted for an oral presentation.

Investigators are notified two to three months prior to the conference. If there are multiple people involved in a research project, only one member of the research team typically will present.

Podium presentations range from 15 to 30 minutes with 5 to 10 minutes of that time dedicated to questions from the audience.[3,4] The structure of the presentation is specified by the organization, but typically follows the IMRAD format: Introduction, Methods, Results, and Discussion.[5] Using this format, the presenter will include: (1) the context of why a particular project was a conducted, (2) background necessary to understand the research, including the conceptual or theoretical framework, (3) the objectives or specific aims, (4) the methods used (e.g., study design, variables, sample, setting, data collection procedures, and statistical analysis), (5) the results, (6) discussion of the results and their implications, including strengths and limitations, (7) conclusion, and (8) next steps for future work.[3-5] At some scientific meetings, students, residents, and fellows often receive feedback on their presentations using an evaluation rubric. If available, the speaker should refer to the rubric when preparing for and practicing their presentation. See Table 23-1 for examples.

Typically, the audience is reflective of the organization's membership. In the case of health-related conferences, such as the American Pharmacists Association Annual Meeting, the audience is comprised of researchers, healthcare professionals, and trainees. The presenter may emphasize specific areas depending upon the profile of the audience.[2,6] For example, if the audience is composed primarily of healthcare professionals, the presenter may emphasize the clinical implications of the results, rather than provide a detailed description of the methods.[4]

Seminar

While podium presentations are quite specific in their purpose and structure, seminars can have a variety of purposes or structures. The purpose of the seminar and/or the profile of the audience drives its structure, or format. One type of seminar is the **research seminar**, which has the same purpose and structure as a podium presentation but is longer in duration. These presentations are usually 45 to 60 minutes in length with 5 to 15 minutes devoted to either questions or discussion. Research seminars often occur at academic institutions and usually have a smaller number of individuals in the audience than at scientific conferences. Attendees are usually students, postgraduate trainees, and researchers.

Researchers often are asked to present their work to stakeholders with non-science backgrounds or the general public. For this type of seminar, the purpose and structure can be quite different than a podium presentation or research seminar. For example, the purpose of presenting one's work for funding would be to inform and persuade, while the purpose of presenting at a community forum would be to educate. The focus is likely on

TABLE 23–1. TWO DIFFERENT ORAL PRESENTATION RUBRICS

Rubric #1: APhA-ESAS Section Best Post Graduate Paper Award Candidate—Podium

Criterion	Noteworthy Comments and Fatal Flaws
1. Background	
Describes the relationship of problem to a theoretical framework, OR previous research, OR to scientific literature.	
Problem is of vital concern to the profession and makes important contributions to the theoretical basis of pharmaceutical sciences.	
2. Research Questions or Objectives	
Questions to be answered or objectives to be met by research are clearly stated.	
3. Methods	
Evaluate the methods considering all of the following *which are* applicable for the type of research being presented:	
hypothesis, research design, sampling strategy, measurement, data collection or sources of data, analysis plan or other appropriate qualitative methods.	
4. Results	
Findings are reported for each study objective or research question.	
5. Implications and Conclusions	
Implications of and conclusions from findings for practice, policy theory or further research are explored and discussed. Conclusions are appropriately stated based on the results.	
6. Presentation	
Oral presentation of research during podium session. Elements include good pace of delivery, no distracting mannerisms, effective audiovisual presentation, and so on.	

Rubric #2: Midwest Social and Administrative Pharmacy Conference

Presenter Name _____   Faculty Reviewer _____

Presentation Title _____   Total Score/12 _____

	Content	Integration of Knowledge	Style/Delivery	Ability to Answer Questions
Excellent **Points: 3**	• Identifies the research question or work • Previous work sets the stage for this study • Has advanced understanding of the experimental approach • Clearly and correctly states the significance of the study • Critically evaluates results, methodology, and/or conclusions • Scientifically rigorous/well researched	• Integrates research findings to broader context • Understands implication of data or method • Identifies future avenues of investigation • Supports arguments or explanation with references	• Uses time wisely • Logical progression • Speaks with good pacing • Makes eye contact and does not read information • Uses engaging tone	• Anticipates audience questions • Understands audience questions • Can integrate knowledge to answer questions • Thoroughly responds to questions
Good **Points: 2**	• Identifies the research question or work • Has basic understanding of the experimental approach • Clearly and correctly states the significance of the study • Critically evaluates results, methodology, and/or conclusions	• Supports arguments or explanation with references • Minimally integrates research findings to broader context • Has some understanding of the implications of data or method • Identifies some future avenues of investigation	• Spends too much time on introduction • Speaks well, but often back tracks • Makes good eye contact and looks at notes occasionally • Uses good vocabulary and tone	• Does not anticipate audience questions • Understands the audience questions • Can integrate knowledge to answer the question • Thoroughly responds to most questions

(Continued)

Rubric #2: Midwest Social and Administrative Pharmacy Conference

Presenter Name _____

Presentation Title _____

Faculty Reviewer _____

Total Score/12 _____

	Content	Integration of Knowledge	Style/Delivery	Ability to Answer Questions
Adequate **Points: 1**	• Research question a bit unclear • Description of experimental approach a bit confusing • Results and conclusions stated but not critically evaluated • No use of outside readings	• Does not integrate the work or method into the broader context • Supports argument or explanation with few references • Makes some errors in interpretation and application of data or method • Makes few connections between data, method, and conclusions	• Presentation poorly timed • Presentation jumping from different topics • Some hesitation and uncertainty are apparent • Makes little eye contact • Monotone and non-engaging delivery	• Does not anticipate audience questions • Makes an effort to address question • Can address some questions • Overlooks obvious questions • Often responds poorly to questions
Inadequate **Points: 0**	• Does not understand research or work • Does not understand experimental approach • Does not understand conclusions or recognize implications for future work	• Does not integrate the work or method into the broader context • Makes little effort to use data to support arguments • Misinterprets information • Makes no connections between data, method, and conclusions • Lacks logic	• Presentation poorly timed • Jumbled with no logical progression • Makes no eye contact and reads from notes • Hesitation and uncertainty are apparent	• Either makes no effort to respond to questions or does so poorly
Score and Comments				

the application or implications of results, rather than the methods of the project. For these seminars, it is particularly important to ask the organizers their expectations regarding the purpose, structure, and duration. In addition, profiling the audience is essential in the development of the presentation.

In-Service or Workshop

The primary purpose of an in-service or workshop is to instruct or provide education, on a particular topic. Research results may be incorporated as part of the presentation, but the focus will be on how results apply to the audience member's professional work or personal life. Though there may be researchers at this type of presentation, the audience is generally composed of community members, healthcare professionals, postgraduate trainees, or students. It is particularly important to profile the audience and their reason for attending when developing this presentation. For example, if the presentation is on the effectiveness of vaccinations, the speaker would include different content when speaking to the general public, as compared to speaking to healthcare professionals. The general public would expect the speaker to emphasize the impact of vaccination individually and in the community, while healthcare professionals would expect more of an emphasis on the data in specific patient populations or practice settings.

Similar to a seminar, an in-service lasts approximately 30 to 60 minutes with 5 to 15 minutes reserved for questions. Workshops vary in length, but typically last longer than 60 minutes and can even occur over multiple days. Two- to four-hour workshops are commonly a part of healthcare professional conferences. Speakers adopt educational principles when developing these types of presentations since they are usually instructional in nature. Individual or group activities, discussion, and/or polling questions are often incorporated to encourage audience members to engage with the content being presented.

TED-Like Talk

In a TED-like talk, the speaker presents an idea to an audience in 18 minutes or less.[7] This format was popularized by its namesake, TED, which originally began as a conference spanning the fields of technology, entertainment, and design. Since this time, TED-like talks have occurred across the globe and in diverse disciplines. Scientific conferences are no exception, where speakers have been asked to adopt TED-like principles for their presentations. Beyond scientific presentations, this format can work well when presenting to the lay public on a variety of health and science topics. One only needs to look at the TED website (www.ted.com) to see the variety of topics being presented, such as how to defend the earth from asteroids[8] to how to use a paper towel.[9]

At the heart of a TED-like talk is the effective communication of *one* idea.[7] Though no speaker is alike in their approach, there is a structure that TED recommends.[7] First, start with a "relatable example" or "intriguing idea". Second, clearly communicate the idea and provide supporting empirical evidence. Third, conclude by telling the audience how they would be affected if they accepted the idea. Slides can be used, but are not necessary for this type of presentation. Consider the content and whether the slides will assist in communicating the idea. The acronym, KISS, or "keep it short and simple" is an appropriate adage for a TED-like talk.

Elevator Speech or Pitch

Traditionally, the elevator pitch was used as a way for entrepreneurs to "pitch" an idea in a short timeframe, such as when traveling in an elevator.[10] However, other disciplines have adopted the elevator pitch to include additional types of short interactions, such as introducing oneself at a conference, talking to a member of a search committee, or describing an initiative for funding.[11,12] Regardless of the purpose, the elevator pitch is a concise and rehearsed statement lasting from one to five minutes.[11,12] The elements of an elevator pitch are: (1) an opening, or hook, to create attention, (2) a statement of a problem or unmet need, and (3) a closing, which often includes an ask, or request. Ultimately, the goal of the statement is to create a memorable first impression.[10-12]

The pitch should be prepared ahead of time, preferably by writing responses to questions specific to the purpose of the pitch. For example, an elevator pitch regarding research would include: (1) personal introduction, (2) the topic of the research, (3) the question that is being investigated, (4) how the question is being addressed with a focus on how its innovative, (5) the goal or purpose of this conversation, and (6) how to follow-up.[11,12] Writing out the responses allows the speaker to reflect upon and improve them. Rather than memorizing the pitch, use bullet points to encourage natural and conversational delivery.[12] Once the pitch is formulated, it should be practiced in front of peers and mentors.[11,12]

Employment Interview Presentation

Depending upon the position, employers may include a formal presentation as part of the interview process. The employment interview presentation gives the employer an opportunity to not only evaluate a candidate's presentation skills but also their ability to conduct research and provide educational content. Employers will dictate what type of presentation the prospective candidate will provide. In some cases, a candidate may be asked to deliver two different presentations: one focused on research and another focused on instructing on a topic either of the candidate's choosing or specified by the employer. Presentations usually last 45 to 60 minutes with 5 to 15 minutes of that time dedicated to questions from the audience. If asked to provide two different types of presentations, they often are shorter in duration, approximately 30 minutes with five minutes of that time for questions. These types of presentations are commonly recorded and shared with employees who were unable to attend.

Part elevator pitch and part seminar, the employment interview presentation incorporates different aspects of the presentation types already discussed. However, the very nature of an interview is an elevator pitch. Candidates are making a "pitch" that they are the best fit for the position. Prospective candidates should have an elevator pitch ready when introducing themselves. Candidates may be interviewing with other employees individually, but there are some institutions that will have candidates meet with small groups of employees. Because candidates may not have an opportunity to meet with all employees during the interview process, candidates should include an overview of their work and how it fits within the institution as part of their formal presentation.

PROFILE THE AUDIENCE

The next step is to profile the audience. Identifying who will be attending the presentation will assist in the development of the presentations.[2,6] Some questions to answer about the audience include: (1) Who are they? (2) What do they know? (3) What are their expectations and preferences? and (4) How do they feel about the topic?[6] Mentors and collaborators should be consulted when answering these questions, as they likely have presented to similar audiences in the past. See Table 23–2 for guidance when profiling the audience.

Who Are They?

The primary audience are those who are directly receiving the content of the presentation.[6] They may be peers, healthcare professionals, researchers, prospective employers, or the general public. In many cases, there may be individuals from all these groups attending a presentation. For example, audience members at a scientific presentation at a pharmacy association conference will likely include peers, researchers, healthcare professionals, and prospective employers. For some presentations, there may be a secondary audience, in which individuals receive information from the presentation indirectly.[6] These individuals may hear a summary of, or messages from, the presentation through those that attended.

What Do They Know?

The background of the audience members will help determine how much they know about the topic being presented. Thinking through how much the audience members know will influence the terminology used, the background information necessary to provide context, and the explanation needed for audience understanding. In many cases, the speaker will be the most knowledgeable person in the room. Scientists and healthcare professionals grounded in the topic of the presentation will need less context and explanation than a lay audience. In the case of trainees, knowledge will likely be somewhere between researchers/healthcare professionals and the lay public. In some cases, the

TABLE 23–2. CHARACTERISTICS AND EXPECTATIONS OF THE AUDIENCE

Who Are They?	What Do They Know?	What Are Their Expectations and Preferences?	How Do They Feel About the Topic?
General public	• Likely limited background knowledge • Unfamiliar with scientific terms and abbreviations	• Relate how a topic relates to society or them as individuals • Use of lay language • Define all terms and abbreviations	Likely some level of interest because they chose to attend presentation
Peers	• Variable depending upon where the peer is in their educational process • Some background knowledge • Some familiarity with scientific terms and abbreviations	• Discuss how research or topic fits within context of current knowledge • Define all terms and abbreviations • Relate how a topic relates to them as individuals or their work	Varies based on whether this was an independent decision to attend presentation or required for a class
Healthcare professionals	• Some background knowledge • Some familiarity with scientific terms and abbreviations	• Discuss how research or topic fits within context of current knowledge • Provide how research or topic has implications for or applies to practice	Interested
Researchers	• Some background knowledge • Familiar with scientific terms and abbreviations	• Discuss how research fits within context of current knowledge • Focus on methods, results, and discussion sections of project • Provide how research has implications for future work	Interested
Prospective employers	• Variable depending upon on the employee classification of audience members	• Focus on fit with institution and department • Highlight knowledge and skills needed to be successful in position	May not be interested in topic, but interested in presentation skills and skills needed or position (teaching and/or research)

audience will be mixed and have different levels of understanding of the topic. For these situations, develop the presentation at a level slightly below the background of an average audience member.[2]

What Are Their Expectations and Preferences?

Audiences have expectations for the format and style of the presentation. Preferences can vary culturally and by discipline. The venue, type, or location of the presentation can provide insight into expectations and parameters for the presentation. For example, as described earlier, there are accepted practices and procedures for presenting at scientific conferences.

How Do They Feel about the Topic?

It is easier to speak to and engage an audience who is interested in a topic. If the purpose or goal of the presentation is not of particular interest to the audience, the speaker should consider how to increase the audience's motivation to care.[6] If the topic or research findings are controversial, the speaker should be prepared for the audience's reactions, as well as the questions they may ask. When presenting on controversial topics, speakers should remember that audience members' reactions and questions are a result of them being placed outside of their comfort zone and generally are not personal in nature.

DECIDE AUTHORSHIP OF THE PRESENTATION

In the academic or research realm, especially for podium presentations at scientific conferences, the speaker often is not the only "author" of a presentation. Authorship refers not only to who should receive credit for the work but also denotes who is accountable and responsible for the conduct of the research. Ideally, authorship and the order in which authors are listed should be discussed among collaborators at the initiation of the research. The order of authors relates to their level of involvement in the project. Each discipline has generally accepted practices regarding authorship, but the first author typically has the most involvement and leads the research endeavor.

There are occasions, however, when the discussion does not take place until it is time to submit an abstract or a manuscript for publication. In the case of presentations, the presenter does not have to be the first author, but should be a part of the research collaboration. There are guidance documents from a variety of organizations to help determine and negotiate authorship based on the role of each author. Two examples include resources from the International Committee of Medical Journal Editors (http://www.icmje.org/recommendations/browse/roles-and-responsibilities/defining-the-role-of-authors-and-contributors.html) and the American Psychological Association (APA) Science Student Council (https://www.apa.org/science/about/psa/2015/06/determining-authorship). Of note, the APA site includes a variety of checklists, worksheets, and agreement forms to facilitate discussion and decision making. Authorship can change during the research process, however, as a rule, decisions regarding authorship and their order should be completed before submitting abstracts to be considered for presentation.

Preparing the Presentation Materials

When faced with preparing a presentation, it is easy to lose sight that this is a learning activity for those watching in the audience. In essence, an effective presenter not only provides information, but also helps others integrate this new information into their current knowledge. Using adult learning theory can help presenters in the preparation of their material in order to maximize the impact of the content. According to Mayer's cognitive theory of multimedia learning, there are three assumptions on how individuals process information. When attending a presentation, individuals: (1) process visual and auditory information using separate channels, (2) have limits to the amount of information they can process at a time, and (3) are more likely to remember information when actively engaged with the material.[13,14] Based on this theory, presenters should use visuals to enhance their presentation, refrain from including extraneous information, and create opportunities for the audience to engage with the material being presented. These principles may be adapted depending upon the purpose of the presentation. For example, there will be less opportunities for the audience to engage with the material in a time-constrained podium presentation as opposed to a seminar.

Further, people are more likely to learn from a presentation when: (1) they find the information relevant or beneficial personally or professionally, (2) the purpose of the presentation is clear, (3) the content matches their needs, (4) they are actively involved, (5) effective visual aids are provided, and (6) it is enjoyable.[1] These assumptions can be used as a guide to preparing materials. The following sections outline best practices in preparing and delivering presentations.

AUDIENCE RESPONSE SYSTEMS

Individuals will be more likely to remember information from the presentation when actively engaged with the material. One way in which to engage the audience is to embed questions or polls into the presentation and allow audience members to respond using an audience response system. There are a wide variety of systems available with varying levels of functionality and price points. Commonly used systems include: Kahoot! (www.kahoot.com/), Pigeonhole (www.pigeonholelive.com/), Poll Everywhere (www.polleverywhere.com/), Slido (www.sli.do/), Turning (www.turning.com/), and Vevox (www.vevox.com/). Many of the systems have a free version or trial period, but there is often a cost associated based on the number of users or for the use of more advanced features. Check with the event organizer to see if they plan to use or have a subscription to an audience response system. Some academic institutions have contracts with companies allowing the use of the system by their faculty and students. If looking for specific features of audience response systems and pricing, Capterra provides product reviews, outlines features for audience response systems, and includes a filter to identify specific system features (www.capterra.com/audience-response-software/).

PRESENTATION SOFTWARE PROGRAMS

In many cases, the presentation software will be dictated by the event organizer rather than chosen by the presenter. However, there are a wide variety of options available to presenters, such as Microsoft PowerPoint (www.microsoft.com/en-us/microsoft-365/powerpoint), Prezi (www.prezi.com), Visme (www.visme.co), Keynote (www.apple.com/keynote/), and Google Slides (www.google.com/slides/about/).[15] If given an option to choose, the presenter should consider the software program's ease of use, the ability for others to collaborate, device compatibility, cost, availability of templates, graphics, or animation, and the ability to embed audio or video.[15] Widely available at academic institutions, PowerPoint is used extensively for presentations of all types. As a result, the following tips for preparing visual materials will be based on using PowerPoint as the software program. However, many of the recommendations are applicable to other software programs. If unfamiliar with presentation software, Wilson and Schwartz have prepared a guide with step-by-step instructions on using PowerPoint, Prezi, and Keynote.[16]

VISUAL MATERIALS

For most oral presentation formats, the speaker is providing an elevated version of "show and tell" or sharing a story using visuals (e.g., slides). The visual materials should be designed to support the story of the presentation regardless of type. Presenters may be advised by the mantra "less is more" both visually and for the number of slides, but it can be difficult to follow when preparing materials. A general rule of thumb is to only include one slide per minute of time allotted.[17-19] If the presentation is 20 minutes, there should be approximately 15 slides, leaving five minutes for questions. This number may vary depending on the structure of the presentation. For example, a slide that is used to create a transition between sections typically will not take 60 seconds to discuss. Staying within the time allotted is critically important. Practicing the presentation helps with timing and is discussed later in this chapter.

Depending on the venue, the background and format of the slides may be provided, which may feel limiting when creating materials. Even when the slide design is predetermined, the speaker can still follow many of the "best" practices for designing visual materials (see Table 23–3). One rule that presenters should always follow is to never show a slide for which they feel they have to apologize.[1] Examples of common mistakes made by presenters include apologizing for figures or tables that are too small, images that are

TABLE 23-3. BEST PRACTICES FOR PRESENTATION OF VISUAL MATERIALS

CONTENT	SLIDE CHARACTERISTICS	FONT
☐ Utilize the eight-second rule—the audience should be able to read text within 8 seconds	☐ Choose simple background	☐ Use only one type of font
	☐ Choose colors that create a contrast between text and background	☐ Choose sans serif fonts, such as Arial, Calibri, and Helvetica
☐ Include three-five items per slide		
○ Utilize short sentences or phrases	○ Dark room: Background dark with lighter text	☐ Use upper and lower case lettering
○ Use active verbs		
○ Create parallelism with text on slide	○ Light room: Background light and darker text	☐ Consider room characteristics when choosing font size
☐ Use visuals and graphics	○ Background and test should be far apart on color wheel	○ Use 32 point or larger for header
○ Place images on left slide of slide to facilitate audience comprehension	☐ Emphasize points using italic or bold fonts	○ Use 28 point or larger for text in the body, if possible
○ Utilize real photos over clip art if possible		
○ Ensure all graphics and charts are labeled appropriately		○ Use 12-14 points for references
☐ Use animations only when emphasizing a point		○ Avoid font sizes smaller than 20 point for text in the body
☐ Create sections for transitions		
☐ Create approximately one slide for every minute of presentation		☐ Avoid red and green font for text to accommodate those with color blindness
☐ Avoid abbreviations		
☐ Check spelling		

Note: See References 5,13,19,21,23,24.

blurry, errors in spelling or content, and excessive content on a slide. As a fail-safe, the slides should be accessible by the presenter from multiple places, including a flash drive, cloud storage, and the presenter's email, almost guaranteeing that the slides will be available when needed.[17]

Presentations typically start with an opening slide. This slide should include the title, name of the speaker, name(s) of collaborators, and date of presentation. During this slide, the speaker usually thanks the audience for attending and/or the conference sponsors for the invitation.[17] Collaborators often are acknowledged as a part of these slides, but they also can be thanked at the end of the presentation.[17] Depending up on the type of presentation, the next slide will either include the learning objectives (for educational presentations) or an overview of the content of the presentation. In many cases, both slides are included so the content of the presentation often does not start until the fourth slide. Refer to the *Determine the Presentation Type* section of this chapter when considering the content to be included in visual materials. Once the general introductory slides are completed, then the presenter can start developing the slides to support the story they are telling.

The key to telling a story is a logical order of supporting materials, which should include a beginning, middle, and end.[20] The body of each slide should include short clusters of information, no more than three to five items per slide, enabling the audience to read the text of the slide in eight seconds or less.[18,19] When there is a choice, presenters should use relevant images and graphics or charts, as opposed to text or numbers.[18] Tables prepared for, or copied from, publications are typically not optimal for oral presentations.[1] Animations can be used, but should be reserved to emphasize or highlight specific points. If the presentation lasts longer than 20 to 30 minutes, breaks or activities should be incorporated in the presentation every 15 to 20 minutes.[18] A blank slide, or one with a discussion question or audience activity, can be used to break up the presentation and promote audience interaction.[18] The speaker should conclude the presentation with the three main points, or takeaways. Many presenters also include a concluding slide specifically inviting the audience to ask questions.[17,20]

If there is flexibility in the design of materials, the assertion evidence approach is a design method that can be used for the bulk of the presentation content. This approach encourages better comprehension and recall by the audience, as well as a deeper understanding of content by the presenter.[19,21] With this approach, the header in the slide is a complete statement, left-justified, and two lines or less. The headline should be 32 point or larger. The body of the slide, which is mostly images with limited text, provides evidence to support the headline. Images and the text should be relevant and directly relate to the statement. If interested in using this approach, Michael Alley, an engineering faculty member, provides example presentations and slide templates on his website.[21]

Practicing and Delivering the Presentation

One of the goals at the beginning of the presentation is to establish a connection with the audience.[19] There are several ways a speaker can do this by how they craft the beginning of their presentation. One way is to create an enticing title for the presentation. For example, *Embracing the Habit: A Prescription for Study Skills* likely sounds more interesting to the audience than *Developing Student Pharmacists' Study Skills* or *Impact of a Workshop on Student Pharmacists' Study Skills*. Another way is for the speaker to share a bit of their background in their opening slides, such as the logo of the institution where they work, or images of them with their students or research team (as long as they have received permission from those individuals).[17]

Typically, a speaker will start the presentation with a personal or professional anecdote on why they are interested in the presentation topic or conducted the research project. For the example provided in the above paragraph, the speaker could relate a conversation they had with a student who was struggling in a course. The next step is to relay to the audience on why they should be interested too.[22,23] When a speaker outlines the "so what" of the presentation, it helps to create the connection to why both the speaker and the audience member are both participating.[24] What is the audience going to learn from the presentation and how does it apply to their lives or work? Why should the audience consider the topic or project important? In this hypothetical audience of professors, outline how they will be able to help their students by listening to the presentation. In addition, some speakers use humor to keep the audience engaged. Before using humor, the presenter should consider if they are comfortable in using it in their daily lives, as well as if it is appropriate for the audience, or venue. If humor is not something they regularly use in their conversations, then they should not use it during a presentation.

VERBAL COMMUNICATION

One of the keys of a successful presentation is to remember that it is a conversation with the audience.[22] The presenter is "telling" a story to the audience, and not "talking" at the audience. The ability to convey enthusiasm or passion about a topic can immediately create a connection with the audience and help them to understand why it is important to listen. Reading the slides does not convey enthusiasm or create a connection.[20,23] In fact, it encourages the audience to engage in other activities, such as looking at their phone. Instead, the speaker can use their voice to convey enthusiasm through inflection and volume. Using a high or low inflection at the end of a sentence, however, should be avoided as it can indicate inexperience or nervousness to the audience.[25] Presenters should speak from the diaphragm rather than the throat because it conveys authority and creates resonance in the voice.[23] Silence also can be used to communicate meaning, as it is a powerful tool to establish the importance of what was said and allows the audience to reflect upon it.

Though a presentation should be conversational, it is not informal. In preparing the presentation, the presenter should consider their natural speaking patterns and habits, such as their rate of speech, enunciation, and word choice. As discussed earlier in this chapter, profiling the audience can help to guide the language used in the presentation. Unfamiliar terms should be defined for the audience. In addition, the speaker should check on the pronunciation of words to ensure they are said correctly. Websites, such as Macmillan Dictionary (https://www.macmillandictionary.com/us/pronunciation/american/medical_1), Merriam Webster Dictionary (https://www.merriam-webster.com/browse/medical/a), and Merck Manual (https://www.merckmanuals.com/home/pronunciations), provide audio pronunciations that speakers can use to practice. Speakers often feel nervous when they first start making presentations. When nervous, the natural inclination is to talk fast, which may affect the enunciation of words and understanding by the audience.[23] Additionally, speakers should avoid using slang or informal language (e.g., gonna instead of going to) or filler words (um, like, uh). Vocal delivery can be refined through preparation and practice, which is covered later in this chapter.

Notes may help a speaker feel more secure in presenting, however, they should be used cautiously because they increase the likelihood of a presentation being read to the audience. If using notes, do not write in complete sentences, but instead use bullet points. Bullet points facilitate the speaker's memory of what is to be said, but discourage reading. Notes can be inputted into the presentation software, or a paper copy can be used. However, when deciding on using notes, the presenter should consider that printed notes often are distracting both to the presenter and the audience.

NONVERBAL COMMUNICATION

Nonverbal communication, such as posture, facial expressions, or eye contact, is just as important as visual materials and vocal delivery. From nonverbal communication, the audience can interpret the speaker's confidence, as well as a passion for the topic, without a word being spoken. If seated in the audience prior to the presentation, the speaker should walk energetically to the podium.[23] Standing tall with chest uplifted projects confidence and assists with breathing and speaking.[23] Start the presentation with a smile. It helps to reduce stress in the speaker and create a connection with the audience.[23] Eye contact also is effective in creating a connection. Looking at different places in the room helps to make eye contact with as many audience members as possible. One approach is envisioning a square within the room to provide a guide for eye contact: look forward, then to the right side of the room, then to the left side of the room, then to the back of the room, then back to starting place.[22] Repeat this process throughout the presentation. In addition, the focus should be on the audience and the speaker should avoid looking back at the screen or stare solely at the computer screen.[23]

Laser pointers should be used cautiously. If it is not necessary, avoid using one. Often, when a speaker is nervous, the laser pointer will shake because the speaker's hands are shaking. In addition, the button can be pushed unintentionally with the light hovering at different places in the room, such as a wall or ceiling, creating a distraction for the audience. However, a laser pointer should be used in instances where it helps in the description of an image or chart. When using a laser pointer, avoid "twirling" the light in circles on the screen.[25]

RESPONDING TO QUESTIONS

Audience questions can feel intimidating to a speaker; however, questions show that the audience listened and is interested in the content. First, the speaker should listen carefully to the question and what is being asked. Second, the speaker should thank the audience member for the question. Third, the question should be repeated or paraphrased to ensure the audience heard the question and the speaker interpreted it correctly. If unsure of what the audience member is asking, the presenter can ask to have it restated or rephrased. After a brief pause, the presenter should answer the question concisely.[16,17] The response should be specific to the question asked and not an elaborate explanation of what all is known about the presentation topic. When uncertain on how to respond to a question, the presenter can say, "This is an interesting question. Let me give it some thought and get back to you" or "This is an interesting question and something I will consider in moving the work forward." The presenter can offer to follow up with the audience member after the presentation for further discussion or contact information.[16,17] If possible, the presenter should ask a colleague to write down the questions.[17]

DRESSING FOR SUCCESS

There are generally unspoken expectations regarding the presenter's apparel.[22] When presenting, the speaker wants the audience to focus on their message and not their clothing. A general recommendation is for a speaker to wear clothing that does not call attention to themselves, allowing the audience to focus on the presentation. At a minimum, the speaker should be dressed better than those sitting in the audience. A suit is often the best choice for presentations at a national conference or venue. Women have a little more flexibility than men in their options, but they should choose clothing that is considered equivalent to a suit. Regardless of choice, the speaker should wear clothing that makes them feel good. Clothing that is not comfortable and does not fit well will be distracting while delivering the presentation for both the speaker and the audience. Just like clothing, shoes should be comfortable, yet professional. Shoes should also "match" the formalness of the clothing. For example, casual shoes with a formal suit can inadvertently make an audience focus on the speaker's feet rather than the presentation. A speaker should consult with their mentors and collaborators on clothing selection as they often have prior experience delivering different types of presentations and at a variety of venues.

ADJUSTING THE PRESENTATION BASED ON FORMAT

Most of this chapter is focused on in-person presentations, rather than those occurring remotely. The best practices outlined for in-person presentations also can be used for those that take place online. However, the speaker has some additional components to consider when preparing materials and delivering the presentation. First, interactive activities are going to be particularly important to keep attendees' attention. Many of the online platforms have a variety of features, including polling, whiteboards, chat, raised hands, and breakout rooms, allowing interaction during synchronous presentations.[26,27] While it can be more difficult to engage a viewer when the presentation is asynchronous, using questions to provoke thought on a topic or creating activities can help keep individuals' attention as they watch the presentation. Answers can be provided in a supplementary document or discussed later in the presentation.

Due to the nature of the presentation being online, there are additional best practices that should be utilized.[28] First, a speaker should include a picture of themselves early in the presentation, especially when not using a camera. If using a camera, ensure that the lighting and background environment is appropriate.[29] Eye contact can be challenging, as the speaker will need to direct their eyes to the camera rather than the slides or attendees.[28] Consider creating a space that encourages direct eye contact, as well as have another person monitor the chat, if possible, for synchronous presentations. Audio quality is particularly important for an online presentation, so the speaker should turn off their phones, use headphones, and minimize any other distractions or noises (e.g., pets).[28] Visual materials also should be adjusted for an online format. Tips include increasing the number and variety of slides, as well as highlight the areas on the slide where attendees should focus. When developing the visual materials, the speaker should consider that individuals could be watching the presentation on their phone rather than a tablet or computer.[26] Presenting online is becoming more commonplace. If presenting online, seek resources and guidance specific to this presentation format.[26–29]

PRACTICING THE PRESENTATION

One of the keys to a successful presentation is to practice giving the presentation multiple times. One of the mistakes presenters make is mentally reviewing what they are going to say rather than practicing the presentation aloud. Saying the words aloud helps the presenter to determine and modify the content and its phrasing. If this is not done, a presenter runs the risk of stumbling or stuttering over their words when the time for the presentation comes. Initially, a presenter may find it helpful to practice in front of the mirror.[19,22] In addition, videotaping practice sessions and reviewing them can help a speaker identify nonverbal and verbal characteristics in which they would like to improve.[20] It also is best to practice the presentation with a microphone, if possible, and a simulated audience, such as family members, friends, peers, and collaborators.[19] However, a presenter is more likely to receive constructive and actionable feedback when practicing the presentation with a mentor who has experience with the type of presentation being delivered. As a part of the practice sessions, the speaker should time the presentation to ensure that they will complete the presentation in the time allotted.

COMBATTING PUBLIC-SPEAKING ANXIETY

It is normal to have anxiety or be nervous presenting. In fact, fear of public speaking is a commonly cited activity as causing anxiety.[30] Fortunately, there are a variety of ways to reduce the anxiety associated with speaking in front of group individuals. First, practicing the presentation in front of others allows a presenter to simulate the experience in a more comfortable setting. Peers and mentors can provide feedback to improve the presentation, as well as prepare the speaker for potential questions from the audience.

When individuals are nervous, such as in the case of public speaking, breathing becomes shallow. Shallow breathing can affect multiple areas in the delivery of the presentation, such as breathlessness while speaking. To combat anxiety, diaphragmatic breathing, sometimes referred to as belly breathing, can be utilized.[22] This breathing technique can be used anytime one is feeling nervous, but it is especially helpful for a speaker to use it while waiting in the audience for their turn to present. First, the speaker should be sitting comfortably with the knees bent and feet on the floor. The head, neck, and shoulders should be relaxed. One hand is placed on the upper chest and the other is placed below the ribcage. As the speaker breathes in slowly through the nose, the stomach should be moving the hand out from the rib cage. The stomach muscles are then tightened on the exhalation through pursed lips. The hand on the stomach should fall inward as the muscles tighten. The hand on the chest should not move during either inhalation or exhalation. See Cleveland Clinic in the Online Resources section for detailed steps and images on diaphragmatic breathing.

Another technique is progressive muscle relaxation, where the speaker would tighten or tense a muscle group, hold the tension, and then release or relax the muscle.[22] In general, this technique starts with tightening the feet first and then moves through the muscle groups upward through the body. As with diaphragmatic breathing, this can be done while sitting in the audience, or anytime when one is feeling anxious. For visual examples or audio guidance, there are multiple infographics and videos demonstrating these techniques online.

Visualization also can be effective in combating public speaking anxiety.[22,23] For visualization, the speaker usually closes their eyes and imagines the presentation. They see themselves delivering the message effectively and answering questions without hesitation. They can "see" the audience and "hear" the applause or the laughter from a joke. They can imagine the positive feelings after the presentation is over. Affirmations and positive self-talk also can help.[2,22,23] The speaker can tell themselves that they will appear confident, do well, and be able to answer questions.

All of these techniques are meant to ease anxiety and improve the confidence of the speaker. The key is for the speaker to try these techniques to see what works for them. Imagining the worst or using negative self-talk will derail these confidence-building techniques and can make one more anxious. If the visualization ends up being about all the disasters that could happen, do not use it. The speaker should select another technique instead. Speakers should discuss their anxiety with their mentors, who can assuage concerns and provide some perspective. In most speaking situations, it is helpful to remember the audience is there by choice and wants to hear what the speaker has to say. For scientific podium presentations, most members in the audience will know that the speaker is a trainee and want to be supportive and help the speaker have a positive experience.

DAY OF PRESENTATION TIPS

On the day of the presentation, arrive at the presentation site early and review the equipment provided. If audio or video is a part of the presentation, check the software and speakers to make sure they are functioning as expected. In addition, the presenter should prepare themselves physically for the presentation, including getting plenty of rest the night before the presentation, eating a healthy meal on the day of the presentation, going to the restroom just prior to the presentation, and having lukewarm water available during the presentation. Plan for clothing the evening before the presentation also helps decrease stress. Prior to the day of the presentation, ask a peer or colleague to attend and be a timekeeper. Arrange for a signal at specific points during the presentation, such as when there are five minutes of time remaining. In many situations, handouts will be available online, but consider the venue and audience in determining if handouts are necessary. Finally, the presenter should have their business cards in the case that an audience member would like to contact them at a later time.

Exemplar of an Oral Presentation by a Learner

Jaclyn, a PhD student who worked with the chapter author, was interested in medication counseling provision in community pharmacy settings. She conducted a qualitative study of pharmacists to explore their perceptions and decision making regarding the provision of medication counseling and communication with patients. She wanted to prepare an abstract to submit to the American Pharmacists Association (APhA) Annual Meeting which typically occurs during March with an abstract deadline of early October. She conducted her interviews with pharmacists during the spring semester. When she and her collaborators started coding data, they quickly realized that analyzing qualitative results is time-intensive and often takes longer than quantitative analysis. The abstract process was stressful because of the short timeline between the completion of the analysis and abstract submission. Jaclyn's first lesson learned was to consider the timeline when planning research and how it fits within the typical abstract deadlines of national conferences.

Jaclyn's abstract was accepted for a podium presentation at the APhA meeting.[31] She was excited about the opportunity to present her work. However, she felt challenged to create her presentation within the restrictions provided by the organization. First, continuing education credit was being provided for this conference session, which required her to develop learning objectives and self-assessment questions beyond her study's specific aims. It was difficult for her to think about the presentation from a learning framework versus a research one. Second, the presentation needed to be reviewed by the conference organizers in order to determine that all continuing education requirements were met. As a result, her presentation slides had to be submitted much earlier than the conference date. Third, the organization provided a PowerPoint template that had to be used for her presentation. She felt her creativity was limited by the template, though she was able to make small adjustments to align with the best practices provided in Table 23–3. These adjustments included: (1) increasing the font size provided in the template, (2) the use of smart art in presenting the theoretical foundation of the study and results, (3) limiting the amount of text on a slide, and (4) utilizing high contrast colors. These changes were made with the goal to make the presentation materials visually appealing and ensure audience members could easily view the slides from any place in the conference room. Jaclyn's second lesson was that adjustments can be made while still following conference guidelines.

An additional challenge Jaclyn faced was presenting a comprehensive review of her project in the 15 minutes she was allotted. Qualitative results are grounded on "text-based" data, which can make it difficult to present concisely. In addition, many projects, such as this one, were based on a theoretical foundation, which often can be complex to explain in a short timeframe. She had to carefully consider what information was essential to understand her project, as well as highlight the key findings from the data. From her perspective, there were many takeaways from the project, but she knew she needed to make the most of her 15 minutes. It was essential for her to identify the findings that she felt would be the most relevant practice of pharmacy, as well as interesting to the audience. She realized she should practice the presentation as she was developing the materials, especially since she had to submit the material well ahead of the conference date. The practice sessions assisted her in determining what should be included in the presentation based on feedback from her peers and mentor. By practicing the presentation while developing the materials, it enabled her to present successfully and confidently within the time allotted. Jaclyn's third lesson was that practice is essential to feeling confident when presenting at a national conference.

Summary and Conclusions

Presenting in front of an audience can feel overwhelming, especially at the national and international levels. The keys to a successful presentation are preparation and practice. Mentors should be consulted in every step of the process, as they can be quite valuable in guiding a speaker on the expectations of the audience and the sponsor, as well as the format of the presentation. When preparing the presentation, it can be helpful for the speaker to remember that they are just telling a story, usually one that they know better than any other person. Using the best practices outlined in this chapter is the first step to successfully storytelling. Creating a visually appealing presentation with audience engagement can be a quite satisfying part of one's career and provide opportunities for future collaborations.

Key Points and Advice

- Presentations are a form of storytelling.
- Rely on mentors and collaborators when developing the presentation.
- Know the audience and consider their characteristics when developing the presentation.
- Visual materials should support the story, but not be the story.
- Audience questions can feel intimidating, but actually are signs of an interesting presentation.
- Preparation is key to a successful presentation.
- Practice the presentation for a mentor prior to the time it is scheduled.
- Remember to breathe when delivering the presentation.
- Deliver the presentation within the allotted time.

Chapter Review Questions

1. How are podium presentations a form of storytelling?
2. What are the characteristics of the different types of presentation?
3. What are some approaches that increase the interest of, and engagement with, the audience?
4. What are the best practices for visual materials for a scientific podium presentation?
5. How should a speaker prepare for giving a presentation at a national conference?

Online Resources

- Audience Response Software. www.capterra.com/audience-response-software/
- Northeastern University: Elevator Pitch Examples. https://onlinebusiness.northeastern.edu/master-of-business-administration-mba/knowledge/elevator-pitch-guide/pitch-examples/
- Chris Anderson on TED's secret to great public speaking. https://www.ted.com/talks/chris_anderson_ted_s_secret_to_great_public_speaking
- Joe Kowan on how to beat stage fright. https://www.ted.com/talks/joe_kowan_how_i_beat_stage_fright
- Cleveland Clinic on Diaphragmatic Breathing. https://my.clevelandclinic.org/health/articles/9445-diaphragmatic-breathing
- Assertion Evidence Approach to Presentations. https://www.assertion-evidence.com/
- Nancy Duarte on The Secret Structure of Great Talks. https://www.ted.com/talks/nancy_duarte_the_secret_structure_of_great_talks#t-1077376
- Asynchronous and Synchronous Webinars: eLearning Learning. https://www.elearning-learning.com/asynchronous/presentation/

REFERENCES

1. Balistreri WF. Giving an effective presentation. *J Pediatr Gastroenterol Nutr.* 2002;35(1):1-4.
2. McConnell CR. Effective oral presentations: speaking before groups as part of your job. *Health Care Manag.* 2009;28(3):264-272.
3. Rogers B. Research presentations. *AAOHN Journal.* 1990;38(4):191-92.
4. Miracle VA, King KC. Presenting research: effective paper presentations and impressive poster presentations. *Appl Nurs Res.* 1994;7(3):147-57.
5. Goldbort R. Professional scientific presentations. *J Environ Health.* 2002;64(8):29-31.
6. O'Rourke JO IV *The Truth about Confident Presenting.* New York, NY: Anthem Press; 2019.
7. TED: TEDx Speaker Guide. Accessed January 19, 2021. http://storage.ted.com/tedx/manuals/tedxspeakerguide.pdf
8. Plait P. How to defend Earth from asteroids. Accessed August 17, 2021. https://www.ted.com/talks/phil_plait_how_to_defend_earth_from_asteroids
9. Smith J. How to use a paper towel. Accessed August 17, 2021. https://www.ted.com/talks/joe_smith_how_to_use_a_paper_towel
10. McCollough BA, Devezer B, Tanner G. An alternative format for the elevator pitch. *Entrepreneurship and Innov.* 2016;17(1):55-64.
11. Dzara K. Going up? Tips for the medical educator's "elevator pitch." *Acad Med.* 2018; 93:1884.
12. Gaffey A. American Psychological Association Science Student Council: The elevator pitch. Accessed January 19, 2021. https://www.apa.org/science/about/psa/2014/06/elevator-pitch

13. Mayer RE. *Multimedia Learning.* 2nd ed. Cambridge, England: Cambridge University Press; 2009.
14. Davis G, Norman M. Principles of Multimedia Learning. Accessed January 19, 2021. https://ctl.wiley.com/principles-of-multimedia-learning/
15. Velarde O. 15 Best Presentation Software for 2021 (Full Comparison Guide). Accessed February 7, 2021. https://visme.co/blog/best-presentation-software/#visme
16. Wilson JH, Schwartz BM. *An EasyGuide to Research Presentations.* Thousand Oaks, CA: SAGE Publications; 2015.
17. Hartigan L, Mone F, Higgins M. How to prepare and deliver and effective oral presentation. *BMJ.* 2014;348:g2039.
18. Michelfelder A. Using Neuropsychology for Effective PowerPoint Presentations. STEM Annual Conference, New Orleans, 2011. Accessed January 19, 2021. https://slideplayer.com/slide/13141416/
19. Wood TJ, Hollier A. Punch up your podium presentations. *J Am Acad Nurse Pract.* 2017;29:470-74.
20. Bourne PE. Ten simple rules for making good oral presentations. *PLoS Comp Biol.* 2007;3(4):e77.
21. Alley M. Assertion-Evidence talks are comprehended better by audiences and project more confidence from speakers. Accessed March 16, 2021. https://www.assertion-evidence.com/
22. Harolds JA. Tips for giving a memorable presentation: Part V. *Clin Nucl Med.* 2012;37(11):1094-1096.
23. Larkin M. How to give a dynamic scientific presentation. Accessed March 23, 2021. https://www.elsevier.com/connect/how-to-give-a-dynamic-scientific-presentation
24. Nosanchuk JD. Effective presentation in medical education and research. Accessed January 3, 2021. http://blogs.einsteinmed.org/effective-presentation-in-medical-education-and-research/
25. Mayer K. Fundamentals of surgical research course: research presentations. *J Surg Res.* 2005;128:174-77.
26. Topor DR, Budson AE. Twelve tips to present an effective webinar. *Med Teach.* 2020;42(11):1216-20.
27. Zoumenou V, Sigman-Grant M, Coleman G, et al. Identifying best practices for an interactive webinar. *J Fam Consum Scien.* 2015;107(2):62-69.
28. Miller O. 18 tips on how to conduct an engaging webinar. Accessed January 21, 2021. https://speakingaboutpresenting.com/presentation-skills/how-to-conduct-engaging-webinar/
29. Clark D. How to give a webinar presentation. Accessed January 15, 2021. https://hbr.org/2018/06/how-to-give-a-webinar-presentation
30. Pull CB. Current status of knowledge on public-speaking anxiety. *Curr Opin Psych.* 2012;25(1):32-38.
31. Myer JR, Rodino A, Plake KS. Cash register counseling: A qualitative study of pharmacists' perspectives on communication across the counter. American Pharmacists Association Annual Meeting, Baltimore, MD, 2016.

Chapter Twenty-Four

Research Manuscripts

Jordan R. Covvey, PharmD, PhD, BCPS and Spencer E. Harpe, PharmD, PhD, MPH, FAPhA

Chapter Objectives

- Describe the format of a typical research manuscript (IMRAD)
- Identify available tools and guidelines for reporting practice-based research in pharmacy
- Describe different types of articles in the practice-based research literature
- Identify the key issues in preparing and writing a practice-based research manuscript
- Discuss ethical issues in writing and publishing research manuscripts
- Describe the process of submitting a manuscript
- Describe the process of selecting a target journal for publication, including open access options
- Describe citation and referencing processes for practice-based research manuscripts
- Describe key considerations in the writing of research manuscripts
- Describe an example of a learner-involved research manuscript

Key Terminology

Abstract, acknowledgment, article processing charges, author-date referencing style, case report, conflicts of interest, corresponding author, cover letter, duplicate publication, duplicate submission, first author, ghostwriting, guest authorship, IMRAD model, keywords, least publishable unit, numerical referencing style, open access publishing, original research article, plagiarize, preprint, redundant publication, review article, salami slicing, secondary publication, senior author, supplemental materials, text recycling, title page

Introduction

Regardless of career stage, authors often ask themselves what makes a good research paper. Some may say that good papers, like beauty, are in the eye of the beholder, or reader in this case. Although there is certainly a wide range of opinions on what makes a good paper, there are a handful of criteria that most would agree are important. In general, good papers make the reader wonder, "Why didn't I think of that?" A good paper focuses on topics that are important, interesting, contemporary, and relevant to the target audience. From a writing standpoint, the paper is crafted such that the title and the abstract draw readers in and make them want to continue reading, contains a clear presentation of data, and presents a compelling discussion. All of these elements are underpinned by the presence of clearly stated aims or objectives and the use of appropriate methods. It is also important to note the role of the target audience based on a journal's scope and readership since what may be a good paper for one journal may not be good for another journal.

Dissemination of findings is a vital step in any research effort, but this is particularly important in practice-based research since the goal is to share information that may improve the provision of care and resulting outcomes. Additionally, dissemination builds the body of knowledge related to pharmacy and serves an important role in advancing the profession. Dissemination should not be limited only to positive or statistically significant findings. After all, negative findings may indeed advance practice. The failure to disseminate negative or nonstatistically significant findings is a major source of publication bias and is a known issue in the scientific literature.[1,2] Publishing results in the scholarly literature may be considered the final step in dissemination, but it should be viewed as one of the several important dissemination routes.

The purpose of this chapter is to provide an overview of the process involved in preparing research manuscripts. The various sections of research articles are discussed, along with typical content for each section. Recommended practices in preparing research manuscripts, guidance on the selection of journals, and selected ethical considerations in the publication are also provided. This chapter concludes with a brief discussion of the process of manuscript submission along with examples of experiences involving learners in writing and submitting research manuscripts.

Types of Articles in Practice-Based Pharmacy Scholarship

A variety of article types are utilized in pharmacy journals. The type that is most familiar is the original research article, which reports the results of research conducted by the author(s). For the profession of pharmacy, this often includes practice-based research and social/administrative research, but other forms of research (laboratory research, simulation studies, etc.) would also fit into this type of article. These original research articles will be the primary focus of this chapter's guidance. Original research articles are often published in either full form or reduced form, sometimes called Research Notes or Brief Communications. Full original research articles usually range in length of approximately 3,000 to 4,000 words, but may be longer depending on the journal. Research notes are often limited to half that length, with restrictions on the number of tables or figures as well. Research notes are generally recommended for studies of limited scope, pilot studies, or studies with notable limitations that preclude broader applicability or generalization.

Review articles are another common type of work submitted for publication by researchers within pharmacy. Review articles focus on providing overviews and analyses of existing and emerging published literature. These also come in various forms. Narrative reviews give a basic, broad, and useful overview of a topic, such as a disease state or medication class, in a manner that is often practice-focused and for introductory learners on a topic. These narrative reviews also can be more advanced in nature, providing updates on new guidelines, strategies, and treatments. They cite relevant literature selected by the author(s), so they may be subject to some level of bias in what they include. Systematic and scoping reviews take a more formalized approach by surveying the literature on a particular topic with a defined set of inclusion/exclusion criteria and search strategies. These provide a qualitative synthesis of relevant literature, but with enhanced rigor and are subject to less bias in terms of what literature is included. Finally, meta-analyses build upon systematic reviews to provide quantitative syntheses of existing literature, combining the results of multiple studies to provide pooled estimates of the effects or harms of some treatment or exposure. Regardless of the type of review, these manuscripts tend to be longer in length than research articles.

Case reports represent another article type commonly accepted by journals. These articles describe the unique clinical course of a single patient or a small series of patients where published literature available on the topic is either nonexistent or extremely limited. Unique cases might include an unusual adverse event, a newly emerging drug interaction, an uncommon set of symptoms, or a novel treatment approach. Case reports add anecdotal evidence to the literature, which often can build in momentum and generate more formalized original research as more individuals encounter similar, but rare experiences.

Publishing reports of the development, implementation, and evaluation of pharmacy services are important ways to advance the profession. These types of articles can provide descriptions of specialized practice roles, sharing unique strategies to approach a workload challenge, or evaluations of new or existing clinical services. Unfortunately, trying to frame these reports in the format of an original research article can be challenging, especially when describing the development and implementation of a new service or practice model. Some journals provide article types that are developed specifically for these practice-focused articles. These types of articles are particularly relevant for practitioners since they provide a mechanism to connect practice with scholarship by providing evidence-based strategies to enhance patient and/or population care. Consulting a journal's author guidelines can provide insight into how these practice-focused articles fit into the journal.

A variety of other article types exist, including commentaries, letters to the editor, perspectives, reflections, and more. Most of these are heavily focused on the informed opinion or experience of the author rather than providing new results through empirical study or synthesis of the literature. Although these provide unique value to the literature, they are not the major focus of this chapter.

General Article Structure

Most research manuscripts prepared for publication follow similar organizational structures. Generally, they follow the IMRAD model, which refers to the sequential progression of sections in a manuscript: Introduction, Methods, Results, and Discussion.[3] As shown in Figure 24–1, this progression can be thought of using an hourglass shape, where the Introduction starts out broadly with the scope of necessary knowledge underlying

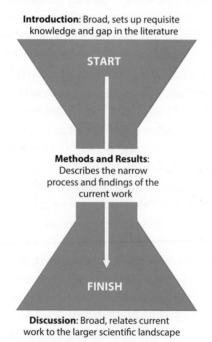

Introduction: Broad, sets up requisite knowledge and gap in the literature

START

Methods and Results: Describes the narrow process and findings of the current work

FINISH

Discussion: Broad, relates current work to the larger scientific landscape

Figure 24–1. Hourglass example. The IMRAD model provides a way to conceptualize the different sections of a manuscript, including broader scope in the Introduction/Discussion, and narrower descriptions in the Methods/Results.

the work. This is then narrowed down to the scope of the specific research conducted, described in the Methods and Results sections. Finally, the manuscript broadens again during the Discussion, where the current research's implications are connected to the broader scientific community. The International Committee of Medical Journal Editors (ICMJE) also provides detailed guidance on the preparation of manuscripts for submission to medical journals, as a part of their larger *Recommendations for the Conduct, Reporting, Editing, and Publication of Scholarly Work in Medical Journals.*[4] This incorporates the IMRAD model and provides useful recommendations on the goals of each manuscript section. The following sections provide additional detail. It should be noted that while these broad recommendations are widely accepted across the medical and scientific communities, each journal will have specific requirements that may complement or deviate from these structures. Authors are strongly encouraged to consult a particular journal's author guidelines at the beginning of the manuscript preparation process to ensure any formatting or content requirements are met. This will help reduce the need for reformatting, restructuring, and rewriting the manuscript later in the process, which can be frustrating, time-consuming, and potentially introduce errors.

TITLE AND ABSTRACT

The title and abstract are the first items that anyone will read for a given study and often serve to help a reader decide if they wish to continue reading forward into the manuscript itself.[5] The title should include key terms that will grab the reader and spark interest while providing a truthful representation of the article's contents.[6] To develop effective titles, Sword[7] recommends that authors simultaneously focus the text of the title (what is being said directly), the paratext (other information that influences the meaning of the title, such as the authors, journal title, or even contemporaneous events), and the subtext (ideas that are implied by the specific wording of the title).

There are two general types of titles used in healthcare research: descriptive titles and informative titles.[5,8] Descriptive titles typically include the study design, study sample, and general area of study and are formulated in a way that describes the study without providing the findings (e.g., "Effects of pharmacist-provided discharge medication reconciliation and counseling on readmission to a community hospital: a randomized trial"). Informative titles, also called more informative titles, provide the overall conclusion directly in the title (e.g., "Pharmacist-provided medication reconciliation and counseling reduced readmissions at a community hospital"). When crafting the title, consider including relevant keywords or terms in the title (e.g., disease state, intervention or exposure, study design) to aid in search engine optimization and the abstracting and indexing process. Furthermore, placing key terms earlier in the title may be beneficial for search engine optimization.[9,10] Some reporting guidelines, such as Consolidated Standards of Reporting Trials (CONSORT),[11] Strengthening the Reporting of Observational Studies in Epidemiology (STROBE),[12] and Preferred Reporting Items for Systematic Reviews and Meta-Analyses (PRISMA),[13] recommend including the study design in the title. Journals may have specific guidance on titles (e.g., whether informative vs. descriptive titles are preferred, the inclusion of the study, word or character count limits). It is also a good idea to develop a short title to accompany the full title. This may be used as a running head in the journal upon final publication.

An **abstract** contains relevant and important summary information regarding the research. Abstracts are generally of two forms: structured and unstructured. Structured abstracts are those that contain specific subheadings that typically map against the IMRAD model, while unstructured abstracts are simply one or more paragraphs without subheadings. Regardless of whether the abstract is structured or not, it should provide a comprehensive summary of the study, including the justification, what was done, what was found, and why it is important. Abstract requirements can vary significantly across journals in terms of structure, size, and format. Because the abstract summarizes all sections of a manuscript, it is usually recommended to write this section last, despite the fact that it is often one of the first items in a manuscript. Most journals will also request keywords alongside abstracts. **Keywords** are terms that are meant to aid in the work becoming discoverable via electronic search engines.

INTRODUCTION

The purpose of the Introduction section of a manuscript is to provide the necessary foundation for the reader to grasp the context of the study. This is commonly achieved using the "problem-gap-hook" approach,[14] where the text clearly identifies a prevalent problem, identifies what is not understood about the given problem, and convinces the reader of the importance of the query. Achieving this generally requires summarization and citation of existing literature, which helps to communicate what has already been done and what the particular contribution of the current manuscript is. A reader should be able to read an introduction and understand the fundamental question of "so what?" regarding the problem being discussed. No data or conclusions from the current work should be included in the Introduction. Think of this section as what knowledge you had as the researcher prior to beginning your own work.

While there are some general recommendations for the length of an Introduction (e.g., three paragraphs) to help new authors visualize their endgame, the more important focus is on whether the appropriate foundation has been laid for the article ahead. While it is important to include relevant background within the Introduction, it is not necessary to examine the problem in its entirety, from basic components to the complex area being investigated.

It is reasonable to assume the reader has some basic level of awareness of the topic. This allows the text to focus on setting up the problem within that preexisting knowledge. A good Introduction is succinct and clear, while giving the reader a clear understanding of why they should continue to read onward. Additionally, it ends with a clear statement of the research objective, question, or hypothesis[15] (see Chapter 4 for more information on research questions, objectives, and hypotheses), which provides a bridging element to the next section of the manuscript, the Methods. Some journals may include the objective or research question as a separate section between the Introduction and Methods.

METHODS

The Methods section provides a comprehensive and clear description of how the research was performed, including an explanation as to why a study was done in a certain way. The section should provide enough detail that would feasibly allow for the work to be replicated by others reading the paper.[16] It is generally written in the past tense, as it describes a process that was previously undertaken by the author(s). This section tends to be more technical than the Introduction, focusing on details and clarity rather than setting up the story the way the Introduction does.

While dependent on the individual journal, the use of subheadings can aid in the organization and synthesis of the information presented. Common subheadings might include: *Sample*, which should detail information on inclusion/exclusion criteria and eligibility of subjects/data for the study; *Measurements*, which should provide information on the methods used to estimate or calculate study variables, such as medication adherence, or specific tools utilized for laboratory-based approaches; *Data sources*, which is important when the study utilizes existing data (such as from electronic health records [EHR] or insurance claims databases), describing the source of data in relation to sample criteria; *Study variables*, which should detail what data were collected, how variables were operationalized, and how outcomes were measured (such as when constructs like quality of life or self-efficacy are being studied); and *Data analysis*, which discusses the analytic and statistical approaches used for the study, inclusive of any necessary software. All of these may not be relevant for every manuscript, so use those that make the most sense for your situation and align with the chosen journal's author guidelines. In the case of research involving humans or animals, it is also essential to include information on the ethics review and approval for the study being described. This is often placed at the end of the Methods.

RESULTS

The goal of the Results section is to provide a curated tour of the findings generated from the study. Like the Methods, this section is often highly technical, with limited incorporation of the "voice" of the author(s). The Results section should not contain any interpretation of the data. Instead, it should provide clear, logical, and concise reporting of the findings. Mechanisms beyond text, such as tables and figures,[17] should be used to enhance a reader's understanding of the results being presented. These can be extremely helpful to help readers visualize trends, compare groups, or understand analyses. While tables and figures are useful strategies, they should only be used in situations where they truly enhance the information provided in the text.

Results can also be divided with subheadings similar to the Methods if the journal allows. Some authors find this useful to enhance the flow of the manuscript, especially for complex projects or those with many objectives. As an example, consider a manuscript involving the use of a questionnaire to measure pharmacists' satisfaction with their job roles. The questionnaire was developed in a sample of physicians, so the authors examined the psychometric properties of the instrument in a sample of pharmacists as part of the analysis. The Results may be divided into separate sections. One might be labeled *Sample characteristics,* where the authors describe the pharmacists who responded to the questionnaire. Another section, *Factor structure,* might provide information on the factor analysis and evaluation of internal consistency in the sample. The final section describing the findings from the main analysis could be called *Job role satisfaction and correlates.*

The first part of the Results section commonly starts with a broad sample description. For patient-oriented studies, this usually includes a description of how many patients met inclusion criteria and participated, a description of how the sample was stratified into groups (if applicable), and a link to a table that provides a descriptive analysis of relevant demographic and clinical attributes of the sample. Study participant flowcharts, such as the ones promoted by the CONSORT guidelines,[11] can be helpful for this purpose. The remainder of the Results should directly correlate to the research objectives and previously detailed methods, making sure that all planned questions and analyses that were described earlier in the manuscript have indeed been addressed.

DISCUSSION

Consistent with the hourglass scheme mentioned previously (see Figure 24–1), the Discussion section is where the manuscript opens up again to allow for the author's interpretation of the findings within the context of the existing body of knowledge. The goal of the Discussion is to synthesize the Results and provide commentary on important findings. This section should *not* include any new information not already included in the Results; rather, it should build on the findings already presented and provide a discussion of their implications.

It is recommended to begin the Discussion with a high-level summary of key findings, perhaps thought of as the main points a reader should walk away with from the manuscript.[18] After this, the Discussion can continue with an examination of potential explanations for the findings, relating them to existing literature. Similar to the Introduction, citation of related work is important here to demonstrate how the current study builds, complements, changes, or challenges current knowledge, practice, or research. The Discussion is also an opportunity to explore future or recommended areas for inquiry or calls to action on a particular topic. These should relate closely to the gaps that were explored in the Introduction. Think of this as a way to answer the "So what?" question that was initially posed.

While Discussion sections are generally unstructured, they should still be focused and maintain a logical flow—starting with what was found, examining what those findings mean, and then concluding with the next steps. Some journals may request a specific subheading for study limitations. Even if not specifically requested, important limitations should still be detailed in the Discussion. All studies are subject to limitations, and authors should be clear in detailing these and discussing the potential implications for the interpretation of their data. This part is usually placed at the end of the Discussion section, just prior to the Conclusions.

CONCLUSIONS

The Conclusions section is generally a single paragraph that provides the final take-home message for the findings. Like the Discussion, it should not include any new findings. Unlike the Discussion, the citation of previous literature is somewhat uncommon in the Conclusions. It is important that this concluding section should be completely and clearly supported by the data collected and findings from the analyses and not overstate findings in an effort to sound more important or impactful. Many research endeavors are designed for incremental gains, and as such, it is perfectly appropriate to keep comments narrowed to this scope.

ADDITIONAL ELEMENTS

Journals will often request additional elements that are necessary for manuscript submission beyond the manuscript itself. A cover letter is commonly requested. The **cover letter** accompanies the manuscript and serves to explain the work's contribution to the literature, describes the fit for the journal, and provides any additional context that may be helpful for the editors. Some journals also require certain statements to be included in the cover letter, such as disclosure of potential conflicts of interest (detailed later), affirmations that the manuscript has not been previously published and is not currently under review elsewhere, or ethical review status. Most journals also require a separate title page to accompany all manuscripts. The **title page** provides descriptive information on author names and affiliations; potential conflicts of interest that might influence the work being presented; details on funding supporting the work; and key manuscript characteristics (word count, number of tables and figures, number of references, etc.). Journals often ask for the unique contributions of each listed author to the work being submitted to be included in an "Author Contributions" section somewhere in the manuscript. Some journals request this as a separate document. Unless directed otherwise by the journal, authors may consider using the CRediT taxonomy to describe the contributions of each author.[19,20] This taxonomy includes a set of 14 roles (conceptualization, methodology, formal analysis, etc.) that are often undertaken by individuals participating in scholarly projects, allowing for each author to have played multiple roles in conducting the project.

Key Considerations for Writing Research Papers

Although there is no one perfect, ideal, or even recommended way to approach writing a research manuscript, there are many best practices that are passed down from previous generations of scientific writers that can help new writers navigate the nuances of expectations, both written and unwritten, within the field. An overview of these practices is provided in Table 24–1, and additional details are provided below. As you gain experience in scientific writing and the manuscript publication process, you will likely develop your own habits and practices that also promote personal success.

JOURNAL SELECTION

Selecting a target journal is a key preparatory element in preparing a manuscript. This is due not only to the need to understand the different technical requirements of each journal so that one can streamline their manuscript preparation process but also to ensure the manuscript eventually reaches the best audience. There are thousands of journals currently available, so choosing the right one is important. Consider the journals that you read for your own practice and/or research development. Check journal websites to identify the journal's overarching aims and scope and read some recently published papers. Identifying any affiliated professional organizations or associations can also help provide a sense of the journal's readership. These can all help give you a sense of a journal's focus and whether your work would be a good fit. While it may sound counterintuitive, avoid focusing too narrowly within your own profession. It is common for pharmacists to think that they have to publish only in pharmacy-centric journals. There are situations where the world outside of pharmacy needs to hear about our work. This is particularly the case with interprofessional practice activities where you may consider a journal in a broader

TABLE 24–1. BEST PRACTICES FOR WRITING RESEARCH PAPERS

Area	Best Practices
Journal selection	• Consider the target audience for the manuscript and match to the readership of a journal
	• Reading past issues and consulting with mentors can help identify the most appropriate journal(s)
	• The publishing approach (traditional vs. open access) may drive journal selection/refinement since open access may involve payment of article processing charges
	• Beware of predatory journals (if it seems too good to be true or looks suspicious, it probably is) and consult the "Think. Check. Submit." initiative for guidance on identifying legitimate journals (https://www.thinkchecksubmit.org)
	• Consider journals outside of pharmacy in your journal selection if they are appropriate to your project
	• Questions about general scope or appropriateness of the manuscript can be asked of journal editors
	• Once a journal is selected, consult the author guidelines and follow them carefully
Sharing research	• Sharing research through nontraditional avenues can complement peer-reviewed publications, increase availability, and broaden reach
	• Consider sharing preprints as a means to facilitate knowledge dissemination
	• Make sure to comply with any applicable copyright laws or licensing agreements
	• Social media postings can allow you to increase the visibility of and extend the reach of your work
Reporting guidelines	• Journals may require the use of certain guidelines and the submission of supplemental material based on those guidelines
	• Even if not required, consider using reporting guidelines when preparing your manuscript
	• Consult the EQUATOR Network (www.equator-network.org)
Manuscript preparation	• Use the general IMRAD structure as a general starting point
	• Once a target journal is selected, carefully follow the author guidelines
	• Ensure that all relevant information is included in each manuscript section (including any additional elements required by the journal)
Authorship	• Discuss authorship (including author order) early in the research process and revisit it regularly
	• Without explicit guidance from a journal, consider the ICMJE criteria for authorship
	• All individuals who meet authorship criteria should be listed as authors
	• Other individuals contributing to the project but not meeting the criteria for authorship should be acknowledgments
	• Avoid guest authorship and ghostwriting
	• Consider using the CRediT taxonomy (https://credit.niso.org) to describe each author's contributions
Presubmission review	• Have another person not serving as an author (e.g., mentor, colleague) review the manuscript prior to final submission
	• Input from colleagues or mentors may help strengthen the manuscript and guide journal selection
	• Avoid seeking input from journal editors about whether your manuscript might be accepted (general questions about potential fit maybe acceptable)

(Continued)

TABLE 24–1. BEST PRACTICES FOR WRITING RESEARCH PAPERS (*CONTINUED*)

Area	Best Practices
Manuscript submission	• Gather all required information and files before starting the online submission process • Verify the names and e-mail addresses of all authors • Ensure the correct version of all required documents are included during manuscript submission

ICMJE: International Committee of Medical Journal Editors; CRediT: Contributor Roles Taxonomy.

disease-focused area (e.g., a diabetes journal) or in another profession (e.g., medicine or nursing). It is more appropriate that you match the work being disseminated with the journal, not the author(s) with the journal. Accordingly, it is appropriate to consider the clinical topic area and methodology used in your work in considering a broad range of potential journals.

There are also tools available to help authors identify potential journals of interest. The Journal/Author Name Estimator, or JANE, tool (https://jane.biosemantics.org/) is a good resource. This website allows authors to enter a title, abstract, or keywords related to their work, which is then used to generate a list of potential journals with similar syntax using PubMed. Some publishers (such as Elsevier, Wiley, and SAGE) also have similar tools available on their websites. Keep in mind that these only search the publisher's own journal catalogs, so they will have more limited reach.

Authors can also contact editors or staff at journals of interest. This strategy is recommended if you have a specific query in determining the fit of your article for the journal and have exhausted other efforts. It is recommended to avoid contacting journals for requests that are in the realm of, "How successful will my article be at getting accepted at this journal?" This is part of the peer-review process and is nearly impossible for a journal to answer based on a simple email. If you do choose to contact a journal, it can be very helpful to provide at least the title and abstract of your paper to provide the editorial staff some idea of the project. Remember that a positive response at that stage in no way guarantees eventual acceptance of your manuscript.

OPEN ACCESS PUBLISHING

It is important to note the difference between traditional and open access publishing models used by journals. This may influence journal selection. In the traditional publishing model, the submission and publication process for authors is free, meaning that there are no fees to pursue the publication of your manuscript. Upon publication, articles published under this model are generally behind a paywall, which either requires a single payment or a subscription to the journal to enable access. Universities and other large organizations typically purchase institutional access to journals via their libraries. This is how journals recover their operating costs. **Open access (OA) publishing** essentially flips the traditional model and involves free access to publications. After acceptance of the manuscript, authors are required to pay a fee, called an **article processing charge** (APC), to have their work published. While the author must pay instead of the reader, this enables free access for everyone who wants to read the article upon publication. OA publishing allows for the potential of a wider readership; however, authors must find ways to cover APCs. Some institutions provide support for these, and researchers can also include potential APCs in grant applications. If such resources are not available, the author must either pay out of their own pocket or request a waiver from the publisher. There is large variability in the APCs charged by publishers. In 2012, Solomon and Björk[21] estimated a range of $8 to $3,900 with a mean of about $900. Using a different set of journals in 2020, Budzinski et al.[22] estimated this range as $15 to over $10,000 with a mean of just under $3,000. A variety of different levels of open access currently exist. These are described briefly in Table 24-2.

TABLE 24-2. OPEN ACCESS APPROACHES

Level	Key Characteristics
Green OA	• No APCs
	• Author can self-archive accepted manuscript in certain places (personal website, institutional repository, approved commercial repositories, etc.)
	• Readers can access accepted manuscript for free
	• Subscription required for final published version
	• Copyright typically retained by the journal/publisher
Gold OA	• Author pays APCs upon acceptance of manuscript (may receive support from institution or grants; waivers sometimes available)
	• Author can self-archive accepted manuscript in certain places (personal website, institutional repository, approved commercial repositories, etc.)
	• Posting of accepted manuscript may be delayed by required embargo periods (often 12-24 months)
	• Readers can access final published version of manuscript for free immediately upon publication
	• Restriction on reuse removed or substantially lowered through flexible licensing approaches (e.g., Creative Commons licenses)
	• Copyright typically retained by the author(s) or shared with author(s) and journal/publisher
Platinum (or Diamond) OA	• No APCs
	• Author can self-archive accepted manuscript in certain places (personal website, institutional repository, approved commercial repositories, etc.)
	• Readers can access accepted manuscript for free
	• Restriction on reuse removed or substantially lowered through flexible licensing approaches (e.g., Creative Commons licenses)
	• Copyright typically retained by the author(s) or shared with author(s) and journal/publisher

APCs: article processing charges; OA: open access.

Early in the OA movement, entire journals used an OA publishing model. These primarily used gold OA approaches and are likely familiar to many researchers, such as the large international publishers like BioMed Central (BMC) and the Public Library of Science (PLoS). Over time, traditional publishers have increasingly offered open access options for authors at the individual article level. The result is that now most journals, particularly those published by large publishing houses, are hybrid open access journals in that some articles are available only via subscription while others are freely available through some OA arrangement.

SHARING RESEARCH

The OA movement spawned additional focus on the ability of researchers to share their research in more open and accessible ways. One relatively recent development is the growth of platforms to share preprints (sometimes called preprint servers) to facilitate the discovery and sharing of preprints. A **preprint** is a preliminary version of a manuscript from some scholarly project. It may be helpful to think of these as a working paper or a paper in progress that has not undergone peer review and has not yet been published. Researchers may post their papers to these servers to share an early version of their research and perhaps get feedback from the scientific or professional community prior to submission and formal peer review. Examples of platforms that facilitate the posting of preprints include medRxiv for medicine and healthcare (https://www.medrxiv.org), bioRxiv for biology and life sciences (https://www.biorxiv.org), Social Science Research Network for the social sciences (https://www.ssrn.com), Research Papers in Economics (https://repec.org), Open Science Framework (https://osf.io), Zenodo (https://www.zenodo.org), and ResearchGate (https://www.researchgate.net). Before posting anything to these sharing services, it is important to ensure that you are following all necessary copyright laws.

An important distinction here is the difference between a preprint, the accepted manuscript, and the final published version. Most journals allow the posting of preprints at any time, although this does need to be disclosed upon article submission. The accepted manuscript is the final version of the manuscript that the author submitted after peer review, which has not been formatted or copyedited by the publisher. Some journals, particularly those allowing green OA options, allow for posting of the accepted manuscript in selected places after an embargo period. The final version is what is seen in the pages of a journal or on the journal website. This contains all the formatting and editing by the publisher to meet the journal's style requirements. Without gold or platinum OA agreements, the final published version typically cannot be posted elsewhere by the author without the permission of the publisher.

Sharing research with the scientific and professional communities has largely been accomplished through traditional avenues like publication and presentation. Social media offers new ways to increase the visibility of you and your work. For example, you could share a recent poster presentation or a new publication through Twitter, Facebook, or LinkedIn. It is also possible to reach considerably more diverse groups of people, such as professionals, researchers, patients, policymakers, and the general public. Furthermore, using social media can generate discussions surrounding your work and even result in potential collaborations for future work. Your local institutional communications department may have additional resources about sharing your work.

PREDATORY PUBLISHERS

Due in part to the role of collecting payment from authors prior to publication in OA publishing and the pressures on academic authors to publish, predatory publishers have emerged. These publishers, or pseudopublishers, may sponsor many journals, books, and even conferences. Some of the journals even look shockingly similar to existing, well-respected journals. These predatory journals typically have peer-review and oversight processes that range from completely nonexistent to poorly implemented. These journals effectively exist to publish anything for which an author is willing to pay. It is important for prospective authors to understand the difference between reputable and predatory journals. The "Think. Check. Submit." initiative (https://www.thinkchecksubmit.org) provides useful resources to help make these determinations. Healthcare or research librarians within your own institution can also be an invaluable resource in making these decisions.

REPORTING GUIDELINES

Clear reporting is an important concept when publishing any scholarly work. Poor reporting can have adverse effects on the success of a submission. Even if accepted, poor reporting can have important implications on the development of the body of literature in an area, particularly when it comes to research synthesis. For example, concerns about insufficient reporting have been raised as reasons for difficulties when including pharmacy services studies in meta-analyses and the resulting inconclusive evidence of the benefit of pharmacists' services.[23,24]

Several reporting guidelines were previously mentioned in Part II of this book. These included CONSORT extension for patient-reported outcomes in clinical trials (CONSORT PRO), STROBE (for observational studies), PRISMA (for systematic reviews), the Survey Reporting Guideline (SURGE), the Standards for Quality Improvement Reporting

Excellence (SQUIRE), the Consolidated Criteria for Reporting Qualitative Research (COREQ), and the Standards for Reporting Qualitative Research (SRQR). The EQUATOR Network (https://www.equator-network.org) provides a comprehensive list of numerous other reporting guidelines. One additional reporting guideline that may warrant special consideration is the Pharmacist Patient Care Intervention Reporting (PaCIR) checklist.[23] This provides guidance on nine critical elements that should be included when reporting studies of pharmacist's patient care interventions.

In addition to reporting guidelines specific to specific study designs or settings, guidance on the reporting of statistical analyses and results is also available. The Statistical Analyses and Methods in the Published Literature (SAMPL) guidelines published by the European Association of Science Editors,[25] the *AMA Manual of Style*,[26] and the *Publication Manual of the American Psychological Association* (APA)[27] all provide general recommendations for reporting statistical analyses. Other useful resources to guide research reporting and writing, in general, are provided in Table 24–3.

TABLE 24–3. RESOURCES FOR REPORTING SCHOLARLY WORKS

Topic	Resources
General guidance	Moher D, Altman DG, Schulz KF, eds. *Guidelines for Reporting Health Research: A User's Manual.* Hoboken, NJ: Wiley Blackwell; 2014.
	Christiansen SL, Iverson C, Flanagin A, et al. *AMA Manual of Style: A Guide for Authors and Editors.* 11th ed. Oxford, UK: Oxford University Press; 2020.
	Publication Manual of the American Psychological Association. 7th ed. Washington, D.C.: American Psychological Association; 2020.
	Council of Science Editors. *Scientific Style and Format: The CSE Manual for Authors, Editors, and Publishers.* 8th ed. Chicago, IL: Council of Science Editors in cooperation with The University of Chicago Press; 2014.
	The Chicago Manual of Style. 17th ed. Chicago, IL: University of Chicago Press; 2017.
Specific research reporting guidance	EQUATOR Network (https://www.equator-network.org): provides a comprehensive list of reporting guidelines and checklist for a wide range of study designs and research approaches
	PaCIR checklist: reporting checklist designed specifically for pharmacists' patient care activities (Clay PG, Burns AL, Isetts BJ, Hirsch JD, Kliethermes MA, Planas LG. PaCIR: a tool to enhance pharmacist patient care intervention reporting. *J Am Pharm Assoc (2003).* 2019;59(5):615-623.)
Reporting statistics	Lang TA, Altman DG. Basic statistical reporting for articles published in clinical medical journals: the SAMPL guidelines. In: Smart P, Maisonneuve H, Polderman AKS, eds. *Science Editors' Handbook.* 2nd ed. Pau, France: European Association of Science Editors; 2013: 175-182.
	Lang TA, Secic M. *How to Report Statistics in Medicine: Annotated Guidelines for Authors, Editors, and Reviewers.* 2nd ed. Philadelphia, PA: American College of Physicians; 2006.

PaCIR, Pharmacist Patient Care Intervention Reporting; SAMPL, Statistical Analyses and Methods in the Published Literature.

AUTHORSHIP

Most research projects involve a team of people to execute the project and bring it to the point of manuscript submission. While authorship on a research manuscript may not seem like a complicated issue at first glance, it can easily become a major issue if not discussed preemptively and transparently. This is because authorship inherently communicates credit for the research. For instance, the order of authors is thought by many to indicate the level of contribution of different parties to the work. As such, some institutions set goals for individuals regarding authorship credit which may influence promotion and tenure decisions or compensation. This may inadvertently push authors toward potential conflict. Additionally, some team members may be involved with projects intermittently, such as helping to generate the idea but not contributing to the actual execution of the research. These individuals may reappear in the lead-up to manuscript preparation, anticipating authorship and potentially causing conflict. Finally, many teams involve members with supervisor-trainee relationships, which have the potential to become coercive through power imbalances. Trainees may be pressured to change author order (e.g., a graduate student making their supervisor first author even though the student contributed the most effort) or inappropriately give authorship to individuals (e.g., a pharmacy resident including a senior pharmacist as the last author when the individual only provided guidance on the initial project idea). These can be particularly problematic since the trainee is likely dependent upon their supervisor or more senior individuals for recommendations and academic progression. Each of these described situations is unfortunate, and in some cases unethical, but can be avoided through proper planning and the use of objective guidance.

It helps to first understand some commonly discussed author roles regarding manuscripts. All submissions require selection of what is known as a **corresponding author**, which is the individual who is responsible for communication with the journal throughout the publication process and from readers should questions arise after final publication. Some individuals further interpret the corresponding author to be the **senior author** (the individual providing oversight and guidance for the work and responsible for it), although this is not necessarily always the case. The **first author** is the individual listed first in the author list and is often considered to receive the most credit for the manuscript as they are generally assumed to have had the bulk of responsibility in executing the work and preparing the manuscript. This role is somewhat coveted and may be a source of conflict among research teams where multiple people invest similar efforts. What can be particularly confusing is that each discipline varies in how the authors are commonly listed and the importance of those placements. They may even change with career stages, where serving as the senior author on papers is expected. In some disciplines, this individual is listed last in the list of authors. Speaking to medical authors, Riesenberg and Lundberg[28] suggested that the first author should be the individual who contributed the most to the work and preparation of the paper, with the remaining authors ordered in decreasing level of contribution.

ICMJE provides guidance to researchers regarding what type of contribution constitutes authorship. This is particularly important since authorship also serves to communicate to readers who hold responsibility and accountability for the research. The ICMJE definition of authorship requires fulfilling four criteria: "(1) substantial contributions to the conception or design of the work; or the acquisition, analysis, or interpretation of data for the work; and (2) drafting the work or revising it critically for important intellectual content; and (3) final approval of the version to be published; and (4) agreement to be accountable for all aspects of the work in ensuring that questions related to the accuracy or integrity of any part of the work are appropriately investigated and resolved."[4] As is evident from these criteria, authors are required to have a presence in the project essentially from the beginning to the end. If individuals involved do not satisfy all four of these criteria, they should be acknowledged rather than listed as authors. These **acknowledgments** typically appear in a separate section within a manuscript that lists individuals who have contributed to the work but have not otherwise met the criteria for authorship. For the sake of clarification, ICMJE provides examples of duties that on their own that rise only to the level of deserving an acknowledgment: general supervision; general administrative support; and assistance with writing, editing, and proofreading. Rather than focusing on authorship, per se, the previously mentioned CRediT taxonomy focuses on contributorship.[20] This may serve as a complementary approach to determining who meets the criteria of authorship. For most journals in pharmacy and the health professions, one must still fulfill the ICMJE criteria to be designated an author.

Overall, it is recommended that research teams discuss authorship near the beginning of a project, so that all expectations are laid out at the start. These discussions should be held regularly, especially when the preparation of the manuscript begins. While there still needs to be some expectation of flexibility in authorship since situations change, this can help to avoid conflict and surprises later in the process when considerable time has been invested.

PRESUBMISSION REVIEW

Prior to manuscript submission, authors may consider some sort of internal peer review. This can be extremely helpful in getting additional feedback on your manuscript before submitting the paper. It is easy for authors to overlook issues in their papers, whether small writing issues or larger conceptual ones. When unresolved, these can cause substantial problems after submission to a journal. This internal review may be informal, such as having a nonauthor colleague or mentor review the paper, or more formal processes like writing clubs, such as the one described by Komperda et al.[29] In addition to providing feedback for the manuscript itself, these internal reviews may also be helpful in determining whether the target journal is appropriate.

Preparing Manuscripts

Even armed with a good understanding of how a manuscript is composed, the most anxiety-inducing step may be starting the writing itself and pulling everything together. Staring at a blank screen can certainly be overwhelming. Keeping some general guidance in mind as you prepare your manuscript can save you a significant amount of time by avoiding major adjustments and changes later.

GENERAL GUIDANCE

One very simple reminder as you start to compose a manuscript is that you are not required to write from top to bottom in the same manner that the manuscript will be read. It is often recommended to start with those sections that you are most comfortable with or can easily complete. Some individuals find it easier to begin with the detailed work of the Methods or Results, while others like to capture the broader frameworks of the Introduction or Discussion first. Either way, beginning where you are most comfortable will help to get the process started. As your pages fill up, your confidence to tackle other sections will increase and help to bring the manuscript to completion.

Outlines are also incredibly useful in mapping the direction of a manuscript. Some authors begin this process during the design phase of their research before they even submit to the project for ethical review and approval. A literature search is necessary for the formulation of good research questions and objectives, so this can be utilized to outline an Introduction. In planning your research, you have to establish what variables you will be collecting and what comparisons are of interest. These can easily be used to create a frame for the Methods and Results sections. While you may wait until the study is completed before outlining the direction of your Discussion, you can think through your hypotheses or research objectives and their importance to the broader field of study early on as a way to prepare for the interpretation of your results. It is important to highlight that you may have the pieces available to formulate a useful outline for your manuscript before you have even started data collection.

Prior to writing, familiarizing yourself with a chosen journal's author guidelines is essential. These guidelines contain important requirements for the submission of the manuscript. While many formatting requirements of journals can be applied at any time during the writing process (e.g., specified margin sizes, line numbering, section headings), other requirements such as page and word count limits may fundamentally guide the composition of the manuscript itself and what can be covered in the allotted space. Generally, authors are expected to adhere to these guidelines closely, although some flexibility in word or page count may be acceptable after consultation with the editor. Even though selecting a journal early in the process is recommended, if a research team has not done this, authors can still use the ICMJE recommendations to create a manuscript that is adaptable to different journal requirements with the understanding that editing will likely be required prior to the submission once a journal has been chosen.

Although many scientific writers crave consistency in submission requirements across journals, this is not the current status of the field. It is the responsibility of authors to be able to adapt to different styles and requirements within their writing. One practice that can help this process is consistently reading journals in your interest area. While often done to keep up with emerging content in your area of experience, it can also serve as a useful reconnaissance in understanding the style and structure of journals that you may consider for your own submissions.

MAIN ARTICLE TEXT

The earlier section on *General Article Structure* provided information on the recommended content for each section of an article. Another general piece of advice is to strive to tell a cohesive story that connects across sections of the manuscript. Readers are most likely to engage with work that fully sets the stage, communicates a clear message, and leaves them wanting to move forward integrating the work.

The use of subheadings within the main sections is a strategy that can be helpful in promoting the readability of a manuscript and helping the reader to partition different aspects of the manuscript. As mentioned previously, they are mostly utilized in the Methods section, but may be used in other sections as well. Journal author guidelines often communicate whether these are allowed (if the author finds them necessary), encouraged (with structure left up to the author), or required (in a prescriptive sense with specific subheadings). There may also be guidance on how these should be incorporated stylistically. Figure 24–2 provides comparative examples of formatting used by the *British Medical Journal* (BMJ)[30] and by the *Publication Manual of the American Psychological Association* (APA).[27] In general, subheadings deeper than three levels are not often needed. Subheadings should only be used when there is a minimum of two subheadings within a given section.[26] Some journals do break from this practice, such as requiring an Introduction section with a single subheading for Study Objective, or a Discussion section with a single subheading for Study Limitations.

Authors may also want to use abbreviations, acronyms, or initialisms (collectively referred to here as abbreviations) to streamline the manuscript. In fact, some journals may require a separate list of these to be included with the manuscript upon submission.

	BMJ	APA
Level 1 (Main section; top level)	**METHODS**	**METHODS**
Level 2	**Study variables**	**Study variables**
Level 3	Dependent variables	*Dependent variables*
Level 4	*Patient variables*	**Patient variables**
Level 5	[No guidance beyond Level 4]	***Patient satisfaction***

Figure 24–2. Examples of subheading formatting. Sample methods sections are separated into several subsections. These show how two different journals may approach formatting.

NOTE: The positioning of the text (flush left, centered, indented) and formatting (bold, plain, italics) reflects the style being demonstrated. Solid lines indicate text.

Within the text, abbreviations should generally be written out in expanded form upon their first use, with consistent use of the abbreviation thereafter. Since the manuscript may not be written top to bottom, authors may find it helpful to write out everything longhand first and then apply abbreviations throughout the manuscript at the end of the writing process. While many authors may utilize abbreviations to navigate word count limits for journals, this should be done with caution as it can be a source of confusion for readers outside the field or across languages.[31] Many fields have standard abbreviations that are commonly used and are appropriate to include. In the field of pharmacy, this might include abbreviations such as T2DM for type II diabetes mellitus or MTM for medication therapy management. The use of nonstandard abbreviations may impede readability through increased mental effort (e.g., PIACS for pharmacists in ambulatory care settings) and can also communicate mixed messages through creating new manuscript-specific abbreviations for those that already have alternative standard uses (e.g., using PE to mean patient education, when many others may instead think pulmonary embolism). While there is no specific definition or list as to what constitutes a standard vs. nonstandard abbreviation, good judgment and input from peers and experienced mentors are usually sufficient to avoid this trap. Another source of abbreviations is the shorthand for a term or phrase used locally within the research group or practice setting. Remember that these may be meaningful locally but may not necessarily translate to other settings. Finally, just because a set of words is used repeatedly in a manuscript does not necessarily mean that an abbreviation is the best solution.

IN-TEXT CITATIONS AND REFERENCING

Although they may feel tedious to assemble, references are essential to provide credit to the existing work and to avoid plagiarism within your own work. Most manuscripts are composed of both a reference list at the end of the manuscript, as well as the use of in-text referencing to connect the reference list to specific statements in the manuscript where that the text is taken from or relates to an outside source. The use of footnotes (i.e., a section at the bottom of each page that can include references, commentary, or other information) is relatively uncommon in pharmacy and biomedical journals.

In general, there are two major approaches to reference lists: author-date and numbered.[32] Author-date referencing (also known as Harvard style) is used primarily in the humanities and social sciences. The reference list is arranged in alphabetical order by author name, and the accompanying in-text references use parentheses to indicate the use of an outside source [e.g., Smith (2020); Johnson et al. (2019)]. The APA referencing format[27] is a well-known citation approach utilizing the author-date style. Numerical referencing (also known as Vancouver style or order of appearance) is more common in the health sciences. The reference list is arranged numerically in the order that references appear in the manuscript. In-text references are denoted with Arabic numerals with varying formats (e.g., enclosed in parentheses or brackets or superscripted). The American Medical Association (AMA) referencing format[26] uses the numbered style. Keep in mind that the author-date and numerical approaches are general groupings. There are various unique styles within each general grouping that differ in terms of areas such as the specific elements included within a specific citation (e.g., requiring issue numbers, including the name of the database, including digital object identifiers) or the formatting of the information (e.g., use of italics for journal or book titles, abbreviations for journal titles, presentation of dates). Although some journals use a specific standardized reference style (e.g., AMA style or APA style), other journals may use a standard style with specific exceptions or may employ their own specialized styles. This highlights the importance of consulting the author guidelines and reviewing previous issues of the journal.

For shorter manuscripts with a limited number of references, many authors choose to manage their reference lists manually. For longer manuscripts (e.g., review articles, theses, dissertations, book chapters), this process can become quite tedious and prone to user error. Additionally, if the manuscript includes multiple authors writing different sections and moving blocks of text around during the writing process, it can be especially difficult to keep up manually with the reference list, particularly when using a numerical citation and reference list style. For these situations, the use of citation manager software is recommended. There are a number of different products currently available (e.g., Zotero, RefWorks, EndNote, Mendeley, JabRef). They vary in terms of cost, portability, sharing capabilities, storage, and operating system compatibility. There are numerous resources available online to help writers choose the software that best fits their needs. Referencing functions are available within word processing applications, such as Microsoft Word, Google Docs, and LibreOffice Writer, but these are much more limited in their capabilities compared to separate citation manager products.

Using citation managers generally requires references to be loaded into the software (manually or using embedded search functions) as a first step. Then the software is used to insert references within the manuscript while writing. The citation manager will auto-generate a reference list for the writer in a variety of selected styles. Although this is a multistep process, the automation provided by citation managers usually results in saved time and fewer errors. Many citation managers offer the ability to update the reference list and in-text citations dynamically as the document is changed. Always be sure to double-check the reference list prior to submission, as some minor fine-tuning is usually required.

TABLES AND FIGURES

Another manuscript element that requires careful consideration is the tables and figures associated with the manuscript. These are often used within the Results, where they help the reader visualize the data and relevant comparisons and trends. It is imperative that tables and figures stand alone without the accompanying manuscript text. This is achieved by constructing meaningful titles for each table and figure and including appropriate footnotes to include important information, such as the meaning of abbreviations. Most journals ask for tables and figures to be submitted separately, although some may ask for them to be embedded within the manuscript text for submission. In either case, it is best practice to submit original editable files. For example, do not submit a table created in a word processing program as an image. Similarly, if you created a figure in a program like Microsoft PowerPoint, then submit that file rather than converting it to a generic image file like a JPEG. This is important so that the journal production office can make small updates to conform to the journal's style. Keeping files in their original editable format is also useful should you need to make any corrections or changes during the review process.

Although tables and figures can greatly enhance a manuscript, it is essential that they are composed correctly in a way that facilitates the display and understanding of the data.[33] For instance, tables should generally list variables of interest in rows, with columns used to represent different groups for stratification or comparison. Each variable row should include units of measurement, especially if there is a mix of categorical and continuous variables within a single table. Columns, when representing different groups for comparison, should usually denote sample sizes within their headers. Figures should be complete with axis labels (if a graph), appropriate and transparent scaling to represent the data, and adequate resolution for reproduction. Additional guidance on when a particular approach (table vs. graph) is useful and tips on how to avoid poorly constructed tables and graphs are available elsewhere.[34,35]

SUPPLEMENTAL MATERIALS

Depending on the nature of the research project, including supplemental materials with your manuscript submission may be necessary. Generally, **supplemental materials** are considered those items that may not be necessary for the main manuscript but can provide useful context and additional details to those readers who are interested in learning more. These materials may include appendices, data sets, additional subgroup analyses, study questionnaires, study protocols, and reporting guideline checklists. Any number of different materials can be included, although the author should keep in mind any relevant copyright issues with supplemental materials. The availability of supplemental material submissions also removes the need for statements like "results not shown" for results that were not included in the main manuscript. The choice of supplemental materials is often author-driven, but some journals may require certain materials to be submitted via this mechanism. Additionally, some reporting guidelines encourage the submission of certain elements, such as the inclusion of explicit search strategies for systematic reviews as recommended by PRISMA.[13] In some situations, journals may request a supplemental element (e.g., a study questionnaire) for peer review purposes, but that will not be included if the manuscript is accepted.

The use of supplemental material can often replace the need for readers to contact the author for further information. This is especially true with respect to data files and study protocols. Additional details about the study protocol and the actual data files along with the manuscript can be deposited in an independent data repository (e.g., Figshare [https://www.figshare.com], Dryad [https://datadryad.org], Dataverse instance [https://dataverse.org], Open Science Framework [https://osf.io]). Researchers can include analysis code as supplemental material, particularly when complex coding is needed for data manipulation or analysis. This supplemental material related to study procedures, data, and analyses ultimately becomes a mechanism to promote reproducibility and enhance transparency in science.

Ethical Considerations When Writing Manuscripts

Many are familiar with the principles of the responsible conduct of research. There are similar principles within the realm of scientific writing and publishing. This area involves a wide range of potential issues, some of which are the focus of active debate and discussion. Running afoul of these questionable writing practices can have real and sometimes serious implications personally and professionally. Minor violations may be associated with a warning or formal reprimand. Consequences for more serious violations range from retractions of published articles or loss of current funding to bans on publishing or the chances to apply for funding, demotion of academic rank, loss of a job, or even civil or criminal charges. The Office of Research Integrity within the U.S. Department of Health and Human Services provides guidance on several issues related to questionable writing practices.[36] This section provides an overview of several common areas that authors should keep in mind when preparing to disseminate their research findings.

AUTHORSHIP CONCERNS

As discussed earlier, authorship is an important consideration when writing a research manuscript. This should ideally be addressed early in the research process and revisited regularly through the point of submission and potential revision. Remember that any individual listed as an author must meet the criteria to be an author. Unless stated otherwise by the target journal, the ICMJE authorship criteria supplemented with the CRediT taxonomy are a useful guide. From the perspective of ethical issues, there are several authorship-related issues to note.

Ghostwriting is when an individual who made contributions to the writing of the paper is not listed as an author or in an acknowledgment. In biomedical research, ghostwriting has been a major concern in studies conducted by the pharmaceutical industry, where there has been a history of using medical writing firms to produce manuscripts and then attach the names of other individuals, such as other medical professionals or researchers, as authors of the paper sometimes with an honorarium for serving as an "author."[37,38] This can be avoided by including all individuals as authors or contributors as appropriate. In situations where writing assistance was obtained, especially in situations with industry funding, disclosing that assistance as an acknowledgment is essential.

Guest authorship is another questionable writing practice. Guest authorship is viewed as the opposite of ghostwriting in that individuals are listed as authors who did not otherwise meet the criteria for authorship.[39] Guest authorship may take a variety of forms. Honorary, gift, or courtesy authorship is sometimes given as a token of appreciation. Including an individual in an attempt to increase the apparent credibility of the work may also be called prestige authorship. Generally speaking, guest authorship is unethical.[40] It is potentially problematic when it is the result of coercion or manipulation of power structures, such as if a research or faculty mentor or senior researcher suggests that a trainee or mentee include them as an author when they did not meet the authorship criteria. If you have reason to believe this is happening, speak to a trusted mentor. You may also consult your institution's research misconduct policies as there may be local policies to deal with this behavior.

Another authorship issue may occur when there is pressure to change the order of authors on a paper. As noted previously, an individual's place in the authorship order may have implications for credit in the academic system. There are also implications for an individual's pride and ego. Maintaining open lines of communication, having realistic expectations of expected contributions, and holding each other accountable can help resolve any potential author order concerns. If the order of authors changes prior to submission, which is perfectly acceptable, this should be done through conversations that are as open and honest as possible. Changes to author order after a manuscript is accepted for publication are discouraged. In limited situations, these may be justified and will require close communication with the editor as journals have varying policies on this issue.

DUPLICATE SUBMISSION

Whenever submitting a manuscript to a journal, you will be asked to confirm that the manuscript is not currently under review at another journal and that it has not been previously published in the same or a similar format. This may be a question encountered during the manuscript submission process or a required statement in the cover letter. Having a manuscript under review at more than one journal simultaneously is called duplicate submission. While it may be tempting to submit a manuscript to multiple journals to hedge your bets against rejection and seemingly gain some efficiency in the publication process, this is a serious ethical violation and must be avoided.

REDUNDANT PUBLICATIONS

Redundant publication involves two distinct scenarios: duplicate (or overlapping) publication and salami slicing. These are somewhat similar in that the motivation behind their use is often to increase the number of publications. Each is described in more detail in the following paragraphs. Redundant publications can have serious implications for the larger body of scientific literature.[41] For example, redundant publications can artificially inflate the number of studies on a given topic and potentially give undue weight to that evidence in meta-analyses or the development of practice guidelines.[36,42,43] In general, these should be avoided without clear justification and appropriate references across related papers.

Duplicate publication, also known as overlapping publication, is defined by the ICMJE as "the publication of a paper that overlaps substantially with one already published, without clear, visible reference to the previous publication."[4] Von Elm et al.[44] proposed different publication patterns that may represent overlapping publication: multiple reports of the same outcomes from the same study sample, reports of different outcomes from the same study sample (this is more akin to salami slicing discussed later), reports from of the same outcomes from a different study sample (e.g., adding or removing subjects, subgroup analyses), and reports of different outcomes from slightly different study samples. In all of these patterns, the study methods were the same, and there was overlap in the authors. The 2015 list of criteria to identify potential overlapping publications endorsed by an international group of cardiothoracic journal editors may also be helpful to consider: similar sample sizes, nearly identical study methods, similar results, at least one common author, and the report in question provides little or no new information.[45]

While duplicate or overlapping publication involves multiple publications from the same study with a substantial overlap of the content of the papers, **salami slicing** involves taking a project and separating it into separate papers (e.g., a separate paper for each research objective).[41,46] The challenge with salami slicing is that it may represent a necessary approach to managing the dissemination of a project's results. When projects have multiple objectives or research questions, authors sometimes encounter difficulty in fitting everything into one paper. As a hypothetical example, assume that you have conducted a project with four research objectives. The target journal you have identified has a strict word limit that prevents you from addressing all objectives in a single manuscript. After consultation with your research team, the first two objectives will be grouped and written separately from the second two objectives. This is not an uncommon problem for many researchers. Unfortunately, this can also be a slippery slope. The increasing pressures to publish peer-reviewed research in certain work settings, notably in academia, has given rise to the idea of the **least publishable unit** where research projects are viewed in terms of the smallest piece that can be published. The major concern when turning one research project into multiple papers is whether the separate pieces (or slices) can stand on their own as independent publications. If so, then separate publications may be acceptable.

Authors may often wonder what constitutes substantially similar or what counts as a previous publication. Journal guidelines are not always clear on these points.[46] It is best to avoid submitting a paper that contains information that has been published previously in full form. The ICMJE recommendations state that the presentation of results, in part or in whole, at a professional meeting should generally not prevent a journal from considering a manuscript.[4] The recommendations also clarify that sharing research through preprint servers and clinical trial registries does not meet the definition of a previous publication. Similarly, the submission of a final report to a funding agency or the submission of a written report or thesis as a degree requirement is not generally viewed as a formal publication.

It is important to note that this discussion of redundant publication is *not* intended to include **secondary publication**, which involves legitimate duplication. Publishing the translation of a paper from another language, republication of a historical work, and the simultaneous publication of a paper across multiple journals represent examples of secondary publication where the duplication is warranted and potentially beneficial. Secondary publication requires prior approval and coordination with the journal(s) involved.

When submitting a manuscript that contains a substantial amount of information that has been presented or published previously, it is vital to include references to demonstrate the link to any previous publication, presentation, or preprint. Similarly, when more than one paper is related to a single project, it is important to describe these relationships within the paper and include any references as appropriate. It is also important to disclose any information related to potential redundancy in the cover letter, as well as in the manuscript itself (e.g., as an acknowledgment or disclosure) to aid reviewers. Journal editors may even request the previous publications to be submitted to allow a more formal assessment of whether the additional publication is warranted.

Unfortunately, the redundant publication does not appear to be an altogether uncommon phenomenon.[44,47,48] Complete duplicate publication (i.e., publishing the exact same paper in more than one journal without prior approval or permission) is a particularly egregious violation since it likely violates copyright laws. Other forms of redundancy, such as publishing a reanalysis after adding new observations to or removing observations from a previous dataset, are generally viewed as unethical. Even with clear references to the related previous publications, authors should give serious consideration to whether the additional manuscripts stand on their own and advance the topic being studied.

PLAGIARISM

The concept of plagiarism is familiar to most individuals as this is a common topic of discussion for students when preparing term papers in high school and university. As Merriam-Webster defines it, to **plagiarize** is "to steal and pass off (the ideas or words of another) as one's own; use (another's production) without crediting the source."[49] The AMA style manual notes four kinds of plagiarism: direct plagiarism, mosaic (intermixing the original words with the author's own words), paraphrase, and insufficient acknowledgment.[26] In all these cases, appropriate attribution of the original source(s) could avoid plagiarism.

With few exceptions (e.g., published under certain open access agreements, certain works of government organizations), the journal, publisher, or professional society typically owns the copyright to any paper that it publishes. This means that plagiarism may also involve a violation of copyright laws. This is in addition to any local violations related to academic, scientific, or professional misconduct.

Another issue that has been proposed to fall under the umbrella of plagiarism is **text recycling**, which is the reuse of text from an author's own previous publications in a subsequent manuscript.[50] Some call this practice "self-plagiarism," but there is considerable debate around the appropriateness of that term.[50-52] It is important to note that this is not the same concept as duplicate or overlapping publications, as noted earlier. A good example of text recycling is when an author is publishing several studies from the same project. (In this case, we can assume that multiple papers are legitimate, so there are no issues with salami slicing.) Since the papers are based on the same methods and data set, there may only be so many ways that a certain research procedure can be described even with rephrasing (e.g., description of questionnaire development and administration, description of statistical procedures, statement of study design). Another example is when a researcher has conducted many studies within an area. Given the similarities in the studies over time, the same background information motivates the studies, so it may be difficult to rephrase previous wording. Guidance for journal editors on text recycling has been developed through a collaboration between BMC and the Committee on Publication Ethics (COPE). Determining when text recycling may be acceptable involves multiple considerations: the amount of text being use verbatim (e.g., one or two phrases or sentences vs. large blocks of text), where in the manuscript the reuse occurs (e.g., methods vs. results), the type of manuscript (research vs. nonresearch), cultural or disciplinary norms, the presence of appropriate attribution or citation, and potential breach of copyright.[53] Since text recycling is still the focus of much discussion in the realm of scholarly publication, authors are best served by trying to minimize text recycling as much as possible. When text is recycled, including a citation to the previous publication is crucial.

A relatively recent area of concern related to plagiarism is the use of preprint servers to share research prior to a peer-reviewed publication. As noted previously in duplicate publications, posting a paper to a preprint server is a legitimate and acceptable form of sharing. While posting a preprint may raise concerns for plagiarism checking software, clearly stating during submission that the paper was posted in preprint form and providing a link to the paper is usually sufficient.

CONFLICTS OF INTEREST

Trust in the biomedical research enterprise is important for the general public, healthcare professionals, and researchers. One way to facilitate that trust is clear disclosure and management of any potential conflicts of interest. Conflicts of interest have the potential to bias or otherwise adversely affect a researcher's attempt to be objective in their work.[26] Conflicts can be both financial, whether direct or indirect, or nonfinancial. Financial conflicts are more frequently discussed since they are likely the easiest to identify. Nonfinancial conflicts are more difficult to identify. For example, consider an author who holds an elected position or appointed membership on an oversight board for an organization. Neither of these positions comes with any compensation, but the organization's work may align with the research efforts of the author. It is possible that the organization could pressure the author to frame the results in a more positive light or even suppress publication altogether if the research results do not favor the work of the organization. Note how there is the potential for the author's actions to be biased through nonfinancial means.

It is not uncommon for pharmacy researchers to have funding from a biopharmaceutical company. Funding from an outside source, even industry, is not necessarily a conflict of interest. To help clarify this, you may be asked to disclose the role of the funder in the design, conduct, analysis, interpretation, and reporting of the study results or affirm that they had no role. There are often processes in place that serve to protect researchers and academic institutions and minimize the potential for conflicts or bias. This is especially true at academic institutions and healthcare institutions conducting research. As part of accepting any outside research support, funding agreements or contracts typically include clauses that allow the industry funder to review the final manuscript prior to submission to provide comments, but the terms of the agreement limit the amount of time the funder has to review (i.e., they cannot have the manuscript under review indefinitely as a way to suppress publication) and state that the final contents of the paper are the sole responsibility of the researchers (i.e., researchers may consider comments provided by the funder, but they are not required to make any changes). If there was no funding for the project being reported in your manuscript, you may be asked to state that explicitly.

The specific elements and processes of disclosing conflicts of interest vary across journals. It is important to consult the journal's website prior to submission. In cases where you have questions about whether a relationship, affiliation, or previous support, may rise to the level of a potential conflict of interest, it is best to disclose this and openly communicate with the journal editor(s) to determine how the potential conflict may be managed.

Submitting the Manuscript

Thankfully, the days of sending multiple hard copies of your manuscript to the journal via postal mail are gone. Almost all journals use online manuscript management systems to receive submissions, conduct the peer review process, and communicate with authors. The first step involves creating an account in the online system by following the appropriate links on the journal website. Look for links labeled "Author information" or "Submit your article." The online system will walk you through the required elements to create your account. This usually involves providing your name, degrees, institutional affiliation(s), mailing address, and personal experience keywords. This last element is important to complete since the journal may ask you to serve as a reviewer in the future. Some journals allow you to link your Open Researcher and Contributor ID (or ORCID iD; https://orcid. org), while others may require that you have an ORCID iD to submit a manuscript.

There is wide variability in the step-by-step process across these online systems, so be prepared to read carefully and follow the directions. It is important to have all documents finalized and ready *before* starting the submission process. Keep in mind that the exact sequence of steps may vary across journals.

The first step in submission typically involves providing basic information about the manuscript. This includes the title (and short title if required), abstract, and article keywords. Be sure to select keywords carefully since these will be used by the editors to identify potential reviewers. You may be asked to enter the authors next, even if the authors are already listed on the title page. It is important to ensure that the authors are listed in the appropriate order and that one is identified as the corresponding author. This individual will serve as the liaison between the journal and all manuscript authors and must be able to respond to any journal correspondence in a timely fashion.

The next step is to upload the manuscript. Some journals will request the manuscript in one complete file, including all tables and figures, while others want each element submitted separately. When submitting separate files, you may be asked to select the type of file (e.g., manuscript text, title page, table) and may be given the option to provide a brief description. Pay attention to acceptable file formats (e.g., *.DOCX or *.DOC files are acceptable while *.PDF files may not be).

One important consideration is the type of review process used by the journal. In double-blind review processes, authors may be asked to prepare two versions of the title page: one with the full author information and one that omits author names. Similarly, some journals require that any reference to the authors or institutions be removed from the text (e.g., replacing institution names with XXX, such as "the study was reviewed by the XXX Institutional Review Board") and possibly even from the references (e.g., replace a reference with a statement like "Redacted to maintain blinding"). Given the potential need to update your manuscript, it is strongly recommended that you consult the author guidelines early in the manuscript preparation process to determine if both a blinded and unblinded manuscript is required for initial submission.

You may also be asked to provide recommended reviewers during the submission process. Consider providing several individuals who have the expertise to review your manuscript and provide objective feedback. Do not suggest those to whom you have close personal connections (your mentor, a close friend you regularly conduct research with, etc.). You may also be asked to identify reviewers that you oppose or prefer *not* to review your paper. Consider listing individuals who may have potential conflicts (e.g., you have asked an individual to provide a prereview of your paper or somebody from whom you received feedback on the project in the early stages). This can be particularly helpful for editors when the paper is in a niche area and the editor may not understand connections among researchers. This is not an opportunity to list individuals because you think they may be too harsh.

After uploading all documents, manuscript management systems typically prepare a final, organized PDF for your review. It is important to review the document carefully to ensure that you have not omitted any necessary files and that the files you did upload are rendered correctly. Since it is common to have multiple versions of manuscript files, be sure to double-check that you have uploaded the correct versions. Also, ensure that your files do not have any embedded tracked changes or comments (i.e., upload a "clean" version, not the marked-up or redlined version). Once you have reviewed the PDF, you can approve it to finalize the submission. You, and perhaps your coauthors, will receive an email confirming the submission. Some journals will email coauthors with a request to verify their contribution to the manuscript and perhaps disclose any potential conflicts of interest (sometimes, this disclosure is done after manuscript acceptance). The corresponding author can check the manuscript status by logging into the journal's manuscript management system page. Journals vary on whether the correspondence is sent to the corresponding author only or all authors and whether authors other than the corresponding author can view the manuscript status. It is good practice for the corresponding author to keep all coauthors informed regarding the manuscript's status.

In situations where a revision is being submitted to the same journal, the process is similar to that of the initial submission. Remember to update the cover letter with any updated information. You should also include a clear response to each and every reviewer and editor comment. Journals may require this information to be copied into a separate field in the online submission system or included as a separate document during resubmission. In some cases, you may be asked for both a clean copy of the revised manuscript and a marked-up version highlighting the changes (i.e., the track changes version). This may be used by the editors or reviewers to clarify what was changed in the manuscript and where. If your manuscript was rejected from a journal and you decide to submit it elsewhere, remember to take the time to incorporate revisions based on reviewer comments. These are meant to improve your paper and may actually increase the chances of acceptance upon submission to another journal. You will then follow the same process to submit your manuscript to the new journal. More information on the peer-review process and responding to the editorial decision can be found in Chapter 25.

Exemplars of Learner Involvement in Research Manuscripts

Students, residents, fellows, and graduate students benefit greatly from "getting their hands dirty" in the writing process early in their careers. They can become more knowledgeable and confident in the process as they gain more experience. As authors of this chapter, we have had the opportunity to work with many learners over time. Preparation of research manuscripts and subsequent publication is an activity that is possible, even preferable, for learners to experience. Below are selected examples demonstrating our experiences when involving learners in writing and submitting research manuscripts.

At one chapter author's (JRC) institution, teams of pharmacy students participate in a five-week research advanced pharmacy practice experiences (APPEs) aimed to provide them with an introductory experience in the basics of research through execution of a project. This APPE provides hands-on experience for important parts of the process, including navigating the institutional review board (IRB), study design, data collection and analysis, use of varying types of software, and composition of abstracts, posters, and manuscripts. Faculty members work together to plan and prepare for the rotation and design the research objectives. The project highlighted here focused on the use of intravenous hydralazine and labetalol for the treatment of asymptomatic hypertension in hospitalized patients. The students and faculty executed the project together, which culminated in the preparation of a manuscript for publication. Students were provided foundational information on the general composition of systematic review manuscripts (similar to guidance in this chapter), and faculty worked with the team to help develop outlines to guide their composition. Authorship was discussed with the students prior to the decision to pursue publication, with the ultimate consensus made to list the students in alphabetical order as the first four authors, followed by the two supporting clinical faculty members, the health outcomes research faculty member supporting the project, and the lead clinical faculty member as the final and corresponding author. The students worked together to generate the first draft of the manuscript, which entered several phases of revision between faculty and students until it was deemed appropriate for submission. Students gained experience in the use of referencing software, the composition of tables, and technical writing throughout the process. As the first publishing experience for these students, the faculty members focused student efforts on the writing aspects of the process, as opposed to the technical aspects of submission and formatting. The manuscript was submitted for publication several months after completion of the research APPE since it required significant work to be completed by the team. Ultimately, the manuscript was returned from the journal with a decision to revise and resubmit. The faculty worked together with students on the project via email to address reviewer concerns and resubmit the manuscript, where it was ultimately accepted for publication.[54]

A second example involves the publication of a residency research project. Pharmacy residencies routinely require the completion of some sort of project. One chapter author (SEH) served as the research mentor for a community pharmacy resident. The project idea involved examining knowledge of used sharps disposal among patients. After several discussions among the resident, research mentor, residency preceptor, and program director, the decision was made to focus the project on patients with diabetes and the disposal of used insulin needles and lancets. As a residency project, the community pharmacy resident took primary responsibility for preparing a study protocol and submitting it for IRB approval. This was done under the supervision of the faculty research mentor. Throughout these early stages in the research process, the importance of gathering relevant background information and preparing useful descriptions in the study protocol and IRB documentation was emphasized as a way to make the final manuscript preparation easier. As with many residencies, the local program required the submission of a final project manuscript that was in publishable form; however, the manuscript did not necessarily need to be submitted. As part of the research process, the faculty mentor and resident had regular discussions about the intention to publish and the necessary effort required. The faculty mentor assisted the resident with the data analysis and framing of the results. The initial draft of the final paper was circulated within the research team that consisted of the resident, the site preceptor, a clinical faculty member in the area of diabetes, and the faculty research mentor falling in that order on the manuscript. After several rounds of revision within the team, the paper was ready to submit. During discussions with the resident, there was uncertainty about the ability to submit and respond to questions in a timely fashion due to changing jobs postresidency. The faculty mentor agreed to be the corresponding author with the understanding that the resident would stay in close contact. Although the paper was rejected by two journals, it was finally accepted.[55] This was an eye-opening experience for the resident to see the persistence needed to see a project through to final publication. The resident was still excited about the topic and was able to publish a continuing education article for the state pharmacy association on the same topic.[56] This was helpful to allow the resident to see the similarities and differences in the two types of writing and publishing processes.

Summary and Conclusions

While the process of preparing and submitting research manuscripts can seem daunting, this is certainly something that learners of all levels can do. There are many resources available to help guide the way. Leaning on the wisdom of mentors with experience is highly recommended as you start. As your career advances and you publish more, confidence in yourself and in navigating the process will undoubtedly grow. It helps to remember that even seasoned authors have to continue working to navigate the ever-changing process of manuscript preparation and submission. Despite these challenges, seeing your work culminate in a publication and adding to the body of literature that shapes the profession of pharmacy and patient care is certainly worth the effort.

Key Points and Advice

- The overall goal of a research manuscript is to describe important, interesting, contemporary, and relevant work to a target audience in a manner that is clear, compelling, and reproducible.
- ICMJE recommendations provide a key unifying framework for the publication process in biomedical fields.
- While many journals follow similar formats, processes, and standards for submission of manuscripts, it is paramount to carefully familiarize yourself with individual author guidelines for each journal you publish within.
- Authors need to take care to avoid ethical issues that can arise in the publication process, such as inappropriate authorship, plagiarism, undeclared conflicts of interest, and utilization of duplicate/overlapping manuscripts.

Chapter Review Questions

1. Briefly describe the main differences between original research articles and review articles.
2. What are the common sections of a research manuscript? Briefly describe the general content of each section.
3. Why is it important to carefully consider the selection of a potential journal for a research manuscript?
4. What are the main differences between the author-date and numerical referencing styles?
5. List three reporting guidelines or checklists and the type(s) of research which they support.
6. Why is redundant publication generally viewed as a potential ethical issue?
7. Describe the different considerations to discuss when deciding authorship order.
8. What are the different forms of guest authorship? Why are these considered unethical?

Online Resources

- *AMA Manual of Style: A Guide for Authors and Editors.* https://www.amamanualofstyle.com
- *Publication Manual of the American Psychological Association.* https://apastyle.apa.org

- *Scientific Style and Format: The CSE Manual for Authors, Editors, and Publishers.* https://scientificstyleandformat.org
- Purdue Online Writing Lab (OWL). https://owl.purdue.edu/
- Directory of Open Access Journals (DOAJ). https://doaj.org/
- Committee on Publication Ethics (COPE). https://publicationethics.org

REFERENCES

1. Dwan K, Altman DG, Arnaiz JA, et al. Systematic review of the empirical evidence of study publication bias and outcome reporting bias. *PLoS One.* 2008;3(8):e3081.
2. Fanelli D. Negative results are disappearing from most disciplines and countries. *Scientometrics.* 2012;90(3):891-904.
3. Sollaci LB, Pereira MG. The introduction, methods, results, and discussion (IMRAD) structure: a fifty-year survey. *J Med Libr Assoc.* 2004;92(3):364-367.
4. Recommendations for the conduct, reporting, editing, and publication of scholarly work in medical journals. International Committee of Medical Journal Editors. Published December 2018. Accessed February 17, 2021. http://www.icmje.org/recommendations/
5. Cals JWL, Kotz D. Effective writing and publishing scientific papers, part II: title and abstract. *J Clin Epidemiol.* 2013;66(6):585.
6. Lingard L. Bonfire red titles. *Perspect Med Educ.* 2016;5(3):179-181.
7. Sword H. *Stylish Academic Writing.* Cambridge, MA: Harvard University Press; 2012.
8. McGowan J, Tugwell P. Informative titles described article content. *J Can Health Libr Assoc.* 2005;26(3):83-84.
9. Writing articles for SEO. Wiley. Accessed February 17, 2021. https://authorservices. wiley.com/author-resources/Journal-Authors/Prepare/writing-for-seo.html
10. Beel J, Gipp B, Wilde E. Academic search engine optimization (ASEO): optimizing scholarly literature for Google Scholar & co. *Journal of Scholarly Publishing.* 2010;41(2): 176-190.
11. Schulz KF, Altman DG, Moher D, CONSORT Group. CONSORT 2010 statement: updated guidelines for reporting parallel group randomized trials. *Ann Intern Med.* 2010;152(11):726-732.
12. von Elm E, Altman DG, Egger M, et al. The Strengthening the Reporting of Observational Studies in Epidemiology (STROBE) statement: guidelines for reporting observational studies. *Epidemiology.* 2007;18(6):800-804.
13. Moher D, Liberati A, Tetzlaff J, Altman DG, PRISMA Group. Preferred reporting items for systematic reviews and meta-analyses: the PRISMA statement. *PLoS Med.* 2009;6(7):e1000097.
14. Lingard L. Joining a conversation: the problem/gap/hook heuristic. *Perspect Med Educ.* 2015;4(5):252-253.
15. Cals JWL, Kotz D. Effective writing and publishing scientific papers, part III: introduction. *J Clin Epidemiol.* 2013;66(7):702.

16. Kotz D, Cals JWL. Effective writing and publishing scientific papers, part IV: methods. *J Clin Epidemiol.* 2013;66(8):817.

17. Kotz D, Cals JWL. Effective writing and publishing scientific papers, part V: results. *J Clin Epidemiol.* 2013;66(9):945.

18. Cals JWL, Kotz D. Effective writing and publishing scientific papers, part VI: discussion. *J Clin Epidemiol.* 2013;66(10):1064.

19. Allen L, Scott J, Brand A, Hlava M, Altman M. Publishing: credit where credit is due. *Nature.* 2014;508(7496):312-313.

20. CRediT – Contributor Roles Taxonomy. National Information Standards Organization. Accessed February 19, 2021. http://credit.niso.org/

21. Solomon DJ, Björk B-C. A study of open access journals using article processing charges. *J Am Soc Inf Sci Tech.* 2012;63(8):1485-1495.

22. Budzinski O, Grebel T, Wolling J, Zhang X. Drivers of article processing charges in open access. *Scientometrics.* 2020;124(3):2185-2206.

23. Clay PG, Burns AL, Isetts BJ, Hirsch JD, Kliethermes MA, Planas LG. PaCIR: a tool to enhance pharmacist patient care intervention reporting. *J Am Pharm Assoc.* 2019; 59(5).

24. Viswanathan M, Kahwati LC, Golin CE, et al. Medication therapy management interventions in outpatient settings: a systematic review and meta-analysis. *JAMA Intern Med.* 2015;175(1):76-87.

25. Lang TA, Altman DG. Basic statistical reporting for articles published in clinical medical journals: the SAMPL guidelines. In: Smart P, Maisonneuve H, Polderman AKS, eds. *Science Editors' Handbook.* 2nd ed. Pau, France: European Association of Science Editors; 2013:175-182.

26. Christiansen SL, Iverson C, Flanagin A, et al. *AMA Manual of Style: A Guide for Authors and Editors.* 11th ed. Oxford, UK: Oxford University Press; 2020.

27. American Psychological Association. *Publication Manual of the American Psychological Association.* 7th ed. Washington, D.C.: American Psychological Association; 2020.

28. Riesenberg D, Lundberg GD. The order of authorship: who's on first? *JAMA.* 1990;264(14):1857.

29. Komperda KE, Griffin BL, Cryder BT, Schmidt JM, Reutzel TJ. Effects of a virtual writing club in a college of pharmacy. *Curr Pharm Teach Learn.* 2010;2(2):68-71.

30. Formatting your paper. BMJ Author Hub. Accessed February 19, 2021. https://authors. bmj.com/writing-and-formatting/formatting-your-paper/

31. Barnett A, Doubleday Z. The growth of acronyms in the scientific literature. *Elife.* 2020;9.

32. Cals JWL, Kotz D. Effective writing and publishing scientific papers, part VIII: references. *J Clin Epidemiol.* 2013;66(11):1198.

33. Kotz D, Cals JWL. Effective writing and publishing scientific papers, part VII: tables and figures. *J Clin Epidemiol.* 2013;66(11):1197.

34. Good PI, Hardin JW. *Common Errors in Statistics (and How to Avoid Them).* 4th ed. Hoboken, NJ: Wiley; 2012.

35. White SE, Dawson B, eds. *Basic & Clinical Biostatistics*. 5th ed. New York, NY: McGraw Hill Companies; 2020.

36. Roig M. Avoiding plagiarism, self-plagiarism, and other questionable writing practices: a guide to ethical writing. US Department of Health & Human Services, Office of Research Integrity. Accessed February 18, 2021. https://ori.hhs.gov/content/avoiding-plagiarism-self-plagiarism-and-other-questionable-writing-practices-guide-ethical-writing

37. Larkin M. Whose article is it anyway? *Lancet*. 1999;354(9173):136.

38. Sismondo S, Doucet M. Publication ethics and the ghost management of medical publication. *Bioethics*. 2010;24(6):273-283.

39. Greenland P, Fontanarosa PB. Ending honorary authorship. *Science*. 2012;337(6098): 1019.

40. Hughes MT. Are honorary authorships ethical? *Virtual Mentor*. 2009;11(4):279-283.

41. Henly SJ. Duplicate publications and salami reports: corruption of the scientific record. *Nurs Res*. 2014;63(1):1-2.

42. Tramèr MR, Reynolds DJ, Moore RA, McQuay HJ. Impact of covert duplicate publication on meta-analysis: a case study. *BMJ*. 1997;315(7109):635-640.

43. Melander H, Ahlqvist-Rastad J, Meijer G, Beermann B. Evidence b(i)ased medicine—selective reporting from studies sponsored by pharmaceutical industry: review of studies in new drug applications. *BMJ*. 2003;326(7400):1171-1173.

44. von Elm E, Poglia G, Walder B, Tramèr MR. Different patterns of duplicate publication: an analysis of articles used in systematic reviews. *JAMA*. 2004;291(8):974-980.

45. Kumar AS, Beyersdorf F, Denniss AR, Lazar HL, Patterson GA, Weisel RD. Joint statement on redundant (duplicate) publication by the editors of the undersigned cardio-thoracic journals. *Eur J Cardiothorac Surg*. 2015;48(3):343.

46. Ding D, Nguyen B, Gebel K, Bauman A, Bero L. Duplicate and salami publication: a prevalence study of journal policies. *Int J Epidemiol*. 2020;49(1):281-288.

47. Schein M, Paladugu R. Redundant surgical publications: tip of the iceberg? *Surgery*. 2001;129(6):655-661.

48. Cheung VWF, Lam GOA, Wang YF, Chadha NK. Current incidence of duplicate publication in otolaryngology. *Laryngoscope*. 2014;124(3):655-658.

49. Merriam-Webster Dictionary. Plagiarize. Merriam-Webster.com. Accessed February 17, 2021. https://www.merriam-webster.com/dictionary/plagiarize

50. Moskovitz C. Text recycling in scientific writing. *Sci Eng Ethics*. 2019;25(3):813-851.

51. Andreescu L. Self-plagiarism in academic publishing: the anatomy of a misnomer. *Sci Eng Ethics*. 2013;19(3):775-797.

52. Bruton SV. Self-plagiarism and textual recycling: legitimate forms of research misconduct. *Account Res*. 2014;21(3):176-197.

53. Text recycling guidelines for editors. Committee on Publication Ethics. Accessed February 17, 2021. https://publicationethics.org/resources/guidelines-new/text-recycling-guidelines-editors-0

54. Cawoski JR, DeBiasio KA, Donnachie SW, et al. Safety and efficacy of intravenous hydralazine and labetalol for the treatment of asymptomatic hypertension in hospitalised patients:
A systematic review. *Int J Clin Pract.* 2021:e13991.

55. Musselman KT, Sicat BL, Thomas MH, Harpe SE. Patients' knowledge of and practices
relating to the disposal of used insulin needles. *Innov Pharm.* 2010;1(2).

56. Musselman KT, Sicat BL, Herbert Thomas M, Harpe SE. Where does this used needle go?
Virginia Pharmacist. 2010;94(6):23, 25-27.

Chapter Twenty-Five

Peer Review and the Publication Process

Shane P. Desselle, RPh, PhD, FAPhA

Chapter Objectives

- Understand the methods of knowing
- Explain the peer review and the publication process
- Describe the roles of reviewers, associate editors, and editors-in-chief of a journal
- Discuss the types of peer reviews and elements of peer evaluation
- Understand best practices for responding to peer review comments
- Describe the decision-making process by the editor after peer evaluation
- Explain the production process, including indexing of the final publication

Key Terminology

Peer review, method of tenacity, method of authority, method of intuition, method of science, desk rejection, editorial board, handling editor, scholarly communication

Introduction

As a prospective author, you have undoubtedly learned much from other chapters in this book. You have considered your own interests, in addition to the topics and conundrums that behoove additional research; conducted appropriate literature review and appraisal; formulated testable hypotheses, selected the appropriate method (or combination of methods) and design; executed the research, analyzed the data, reached logical and defensible conclusions; and perhaps you have also shared the results in poster or presentation form at a conference. You have begun to prepare or at least have thought about how you will prepare a manuscript, particularly in accordance with the knowledge and wisdom provided to you in the previous chapter. As you begin to bring that publication plan to fruition, there are some additional elements to consider in maximizing your success in getting the paper published and also in bolstering the paper's impact following its publication, if indeed you have a good fortune (and skill and perseverance) to have made that happen.

This chapter will discuss these strategies, provide a historical account of peer review, how peer review has evolved into what it is currently, and how it coincides with the scientific process, in contrast with other methods of knowing, to advance knowledge. It will discuss peer-reviewing not only from a conceptual but also in a mechanistic way, i.e., the things that you do as an author and the things that reviewers and editors do. This chapter also features best practices for success in regard to each component of a manuscript through the eyes of editors and reviewers, as well as provides suggestions for revising manuscripts and handling rejection. It concludes with some discussion of things to do after your paper has been accepted, including boosting the paper's visibility and readership.

Peer Review: Historical Context

Dissemination of research findings through conference presentations and even more so through publication in peer-reviewed journals is at the crux of scholarly communication. Scholarly communication involves the publication and dissemination of findings from research abiding by the scientific process. Publishing in peer-reviewed journals represents not only our way of documenting what we have accomplished but the mechanism by which scientific knowledge is advanced as well. Conference presentations represent a way to communicate our findings (and our scholarly viewpoints) and particularly garner feedback to hone our message, have a sounding board from which to bounce ideas, and forge potential collaborations moving forward. However, beyond an abstract that might be published, there is little to actually document those findings so that researchers and other readers can apply them to practice or to future research. Research communicated at conference presentations and/or in peer-reviewed journals might also find its way into the lay press, professional media, and magazines, or other places in the grey literature, such as in technical reports, white papers, government documents, task force findings/proceedings, and other. This occurrence will depend on the topic and the field in which you work and might end up having a momentous impact in some form or another. The grey literature is not to be discounted and often should be searched as part of your literature review; however, publication in peer-reviewed journals is the primary currency by which we measure the productivity of a scholar and the primary means by which we advance knowledge in the field, as well as propel a discipline or entire profession forward.

In the midst of reading other chapters in this book, you have encountered the concept of peer review. Here, we discuss peer review in more detail and how it relates to your success in publishing and in your entire stream of research. Historically, perhaps the first documented description of a peer-review process is in a book called *Ethics of the Physician*.[1] This work stated that it was the duty of a visiting physician to make duplicate notes of the condition of the patient on each visit. When the patient had been cured or had died, the notes of that doctor were examined by a local council of physicians, who would adjudicate as to whether the doctor in question had performed according to the standards that then prevailed. A universal method for the generation and assessment of new science was enunciated by Francis Bacon in 1620. This work inspired many European scholars, some of whom engaged in an informal pattern of meetings to discuss and debate their varied views and opinions on emerging science.[2] In the mid-1800s, there was more journal space than there were articles to print. The primary responsibility of editorial boards was to solicit papers, and for the next century, peer-review mostly comprised the editors' and these boards' opinions.[2] It was the increasing diversity and specialization of material presented to journal editors that made it necessary for them to seek assistance outside that board. This happened at different times for different journals. *Science* and the *Journal of the American Medical Association* did not use outside reviewers until after 1940.[3] Around this time, the number of people working worldwide to generate new science increased considerably, so that the previous excess of space in journals vanished, and there was an increased need to be more discriminating as to what was published.

Peer review is the evaluation of work by one or more people with similar competencies as the producers of the work. It functions as a form of self-regulation by qualified members of a profession within the relevant field. Peer review methods are used to maintain quality standards, improve performance, and provide credibility.[4] Peer review serves as the backbone not only of journal publishing but also for the entire scientific process and all that it embodies. Peer review is used to discern the quality of grant applications and the basis by which to award funding, determine the papers prioritized for presentation at conferences, awards given to scientists, and even in discerning the quality of teaching in institutions of higher learning. This is due at least in part to the recognition of the peer review process as being tantamount to adjudication of questions of rigor, quality, and objectivity.[5] Having experts in the field often (though not always) blinded to the identity of the contributor(s)/author(s), whose recommendations are weighed by a panel, an editor, or some other authority, is a process that inherently improves the quality of information and the processes used to generate that information, even if biases inherent to any human process render it imperfect.[6]

Methods of Knowing and the Scientific Process

As peer review serves as the backbone of scientific inquiry, it is important to understand more about science as a "method of knowing" versus other methods. It is argued that there are four basic ways of knowing—(1) the method of tenacity, (2) the method of authority, (3) the method of intuition, and (4) the method of science.[7]

The **method of tenacity** refers to the fact that people hold to certain beliefs because they have always "known" these beliefs to be true, whether actually true or not. When people believe in something, they look for evidence to confirm that belief and ignore disconfirming instances, thus reinforcing confirmation bias. Even in the face of facts to the contrary, they hold tenaciously to their beliefs and build new knowledge from assumptions that might be false. The **method of authority** is that which is derived from experts in the field. Individuals turn to those in authority positions for knowledge and truth, for example, from education, business, clergy, and others. It might appear superior to the method of tenacity; after all, those in authority presumably acquired such a position at least in part due to knowledge and wisdom. However, some persons in authority have tendencies to project greater knowledge or convey information outside of their more immediate expertise and will also have their own biases.[8] Additionally, there is always some debate as to whom persons should turn with respect to authority, or which individuals are in fact, the most authoritative in a given subject. Some might assume someone is a source of authority due to a position they hold; however, these persons are not necessarily the most knowledgeable on a given topic. The **method of intuition** is a method of knowing that is built on assumptions that are obvious or deemed self-evident. They may agree with a reason (logic) but not necessarily with experience (and thus, truth). The idea seems to be that individuals can discover the truth by using reason and logic because there is a natural inclination toward truth. However, this method of knowing is as limited as the person behind the reasoning. Two very sincere and intelligent persons can come to completely opposite conclusions about a given problem or phenomenon. For much of the history of mankind, for example, it was regarded as self-evident that the earth was flat because it "stood to reason."

The **method of science**, or reflective inquiry, requires investigation, critical thinking, and discourse to support the most reliable way of knowing. It provides a means to affix data and findings in such a way that the "ultimate conclusion of every man must be the same . . . There are real things, whose characters are entirely independent of opinions about them."[9] Thus, the scientific approach has two unique characteristics absent in the other methods of knowing. Science is self-critical and self-correcting, i.e., the "reflective" component of reflective inquiry. It has within it safeguards to verify procedures and produce dependable and reproducible outcomes. Even if a hypothesis is supported, the researcher is skeptical and seeks rival hypotheses in an attempt to find counterexamples and refine the findings.

When using the scientific approach, no explanation is final because a better one may be devised at any time; science is open. Nothing is irrevocably proved; in fact, those with a scientific temper stay clear of the term "proved"; instead, they suggest that currently, the evidence supports the conclusion. Incidentally, suggesting that your research proves something or speculating on implications beyond what you have tested not only violates the very nature of science but also is likely to lessen your paper's likelihood of publication. Thus, the scientist employs a stance that is impersonal, external, and even "disinterested," which thus fosters greater objectivity.[10]

OBJECTIVITY AND PEER REVIEW

While perhaps not possible to attain complete objectivity, it is the aim of science (and the scientist) to do so. Scientists attempt to design their research such that the methods are apart from themselves, their influence, their predilections, and their biases. The goal is to find a method of knowing that stands the test of independence from the researcher—in other words, one that is objective such that any observer with minimum competence will agree on a study's observation and its findings. The study's results are said to be reproducible. When researchers carry out their studies, they aim for objectivity by making their procedures, measures, and controls clear, explicit, and replicable, even while this often is more challenging in the behavioral and even clinical sciences than in the physical sciences.[10,11] Objectivity is more a characteristic for a procedure or process than it is a description for individual researchers. Peer review brings that into focus by the careful evaluation of scientific work by impartial referees who discern not only the quality of the work, but its clarity and contribution to the known world, or extant literature. Peer review serves as the ultimate judge insomuch as these impartial evaluators often work independently of one another in deriving conclusions about the work under question, and whose similarities and differences in opinion are adjudicated by the editor, editorial board, or some other body. Peer review does have its critics, and many point to the need for reforms. Even the fundamental basis of "when do we know what we know?" has been questioned.[12] This will be addressed; however, doing so first merits a deeper exploration into the concept and process(es) of peer review itself.

Peer Review: Journal Workflow

While each peer-review journal and other peer review mechanisms (e.g., for awards, grants, teaching) might have some varied particulars for its conduct, the overall process is quite similar conceptually (see Figure 25–1). An author(s) submits their paper to the journal, and it is received by an editor. Some journals are large and have an editor-in-chief (EIC) along with managing or deputy editor(s). In this case, the EIC often makes overarching policy decisions and sets the direction for the journal, in addition to other administrative tasks such as negotiating publication rights with conferences, dealing with the journal's publishing company, and soliciting feedback from key stakeholders in the scientific community. The EIC might field papers initially for handoff to one of the managing or

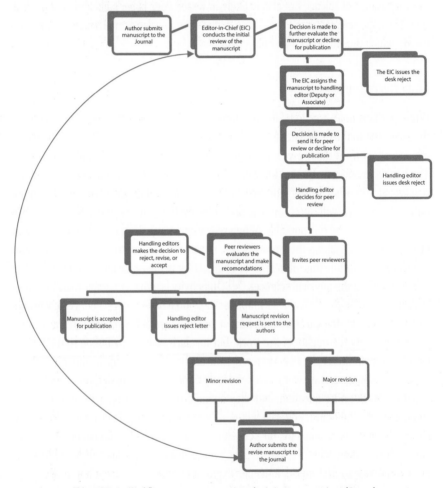

Figure 25–1. Workflow process—manuscript submission to peer-reviewed journal.

deputy editors, particularly if the journal's total volume of papers and its scope of topics might be expansive. Otherwise, papers might come directly to a managing or deputy editor. The workflow of a journal will determine these processes. Most journals are large enough to where there are also associate editors. Associate editors often will be the ones who ultimately "handle" a submission, whether that submission is assigned by the EIC or by a deputy/managing editor. Thus, the associate editor or whoever is assigned that paper might be referred to as the "handling editor," which is not a title but who, on an individual basis, is responsible for seeing the paper through the process. Depending on the journal's workflow, the EIC, managing/deputy, or associate editor can offer a **desk rejection** of the paper, meaning that the paper has been precluded from further consideration for publication without peer review. Reasons for a desk rejection, along with rejection following review, are addressed later in this chapter.

Most journals also have an editorial advisory board or simply "editorial board." **Editorial boards** of a journal offer expert advice on content, policy, and scope, and other activities to strengthen and promote the journal. The boards vary in size and level of responsibility. Editorial board members for most journals, at the minimum, can expect to conduct several peer reviews per year during their term on the board, which might range from one to two up to several years. Editorial board members, in fact, may be selected at least in large part due to their own contributions as an author and for the quality of their reviews undertaken for that journal prior to becoming a member of the editorial board. Editorial board members might also be asked to weigh in on certain policy and strategic positions of the journal as well as to recruit and solicit papers and advocate for the journal. Some editorial board members of certain journals might be asked to serve on an ad hoc committee.[13]

Peer Review: The Process

When a paper is submitted, appropriate personnel with the journal (usually the editor-in-chief) is/are notified through the journal's electronic platform using automated email messaging. Depending upon the workflow, the editor either handles the submission or assigns it to an associate or deputy editor if the paper is not desk rejected by the chief editor. The **handling editor** is the person who will seek peer reviews and use those make recommendations from peer reviewers in making a publication decision; that is, whether or not to pursue publication, often in revised form. Depending upon the journal, the handling editor might also have the prerogative to render a desk rejection without seeking peer review. The handling editor will typically use the assistance offered by the journal's electronic platform, which offers various services such as identification of similar papers previously published and/or providing directly the names of individuals with similar areas of expertise as those in which the paper resides. Nonetheless, the handling editor often will also use some intuition, know which peer reviewers are "good" reviewers and which will have particular expertise in another facet of the paper. For example, the paper's study might employ a certain type of statistical procedure wherein the handling editor might seek someone with expertise in use of that procedure, or in statistics, in general.

The handling editor will call upon the journal's editorial advisory board more frequently to serve as peer reviewers. The handling editor will balance the need for various types of expertise and also other considerations, such as whether a potential reviewer has previously published with the journal. The handling editor will invite reviewers through the journal's platform and usually seek two to three reviewers, depending upon journal policy and the type of submission category (i.e., whether the paper is original research, an editorial, letter, commentary, review, or other). The handling editor will typically have to input replacement reviewers should initially invited reviewers to decline or fail to respond. The handling editor will then, through the journal's electronic platform, perhaps send out reminders to those accepting the invitation to review every so often so as to try to keep the schedule. Depending upon the journal, reviewers might be given three to six weeks to submit their review. When all the peer reviews have been submitted, the handling editor is notified, and then they will study the reviewers' recommendations and make a decision. The reviewers will have likely submitted both qualitative comments as well as a recommendation to pursue publication with either minor or major revisions. The handling editor will either reject the paper or pursue a publication of a revised version of the paper, provide the reviewers' comments in the decision letter, and might add comments of their own.

The authors will be given a date by which to address the comments and recommendations of the reviewers in a revised draft and also to point out in a letter notifying the editor and reviewers of the changes/edits they made to the paper, offering a response to each of the reviewers' recommendations. Of course, authors might feel as though they are unable to address all the comments and withdraw the paper to submit it elsewhere. More often than not, authors will attempt to address the reviewers' comments and submit a revised paper. The handling editor will then decide if the paper is to be published as-is, possibly reject (less likely at this point), or pursue another round of peer review, usually by the same, but sometimes by different persons, particularly if the initial reviewers are not available. This iterative process might end at this point with an accept decision, or it could go on for another round or two.

Peer Review: Types of Submissions

Many of the journal submissions are research papers, or perhaps a category within an original research paper such as a brief report, research note, or methods paper. Some journals publish research protocols or similar such, wherein the manuscripts describe the impending conduct of a competitively funded study or trial. Other types of papers may include reviews, either systematic or narrative or scoping, thus not necessarily inclusive of the entire literature and aiming more toward a general description of the topic of interest.[14] Also, journals might publish letters to the editor, often in response to a paper previously published, editorials that signify a succinct opinion or call to action, and also perhaps extended commentaries which take a scholarly approach to evaluating a particular phenomenon or topic of interest with greater depth of treatment than a letter or editorial. More information on the type of manuscript categories can be found in the previous chapter of this text.

Peer Review: Mechanics

Regardless of submission type, except for perhaps some editorials and letters to the editor, your submission will likely undergo the process of peer review if it does indeed make it past the hurdle of an editor's desk rejection. While potential pitfalls for rejection of the paper will be discussed later, it is worth mentioning here that desk rejections are likely to occur if the lack of quality or scientific rigor in the methods and/or paper is readily apparent if the writing is of very poor quality if the topic does not fit within the scope of the journal, and/or there are many errors either typographical in nature or via the paper not conforming to journal stylistic guidelines. The number of papers submitted to most pharmacy journals continues to be on the upswing, and editorial staff and peer reviewers are stretched thin. If a paper appears as though it is simply too much of a project for the editorial staff or that the errors convey an air of sloppiness or lack of diligence, the paper might likely meet the unwanted fate of a desk rejection, thus not even acquiring the beneficial feedback of peer review.

Journal editors will often seek two to four reviewers for your paper, depending on the journal, type of submission, and availability of reviewers. These are mostly gathered upfront; however, journals might acquire an additional reviewer if there is no clear-cut recommendation for the handling editor from the recommendations of the initial reviewers. Editors often seek a review from at least one member of their editorial board as well as a review from someone outside the board with particular expertise in the subject matter of interest. Reviews might be sought from persons with different sets of expertise for a particular paper so as to cover various aspects. For example, a paper describing the validation of a new instrument to measure health-related quality of life in diabetes patients might solicit peer reviews from a clinician with expertise in diabetes, someone well versed in psychometrics or measurement so as to discern the rigor and quality of the methods used, and perhaps an expert specifically in quality of life measurement, statistical analysis, or some other aspect of the paper.

Peer reviewers are usually given two to four weeks to submit their completed reviews; however, some reviewers will be late. Additionally, it is becoming more difficult and time-consuming for editors to acquire peer reviewers. As such, you might expect to wait at least several weeks or months before you hear back from the journal with an initial decision; however, the amount of time it takes can vary quite a bit by journal or sometimes by the time of the year, the nature of your paper's topic, and sometimes other circumstances beyond any one person's control.

Peer Review Recommendations and the Editorial Decision

Authors might be surprised by the feedback they receive from peer reviewers, and that underscores the strength of the peer review system because, as an author, you have come to see the project and paper with your vision, appreciation for, and level of understanding of the research and topic area. However, even venerable scholars might not see it so clearly in their minds and usually can offer substantial recommendations for how the paper might be made better, stronger, clearer, better organized, less speculative, or inclusive of additional tests and considerations. Thus, it is easy to become "lost" in your work without seeing the proverbial forest through the trees. And peer reviewers can help.

Peer reviewers are often asked to provide quantitative and qualitative feedback. The quantitative feedback might include their responses to scaled questions regarding various aspects of the paper, such as its scope, study design and methods, breadth of literature review, appropriate analysis plan, discussion, and conclusions. They will also make a recommendation as to whether the paper should be rejected or pursued for publication following appropriate revisions. The ratings might assist the editor; however, more can be gleaned by the author from the reviewers' qualitative feedback. It is here that peer reviewers proffer recommendations and questions to the author for improving the paper. Some journals have provided their own commentary, well beyond instructions for authors found on nearly every journal's website, with an aim to assist both peer reviewers and authors. For example, the Journal of Clinical Epidemiology provides a rather comprehensive guide to conducting a proper peer review that includes considerations/actions prior to getting started; the structure of the review; general rules for good reviews; and a final check on items such as overall strength of the paper, the relevance of the research question, important discussion points, and data-supported conclusions.[15] This resource provides reviewers with excellent direction on providing specific comments to improve a paper rather than making generally negative statements upon which the authors cannot really take substantive action. A pharmacy journal published a paper on what peer reviewers often look for, what they should be looking for, how they should comport themselves, and thus how authors can anticipate potential pitfalls and ways to make their paper as strong as possible upon submission.[16] Following are some recommendations for consideration by authors as acquired from this resource:

JOURNAL SELECTION

Select the most appropriate journal and type of submission for your paper. Balance your potential desire to publish in a journal with the highest impact versus the journals' aims/scope and its readership. While it is a good idea to identify reputable journals with at least a fair amount of impact (as per its impact factor score[17]), the best strategy is not necessarily one where you identify the journal with the highest impact, without a really good fit. An impact score is a measure of the frequency with which the average article in a journal has been cited in a particular year. It is used to measure the importance or rank of a journal by calculating the times its articles are cited and is often the currency used to measure a journal's clout, even in spite of the limitations associated with calculating an index of any sort. So, while an author would like their work published in a reputable journal, seeking the one with the highest impact without regard to fit and most appropriate audience (readership) reached is counterproductive. Moreover, if a paper is rejected, you can and most likely will submit it elsewhere, which is perfectly acceptable. However, the "pharmacy world" is a small one, and there are only so many experts in a given area. It is not uncommon for two different journals to seek the same reviewers. If a reviewer sees the paper has been submitted elsewhere and rejected, particularly if you made no changes to the paper-based upon the initial journal's review, then the likelihood of rejection at the second journal rises dramatically. After two to three rejections, a paper begins to carry a certain stench with it. While the presence of Google Scholar and other services are to at least an extent obviating the necessity of highly regarded indexing services, it still is important to identify a journal that is indexed in the type of databases that you want people to find your article should they be conducting a search of your paper's topic, or a similar one.

PRE-SUBMISSION

Competition for journal space, especially in clinical and social pharmacy, has become increasingly fierce. Besides assuring proper fit, make sure that your paper comports with the journal's stylistic guidelines and considerations. Authors should understand that, for the most part, journals receive a relatively small proportion of papers that are absolutely outstanding. They receive a larger but still not majority of papers that are very weak scientifically and will invariably face desk rejection. Many submissions are within a certain range of quality. Thus, the "competition" between them for journal space is tightly contested, and sometimes not paying attention to "the little things" such as failure to comport with the journal's stylistic considerations, or submitting a paper with "adequate" scientific merit but rife with errors can spell its doom.

INTRODUCTION/BACKGROUND

This section, which may include the stated objectives/hypotheses, is often said to be the most difficult to write, since the methods are a factual account of what processes you undertook in executing the project, and the results are also *relatively* straightforward. Peer reviewers will be looking for you to have established a compelling rationale for the study's conduct, i.e., that the answers to questions you raise merit deriving an answer and that those answers have not already been reported elsewhere. They are also looking for concise, cogent, and well-organized background material that appropriately establishes your study by providing the right context for study objectives/hypotheses. A mistake that even experienced authors make is to include additional material not entirely germane to the research question(s), and this might begin as soon as the opening statement of the paper. For example, a paper on the need to establish a new health-related quality of life (HRQoL) instrument for patients with diabetes need not and SHOULD NOT begin with a discussion of the incidence, prevalence, and extraordinary morbidity of diabetes and it is a "worldwide problem." This type of information can be found in any tertiary source or even quite easily from the internet, on such sources even like Wikipedia. Rather, the opening sentence should be more straightforward and state to the effect that existing measures of HRQoL for diabetes patients have shortcomings that limit their viability and applicability, while the remainder of the introduction expounds upon that narrow but salient focus in establishing the study's objective(s). In regard to the study objectives, there is no rule for the number of them, but an original research paper will probably have two to four. The objectives should be clear and written in a manner so that they suggest being testable. They are to be concise and specific as to what you are attempting to accomplish and not overstate your endeavor or what problems/questions you aim to solve/answer.

METHODS

As mentioned previously, some might argue this is the "easiest" component to write. Indeed, there are probably fewer word choice nodes and less conjecture and ambiguity inherent to writing the methods section. However, it should be noted that this section often drives reviewer recommendations in pursuit of publication. Not only should the methods be sound and appropriately rigorous to include validity, reliability, and entrust ability checks where appropriate, but the manner in which you communicate these should also be clear. A reviewer "frustrated" after reading the methods section several times and still unclear on precisely what was done might offer you the benefit of the doubt and request further clarification; however, if there are substantial problems here and particularly if there are other problems with the paper, a "reject" recommendation is likely forthcoming. The methods section should clearly delineate various components, i.e., the design of the study, the methodological procedures undertaken, and the analysis plan, perhaps in addition to how the methods comport with foundational principles or theory upon which they were framed. An appendix illustrating a copy of a survey used, a focus group interview guide, a flow chart for a review, data fields for a secondary base research project, or similar is generally appropriate to include and can always be removed later upon request. Some authors make the mistake of failing to articulate the analysis plan, then write the results section with myriad "p-values," thus leaving reviewers scratching their heads. A good principle to follow is that the analysis plan describes which tests will be used to discern the specific objectives/hypotheses described in the introduction section.

RESULTS

The results section likewise appears to be straightforward, and it should be if we do not allow ourselves to get overly distracted or over-awed with ourselves for all the numbers that we could putatively proffer. Again, in keeping your paper on track, cogent, and clear, it is good practice to provide the results according to the objectives. So again, objectives are presented in the introduction, the data analysis plan discusses the specific statistical tests and thresholds used to discern those results, and the results section states very clearly the results of those tests corresponding to the particular objectives. Reviewers are looking to see if you have addressed the study objectives. The presentation of results from tests not in the analysis plan, an overabundance of p-values, and ex post facto hypothesizing (e.g., "we have the data, so here are some more tests—why not?") will not be met with enthusiasm by reviewers; rather, they detract from the paper's clarity, and reviewers will almost invariably accuse you of throwing up everything possible onto the wall to see what sticks. Clarity is the key, and to the extent possible, notwithstanding limits on such, the results of tests should be placed in clearly illustrated tables that are titled appropriately and just briefly highlighted in the text portion of the manuscript.

DISCUSSION AND CONCLUSIONS

There are a number of ways to "tackle" the discussion section. However, some basic guidance exists that should, in large part, be followed. The discussion can begin with a brief summary of the principal findings and the extent to which the objectives were met and hypotheses tested. The critical part of the discussion is providing the proper context for the results. It is not uncommon (though not mandatory) for a discussion section to have as many or even more references as the introduction. The results should be compared and contrasted with similar studies and with studies showing a different but related angle of the same phenomenon of interest. Peer reviewers are looking for the unique contribution made by your study, so contextualizing it against what is already known and what it adds to the extant knowledge is absolutely paramount. That being said, a common mistake by authors is to go off on unrelated tangents and speculate what their findings MIGHT mean and then cite unrelated literature. Another common mistake is to overstate the findings. Remember, there have been literally millions of papers published, and many of them very good papers. The idea that your paper should somehow end the need for additional research and solve all problems borne of the profession or society is not only fallacious but also narcissistic. Reviewers will be quick to catch you on that. To that end, the best research papers are those that answer a very limited set of questions then raise additional ones for further testing. Those questions should be raised and might be included in a strong limitations section that cautions readers about the caveats to be taken into account when they are attempting to glean what they can from the results and perhaps extrapolate them. Finally, the conclusion section places into a final paragraph or two the nature of the study, its critical findings, and salient points for learning from it and in moving forward. It does not simply rehash the results and certainly does not introduce new concepts and likely should avoid additional citations. Also, it is important to avoid statements like the research being "the only one" to have done (so-and-so) and avoid using adjectives and superlatives about the uniqueness and quality of the work. In fact, adjectives should be used quite judiciously throughout a research paper. Let the reader make their own judgment about the salience and contribution of your work.

In addition to these suggestions, other pharmacy journals have opined on the peer review system and best practices for reviewers and authors.[18-22] These papers offer criticisms of how the peer review system can be improved, and there are journals now beginning to offer more recognition of reviewers, as well as even list them post-publication as helping to shape the paper, and fewer still offering at least nominal remuneration for their service. However, while evolving, the peer-review system as described in this chapter should provide you a good sense of how the mechanism works. It should also be noted that journals, and in particular pharmacy journals, are doing more and more to make their mechanisms as transparent as possible and publishing more papers from their editorial staff to offer guidance on specifically what they are looking for, ranging from topics and helpful hints, even as specific as to how to report the findings of statistical procedures.[23,24]

All of this should be helpful to authors and even to reviewers. Following the process, ultimately the handling editor will make a publication decision, which is very rarely "accept as is," but perhaps the pursuit of publication with revisions, or unfortunately, rejection. The editor will base this decision in large part on the recommendations of the reviewers. Editors will seldom reject a paper if all reviewers recommended the pursuit of publication, and likewise will seldom pursue publication if all reviewers recommended rejection. However, it is possible that they do so. For example, if reviewers recommended rejection due to lack of clarity in the paper or some other reason that the editor deems can be addressed in a revision, the editor might still pursue it. Or, if reviewers point out a "fatal flaw" but still suggest that the paper is "salvageable," the editor might disagree and reject it. All of this comes especially into play when there is not a consensus among reviewers; i.e., that one to two of the three to four who have reviewed it comes up with different recommendations for the pursuit of publication, even if they found similar strengths and weaknesses in the study and its resultant manuscript.

The editor will consider these in light of other environmental issues. It is folly to think that a journal's decision on a particular paper would be the same if the same paper were submitted at some other time. Journals sometimes face a backlog of accepted papers, have an extraordinary number of papers recently submitted, and at times might be looking to shape a particular direction in which they intend to evolve. These conditions will impact the likelihood of success of a paper. Recall earlier in the chapter when it was stated that many papers fall into a category where they could be accepted or rejected and thus "straddle the fence." This underscores the need for the paper to conform to stylistic considerations, be well written, and pose a unique contribution to the literature, as it is more likely to be on the positive side of said fence. That is why it is also important to establish a positive rapport with a journal and its editorial staff. Journals will not willfully publish bad research nor reject really good papers. But again, for those straddling the fence, it does make a difference, i.e., provide a more positive inclination for editors, if you have reviewed papers for them when invited, been timely with your communications, including your peer reviews of others' work, and have maintained professional comportment and demeanor with editorial staff and perhaps even advocated for the journal through word of mouth and on social media. Again, this is not a matter of a quid pro quo, but "doing all the little things" that help tilt the odds in your favor.

Moving Past the Editor's Decision: Revising a Manuscript

If you have the good fortune of being invited to submit a revised paper, there are few things to note in maximizing the likelihood of success. For one, read all of the comments from the reviewers and think about them as a whole. Our egos dictate our thinking that the paper we submitted is near perfect. In an attempt to assuage our ego, it is tempting to isolate each comment from each reviewer and get defensive or angry, calling the comments "nit-picky" or assuring ourselves that the reviewer(s) "just don't get it." For sure, reviewers can make errors and be predisposed to any of various negative biases just like anyone else can. But in all likelihood, the reviewers took the time (usually at least several hours or more, unpaid, as a service) to think about your paper very conscientiously and provide recommendations on how you might improve it. Rather than focusing on each comment initially, stand back and look at the sum of those comments and attempt to discern what they tell you. Perhaps greater clarity is needed in some sections, as things apparent to you IN YOUR MIND were not necessarily made that clear to a first-time reader. Look for commonalities in the reviewers' recommendations, even if they expressed them in different ways. Thus, strategize on revisions, sometimes even small tweaks that you can make to the paper that will assuage more than one reviewer and even several comments, concomitantly. Sometimes even the deletion of a few sentences or a couple of paragraphs that, upon further thought, are either extraneous or were written poorly can provide greater clarity and focus, and thus address several reviewer comments and concerns with merely a few keystrokes (or use of the cut or delete button). Again, think about the gestalt of the reviews and how you might make modifications that affect the entire tone of the paper. Let the comments percolate for a bit prior to addressing each one of them. Some might argue to make the little fixes first, but in addressing the gestalt of the comments with some modest modifications, some of the little fixes will have inherently been remedied. As you are addressing the comments in a revision, think about how defensible your changes are and how you are going to describe them to the editor. If you cannot in good faith provide an excellent defense of the changes you are making (or not making), then you need to rethink how, or what remedies you are proffering to improve the paper.

In some cases, you will have evidence on your side that a recommended change is unnecessary or even ill-advised, for it might actually weaken rather than strengthen the paper. In this case, you will need to prepare a carefully worded and thoughtful "defense" of why you are not making the changes, conducting additional tests, or whatever was recommended; however, even if not making a major change, it might be wise to offer in the paper, itself (not just in your response to the recommendations) some new language that might make a particular point more clear. When opting not to make changes, it is often a good idea to provide citations and the best evidence possible as to why those recommended changes would not strengthen the paper.

The letter of response you provide to a journal to accompany your revised submission can greatly impact your likelihood of success for publication. Best practices would indicate that you list each point/recommendation/criticism of every reviewer and provide a response. Indicate what you have done to comply or comport with their recommendation, thank them for pointing out issues and statements you have made in the paper where a fix greatly improved the paper's clarity and strength. Provide evidence when you did not make a change, and through it, all, be very professional and courteous. It might be tempting to do otherwise. Even if a reviewer happened to be unkind or unprofessional, doing the same in return will not curry you any favors with the editor nor with other reviewers should the editor decide to send it for the second round of review. Even though your paper might not get subjected to the second round of review and might be accepted (or rejected) by the editor upon the submission of your revision, you should write the letter with the expectation that it will be.

There are many other tips and strategies for success in publishing a particular paper and for publishing, in general. Authors should seek counsel from well-published authors and mentors, but understand if their availability is limited. Be professional, courteous, and patient. Occasionally, a paper might "slip through the cracks," but generally, multiple emails to the editor if a paper's decision is running behind or later than your expectation for a decision will not bode well. When you are prepared to submit, carve out some time. It will take a while to go through the process of submitting, even if you have all the necessary documents aligned and in the right format, including the title page, cover letter, appendices, and so on. Avoid working feverishly at late hours, Friday evenings, and so on merely to get the submission "off your plate." This usually results in errors on your part during the process that makes your submission all the less impressive. Be aware that journals might take longer to render a decision if you submit at certain times, such as during the Holiday season, or perhaps in the middle of summer when many prospective reviewers might be on vacation.

Moving Past the Editor's Decision: Facing a "Reject" Decision

Invariably, even the best researchers and writers face a reject decision on occasion. This is an opportunity for further growth, development, and decision making. One highly ranked journal conducted an analysis of the Ovid database to determine the fate of papers they rejected and found that 47% had been published elsewhere, which they estimated to be lower than the true proportion, given that some papers will have been published in journals not indexed in Ovid.[25] A rate of publication exceeding 50% for initially rejected papers has been further confirmed, with the additional note that in the end, papers are improved as a result of rejection, and that persistence of authors indeed pays off.[26] Along with persistence, effective coping with rejection, resilience, and learning from your mistakes are key not only in getting that particular paper published but also in having a successful and productive career.[27] Indeed, research has uncovered that persons facing rejection of their manuscript or grant application handle this rejection in highly varied ways, and mechanisms of coping can mean the difference between a venerable and decorated researcher versus someone who has completely abandoned an academic and/or research career, entirely.[28]

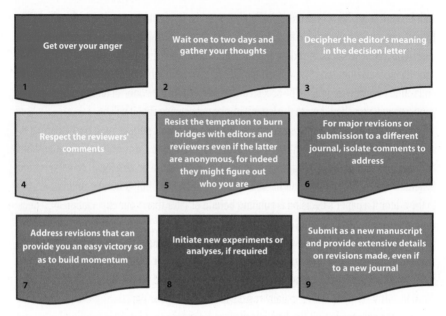

Figure 25–2. A "Step Program" of coping with a "Major Revision" or "Reject" decision.

Assuming that an author will choose to submit the paper elsewhere, the author of this chapter has long proposed a "step program" of coping (see Figure 25–2). These steps assume that you will pay mind to the reviewers' recommendations even though you are submitting them elsewhere. Again, one of the reviewers might end up being the same who reviewed the previous submission elsewhere, and journal editors will actually look upon favor the idea of you expressing candor in the paper having been rejected elsewhere and what you have done to address the reviewers' comments from that first journal. In fact, some journals are now requesting this sort of information (i.e., past history) for papers that you newly submit to them. Humility throughout the entire process will enable you to do this without a problem, and humility meshes quite well with persistence and resilience.

Post Acceptance of Your Paper

On a more positive note, you may have found yourself with the good fortune of having your paper accepted for publication. Currently, most journals publish electronically, even while some of the more traditionally established and venerable journals also publish a hard copy or at least a digital version of a hard copy. As such, you might expect a digital copy of your article out perhaps even as quickly as a few weeks from its acceptance. In fact, some journals are now publishing uncorrected proofs of your paper even within days after its acceptance for publication.

As such, it is important that you try to have your paper looking as polished as possible in what you might anticipate is its final round of revision. Further, you certainly want to look carefully over galley proofs offered you by the publisher. The galley proofs look much the same as the actual article will appear in print and/or online. There will likely be minor author queries for you to attend, and your delay in responding to those will only serve to delay the publication of your paper. Unfortunately, some authors just address those queries and do not take a really close look at the paper during the galley proofing stage. In spite of all the channels and hoops that the paper has gone through, there still can be errors in the final paper, ranging from a typographical one to even having a co-author's name or institution, title, or degrees misspelled. An error could possibly detract from the quality of the paper, though probably not at this stage. It could result, however, in an embarrassing or uncomfortable situation if someone's name has been misspelled, an acknowledgment was not provided, a source of funding was inadvertently excluded, or the wrong institution was listed with you and/or one of your co-authors. If there are multiple typographical errors (which is possible, given how many journals' editorial staffs are currently stretched very thin), then it does detract from the paper.

It is important to remember that for most journals, the publisher has copyright over your printed material (you typically sign a document or check a box upon submitting your paper indicating your agreement with this), not you, the author. This has a number of implications. For one, you do not have the right to unlimited free copies of your article. Typically, the publisher will offer you a few free copies or a certain length of time to access your article electronically for free as a result of publishing with them. Of course, if the journal you published in can be accessed for free utilizing your institution's library resources, you have access to it in no different way than you do other journals and articles it provides similar access to. As with any article (including those not your own), there are restrictions that limit your ability to distribute it widely. Exceptions are typically made for the article's use for educational purposes, such as in teaching students, but not necessarily if you are using it for distribution at a conference or at a continuing education seminar in which you are being paid. You also may not use the same table or illustration in a different publication, even if they are for different purposes, for example, in a chapter of a book you may be writing. There are myriad potential instances not so "cut-and-dry" where copyright comes into play, and it is simply best to contact the appropriate person at the journal and/or the Copyright Clearance Center[29] to resolve any questions you might have and also obtain the necessary permissions. While the copyright is owned by the publisher, many journals are generally flexible to the extent they can be if you have published your work with them and especially if you have established a good rapport with journal editorial staff, as described above.

The journal maintains copyright and has a role to play not only in serving as a repository for your work but also in helping to disseminate information about your publication. Journals are working more closely than ever with authors to help spread the word about your paper, as this helps create more visibility for both you and the journal. This is very much the case in our era of social media. One study found a significant and positive correlation between the number of times articles have been Tweeted and their number of citations,[30] and still another uncovered the sustaining effect, or durability, of the impact of the Twitter activity on a paper's attention and citations.[31] Even while the latter-mentioned study has since drawn criticism and some equivocation about the effectiveness of tweeting,[32] there is little doubt by its very nature that some followers of the journal on Twitter, Facebook, and other social media platforms, as well as friends and colleagues of your own, will become more quickly and thoroughly aware of your paper and its contributions. Even if this does not ultimately improve its number of citations, it almost ensures more reads immediately upon publication and lets others know of your expertise in an area of which they might not have been aware previously. This could result in you being invited to collaborate on similar projects, being asked to contribute to a scholarly book or book chapter, or be recognized by a professional organization if the work is salient to them and to their mission.

Thus, working with a journal/publisher to market your work serves to benefit the journal's readership, helps to create awareness of study results that will be important at least to certain persons and audiences, thus helping to advance the science and profession, and ultimately assists you with invaluable networking opportunities. This is important not only for that particular paper but also for your entire research career. Productivity and success breed additional productivity and success. One can carry to the extreme, boasting about one's accomplishments and making declarative statements about how great of a researcher you are. Similar to the aforementioned advice about keeping superlatives and braggadocio to a minimum (as it will have just the opposite effect on your networking opportunities), there is absolutely nothing wrong with Tweeting or Facebooking an accepted publication in working with the journal to facilitate dissemination of your work. The work is hopefully part of a "stream" of research where you are working on different facets or angles of a phenomenon or hypothesized relationship and establishing your credibility and expertise in that area. The better your work is known and recognized, the more doors it will open for you.

Summary and Conclusions

Peer review serves as the backbone of the scientific process and is commensurate with that process being superior among the methods of knowing and advancing a profession and, in the case of pharmacy, advancing patient care processes and education. Authors, peer reviewers, editors, publishers, and other stakeholders all have a role to play in this endeavor. The peer-review process is one that is a human process and thus imperfect, but one that invariably produces higher quality work in the end. Editors seek publication recommendations from reviewers who have expertise in matters related to the submitted paper, who offer advice on how to strengthen the paper, regardless of whether it is ultimately accepted or not. The process is a meticulous one and is one that requires patience, persistence, and resilience for authors. Editors make decisions based upon the quality of the paper and the opportunity for it to advance the science and/or profession. Appropriate coping strategies will facilitate your success in publishing and your journey as a scholar. Working with publishers and using contemporary forms of communication such as social media will help enhance the visibility of your work and open doors for you throughout your career.

Key Points and Advice

- There are four basic ways of knowing—(1) the method of tenacity, (2) the method of authority, (3) the method of intuition, and (4) the method of science. The method of science is the method in which we place the most trust and produces more accurate and less biased observations.
- Peer review serves as the backbone of scientific processes, thus inspiring greater confidence that we are advancing knowledge and/or selecting the appropriate criteria upon which to make decisions and direct further inquiry.
- A peer-reviewed journal is one that employees the peer review process and involves multiple stages of quality assurance, involving evaluations by a chief editor, associate editor(s), and peer reviewers. A journal's editorial board assists with peer reviews and setting direction and policy for a journal. Publication in peer-reviewed journals is the primary means by which scholars communicate and advance science.
- Authors, peer reviewers, and editors thusly have important roles to play. Reviewers and authors have a number of sources they can turn to for best practices. For authors, journal fit is important in the selection of a journal to submit your scholarly work. There are also a number of details which they should attend. Reviewers must provide constructive criticism rather than vague, negative statements.
- Authors facing a "reject" decision should consider it as an opportunity for further growth, development, and decision making and are advised to cope with this in a healthy manner.
- Authors can seek to leverage their own networks and the journal's social media outlets to help disseminate their research findings and manuscripts.

Chapter Review Questions

1. How has the concept or phenomenon of peer review evolved from its origins to what it is today?
2. What is the relationship between peer review and the scientific process in regard to methods of knowing?
3. How does the peer review process essentially work, or what are its mechanistic and its conceptual underpinnings and its ramifications?
4. What are some things to think about in each component of a research paper that reviewers might be looking for, as well as things to avoid doing in consideration that the paper will undergo peer review?
5. What are some things you should do (and avoid) when having a paper accepted or rejected into a peer-reviewed journal? What should be some commonalities in your reaction and response regardless of the particular publication decision?

Online Resources

- Stoop J. Tips & Tricks for Managing the Peer Review Process with Editorial Manager—Part 1. Elsevier Connect. https://www.elsevier.com/connect/editors-update/tips-and-tricks-for-managing-the-peer-review-process-with-editorial-manager-part-1
- Stoop J. Tips & Tricks for Managing the Peer Review Process with Editorial Manager—Part 2. Elsevier Connect. https://www.elsevier.com/connect/editors-update/tips-and-tricks-for-managing-the-peer-review-process-with-editorial-manager-part-2
- How to Write a Peer Review. PLOS. https://plos.org/resource/how-to-write-a-peer-review/
- Top 10 Tips for Peer Review. JBJS Journal. https://journals.lww.com/jbjsjournal/Pages/Top-10-Tips-for-Peer-Review.aspx

REFERENCES

1. Al Kawi MZ. History of medical records and peer review. *Ann Saudi Med.* 1997;17(3):277-278.
2. Spier R. The history of the peer-review process. *Trends Biotechnol.* 2002;20(8):357-358.
3. Burnham JC. The evolution of editorial peer review. *JAMA.* 1990;263(10):1323-1329.
4. Chimanski LA, Alperin JP. The evaluation of scholarship in academic promotion and tenure processes: past, present, and future. *F1000Research.* 2018;7:1605.
5. Marsh HW, Jayasinghe UW, Bond NW. Improving the peer-review process for grant applications: reliability, validity, bias, and generalizability. *Am Psychologist.* 2008;63(3):160-168.

6. Lee CJ, Sugimoto CR, Zhang G, Cronin B. Bias in peer review. *J Am Society Info Sci Technol.* 2013;64(1):2-17.

7. Buchler, J, ed. *Philosophical Writings of Peirce.* New York, NY: Dover; 1955.

8. Kerlinger FN. The influence of research on education practice. *Educ Res.* 1977;6(8):5-12.

9. Boghossian P. Behaviorism, constructivism, and Socratic pedagogy. *Educational Philos Theory.* 2006;38(6):713-7122.

10. Kerlinger FN. *Foundations of Behavioral Research.* 3rd ed. New York, NY: Holt, Rinehart and Winston; 1986.

11. Lodahl JB, Gordon G. Differences between physical and social sciences in university graduate departments. *Res Higher Educ.* 1973;1(1):191-213.

12. Cutcliffe JR, McKenna HP. When do we know that we know? Considering the truth of research findings and the craft of qualitative research. *Intl J Nurs Studies.* 2002;39(6):611-618.

13. Elsevier. Editorial Boards. Accessed March 29, 2021. https://www.elsevier.com/editors/editorial-boards

14. Peterson J, Pearce PF, Ferguson LA, Langford CA. Understanding scoping reviews: definition, purpose, and process. *J Am Assoc Nurse Practitioners.* 2017;29(1):12-16.

15. Spigt M, Arts ICW. How to review a manuscript. *J Clin Epidemiol.* 2010;63(12):1385-1390.

16. Desselle SP, Chen AM, Amin M, et al. Generosity, collegiality, and scientific accuracy when writing and reviewing original research. *Res Social Adm Pharm.* 2020;16(2):261-265.

17. Measuring Your Impact: Impact Factor, Citation Analysis, and Other Metrics: Journal Impact Factor (IF). Subject and Course Guides. Accessed March 23, 2021. https://researchguides.uic.edu/if/impact#:~:text=The%20impact%20factor%20(IF)%20is,times%20it's%20articles%20are%20cited

18. Malcolm DL. It's time we fix the peer-review system. *Am J Pharm Educ.* 2018;82(5):Article 7144.

19. Haines ST, Baker WI, DiDominico RJ. Improving peer review: what journals can do. *Am J Health Syst Pharm.* 2017;74(24):2086-2089.

20. Hasegawa GR. An editor's perspective on peer review. *Am J Health Syst Pharm.* 2017;74(24):2090-2094.

21. DiDomenico RJ. Improving peer review: what reviewers can do. *Am J Health Syst Pharm.* 2017;74(24):20880-22084.

22. Janke KK, Bzowyckyk AS, Traynor AP. Editors' perspectives on manuscript quality and editorial decisions through peer review and reviewer development. *Am J Pharm Educ.* 2017;81(4):Article 73.

23. Schreiber JB. New paradigms for considering statistical significance: A way forward for health services research journals, their authors, and their readership. *Res Social Adm Pharm.* 2020;16(4):591-594.

24. Desselle SP, Amin M, Aslani P, et al. Moving the needle—what does RSAP look for and what does it aim to do? *Res Social Adm Pharm.* 2019;15(1):1-2.

25. Opthof T, Ferstner F, van Geer M, Coronel R. Regrets or no regrets? No regrets! The fate of rejected manuscripts. *Cardiovas Res.* 2000;45(1):255-258.

26. Venkatesh S, Maymone MCB, Vashi NA. Peer reviews: the dreaded rejection. *Derm Online J.* 2018;24(3):1-3.

27. Fahed R, Shamy M, Dowlatshahi D. "It's about how hard you can get hit and keep moving forward": how to survive rejection and get your paper published. *Stroke.* 2020;51(5):e71-e74.

28. DeCastro R, Sambuco D, Ubel PA, Stewart A, Jagsi R. Batting 300 is good. Perspectives of faculty researchers and their mentors on rejection, resilience, and persistence in academic medical careers. *Acad Med.* 2013;88(4):497-504.

29. Copyright Clearance Center. Copyright & Licensing Experts website. Updated May 27, 2020. Accessed March 26, 2021. https://www.copyright.com/

30. Klar S, Krupnikov Y, Ryan JB, Searles K, Shmargad Y. Using social media to promote academic research: identifying the benefits of Twitter for sharing academic work. *PLOS One.* 2020.

31. Luc JGY, Archer MA, Arora RC, et al. Does tweeting improve citations? One-year results from the TSSMN prospective randomized trial. *Ann Thor Surg.* 2020.

32. Davis P. Reanalysis of tweeting study yields no citation benefit. The Scholarly Kitchen—Official blog of the Society for Scholarly Publishing. Accessed September 6, 2020. https://scholarlykitchen.sspnet.org/2020/07/13/tweeting-study-yields-no-benefit/

Index

Page numbers followed by "f" denote figures; those followed by "t" denote tables.